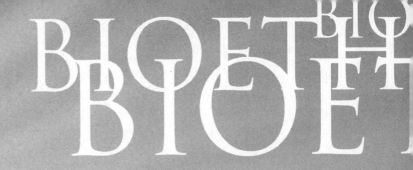

Bioethics: a nursing perspective

fourth edition

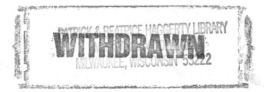

You should not decide until you have
heard what both have to say.

Aristophanes, *The Wasps*

Nobody is infallible; and for that reason
many different points of view are needed.

Mary Midgley, *Can't we make moral judgements?*

Bioethics: a nursing perspective

fourth edition

Megan-Jane Johnstone

RN, BA, PhD, FRCNA, FCN (NSW)

Professor of Nursing
RMIT Nursing and Midwifery
School of Health Sciences
RMIT University, Melbourne

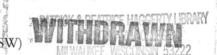
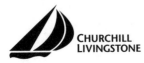

CHURCHILL
LIVINGSTONE

Sydney   Edinburgh   London   New York   Philadelphia   St Louis   Toronto

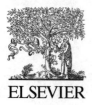

ELSEVIER

First edition published 1989
Second edition published 1994
Third edition published 1999

National Library of Australia Cataloguing-in-Publication data

Johnstone, Megan-Jane
Bioethics: a nursing perspective

4th ed.
Bibliography.
Includes index.
ISBN 0 7295 3726 9.

1. Nursing ethics. 2. Bioethics. 3. Medical ethics.
I. Title.
174.2

Publishing Editor: Meg O'Hanlon
Developmental Editor: Rhiain Hull
Publishing Services Manager: Helena Klijn
Project managed, edited and indexed by: Forsyth Publishing Services

Designed and typeset by The Modern Art Production Group
Printed in Australia by Southwood Press

Contents

Preface

It is over 15 years since the first edition of this book was published, and it is no small measure of the importance of the topic that there now exists a demand for this fourth revised edition. In 1989, when the first edition of this work was published, very little had been written on bioethics from a nursing perspective, and nursing ethics itself was largely invisible and poorly understood. This situation made it very difficult for nurses to have their concerns about ethical issues heard, let alone addressed, and to fulfil their professional responsibility to advocate for the needs and moral interests of the individuals, groups and communities for whose health care they shared responsibility.

At the time of its 1989 publication, *Bioethics: a nursing perspective* stood as the first text of its kind to be written from an Australasian perspective, and attempted to give 'visibility' to nursing concerns about ethical issues in health care domains and to remedy the palpable lack of understanding about nursing ethics that existed at the time. It also attempted to give nursing a much needed 'voice' in both the health professional and bioethics literature, and to 'defend' the legitimacy of a nursing point of view. To this end, a key aim (and focus) of the first and second editions was to demonstrate that bioethics was a legitimate professional concern for nurses and one that warranted serious attention by all concerned. In this aim, the first two editions succeeded beyond all expectations.

At the time the third revised edition was prepared, much had changed. Nursing ethics had gained legitimacy and respect as a distinctive field of inquiry in its own right and the 'defensive' position taken in the first two editions was no longer warranted. Although retaining Chapter 2 ('Be good women but don't have a code of ethics') in which a number of important historical examples of the marginalisation of nursing ethics were discussed, the third edition thus largely abandoned the emphasis on 'defending' the legitimacy of nursing ethics evident in the previous two editions.

In response to new and emerging developments in the field, the third revised edition included new and/or expanded discussions on a range of issues including, but not limited to: the changing moral world and its implications for nurses (including the problems of moral pluralism, postmodern ethics, and the demise of traditional moral certainty in health care domains); the history and nature of mainstream bioethics and its relationship to nursing ethics and the nature and implications of nursing ethics (including a new and more substantive definition of what constitutes and distinguishes nursing ethics from other branches of ethics). The third revised edition also included new material on human rights and the mentally ill; ethical issues associated with the reporting of child abuse; and the promotion of ethical practice in nursing. In regard to the latter, particular attention was given to a range of issues, including: the formulation and enactment of meaningful standards of ethical nursing conduct, providing preventive and remedial nursing ethics education programs, ethical management and improving the moral culture of the organisations in which nurses work, supporting nursing research and scholarship, and taking political action aimed at achieving public policy and law reforms to facilitate the ethical practice of nursing.

This fourth revised edition of *Bioethics: a nursing perspective* marks a significant turning point in nursing ethics in that it serves not only to inform but to revitalise and progress debate on the issues presented. To this end, several chapters are entirely new or contain entirely new material, and others have been greatly rewritten; still others have been removed altogether since, over the past decade, their relevance has declined or they are being addressed appropriately and comprehensively in other forums.

Notable among the revisions made in this fourth edition (and which distinguish this edition from its previous editions) are those contained in the entirely new chapters: Chapters 1, addressing the topic 'Professional standards and the requirement to be ethical'; Chapter 14, raising the issues of nursing ethics futures and the need for nurses to engage in moral activism; and Chapter 15, in which the challenges posed by considering the concerns of indigenous peoples are presented as a 'final word' to this edition. Meanwhile, the discussions on the popular issues of: transcultural ethics, patients' rights (especially in regard to informed consent and competency to decide, and quality of life), mental health ethics (including new material on the use of psychiatric advanced directives or 'Ulysses contracts'), abortion (and the 'new abortion ethics'), euthanasia and assisted suicide (including the issue of withholding/withdrawing food and fluids from sedated patients), end of life decision-making (including new material of medical futility, advanced directives, and quality of life) and clinical ethics committees, have all been substantially updated and, where relevant, expanded. The theoretical underpinnings of these issues have, in turn, been modified to ensure that they are articulated succinctly and in a manner that can be readily understood and applied. In this regard, the more complex discussions on ethical theory contained in the earlier editions have been removed. Despite these major changes, the essence and methodological starting point of this work has not changed, that is: *the lived realities of nurses and nursing practice*. Accordingly, the fourth edition has increased significantly its collection and discussion of case exemplars pertinent to every day nursing practice and the ethical practice of nursing.

In making the revisions to this fourth edition, it is hoped that nurses (as well as those with whom they work) will be assisted further in their quest to gain knowledge and understanding about the ethical issues affecting nursing practice, to use this knowledge and understanding to challenge and change the status quo in health care contexts — particularly where this is not conducive to the welfare and wellbeing of patients — and thereby to make a difference to the moral world in which they live and work.

Megan-Jane Johnstone

Acknowledgments

In writing and revising this book I have become indebted to a number of people. Foremost among them are the many nurses, students, patients/clients, colleagues and others whose generosity in sharing their experiences and views has, in many ways, made this book possible. A special thanks is also due to my good friends and colleagues Professor Olga Kanitsaki, AM, and Dr Bill McArthur who, as in the case of all the previous editions, have been stalwart supporters of my work and have served as ready sounding boards for my ideas and 'ally readers' of my revised chapter drafts. And thanks is due to my good friend and colleague Dr Sally Goold, OAM, for so generously agreeing to provide the poignant 'last word' to this work.

Finally, these acknowledgments would not be complete without thanks being given to Meg O'Hanlon, Rhiain Hull, and Helena Klijn, at Elsevier Australia, and Jon Forsyth, at Forsyth Publishing Services, for their contribution to the successful production of this book. The final work is, however, my own as are any weaknesses and omissions.

Permissions acknowledgments

The author and publisher would like to thank the following for granting permission to reproduce material:

- Oxford University Press, New York: Beauchamp T. and Childress J. (2001). *Principles of biomedical ethics*, 5th edition.
- The Hastings Center Report, New York: Benjamin M. 'Between subway and spaceship: practical ethics at the outset of the twenty-first century', *Hastings Center Report* 31(4):22–31.
- Martin Benjamin: Benjamin M. 'Between subway and spaceship: practical ethics at the outset of the twenty-first century', *Hastings Center Report* 31(4):22–31.
- Cambridge University Press, Melbourne: Buchanan A. and Brock D. (1989). *Deciding for others: the ethics of surrogate decision making.*
- BMJ Publishing Group, London: Craig G. (1994). 'On withholding nutrition and hydration in the terminally ill: has palliative medicine gone too far?' in *Journal of Medical Ethics*, 20(3):140–2; and Wyatt (2001). 'Medical paternalism and the fetus' in *Journal of Medical Ethics*, 27(suppl ii):ii15–ii20.
- University of Chicago Press, Chicago: Wong, D. (1992). 'Coping with moral conflict and ambiguity' in *Ethics*, 102(4):763–84.
- eContent Management Pty Ltd, Queensland: Johnstone M. (2002). 'The changing focus of health care ethics: implications and challenges for the health care professions', *Contemporary Nurse* (*www.contemporarynurse.com*), 12(3):213–24.

Chapter 1

Professional standards and the requirement to be ethical

LEARNING OBJECTIVES

Upon the completion of this chapter and with further self-directed learning you are expected to be able to:

- Locate the code of conduct, code of ethics and competency standards developed by the relevant peak nursing organisations in the jurisdiction/state/country of your practice, and which you are expected to uphold as a professional nurse.
- Identify the ethical standards and ethical competencies expected of professional nurses in the country of your practice.
- Discuss why, if at all, nurses should uphold the standards of ethical conduct prescribed by peak nursing organisations.
- Reflect critically on why, if at all, the practice of nursing is a moral undertaking.

KEYWORDS

- Ethical competencies/capabilities
- Ethical conduct
- Ethical practice
- Ethical safety
- Professional boundaries
- Professional conduct
- Professional practice
- Professional standards

Introduction

From the moment a nurse enters into professional practice she or he is bound by strict standards of professional conduct. The standards of conduct expected of professional nurses are stated publicly in a range of documents including formally endorsed professional codes of conduct, codes of ethics, competency standards, and guidelines and position statements formulated on a range of issues relevant to the profession and practice of nursing. For example, nurses in Australia are bound by the standards of conduct expressed in the following documents published by the Australian Nursing Council:

- *Code of Professional Conduct for Nurses in Australia* (2003)
- *Code of Ethics for Nurses in Australia* (2002)
- *National Competency Standards for the Registered Nurse and the Enrolled Nurse* (2002) [available at: *www.anc.org.au*].

Depending on the jurisdiction in which they are registered, nurses are also obliged to follow various guidelines as set down by their local nurse registering authority. For example, nurses in the Australian states of New South Wales, Queensland and Victoria are bound respectively by the following guidelines on professional boundaries:

- *Guidelines for Registered Nurses and Enrolled Nurses Regarding the Boundaries of Professional Practice* (approved for use in Queensland by the Queensland Nursing Council) (Nurses Registration Board of NSW, 1999) [available at: *www.nursesreg.nsw.gov.au*];
- *Queensland Nursing Council and Health Practitioners Boards' Statement on Sexual Relationships Between Health Practitioners and their Patients* (Queensland Nursing Council, 2000) [available at: *www.qnc.qld.gov.au*];
- *Professional Boundaries Guidelines for Registered Nurses in Victoria* (Nurses Board of Victoria, 2001) [available at: *www.nbv.org.au*].

Similar guidelines exist for nurses in other Australian states and territories.

Nurses in other countries are likewise bound by the standards of conduct developed, endorsed and published by their respective peak nursing organisations. Nurses in New Zealand, for example, are bound by the Nursing Council of New Zealand's *Code of Conduct for Nurses and Midwives* (2001) [available at: *www.nursingcouncil.org.nz*] and by the standards expressed in the following documents published by the New Zealand Nurses Organisation (NZNO):

- *Code of Ethics* (1995);
- *Social Policy Statement* (1993);
- *Standards for Nursing Practice* (1993) [available at: *www.nzno.org.au*].

Nurses in Singapore, meanwhile, are bound by practice standards set by the Singapore Nurses Association (*www.sna.org.sg*), Hong Kong Nurses by standards set by the Nursing Council of Hong Kong (*www.nchk.org.hk*), and nurses in other countries (for example, the United States of America, Canada, the United Kingdom, and so on) are bound by the standards set by their respective peak nursing organisations.

Australian, New Zealand, Singaporean and Hong Kong nurses, like their counterparts in other countries, are also bound by the codes, policy and position statements published and endorsed by the International Council of Nurses (ICN) Code. Of particular note are the ICN's:

- *Code of Ethics for Nurses* (2000);

- *Framework of Competencies for the Generalist Nurse* (2003);
- Position and policy statements on a range of issues relating to:
  - nursing roles in health care service
  - nursing profession
  - socio economic welfare of nurses
  - health care systems
  - social issues [available at: *www.icn.ch*].

A central and important requirement of these and other codes and related policy and position statements is the fundamental expectation that, when practising in a professional capacity, nurses in all levels and areas of practice will uphold the highest standards of *ethics* and indeed be 'exemplars' (models) of excellent *ethical* behaviour in professional and related contexts.

The requirement to be ethical

The requirement for nurses to be ethical and to uphold the highest standards of ethical conduct when practising in a professional capacity is not unique to nursing. It is generally expected that when performing their duties and conducting their affairs, professionals (of all fields) will uphold *exemplary* standards of conduct — commonly taken to mean standards that are higher than and not generally expected of lay people or of the 'ordinary person on the street'. A key reason underpinning this expectation relates to the potential vulnerability of clients and an associated expected 'special obligation' on the part of professionals to reduce this vulnerability by conforming to 'particularly high ethical standards both in their professional and non-professional lives' (Freckelton 1996, p. 142; Johnstone 1998). Such is this expectation that exemplary standards of ethical conduct have historically been cited as one of the key hallmarks of professionalism and indeed as a necessary feature of professions generally (Bayles 1981).

Questioning the requirement to be ethical

The demand placed on nurses to be ethical and to uphold exemplary ethical standards of conduct is not without controversy. One reason for this is that the expectation to be ethical seems to assume (without supporting evidence) that nurses, like other professionals, should *as a matter of fact* be ethical. This assumption raises a number of important questions, such as:

- What is ethics and ethical professional conduct?
- Is it the case that nurses *should* be ethical?
- What does it mean to be an 'ethical practitioner'?
- Is it possible to be an ethical professional in health care environments, situations, and circumstances that are not supportive of ethical conduct?
- How should ethics be practised in professional (nursing and health care) contexts?
- What ethical 'competencies' and 'capabilities' does a professional person need in order to be able to practice ethics safely and effectively as an accountable and responsible professional?

Whatever the possible answers to these and related questions (and there are many), one thing is clear: *nurses may be able to accept or reject the different viewpoints expressed, but they cannot ignore them.* This is because, so long as nurses continue to work with and care for people — and strive to promote the health and wellbeing of people (a core purpose of nursing practice) — they will not be able to avoid the many and complex moral problems that will inevitably arise during the course of their work. Neither will nurses be able to avoid making decisions and taking action (including the 'action' of deliberately not taking action) in response to the problems they encounter. As Hinman (1994, pp. 1–2) explains in another context:

> We cannot avoid confronting moral problems, because acting in ways that affect the wellbeing of ourselves and others is as unavoidable as acting in ways that affect the physical health of our own bodies. We inevitably face choices that hurt or help people, choices that may infringe on their rights or violate their dignity or use them as mere tools to our own ends. We may choose not to pay attention to the concerns of morality such as compassion or justice or respect, just as we may choose to ignore the concerns of nutrition. However, that does not mean we can avoid making decisions about morality any more than we can evade deciding what foods to eat. We can ignore morality, but we cannot sidestep the choices to which morality is relevant, just as we cannot avoid decisions to which nutrition is pertinent even when we ignore the information that nutritionists provide for us. Morality is about living, and as long as we continue living, we will inevitably be confronted with moral questions – and if we choose to stop living that too is a moral issue.

Nursing as a moral project

Nursing is, without question, a moral undertaking. Its practice never occurs in a moral vacuum and is never free of moral risk. Even nursing care practices and procedures that might seem 'simple', 'basic' or 'trivial' (e.g. placing a person on a bedpan; administering an aspirin tablet) could, potentially, have morally significant, harmful consequences. It is because of the potential to cause morally significant harm to others — not to mention the breach of trust that could occur as a consequence of such harm being caused — that nursing practice and the conduct of nurses warrants attention from an ethical point of view. It is the purpose of this book to provide such attention and to advance a critical examination of the moral role, responsibilities and rights of nurses as accountable and responsible health care professionals. To this end, in the chapters to follow, particular attention will be given to explaining what ethics is and why nurses 'should' be ethical — even in contexts which are not supportive of ethical conduct and where being ethical may be difficult. Issues and examples will be discussed critically to show that it is not enough just to be 'sensitive' to and to have knowledge of certain ethical issues, but also to know *how* to deal with them safely, competently and effectively and, equally important, to have the capacity to act in order to achieve morally desirable outcomes.

Conclusion

Nurses in all levels and areas of practice are bound by strict standards of professional conduct and are expected publicly to uphold the highest ideals of ethical professional practice. However, just why nurses should uphold the standards expected of them and how best to do so remains an open question. It is important, therefore, for nurses (whether beginning or advanced practitioners) to critically examine and reflect on such questions as:

- What is ethics?
- What is ethical professional conduct?
- Why should I be ethical?

- What should I do in situations where I know what the 'right' thing to do is, but I have no support to act on my judgment?
- Do I know enough about ethics in order to practise ethics safely and effectively as an accountable and responsible professional?
- What ethical 'competencies' and 'capabilities' do I need to develop in order to fulfil my responsibilities as an ethical practitioner?

CASE SCENARIOS AND CRITICAL QUESTIONS

Case scenario 1

While undergoing treatment in a public hospital over a six week period an 81-year-old man was robbed of $33 000 by a nurse working at the hospital. The robbery took place after the nurse in question allegedly stole the man's bank keycard and personal identification number (PIN) from his wallet on the night that he was admitted to the hospital (Rogers 2000, p. 3). The money was stolen from the man's bank account in '59 separate transactions over a six-week period'. It was reported that the man 'only realised that the money was missing from his account when he received a letter from his bank advising him that his account was overdrawn' (Rogers 2000, p. 3). The nurse, who subsequently resigned from the hospital and moved interstate, was later summonsed on '59 counts of obtaining a benefit by deception' and arrested to face charges in the local court of the town where the offences allegedly took place.

Case scenario 2

Nurse D became the subject of disciplinary action by the state's nurse registering authority after he was reported for the assault of four elderly residents in his care. The assaults included Nurse D:

placing his hands around the neck of a resident, hitting a dementia patient who had struck out accidentally at him, and showering a patient on the floor where she had fallen (Peisley 2002, p. 15).

In another incident, a resident in Nurse D's care was 'found naked, restrained and unattended on a toilet by another staff member' whilst Nurse D was working at a computer (Peisley 2002, p. 15). It was also reported that one resident was so afraid of Nurse D that she barraged herself in her own room as a means of self-protection.

Nurse D was found by the nurse registering authority to have engaged in unprofessional conduct of a serious nature and had his registration suspended for two years. The nurse registering authority also determined that Nurse D undergo counselling 'with particular attention to anger and stress management' and that, when he returned to work, 'a condition be imposed that he not work in aged care' (Peisley 2002, p. 15). During the course of the disciplinary proceedings, however, Nurse D indicated to the nurse registering authority that he intended never to work in nursing again and 'chose not to attend the hearing into his conduct' (Peisley 2002, p. 15).

In reaching its findings the nurse registering authority acknowledged that 'there is a tendency in Australian work places not to "dob in" a fellow worker', but that nonetheless, 'nurses are professionals with a duty of care to residents, patients or clients' and that the duty of care 'must override this reluctance' to report unprofessional conduct (Peisley 2002, p. 15).

Critical questions

1. What standards of ethical professional conduct did the nurses breach in these scenarios?
2. If you were a nurse working in a hospital or a residential home care setting and you suspected or knew that a nurse was abusing or defrauding a patient or resident what, if any, action would you take?
3. Upon what basis would you justify your actions (or non-actions, as the case may be)?
4. What might be the consequences both to the patients/residents and to yourself, in either case, of you taking action or not taking action?

Chapter 2

Ethics, bioethics and nursing ethics: some working definitions

LEARNING OBJECTIVES

Upon the completion of this chapter and with further self-directed learning you are expected to be able to:

- Define the following concepts:
  - ethics
  - morality
  - bioethics
  - nursing ethics.
- Discuss why it is important to have a correct understanding of the terms commonly used in discussions and debates about ethics and ethical issues in nursing and health care.
- Discuss why each of the following processes cannot be relied upon to guide sound and just ethical conduct in nursing and health care contexts:
  - law
  - codes of ethics
  - hospital or professional etiquette
  - hospital or institutional policy
  - public opinion or the view of the majority
  - following the orders of a supervisor or manager.

KEYWORDS

- Bioethics
- Codes of ethics
- Ethics
- Etiquette
- Law
- Moral issue
- Morality
- Nursing ethics

Introduction

Understanding the basis of ethical professional conduct in nursing requires nurses to have at least a working knowledge and understanding of the language, concepts and theories of ethics. One reason for this, as explained by the English philosopher, Richard Hare (1964, pp. 1–2), is that:

> in a world in which the problems of conduct become every day more complex and tormenting, there is a great need for an understanding of the language in which these problems are posed and answered. For confusion about our moral language leads, not merely to theoretical muddles, but to needless practical perplexities.

At first glance it might seem cumbersome spending time on clarifying and developing an understanding of the language, concepts and underpinning theories used in discussions and debates on ethics. Upon closer examination, however, it soon becomes clear that such an undertaking is crucial if nurses and their associates are to engage in a meaningful inquiry into what ethics is, what constitutes 'nursing ethics' and how, if at all, nursing ethics differs from other fields of ethics, what it means to be an 'ethical practitioner', why nurses have an obligation to practice their profession in an ethical manner, and how to *be* an ethical practitioner. Furthermore, and not least, how best to proceed with the difficult task of identifying and resolving the many moral problems that nurses (like others in the health care team) will inevitably encounter during the course of their everyday practice.

The importance of understanding ethics terms and concepts

The terms 'ethics', 'morality', 'rights', 'duties', 'obligations', 'moral principles', 'moral rules', 'morally right', 'morally wrong', 'moral theory', to name some, are all commonly used in discussions about ethics. Nurses, like others, may use some of these terms when discussing life events and practice situations that are perceived as having a moral dimension. These terms are not always used correctly, however, with the unfortunate consequence of communication and discussions about ethical issues sometimes becoming distorted and, as a consequence, giving rise to problems and perplexities that did not exist previously or which could otherwise have been avoided had they been dealt with more competently.

One notable example of the incorrect use of ethical terms can be found in the tendency by some nurses (scholars included) to treat the terms 'rights' and 'responsibilities' or 'duties' as being synonymous, and thus able to be used interchangeably. An example of this is found in the International Council of Nurses (ICN) position statement on the 'rights and duties of nurses', adopted at the ICN's Council of National Representatives meeting in Brazil in June 1983: 'Nurses have a *right* to practise within the code of ethics and nursing legislation' (Keireini 1983, p. 4, emphasis added). When the nature of rights and duties is examined later, it will become clear that the term 'right' in this example should, in fact, read 'duty'. The implications of confusing the meanings of the terms 'rights' and 'duties' and treating these two terms as being synonymous will be explored more fully in the chapters to follow.

Another common mistake is the tendency by some nurses to draw a distinction between the terms 'ethics' and 'morality'. They draw a distinction on the grounds that, in their view, morality involves more a personal or private set of values whereas ethics is more concerned with a formalised, public and universal set of values (see, for example, Thompson et al. 2000; Leininger 1991; Kelly 1985). As will be shown shortly, there is, in fact, no philosophically significant difference between the terms 'ethics' and 'morality' and to distinguish between them is both unnecessary and confusing.

The need for a critical inquiry into ethical professional practice

It is acknowledged that most people brought up in a common cultural context share what Beauchamp and Childress (2001, p. 3) call a 'common morality'; that is, a set of core norms and dimensions of morality that most people accept as being relevant and important (e.g., respect the rights of others, do not harm or kill innocent people, it is wrong to steal, it is wrong to break promises, and so forth) and about which philosophical debate 'would be a waste of time' (Beauchamp and Childress 2001, p. 3). It would be a mistake, however, to assume or to accept that 'common morality' or 'common sense morality' is in and by itself sufficient to enable nurses to deal with the many complex and complicated ethical issues that they will encounter in their practice. As examples to be presented in the following chapters will show, while our 'ordinary moral apparatus' may motivate and guide us to behave ethically as people, it is often quite inadequate to the task of guiding us to deal safely and effectively with the many complex ethical issues that rise in nursing and health care contexts. A much more sophisticated moral competency and capability is required than that otherwise provided by a 'common sense' morality.

If nurses are serious about ethics and about practising ethically, then they must engage in a critical inquiry about what ethics is and how it can best be applied in the 'real world' of professional nursing practice. It cannot be assumed that just because we know of and use certain ethical terms in our conversations that we know what they mean or that we are using them correctly. As Warnock warns in his classic work *Contemporary moral philosophy* (1967, p. 75):

> When we talk about 'morals' we do not all know what we mean; what moral problems, moral principles, moral judgments are is not a matter so clear that it can be passed over as simple datum. We must discover when we would say, and when we would not, that an issue is a moral issue, and why; and if, as is more than likely, disagreements should come to light even at this stage, we could at least discriminate and investigate what reasonably tenable alternative positions there may be.

Understanding moral language

When discussing and advancing debates on ethical issues in nursing and health care it is vital that all parties involved have a shared working knowledge and understanding of the meanings of terms and concepts that are fundamental to the issues being considered. This imperative is captured by the philosophical adage 'there must first be agreement before there can be disagreement'. The reasoning behind this imperative is that unless there is a shared understanding of core terms and concepts it will be extremely difficult if not impossible to develop insight and understanding of the issues at stake and address if not resolve the disagreements and conflicts that may have arisen in relation to them. For example, if two dissenting parties do not share a common understanding about the nature and content of human rights (what these entail, the moral authority they have, what entities can validly claim human rights, and so forth) they cannot even begin to debate the conditions under which human rights ought to be respected and when they might justifiably be overridden, and to take action accordingly. Similarly, if two dissenting parties do not share a common conception of what nursing ethics is, then they cannot meaningfully debate whether or not nursing ethics ought to be recognised as a distinctive field of inquiry and practice in its own right, or whether nurses are obliged to uphold the standards of ethical conduct developed as a result of focussed nursing ethics inquiry.

In developing a shared understanding of core terms and concepts used in discussions and debates on ethical issues it is important for nurses to be aware that, contrary to expectations, many of the terms commonly used in ethical debates are themselves 'ethically loaded' and thus, paradoxically, at risk of distorting if not corrupting the debates. The notion of 'quality of life' is a good example. Many writers on bioethics assume that when a life ceases to be 'independent' it has diminished worth. In instances where quality of life has been a criterion for decision-making at the end stage of life, euthanasia might be considered a right and proper course of action to take. Here the ethically loaded notion of 'dependence' imparts a sense of the permissibility of the euthanasia option and limits thought of, say, pursuing a rehabilitation option. It also overrides thought of the possibility that for some people dependence may be quite irrelevant to the notion of a worthwhile life. Kanitsaki (1989, 1993, 1994), for example, has shown that in some traditional cultural groups, familial and friendly relationships are characteristically *collective and interdependent*, and that any thought of *individual independence* is quite irrelevant to the assessment of 'a life worth living'.

Poorly or inappropriately defined ethical terms and concepts can seriously impinge upon and limit people's moral imagination, and the moral options and choices that might otherwise be identified, considered and chosen in the face of moral disagreement, conflict and adversity.

What is ethics?

It is appropriate to begin the task of defining commonly used ethical terms and concepts by first examining the terms 'ethics' and 'morality', and clarifying from the outset there is no philosophically significant difference between the terms 'ethics' and 'morality'. If a distinction is to be drawn between these two terms it is one that is based on etymological grounds (the study of the origin of the words), with 'ethics' coming from the ancient Greek *ethikos* (originally meaning 'pertaining to custom or habit'), and 'morality' coming from the Latin *moralitas* (also originally meaning 'custom' or 'habit'). This means that the terms may be used interchangeably, as they are in the philosophic literature and in this work. With respect to deciding which terms should be used in ethical discourse (i.e. whether to use the term 'ethics' or the term 'morality'), this is very much a matter of personal preference rather than of philosophical debate, noting, however, that the terms ethics and morality have come to refer to something far more sophisticated than 'custom' or 'habit' as will soon be shown.

Having clarified that there is no philosophically significant difference between the terms 'ethics' and 'morality', it now remains the task here to define what 'ethics' is?

For the purposes of this discussion ethics is defined as a generic term that is used for referring to various ways of thinking about, understanding and examining how best to live a 'moral life' (Beauchamp and Childress 2001). More specifically, ethics involves a critically reflective activity that is concerned with a systematic examination of living and behaving morally and 'is designed to illuminate what we ought to do by asking us to consider and reconsider our ordinary actions, judgments and justifications' (Beauchamp and Childress, 1983, p. xii). For example, a nurse may make an 'ordinary' moral judgment that abortion is wrong and conscientiously object to assisting with an abortion procedure. Whether her conscientious objection ought to be respected, however, requires a critical examination of the bases upon which the nurse has made that judgment and a consideration of the justifications (moral reasons) she has put forward to support the position she has taken.

Ethics, as it is referred to and used today, can be traced back to the influential works of the Ancient Greek philosophers Socrates (born 469BC), Plato (born 428BC) and Aristotle (born 384BC). The works of these ancient Greek philosophers were especially influential in seeing ethics established as a branch of philosophical inquiry which sought dispassionate and 'rational' clarification and justification of the basic assumptions and beliefs that people hold about what is to be considered morally acceptable and morally unacceptable behaviour. Ethics thus evolved as a mode of philosophical inquiry (known as moral philosophy) that asked people to question why they considered a particular act right or wrong, what the reasons (justifications) were for their judgments, and whether their judgments were correct. This view of ethics remains an influential one and, although the subject of increasing controversy over the past two decades, retains considerable currency in the mainstream ethics literature.

It is important to clarify that ethics has three distinct 'sub-fields', namely: *descriptive ethics*, *metaethics* and *normative ethics*. *Descriptive ethics* is concerned with the empirical investigation and description of people's moral values and beliefs (that is, values and beliefs concerning what constitutes 'right' and 'wrong' or 'good' and 'bad' conduct). *Metaethics*, in contrast, is concerned with analysing the nature, logical form, language, and methods of reasoning in ethics (for example, it gives consideration to meanings of ethical terms such as 'rights', 'duties', and so on). *Normative ethics*, in turn, is concerned with establishing standards of correctness by identifying and prescribing certain rules and principles of conduct and developing theories to justify the norms established. Unlike descriptive ethics and metaethics, normative ethics is evaluative and prescriptive (hortatory) in nature. In the case of the latter, ethics inquiry is not so much concerned with how the world is, but with how it *ought* to be. In other words, it is not concerned with merely *describing* the world (although, of course, a description of the world is necessary as a starting point for an evaluative inquiry), but rather in *prescribing* how it should be and providing *sound justification* for this prescription. Just what is to count as a 'sound justification', however, is an open question and one that will be considered in the following chapter. In this book, all three sub-fields are drawn upon in varying degrees to advance knowledge and understanding of ethical issues in nursing and health care.

What is bioethics?

Bioethics is a relatively new field of inquiry and can be defined as 'the systematic study of the moral dimensions — including moral vision, decisions, conduct and policies — of the life sciences and health care, employing a variety of ethical methodologies in an interdisciplinary setting' (Reich 1995a, p. xxi). The term 'bioethics' (from the Greek *bios* meaning 'life', and *ethikos*, *ithiki* meaning 'ethics') is a neologism which first found its way into public usage in 1970–71 in the United States of America (Reich 1994). Although originally the subject of only cautious acceptance by a few influential North American academics, the new term quickly 'symbolised and influenced the rise and shaping of the field itself' (Reich 1994, p. 320). Significantly, within three years of its emergence, the new term was accepted and used widely at a public level (Reich 1994, p. 328). Interestingly, it is believed that the term 'bioethics' caught on because it was 'simple' and because it was amenable to exploitation by the media which had placed a great premium 'on having a simple term that could readily be used for public consumption' (Reich, 1994 p. 331). It is worth noting that initially the term 'bioethics' was used in two different ways reflecting both the concerns and ambitions of two respective academics who, it is suggested, quite possibly created the word independently of each other. The first (and later marginalised) sense in which the word was used had an 'environmental and evolutionary significance' (Reich 1994, p. 320). Specifically, it was intended to advocate attention to 'the problem of survival: the questionable survival of the human species and the even more questionable survival of nations and cultures' (Potter 1971 — cited by Reich 1994, p. 321). In short, it advocated long-range environmental concerns (Reich 1995b, p. 20). Reich (1994, pp. 321–2) explains that the key objective in creating this term was:

> to identify and promote an optimum changing environment, and an optimum human adaptation within that environment, so as to sustain and improve the civilised world.

The other competing sense in which the word 'bioethics' was used referred more narrowly to the ethics of medicine and biomedical research. The primary focus of this approach was (Reich 1995b, p. 20):

1. the rights and duties of patients and health care professionals;
2. the rights and duties of research subjects and researchers;
3. the formulation of public policy guidelines for clinical care and biomedical research.

Significantly, it was this latter sense which 'came to dominate the emerging field of bioethics in academic circles and in the mind of the public' — and which remains dominant today (Reich 1994, p. 320). There are a number of complex reasons for this, not least, the climate at the time which saw the rise of the civil rights movement (including women's rights and the legal right to abortion which helped to keep bioethical issues 'before the public'). Given the significant shift in social and moral values that was occurring at the time, however, it is perhaps not surprising that this essentially medical/biomedical sense of bioethics prevailed (Jonsen 1993; Singer 1994). For instance, it is now almost certain that the ideas behind the development of the field of bioethics in its medical/biomedical sense had been simmering for almost a decade before the field was eventually named (Jonsen 1993, S3). Notable among the events inspiring the development of the field were: the dialysis events of the early 1960s, the publication in 1966 of Henry Beecher's legendary and confronting article on the unethical design and conduct of 22 medical research projects, the heart transplant movement, and later the now famous 1975 Karen Ann Quinlan case (Jonsen 1993; see also Singer 1994; McNeill 1993; Pappworth 1967; Beecher 1966).

Today, the dominant concerns of mainstream Western bioethics are still essentially medically orientated, with the most sustained attention (and, it should be added, the most institutional support) being given to examining the ethical and legal dimensions of the 'big' issues of bioethics, such as abortion, euthanasia, organ transplantation (and the associated issue of brain-death criteria), reproductive technology (for example, in vitro fertilisation (IVF), genetic engineering, human cloning, and so forth), ethics committees, informed consent, confidentiality, the economic rationalisation of health care, and research ethics (particularly in regard to randomised clinical trials and experimental surgery). Not only has mainstream bioethics come to refer to and represent these issues, but, rightly or wrongly, has given legitimacy to them as *the* most pressing bioethical concerns of contemporary health care across the globe.

It is alleged that Potter (one of the authors of the term 'bioethics') was himself very frustrated with this narrow conception of bioethics and is reported as responding that 'my own view of bioethics calls for a much broader vision' (Reich 1995b, p. 20). Indeed, Potter feared (prophetically as it turned out) that 'the Georgetown approach would simply reaffirm medical professional inclination to think of issues in terms of therapy versus prevention' (Reich 1995b, pp. 20–1). Whereas Potter viewed bioethics as a 'new discipline' (of science *and* philosophy) emphasising a search for wisdom, the Georgetown group saw bioethics as an old discipline (applied ethics) to resolve concrete moral problems; that is, 'ordinary ethics applied in the bio-realm' (Reich 1995b, p. 21; see also Clouser 1978).

It has been claimed that 'bioethics is a native-grown American product' reflecting distinctively American concerns and offering distinctively American solutions and resolutions to the bioethical problems identified (Jonsen 1993, S3–4). Whatever the merits of this claim, there is little doubt that bioethics in its medical/biomedical sense has become an international movement. This movement (propelled along by a variety of processes) has witnessed a number of spectacular achievements, including:

- the development of an awesome international body of literature on the subject of bioethics (including the publication in 1978 of the first *Encyclopaedia of bioethics*, and in the 1990s the development and dissemination of the CD-ROM 'Bioethics Line');
- the global establishment of research centres devoted specifically to investigating ethical issues in health care and related matters;
- the emergence in the 1990s of a new profession of hospital ethicists/consultant ethicists;
- the establishment of prestigious university chairs in applied ethics;
- the rise of a commercially viable and even lucrative bioethics education industry; and, not least,
- the stimulation of public and political debate on 'life and death' matters in health care which, in many instances, has had a positive effect on influencing long overdue social policy and law reform in regard to these matters.

The medical/biomedical senses of the term 'bioethics' have indeed dominated intellectual and political thought over the past three decades. Nevertheless, there are signs that this dominance is being called into question (see, in particular, the introduction to the second edition of the *Encyclopaedia of bioethics* [Reich 1995a]). At present, there is considerable room to speculate that in the not too distant future the term 'bioethics' might once again hold an environmental and evolutionary significance, and have a much broader focus than it has up until now.

What is nursing ethics?

Nursing ethics can be defined broadly as the examination of all kinds of ethical and bioethical issues from *the perspective of nursing theory and practice* which, in turn, rest on the agreed core concepts of nursing, namely: person, culture, care, health, healing, environment, and nursing itself (or, more to the point, its ultimate purpose) — all of which have been comprehensively articulated in the nursing literature (too vast to list here). In this regard, then, contrary to popular belief, nursing ethics is not synonymous with (and indeed is much greater than) an ethic of care, although an ethic of care has an important place in the overall moral scheme of nursing and nursing ethics. Unlike other approaches to ethics, nursing ethics recognises the 'distinctive voices' that are nurses, and emphasises the importance of collecting and recording nursing narratives and 'stories from the field' (Benner 1994, 1991; Hodge 1993a, 1993b; Bishop and Scudder 1990; Parker 1990). Collecting and collating stories from the field are regarded as important since issues invariably emerge from these stories that extend far beyond the 'paramount' issues otherwise espoused by mainstream bioethics. Analyses of these stories tend to reveal not only a range of issues that are nurses' 'own', as it were, but a whole different configuration of language, concepts and metaphors for expressing them. As well, these stories often reveal issues otherwise overlooked in mainstream bioethics discourses. Given this, nursing ethics can also be described as *methodologically and substantively, inquiry from the point of view of nurses' experiences*, with nurses' experiences being taken as a more reliable starting point than other locations from which to advance a rich, meaningful and reliable system and practice of nursing ethics.

Like other approaches to ethics, however, nursing ethics recognises the importance of providing practical guidance on how to decide and act morally. Drawing on a variety of ethical theoretical considerations (what Beauchamp and Childress 2001, p. 400 call a 'coherentist' approach, and Benjamin, 2001 calls a 'pragmatic reflective equilibrium' approach), nursing ethics at its most basic could thus also be described as a practice discipline which aims to provide guidance to nurses on how to decide and act morally in the contexts in which they work.

The project of nursing ethics has many aspects to its nature and approach. Among other things, it involves nurses engaging in 'a positive project of constructing and developing alternative models, methods, procedures [and] discourses' of nursing and health care ethics that are more responsive to the lived realities and experiences of nurses and the people for whose care they share responsibility (adapted from Gross 1986, p. 195). In completing this positive project, nursing ethics has had — and continues to have — the positive consequence of allowing other 'weaker' viewpoints (including those of patients and nurses themselves) to emerge and be heard. In this respect, nursing ethics is also intensely political — although, it should be added, no more political than other role-differentiated ethics.

As in the case of moral philosophy, nursing ethics inquiry can be pursued by focusing on one or all of the following:

- *descriptive nursing ethics* (describing the moral values and beliefs that nurses hold and the various moral practices in which nurses engage across and within different contexts);
- *meta(nursing) ethics* (undertaking a critical examination of the nature, logical form, language, and methods of reasoning in nursing ethics); and

- *normative nursing ethics* (establishing standards of correctness and prescribing the rules of conduct with which nurses are expected to comply).

(Johnstone 1998, pp. 39–69)

It is important to remember (as discussed in the previous edition of this work [Johnstone 1999a]) that nursing ethics has not always enjoyed the status that it has today. Its development, legitimation and recognition as a distinctive field of inquiry is testimony to the reality that nursing ethics is both necessary and inevitable. It is necessary because 'a profession without its own distinctive moral convictions has nothing to profess' and will be left vulnerable to the corrupting influences of whatever forces are most powerful (be they religious, legal, social, political or other in nature) (Churchill 1989, p. 30). Furthermore, as Churchill (1989, p. 31) writes, 'Professionals without an ethic are merely technicians, who know how to perform work, but who have no capacity to say why their work has any larger meaning'. Without meaning, there is little or no motivation to perform 'well' (see also Johnstone 1998, pp. 74–6).

In regard to the inevitability of nursing ethics, as Churchill (1989, p. 31) points out, the 'practice of a profession makes those who exercise it privy to a set of experiences that those who do not practice lack'. By this view, those who practise nursing are privy to a set of experiences (moral experiences included) that others who do not practise nursing lack. So long as nurses interact with and enter into professional caring relationships with other people, they will not be able to avoid or sidestep the 'distinctively nursing' experience of deciding and acting morally while in these relationships. It is in this respect, then, that nursing ethics can be said to be *inevitable*.

What ethics is not

To further our understanding on what ethics (and its counterparts bioethics and nursing ethics) is, it would be useful to also give some attention to what ethics is not. For instance, ethics is not the same as law or a code of ethics. Neither is ethics something that can be determined by public opinion, or following the orders of a supervisor or manager. Failing to distinguish ethics from these kinds of things could result in otherwise avoidable harmful consequences to people in health care domains.

Law

Ethics and legal law overlap in significant ways, but they are nevertheless quite distinct from one another. This distinction becomes particularly clear in instances where what the law may require in a given situation, ethics might equally reject, and vice versa. Consider, for example, the issue of active voluntary euthanasia and the plight of patients suffering intractable and intolerable pain who request euthanasia as a 'treatment' option (Lanham 1993). Current Australian legal law prohibits voluntary active euthanasia. As the law stands, it is quite clear that any nurse or doctor who administers a lethal injection to a patient with the sole intention of bringing about that patient's death would probably be charged with murder. The fact that such an act was demonstrably in accordance with the patient's autonomous wishes would not be a legitimate defence. Regardless of the benevolence and voluntariness of an act of euthanasia, it would still be deemed by law as illegal, and thereby *legally wrong*. This legal wrongness, however, is in no way synonymous with moral wrongness. Consider the following.

Ethics essentially requires that people be respected as self-determining choosers, and further that the considered preferences of autonomous persons be maximised. This requirement holds even in instances where a person's individual preferences might be considered mistaken or foolish by others. Ethics also requires that otherwise avoidable harm (such as the needless suffering of intractable and intolerable pain) should be prevented where this can be done without sacrificing other important moral interests. Returning to our euthanasia example, it soon becomes clear that an application of ethics (or, more particularly, the principles of bioethics) in this instance would probably permit the administration of a lethal injection to a suffering patient who has autonomously requested it. Not only would ethics permit such an act; it would most likely require that it be done. Given the benevolence and voluntariness of the act, it would be deemed as having accorded with the principle of ethics and thereby as being *morally right*.

Other compelling examples illuminating the difference between law and morality can be found by considering the laws enforced during wartime (such as those upheld by the Nazi regime), and the laws used to enforce apartheid (such as those upheld in early North America, and, until recently, in South Africa). The legal laws of the Nazis and of the apartheid-supporting regimes, although evil, still stand as constituting valid *legal* law (Hart 1958). We would presumably want to resist condoning the *morality* of these laws, however.

Law and ethics are quite separate action-guiding systems, and care must be taken to distinguish between them. Making this distinction may not only help to prevent moral errors, but may also enforce moral and intellectual honesty about the undesirability of morally bad (evil) law (Hart 1958). Further, if we do not make this distinction we will not have an independent value system from which to judge the moral acceptability or unacceptability of valid legal law. For instance, if morality were not distinct from legal law, we could not judge certain laws (e.g. Nazi laws) to be morally bad and wrong.

The question remains, however, of how the distinction between law and ethics can be made, and, equally important, what the essential differences are between a legal decision and a moral/ethical decision, and, indeed, a clinical decision.[1]

A very traditional view of law is that it is the command or order of a sovereign (for example, a government) backed by a threat or sanction (for example, punishment) (Hart 1961). For instance, governments around the world have formulated laws which command their citizens to pay taxes; if the citizens in question fail to pay their taxes, they can expect to be punished in some way, such as by being fined or even sent to prison. The mere fact that they have not complied with the command — in essence, have broken the law — would probably be deemed sufficient justification for a sanction or punishment to be directed against them. Although this view of law does not capture its more political nature (see, for example, Johnstone 1994; Fineman and Thomadsen 1991; Thornton 1990; Kairys 1982), it is nevertheless sufficient for the purposes of this discussion in regard to distinguishing between law and ethics.

Accepting the above view of law, there is a fundamental sense in which the concept 'legal decision' as it is used by nurses probably refers to a type of decision that is made on the basis of what is required or prohibited by law — together with a desire to avoid a legal sanction or punishment for non-compliance. In this respect, the notion 'legal decision' is probably more aptly described as a 'legally defensive' decision. Consider the following example. A nurse who regards voluntary euthanasia as morally justified in cases of intolerable and intractable suffering may nevertheless decline a patient's considered request for assistance to die in order to avoid any risk of receiving the penalty that would almost certainly be applied for murder should her actions be discovered. In this instance, the nurse's decision not to comply with the patient's request could be described as a 'legal decision' rather than a moral or clinical decision, and also as being 'legally defensive'. This is because her decision was influenced predominantly by considering the legal consequences of complying with the patient's request, rather than the moral or clinical consequences of doing so.

The question remains, however, of how a legal decision differs from an ethical decision. As is discussed more fully in the following chapter, ethics can be defined as a system of overriding rules and principles which function by specifying that certain behaviours are either required, prohibited or permitted. These principles are chosen autonomously on the basis of critical reflection, and are backed by autonomous moral reason (generally recognised in moral philosophy as the central organising principle of morality) and/or by feelings of guilt, shame, moral remorse and the like which operate as kinds of moral sanctions. For example, we may choose autonomously to follow a moral principle which demands truth telling; if we fail to tell the truth in a given situation, we may then reason the act to be wrong and/or experience feelings of guilt, shame or moral remorse accordingly. Unlike what happens in instances involving a breach of legal law, however, we are not generally 'punished' for lying — for example, by being fined or sent to prison — unless, of course, our lying entails an outright act of perjury in a court of law.

Accepting this view of ethics, it is probably correct to say that the concept 'ethical decision', as it is used in health care contexts, refers to a type of decision which is guided by certain moral principles of conduct or other moral considerations (rather than by punitive legal laws) and a desire to achieve a given moral end. Thus, a doctor or a nurse tempted to tell a lie to either a colleague or a patient may choose instead to tell the truth in order to achieve some predicted overriding moral benefit and thereby also preserve her or his integrity as a morally autonomous person (as distinct from, say, a law-abiding citizen).

In light of these basic views on law and ethics and legal and ethical decision-making, what then is the nature of clinical (nursing and medical) decision-making? Primarily, nursing and medicine involve the skilful practice and application of tested principles of applied science and care to prevent, diagnose, alleviate or cure disease, illness and sickness and restore a person's health and sense of wellbeing. The practices of nursing and medicine are backed by legal and professional sanctions. For example, doctors and nurses can be found financially liable for negligence, and can be deregistered for professional misconduct, or even for civil misconduct unbefitting a professional person (see, for example, Pyne 1981; Johnstone 1998).

Given this, to say of a decision that it is a 'nursing decision' or a 'medical decision' in this context is probably to say little more than that it has been made by a nurse or a doctor respectively, and is based on an established body of knowledge and 'reasonable' professional opinion on how this knowledge should or should not be applied in a clinical situation. For example, a doctor may venture the 'reasonable' medical opinion that if a certain life-saving treatment is stopped the patient will surely die. Or a nurse may venture the 'reasonable' nursing opinion that if a certain nursing care is not given the patient will suffer a particular type of harm. It must be understood here, however, that neither of the clinical opinions expressed in these instances is tantamount to expressing a valid moral judgment. For example, to say that a patient 'will die' if a certain drug or other treatment (for example, surgery) is given or withheld says nothing about the moral permissibility or imperatives of giving or withholding the drug or other treatment in question. The morality of a given clinical act is not implicit in the act itself; this is something which can be determined only by independent moral analysis.

Given these rough comparisons, it can be seen that legal, ethical and clinical decisions can be readily distinguished from one another (see Figure 2.1). What is also obvious is the enormous potential for the respective demands of each of these three types of decisions to come into conflict. For example, a medical decision not to resuscitate a patient in the event of a cardiac arrest (on the grounds that the patient's condition is 'medically hopeless') may be supported by an established body of medical opinion, but nevertheless be deemed morally unsound or even illegal, or both. For instance, the patient's autonomous wishes may not have been established before the medical decision was made, or the patient's legally valid consent may not have been obtained to withhold cardiopulmonary resuscitation (CPR) in the event of a cardiac arrest. Or, to take another example, a medical decision to continue treating a patient may accord with a 'reasonable body of medical opinion', be legal (as in cases where patients have been deemed rationally incompetent under a mental health act), yet be quite unethical if the patient has expressly stated a wish not to be treated, and if this expressed wish, contrary to popular medical opinion, is not 'irrational'. We can also imagine cases where a medical decision to cease treatment accords with moral principles but may nevertheless invite legal censure — as in the case of withholding unduly burdensome life-prolonging treatment from severely disabled newborns or severely brain-injured adults.

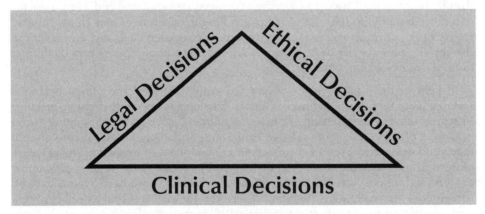

Figure 2.1 Types of decisions in clinical settings

Although there is potential for conflict between ethical, legal and clinical decisions, it is not the case that these are always on a direct collision course; indeed, they may even be in harmony with each other, as examples given in the chapters to follow show.

In drawing comparisons between legal, ethical and clinical decisions, there remains another crucial point to be observed: that it is conceptually incorrect to regard nursing or medical decisions per se as synonymous with either legal or moral decisions. This is not to say that we cannot meaningfully speak of nursing or medical decisions as being legally or morally correct or incorrect. On the contrary, it makes the point that, in asserting the legal or moral status of a given clinical (nursing or medical) decision, a judgment *independent* of the generally accepted scientific or indeed conventional standards of nursing or medicine must be made. In the case of ethics, the moral status of a clinical decision requires independent *philosophical/moral* analysis and judgment based on relevant moral considerations (e.g. moral rules and principles); and in the case of law, the legal status of a clinical decision requires an independent *legal* analysis and judgment based on relevant legal considerations (e.g. legal rules and principles).

Codes of ethics

A code may be defined as a conventionalised set of rules or expectations devised for a select purpose. A code of professional ethics by this view could be described as a document that sets out a conventionalised set of moral rules and/or expectations devised for the purposes of guiding ethical professional conduct. It is important to understand, however, that codes of ethics are not ethics per se since they are not a fully developed system of ethics. Nevertheless, codes of ethics tend to reflect a rich set of moral values that have been expressed through a process of extensive consultation, debate, refinement, evaluation and review by practitioners over a period of time, and thus are well situated to function as meaningful action guides (Johnstone 1998, pp. 7–15).

It is important to state at the outset that codes of ethics can be either *prescriptive* or *aspirational* in nature. In the case of *prescriptive codes*, provisions are 'duty-directed, stating specific duties of members' (Skene 1996, p. 111). In contrast, *aspirational codes* are 'virtue-directed, stating desirable aims while acknowledging that in some circumstances conduct short of the ideal may be justified' (Skene 1996, p. 111). Either way, codes of ethics have as their principal concern directing:

> what professionals ought or ought not to do, how they ought to comport themselves, what they, or the profession as a whole, ought to aim at ...
>
> (Lichtenberg 1996, p. 14)

Codes of ethics are not, however, without difficulties — a point noted almost 100 years ago by the distinguished North American nurse leader and scholar, Lavinia Dock.

In a little-known but important essay entitled 'Ethics — or a code of ethics?', Dock (1900, p. 37) challenged:

> What, exactly, could a Code of Ethics be? ... What are ethics and can they be codified? Do we aim at ethical exclusiveness and shall our ethical development be bounded or limited by a code? 'Code' suggests statutes, infringements, penalties, antagonisms. If we have the ethics, we will not need a code. The code is to regulate those who have no ethics, and in proportion as ethical principles are made a part of our natures and lives, our codes and restrictions will shrivel away and die the death of inanition.

Dock goes on to explain that she is not advocating the total rejection of rules and regulations of professional conduct — to the contrary, particularly since such rules and regulations, as given in a code, could serve as helpful mechanisms 'to prop up the steps of those who are young in self-government or feeble in self-control' (p. 38). Rather, the issue was not to call codes of rules and regulations *ethics*, since, as she argued persuasively, there was a real risk that (p. 38):

If we call them ethics we may perhaps come to believe that they are all there is of ethics, and presently be worshipping the code rather than the thing, so unreasoning a reverence is there in our souls for statutes, fines, and punishments; so exaggerated a notion of the potency of drafted laws; so strong a tendency to make rules the end and aim of life rather than simply conveniences, changeable contrivances.

Although written over a century ago, Dock's visionary words are applicable today. Nurses globally would be well advised to be cautious in their use of formally stated and adopted codes of ethics, and to be especially vigilant not to fall prey to 'worshipping the code' at the expense of *being* ethical — and not to fall into the trap of treating the requirements of a code as absolute, and as ends in themselves, rather than as prima facie guides to ethical professional conduct.

It has long been recognised that a professional code of ethics is an important hallmark of a profession (Bayles 1981; Goldman 1980). Whether professional codes as such have succeeded in fulfilling their intended purpose of 'formulating the norms of professional ethics' (Bayles 1981, p. 25) and guiding ethical professional conduct is, however, another matter. Some have argued that codes of ethics have failed to ensure this; instead, codes of ethics have served to protect the interests of the professional group espousing them, rather than the interests of the client groups whom the professionals are supposed to be serving (Beauchamp and Childress 2001, pp. 5–7; Kultgen 1982, pp. 53–69).

Despite the demonstrable shortcomings of professional codes of ethics, it is evident that many professional codes of ethics have been written with the noble intention of guiding ethically just professional practice. What needs to be understood, however, is that even the most scrupulously formulated and well-intended professional code of ethics is not without its limitations and, in the final analysis, may do little to either guide moral deliberation or ensure the realisation of morally just outcomes in morally problematic situations. In the case of the nursing profession, neither will following a code of ethics necessarily protect nurses when they are called upon to defend their actions, say, in a court or disciplinary hearing (see Johnstone 1994b, pp. 251–67; 1998).

In a 1990 Australian case, for example, involving the alleged unfair dismissal of a registered nurse involved in a case of suspected child sexual abuse, the deputy president of the Industrial Relations Commission of Victoria (where the case was heard) rejected the authority of the International Council of Nurses (ICN) (1973) *Code for Nurses*, which was referred to in defence of the nurse's actions (*In re alleged unfair dismissal of Ms K Howden by the City of Whittlesea* 1990). In this case the deputy president of the Commission pointedly criticised the ICN Code as being 'imprecise' and lacking the ability to provide 'clear guidance' in matters requiring fine discretionary professional judgment. He also pointed out that the 'code in its terms cannot stand alone' and must be considered in relation to the guidance which is also offered by the law (*In re alleged unfair dismissal of Ms K Howden by the City of Whittlesea* 1990). The fact that the ICN Code is widely accepted by professional nursing organisations around the world had little bearing on the deputy president's views in this case.

The legal status of the acclaimed *Code of Professional Practice* of the United Kingdom Central Council for Nursing, Midwifery and Health Visiting (1984) is also uncertain, its authority having been rejected by at least one court since its adoption in the early 1980s (Rea 1987, p. 534).

One question which arises here is that, if codes of ethics are problematic, and have only limited legal (and, it should be added, moral) authority, should nurses adopt them? The short answer to this question is yes. One justification for this is that, despite their limitations, codes of ethics have an important role to play in the broader schema of professional nursing ethics insofar as they can provide a public statement on the kinds of moral standards and values that patients and the broader community can expect nurses to uphold, and against which nurses can be held publicly accountable. Second, they can also inform those contemplating entering the profession of the kinds of values and standards which they will be expected to uphold, and which, if not upheld, could result in some sort of professional censure. For example, the ICN (2002) *Code of Ethics for Nurses* makes explicit that a nurse's 'primary responsibility is to people requiring nursing care', and that, in providing care, the nurse will promote 'an environment in which the human rights, values, customs and spiritual beliefs of the individual, family and community are respected'. If people contemplating entering the profession of nursing are informed of these prescriptions, and do not agree with them, they will be in a better position to make an informed choice about whether or not to enter the profession.

Another justification is that codes of ethics can help with the cultivation of moral character (Johnstone 1998, pp. 7–15). They can do this by 'increasing the probability that people will behave in some ways rather than others' — specifically that they will behave in 'the right way' and, equally important, 'for the right reasons' (Lichtenberg 1996, p. 15). As already stated, although codes of ethics do not constitute a system of ethics (at best, they comprise only a list of rules that have been derived from systematic ethical thought), they nevertheless provide people with a reason to think and act ethically, not least by reminding them 'of the moral point of the sorts of activities they are involved in *as* members of the particular profession or group' (Coady 1996, p. 286). On this point, Lichtenberg (1996, p. 18) contends:

> A code of ethics can increase the probability that people will think about it [what one is doing] — can make it more difficult to engage in self-deceptive practices — by explicitly describing behaviour that is undesirable or unacceptable.

Crucial to the cultivation of moral character, is self-conscious moral reflection. And, as Freckelton (1996, p. 130) suggests controversially, codes of ethics 'are a means to this end'. He states (p. 130):

> They [codes of ethics] have the potential to articulate the characteristics and ideals of a profession and to facilitate consciousness of and discourse about ethical issues. Through the process of moral deliberation thereby engendered, they may operate as the catalysts for ethical conduct both by heightening awareness of ethical priorities and by providing guidance from experienced professionals for the resolution of ethical conundra encountered at a practical level by practitioners ... By articulating the parameters of a profession and of acceptable professional conduct by its practitioners, a code defines what a profession is and is not, as well as the limits of proper conduct.

Self-conscious moral reflection and discussion about ethical issues are facilitated by codes of ethics in at least one other important way, namely, by what Fullinwider (1996, p. 83) describes as supplying a vocabulary (which can be used for the purposes of stimulating 'moral self-understanding') and helping to '*create* a community of users'. To put this another way, by expressing a given set of ethical values, a code of ethics makes discussion and debate of ethical issues possible within a given professional group (community); it provides a (common) moral language, which can be used meaningfully by subscribers to a given code, to identify and discuss matters of moral importance and to advance the task of professional ethics generally in their milieu.

The point remains, however, as already argued, that codes of ethics have only prima facie moral authority (that is, they may be overridden by other, stronger moral considerations), and hence can only *guide*, not mandate, moral conduct in particular situations. Further, as Seedhouse (1988, p. 65) points out, it is important to understand that a code cannot inform a nurse which principles to follow in a given situation, how to interpret chosen principles, how to choose between conflicting principles, or 'how to decide when it is most ethical to disregard the rules and deliberate instead as a unique and independent individual' as is sometimes required. Accepting this, and as the examples given in the following chapters show, it can be seen that no code of professional nursing ethics should be regarded as an authoritative statement of universal action guides. Rather, it should be regarded only as a statement of prima facie rules which may be helpful in guiding moral decision-making in nursing care contexts, but which can be justly overridden by other, stronger moral considerations.

Hospital or professional etiquette

Nothing could be more different from ethics than etiquette. Although both seek to guide behaviour and conduct, they do so in quite different ways and for quite different purposes. Ethics, for example, speaks to morally significant rights and wrongs, with behaviour being guided by critically reflective moral thought and the application of sound moral values which seek to maximise the moral interests of all people equally. Etiquette, by contrast, speaks more to maintaining style and decorum, with behaviour being guided by the unreflective and arbitrary requirements of custom and convention. In application, etiquette paves the way for coordinated, consistent, predictable and, where possible, aesthetically pleasant practice and conduct, and serves only the interests of particular persons in particular circumstances (May 1983). As with legal law, what etiquette might demand in one situation, ethics might reject, and vice versa.

The extent to which the notions of ethics and etiquette can be confused in health care settings is well illustrated by the following case — which demonstrates the reluctance by some health professionals (including nurses) to advise patients to seek a second medical opinion, in the mistaken belief that doing so would constitute a serious breach of ethics.

The case (personal communication) involves a middle-aged woman suffering moderately severe retrosternal chest pain and shortness of breath who presented to the accident and emergency department of a large city hospital. The nursing staff admitted the woman into a cubicle equipped to deal with 'cardiac emergencies' and proceeded to perform an electrocardiograph (ECG). The ECG showed a number of cardiac arrhythmias, all of which were suggestive of an acute cardiac condition warranting immediate specialised medical and nursing care. Upon further questioning, it was revealed that the woman was also suffering a mild pain in her left arm (a pain she had 'never had before'), which is characteristic of cardiac disease. The pain improved, however, while she rested in the casualty department. Her past medical history indicated no known heart disease or any previous incidence of chest pain. This was the first time she had ever experienced such symptoms — symptoms which were indicative of significant underlying cardiac disease.

A junior first-year medical resident examined the woman and decided she should be admitted immediately into the coronary care unit for further cardiac monitoring and tests. As required by the hospital's admission policy, he contacted the registrar 'on call' to have his diagnosis confirmed and to arrange the woman's admission formally. Upon examining the patient, however, the registrar declined to admit her, since there were no 'cardiac beds' available in the hospital and he was not convinced that the ECG findings indicated a life-threatening cardiac condition. He discharged the woman, advising her to see her own general practitioner the following morning. He gave her a medical note and a prescription for an oral cardiac anti-arrhythmic agent.

The nursing staff were very concerned, as was the first-year medical resident. All felt the patient should have been seen by another doctor for a 'second opinion', but could not decide whether to advise the woman to go immediately to another hospital. After some 20 minutes of deliberation, the attending nursing supervisor concluded it would be 'unethical' to advise the patient to go to another hospital for a second examination. The nursing staff and junior doctor involved agreed. The patient walked out of the door and was not informed that it would be in her interests to seek a second medical opinion. At this hospital, it was not 'standard practice' to advise patients to seek second medical opinions.

What was at issue here, however, was breaching hospital *etiquette*. Advising the woman to seek a second medical opinion, in this case, would not have been unethical; indeed, there is considerable scope to suggest that offering such advice was morally obligatory in this case.

Etiquette obviously has its place in the professional and health care arena; it is not without limits, however. Unfortunately, as Blackburn (1984, p. 189) points out, people do 'often care more about etiquette, or reputation, or selfish advantage, than they do about morality'. The lesson to be learned here is that acting in accord with hospital or professional etiquette might sometimes be tantamount to acting unethically or immorally — or, in some instances, even illegally. It is, therefore, important that nurses learn to distinguish between the demands of etiquette and those of ethics.

Hospital or institutional policy

Hospital policy or institutional policy is often appealed to in order to legitimise a worker's actions and, in some cases, to settle a conflict of opinion about what course of action should be taken in a particular situation. In this respect, institutional or hospital policy plays an important practical role — it helps to coordinate 'the running of the system' and to make institutional practices consistent and predictable; nevertheless, it also paves the way for uncompromising control. Like legal law and etiquette, institutional policy can be morally bad and in application can seriously conflict with the demands of ethics. The following case (taken from the author's personal observations) is a good example of how institutional policy can be at odds with ethics.

A 20-year-old woman in advanced premature labour was admitted to the casualty department of a city hospital. She was of a traditional Maori background, married, and the pregnancy had been planned. This was her third premature labour. On the two previous occasions she had spontaneously aborted at around 20 weeks' gestation. Her current pregnancy was also of approximately 20 weeks' gestation.

The obstetrics registrar was notified, but failed to appear before the young woman delivered her fully formed male fetus. The fetus was active upon delivery and was noted by nursing staff to have breathed, emitting a faint but audible high-pitched 'rasp' as it did so. In accordance with 'standard hospital procedure' the fetus was placed in a stainless steel kidney dish, taken immediately away from the mother's view, and placed, covered with a bed pan sheet, in the sluice room to die. The mother and her family, however, wanted to have 'the baby' near, not only to see it but more importantly to perform *karakia* (a kind of incantation or prayer), as stringently required by ancient Maori custom.[2]

Maori Enrolled Nurses working in the casualty department were greatly distressed by what was happening. As the mother and her family (one of whom was a *Tohunga* [priest]) were pleading to have the fetus returned, one of the Maori enrolled nurses went to the fetus in the sluice room 'to be with it, so that it would not die without knowing love'. Crying softly, she also admitted to a registered nurse involved in the case that she was going to offer a prayer 'for the child as he goes on his way ...' (Makereti 1986).

The doctor had, meanwhile, arrived in the department and examined the mother. He explained to her and her family that the fetus could not be released to them because 'tests had to be done on it'. He later explained to protesting nursing staff that fetuses delivered at the hospital were generally regarded as 'hospital property' and that it was 'hospital policy to send all aborted fetuses to the laboratory for analysis'. He also explained that the present case was particularly complicated because the fetus was of 20 weeks' gestation, and had breathed. It was therefore, technically speaking, a 'live birth', and thus an autopsy would have to be performed. This, he further claimed, was a legal requirement. Whether in fact this was correct was not known by those present at the time; informal sources subsequently indicated that autopsies cannot be performed without consent, and it is likely that the parents' claim to the fetus could have been legally upheld. Most of the registered nurses present nevertheless accepted the doctor's explanation and resigned themselves to 'hospital policy'.

One registered nurse, however, pressed the matter further and explained to the doctor that the 'hospital policy' in this instance was quite inappropriate given the situation at hand, and that to uphold the policy so rigidly stood to violate the Maori family's rights and interests. At the same time, the fetus had meanwhile been mistakenly submerged in the liquid preservative formalin and taken by a hospital orderly to the laboratory.

Fortunately, the doctor was sympathetic and sought to resolve the difficulties he perceived he would have with the hospital authorities by registering the fetus as being of less than 20 weeks' gestation, and as not having breathed. Nevertheless, the fetus was not retrieved from the laboratory for another 24 hours, by which time, sadly, considerable damage had already been done. The most the family and the *Tohunga* could now do was to try and appease the *wairua* (spirit) through *karakia*, and to try and persuade it to travel without taking harm with it. The mother's single room was turned into a *marae* (meeting place) setting, and a *tangi* (funeral) commenced. This was an act of sheer desperation, and in part an attempt to explain to the *wairua* why the violation and act of cruelty had occurred. It was also to grieve for what they had lost, and what would be lost to them forever.

Upholding hospital policy in this case resulted in an unacceptable level of human suffering — suffering which could have been avoided by a more critically reflective approach to the situation. Had those present been more aware of their moral obligations to respect the wishes of the mother and her family, a morally tolerable outcome could have been achieved. Fortunately, as a result of this particular incident, the hospital policy was revised, making it easier for Maori mothers to claim their fetuses lost through miscarriages.

This case demonstrates a situation where ethics is quite distinct from institutional policy, and where a review of ethical considerations may prompt reform of policy. It also shows how respect for hospital policy is not sufficient to ensure the realisation of morally desirable or morally tolerable outcomes.

Public opinion or the view of the majority

Public opinion is often cited in defence of the 'ethics' of something such as the moral permissibility of abortion, euthanasia or the use of fetal tissue for research. For example, those in favour of the legalisation of euthanasia will commonly cite public opinion polls favouring the legalisation of euthanasia to support their stance.

Ethics is not something that can be determined or decidedly reliably by public opinion, however. If ethics were merely a matter of public opinion, all we would have to do is conduct an opinion poll and establish a 'majority view' on a matter to find out whether it was morally right or wrong. If ethics was determined by mere public opinion, our moral standards would be rendered hopelessly and unacceptably changeable, making it extremely difficult to practice ethically. Consider the following example.

In 2002 it was reported that most Australians (including Catholics) supported the use of fetal tissue in medical research (Kissane 2002, p. 7). A survey of 9293 people (including 2120 Catholics) found that 36 per cent strongly approved and 40 per cent approved (that is, a total of 76 per cent approved) the use of cells from a fetus for 'testing new ways to treat cancer or Parkinson's or other serious diseases' (Kissane 2002, p. 7). The survey also found that 19 per cent of respondents believed that *human life* began at conception, but that most believed the fetus was not human until two–three months of gestation and 83 per cent believing the fetus was not human until four or five months, 'when the mother could feel it move' (Kissane 2002, p. 7). It was suggested that these findings had enormous implications for the abortion debate (Kissane 2002, p. 7) — the main implication being that if it is permissible to experiment on fetuses (at least before the third month of gestation), then it is also permissible to perform abortions (at least before the third month of gestation).

If ethics was just a matter of public opinion, in this example we would be committed to accepting that the fetus is not 'human' until the second, third, fourth or fifth month of gestation and that it is morally acceptable to experiment on fetuses (at least before the third month of gestation) since it is not 'human'. The human fetus is, of course, *genetically human* from the moment of conception even though public opinion, in this instance, would however have us believe otherwise and, inconsistently, across a continuum of time, that is, of two, three, four and five months. The issue of when the fetus becomes a *human being* is, however, a different matter entirely and, unfortunately, not covered in the report. Nevertheless, even if this question was settled in favour of 'humanhood', it is not clear whether this would be sufficient to change public opinion. If public opinion were to change — and it turned against the permissibility of using fetal tissue for research purposes — we would be committed to accepting the impermissibility of using fetal tissue for research purposes even when this could result in finding a cure for terrible diseases. A public opinion view of ethics, in this instance, could therefore result in a change in the judgment on the rightness or wrongness of using fetal tissue for research purposes from one day to the next.

A public opinion or majority view of ethics is open to serious objection. On a philosophical level, it violates a formal and necessary requirement for sound moral judgments, notably the requirement for *internal consistency* (Kuhse 1987, p. 25). Its findings are liable to reflect sudden and unpredictable changes in attitudes and opinions, and thus are morally unreliable. As well as this, on a more pragmatic level, there is the distasteful possibility that public opinion might be mistaken or wrong or misguided — particularly where it has been manipulated by pressure groups, politicians or by the media, as occurred in the much publicised 'Kids Overboard' incident that occurred in Australia in the lead up to the 2001 Federal election. The incident involved the public misrepresentation of photographic images and false claims by Federal government politicians that asylum seekers, who were attempting to enter Australian territory illegally by sea, had 'deliberately' thrown their children overboard from the boat they were on in order to force their rescue and subsequent entry into Australia via the HMAS *Adelaide*, a nearby Naval ship. It was later revealed, however, and subsequently verified by a Senate Inquiry into the matter, that *no* children had, in fact, been thrown overboard (Senate Select Committee on a Certain Maritime Incident, 2002). In the lead up to the Federal election on 10 November, this incident was used along with other incidents (e.g. the *Tampa* rescue of Afghan refugees) to support the Federal government's 'hardline political response to unauthorised arrivals' and to sway public opinion against asylum seekers seeking refuge in Australia by portraying them (demonising them) as 'faceless, violent queue jumpers' (ABC 2002) and as people of poor moral character ('What kind people throw their children overboard?', Senate Select Committee on a Certain Maritime Incident 2002). Post election analyses indicated that the 'Kids Overboard' incident had influenced public opinion in favour of the Federal government's tough (some would say, inhumane) policies on the admission and detention of refugees and asylum seekers in Australia and contributed to the Federal government's re-election in 2001.

There is also the risk of opinion polls being fraudulent. As one woman wrote in a letter to the editor of *The Age*:

> If I felt strongly enough about the issue at hand [television phone-in polls] I could have spent the evening by my phone and, with the simple touch of one button, registered votes almost continuously without anyone being any the wiser to my hundreds and possibly thousands of votes …
>
> … Unfortunately many people never question the validity of opinion polls and instead take them at face value. I suspect that many think they represent general opinion, otherwise why conduct them.

(Romanin 1988, p. 12)

It is not being denied here that public opinion is an important and relevant consideration that warrants some attention when deciding ethical issues. On the contrary, public opinion which reliably indicates a certain view on a given matter might well be a useful tool in guiding beneficial social policy and law reforms. However, public opinion is not infallible in matters of morality and mere *common acceptance* does not imply validity (Brandt 1959, p. 57). The moral rightness or wrongness of an act can be decided only by sound critical reflection, not merely by public opinion or 'collective desire' or 'collective preference'.

Following the orders of a supervisor or manager

Following the moral commands of another is quite incompatible with the notion of ethics and the autonomous moral thinking that underpins it (for reasons that will be explained in Chapter 3). Moreover, it paves the way for the abdication of moral responsibility and accountability. Supervisors have supervisors, and these supervisors have still more supervisors. A hierarchical system of authority may mean in practice that, because everyone is accountable for a given action, it is difficult or impossible to decide who is to be held ultimately accountable (Barry 1982, p. 13).

A classic example of this occurred at Waikato Hospital, New Zealand, in 1982. The incident in question involved a 28-year-old woman who died after being given an incorrectly prescribed dose of morphine. At the coronial inquiry into her death, it was revealed that the charge nurse who administered the 50milligram intramuscular dose of morphine did so on the insistence of the prescribing 'doctor' (who was in fact a final-year medical student from Australia). The prescribing 'doctor' in turn insisted that she 'did not prescribe the morphine, but simply passed on [the covering registrar's] prescription for the nurse to administer' (*Waikato Times* 1984b, p. 3). The medical registrar, in turn, claimed that he had worked from eight in the morning on Saturday to midday Sunday, and had only had four hours' sleep during that time — implying that 'the system' was to blame. The medical consultant under whom the registrar was working meanwhile stated that 'if he was asked' he would not regard the duties of the medical student as being 'those of a house surgeon' (the New Zealand term for medical resident) — implying that his registrar was ultimately responsible (*Waikato Times* 1984a, p. 1). The medical superintendent, in turn, stated that the registrar 'should have been in charge of prescribing narcotics' (*Waikato Times* 1984a, p. 1), while the Waikato Hospital Board suggested that 'no one person be blamed for the overdose' (*Waikato Times* 1984b, p. 3).

The coroner is reported to have concluded that it would be quite 'unfair, unkind and not based on the evidence' to blame the medical student who prescribed the morphine for the woman's death. On the basis of the coroner's overall findings, the police did not press charges.

Admittedly this case emphasises more the issues of legal responsibility and accountability than those of moral responsibility. Legal and moral responsibility and accountability, however, travel a common path, as made evident by the much noted *Bormann defence*, named after Martin Bormann, third deputy under the Nazi regime of World War II, who argued in defence of his involvement in wartime atrocities that he was 'just following orders' (Barry 1982, p. 13). This kind of defence is a convenient 'moral cop-out' for those who have no sense of moral accountability, or a poorly developed sense, and who ordinarily try to justify their behaviour as Bormann did: 'I was told to do it'; 'I was expected to do it'; 'I was just doing my job'; 'That's how things operate around here'; and so forth (Barry 1982, p. 13).

The outcome of the 1945–46 Nuremberg trials made it abundantly clear that a plea of following the orders of one's superiors was not an acceptable or a legitimate defence in the eyes of the law. Such a precedent had already been well established for nurses as early as 1929, however, with the successful prosecution in the Philippines of a newly graduated nurse by the name of Lorenza Somera, who was found guilty of manslaughter, sentenced to a year in prison, and fined 1000 pesos because she had followed a physician's incorrect drug order (Grennan 1930). In court it was proved that the physician had ordered the drug, that Somera had verified it, and that the physician had administered the injection. But, as Winslow (1984) writes, 'the physician was acquitted and Somera found guilty because she failed to *question* the orders'. The case stunned nurses around the world. A campaign of protest was organised, and Somera was given a conditional pardon before serving a day of her sentence.

In an institutional setting, it is very easy to rationalise moral 'unaccountability':

> So many people, even institutions, can get involved at so many levels that moral buck-passing can become the order of the day. The blind pursuit of prestige and profits also blurs moral accountability. And most important, the intense pressure to keep one job and to secure promotions can be used to justify almost anything. The point is that working within an organisation provides easy excuses for abdicating personal moral accountability for decisions and actions.
>
> (Barry 1982, p. 13)

One way of avoiding this abdication is to draw a firm distinction between ethics and following the orders of a supervisor or manager, and to recognise that moral demands are always the overriding consideration, irrespective of a supervisor's or a manager's orders.

The task of ethics, bioethics and nursing ethics

In considering what ethics is, and what it is not, it is also important to have some understanding of exactly what ethics, in its broadest sense, is attempting to achieve; in short, what is the task of ethics and to what extent do bioethics and nursing ethics respectively contribute to this task?

In identifying and exploring the task of ethics, it is necessary to give a brief historical overview of the development of Western moral thinking. The task of ethics has been the subject of rigorous philosophical debate for almost 3000 years. In the Platonic dialogues, for example, we are told that the ultimate task of morality is to find out 'how best to live' or, in other words, how to lead 'the good life' and enjoy supreme wellbeing (Allen 1966, pp. 57–255). For the British philosopher Thomas Hobbes (1588–1679), the task of morality is a little different: notably, to find a device that will ensure mutual agreement and cooperation among each of society's members. It was Hobbes' view that, without such a device, the prospects of human survival would at best be slim (Hobbes 1968, p. 205).

Hobbes' concerns were echoed almost a century later by the Scottish philosopher David Hume (1711–76), who insisted, among other things, that morality was a subject of supreme interest since its decisions had the very peace of society firmly at stake (Hume 1888, p. 455). Like Hobbes, Hume recognised that the human mind was more than capable of courting the undesirable qualities of 'avarice, ambition, cruelty [and] selfishness'; and, like Hobbes, he recognised that society's hope for peace depended very much on the formulation of certain rules of conduct (Hume 1888, pp. 494–6). These rules of conduct need to be developed and enforced precisely because people fail to pursue the public interest 'naturally, and with a hearty affection' (Hume 1888, p. 496).

The influential German philosopher, Immanuel Kant (1724–1804) took a slightly different view from his predecessors. Unlike Hobbes and Hume, he saw the task of ethics (or rather, moral philosophy) as being 'to seek out and establish the supreme principle of morality' (Kant 1972, p. 57). Like those before him, Kant recognised that persons were vulnerable to being 'affected … by so many inclinations and lacked the power to conduct their life in accordance with practical reason'. Kant went on to argue that as long as the 'ultimate norm for correct moral judgment' is lacking, morals themselves will be vulnerable to corruption (Kant 1972, p. 55).

Kant's overall investigation succeeded in providing a supreme, although not uncontroversial, principle of morality for guiding human actions. Upholding the tenets of *ethical rationalism* (now regarded as a controversial thesis), this principle took the form of a *categorical imperative* which essentially commands that rational autonomous choosers should 'act only on that maxim through which you can at the same time will that it should become universal law' (Kant 1972, p. 84). In other words, act only on those moral rules and principles which you are prepared to accept apply to all other people as well. His final analysis made clear that the influences of self-interest and/or of individual 'feelings, impulses and inclinations' could have no place in a system of sound morality (Kant 1972, p. 84). If 'rational agents' are to act morally, they must act in strict accordance with the dictates of 'rational moral law'.

The moral law was seen by Kant as providing ultimate, overriding principles of conduct and ones which all rational agents ought to respect. He was optimistic that if all rational persons lived absolutely by the moral law then they could hope to live in a world (or rather 'a kingdom', as he called it) where rational agents would be respected as ends in themselves and not as the mere means to the ends of others (Kant 1972, p. 96).

The influential views of Plato, Hobbes, Hume and Kant concerning the task of ethics continue to have force in modern moral philosophy. For example, the Australian philosopher John Mackie (born in Sydney in 1917) argues that so-called 'limited sympathies' exist as a profound threat to what might otherwise be regarded as the 'good life' (Mackie 1977, p. 108).[3] Mackie echoes the view that if an all-enduring and decent (harmonious) life is to be secured, the problem of limited sympathies needs to be counteracted. The only way this can be done is by finding something which will coordinate and marry together individual and differing choices of action. In other words, what is needed is a device which could act as a kind of 'invisible chain' keeping together many sorts of 'useful agreements' (Mackie 1977, pp. 116, 118).

The solution for Mackie lies squarely at the feet of morality, which he interprets as (1977, p. 106):

> a system of a particular sort of constraints on conduct — ones whose central task is to protect the interests of persons other than the agent and present themselves to an agent as checks on his [or her] natural inclinations or spontaneous tendencies to act.

Mackie argues further that a morality applied appropriately is a morality which will help to facilitate the realisation of the overall wellbeing of people. In order for morality to work in this way, however, it must have at its core the vital component 'humane disposition' (Mackie 1977, p. 194). A humane disposition in this instance is that which 'naturally manifests itself in hostility to and disgust at cruelty, and in sympathy with pain and suffering whenever they occur' (p. 194). People who are of humane disposition, suggests Mackie, 'cannot be callous and indifferent, let alone actively cruel either toward permanently defective human beings or toward non-human animals' (p. 194).

The English philosopher Richard Hare also views the task of ethics in terms of imposing stringent requirements on persons to act in morally just ways. On this, Hare argues that (1981, p. 228):

Morality compels us to accommodate ourselves to the preferences of others, and this has the effect that when we are thinking morally and doing it rationally we shall all prefer the same moral prescriptions about matters which affect other people ...

Hare ultimately advocates morality as a form of compelling 'rational universal prescriptivism', and concludes that 'moral reason leaves us with our freedom, but constrains us to respect the freedom of others, and to combine with them in exercising it' (Hare 1981, p. 228).

The notion that the task of ethics is to supply a system of ultimate, overriding principles of conduct is also supported by the American philosopher Stephen Ross (1972, p. 283), who argues that the goal of morality is 'to reach a common set of moral ideals which everyone can follow' or, rather, to 'seek principles of conduct which everyone can live by'. According to Ross, moral principles are needed to regulate our moral decisions and to help settle competing alternatives. Moral principles remind us of our overriding duties to others and of the merits of morally principled action. Principles of morality also lend people 'tools' which can be used to deal appropriately and effectively with moral crises and dilemmas in both everyday and special (e.g. professional) worlds. They remind us that, without secure, ultimate and overriding rules of conduct, people may find it all too easy to abdicate their moral responsibilities and to commit atrocities. (The My Lai massacre during the Vietnam War is a poignant example of how unclear and unstable rules of conduct can contribute significantly to the realisation of atrocious human behaviour [see in particular Peers, 1979, p. 33; Bilton and Sim, 1992; Kelman and Hamilton, 1989].)

Other American philosophers such as John Rawls, Tom Beauchamp and James Childress, David Gauthier, and H. Tristram Engelhardt Jr have described the task of modern moral philosophy in similar terms again. Rawls (1971) for example, sees the task of ethics as to validate the conception of morality 'as a set of rational, impartial constraints on the pursuit of individual interest', and to adjudicate cases in which there are conflicts of interest. Beauchamp and Childress, on the other hand, suggest that the task of ethics is to supply an 'ideal code consisting of a set of rules that guide the members of a society to maximise intrinsic value' (1983, p. 40). Gauthier (1986, p. 6), describes the task of ethics as that of developing a way of ordering interests. Engelhardt (1986, pp. 67–9), meanwhile sees the task of ethics as searching for common grounds to bind consenting individuals in a peaceable community — in short, to achieve peaceable bonds among persons without brute force. He also sees the task of ethics as being that which (p. 26):

aspires to provide a logic for a pluralism of beliefs, a common view of a good life that can transcend particular communities, professions, legal jurisdictions, and religions, but whose grounds for authenticity are immanent to the secular world.

Both bioethics and nursing ethics share the task of ethics.

Conclusion

Advancing ethics, bioethics and nursing ethics inquiry and practice requires at least a basic knowledge and understanding of the definitions and meanings of such terms as 'ethics', 'bioethics' and 'nursing ethics'. In this chapter, working definitions of these notions have been provided (the definitions of other commonly used moral terms such as 'rights', 'duties' and 'obligations' will be given in Chapter 3). In providing these working definitions, attention has also been given to demonstrating what ethics (bioethics and nursing ethics) *is not*. For example, ethics, bioethics and nursing ethics are not: legal law, codes of ethics, hospital or professional etiquette, hospital or institutional policy, public opinion or the view of the majority, or following the orders of a supervisor or manager.

A brief examination has also been made of the task of ethics; namely, to find a way to motivate moral behaviour, to settle disagreements and controversies between people, and to generally bind people together in a peaceable community. Both bioethics and nursing ethics share in this task, acknowledging, however, that such a task has been and remains a complex and complicated one. To help understand the complexity of this task and how it might be achieved, it is necessary to first gain some understanding of the theoretical underpinnings of Western ethics generally and of bioethics and nursing ethics which have been strongly influenced by it. It is to examining these theoretical underpinnings and their influences on the development of contemporary bioethics and nursing ethics that the next chapter will now turn.

CASE SCENARIO AND CRITICAL QUESTIONS

Case scenario

Nurse B, an experienced registered nurse working in aged care, formed the view that an elderly resident for whom she was caring 'was not receiving sufficient treatment for pain' (*Nexus* 1996, p. 9). Although the resident had been prescribed morphine 'when needed', this was cancelled by the resident's attending medical practitioner when he became concerned that 'the resident was only receiving the morphine when Nurse B was on duty'. Instead, he asked to be called if and when the resident was in pain so that he could make a direct assessment and tailor an appropriate prescription for pain treatment. Subsequently, however, when the resident experienced what Nurse B believed to be a 'cardiac episode', Nurse B contacted a locum medical practitioner (not the resident's usual medical practitioner) who ordered a 'once only' dose of morphine (*Nexus* 1996, p. 9). Nurse B administered the 'once only' prescribed dose of morphine. Later in the evening, however, Nurse B believed the resident experienced further pain and decided to independently write an order for 10 mgms of morphine, sign it as the prescribing medical practitioner and administered it to the resident (*Nexus* 1996, p. 9). The incident was later discovered and Nurse B was reported to the nurse registering authority and disciplined. The specific allegations against her (and subsequently substantiated by the disciplinary panel hearing her case) were:

- writing an order for morphine 10 mgms for a nursing home resident;
- forging the signature of a registered medical practitioner on that order; and

- administering morphine 10 mgms to the resident when she was not authorised to do so (*Nexus* 1996, p. 9).

Critical questions

1. What standards of professional conduct were breached in this case?
2. Did what the nurse do necessarily constitute a breach of *ethical* standards (give reasons for your answer)?
3. What, if any, ethical issues are raised by this case?
4. If you had discovered the medication fraud by this nurse, how would you have responded?
5. What if the resident did have a genuine pain state that was not being assessed and treated appropriately?
6. Would you have reported her to the Nurses Board (whether yes or no, provide a sound justification for your response)?

---

1   The following discussion of these distinctions is drawn from Johnstone 1994a.

2   The Oxford scholar Makereti (otherwise known as Maggie Papakura), the first Maori scholar to publish a comprehensive ethnographic account of Maori life, offers an illuminating explanation of this custom. In her celebrated work *The Old-Time Maori*, first published in 1938, she wrote (pp. 121–2):

> A case of premature birth seldom happened in the old days, and when it did, was supposed to be caused by the mother's breaking the laws of tapu [taboo]. A *Tohunga* [priest] then had to perform a *karakia Takutaku* over the woman to send away the *wairua* [spirit] of the unformed child, which was supposed to fly about in space — or it might enter a *mokomoko* [lizard] — and do harm to living people. A wairua of this kind, having never been properly formed, would never know any feelings of affection or love, and so would only try to do harm ... to living men, women and children ...

3   Quotations from J.L. Mackie (1977), *Ethics: inventing right and wrong*, Penguin Books, Harmondsworth, Middlesex, are reproduced by permission of Penguin Books Ltd.

Chapter 3

Moral theory and the ethical practice of nursing

LEARNING OBJECTIVES

Upon the completion of this chapter and with further self-directed learning you are expected to be able to:

- Explain moral justification.
- Discuss critically the importance of moral justification to moral decision-making and action.
- Outline the relationship between moral justification and moral theory.
- Define ethical principlism.
- Discuss critically how the moral principles of autonomy, nonmaleficence, beneficence and justice might be used to guide decision-making in nursing and health care contexts.
- Outline a moral rights theory of ethics and its application to nursing.
- Discuss critically virtue ethics and its particular significance to nursing ethics.
- Distinguish between deontological and teleological ethics.
- Differentiate between a moral right and a moral duty.
- Discuss critically the limitations and weaknesses of contemporary moral theory.

KEYWORDS

- Deontology
- Ethical/moral theory
- Ethical principles
- Ethical principlism
- Moral duties
- Moral justification
- Moral obligations
- Moral rights
- Teleology
- Virtue ethics

Introduction

When encountering an ethical problem during the course of their work nurses are confronted by at least three basic questions:

1. What should I do in this situation?
2. What is the 'right' thing to do?
3. How can I be sure (and be reassured) that my decisions and actions in the situation at hand are 'morally right' all things considered? In short, how can I be sure that I am behaving ethically and doing the 'right thing'?

In seeking answers to these questions, it would be natural for a nurse to incline toward and draw on his or her own personal values, beliefs, professional knowledge and life experience. Whether this would be sufficient to provide the moral warranties or 'moral authorisations' being sought is another matter, however. Deciding the 'morally right' thing to do in a situation and taking moral action accordingly is rarely a straightforward process. Among other things it requires a broadly informed, systematic and deeply experienced approach to thinking about the issues at stake and how best to resolve them. This, in turn, requires 'mastery' and 'not just surface competence' of relevant ethical concepts and principles as well as 'the skill to navigate them when they tangle together in concrete situations' (Little 2001, p. 35).

Most people have strong beliefs and opinions about the world. No matter how sincerely held, however, beliefs and opinions can sometimes be mistaken. For example, there was a period in history when people sincerely believed that the world was square and that if they sailed to the edge of it they would drop off. Although a sincere belief, the view that the world was square was obviously mistaken, as explorers and scientists later proved. People now hold very different beliefs about the shape and geology of the world and it is conceivable that these too may be challenged and changed in the future.

Most people also have strong beliefs and opinions about what constitutes 'right' (good) and 'wrong' (bad) conduct. Moral beliefs, like other kinds of beliefs, can be mistaken, however, as centuries of moral inquiry have shown. Indeed, the philosophic literature is full of examples demonstrating convincingly (and giving good reasons for accepting) that some moral decisions and actions are clearly better than others (e.g. acts of compassion are better than acts of cruelty), and that some moral beliefs and theories seem manifestly 'wrong' and ought to be rejected (e.g. women lack moral capacity, black people have no moral worth, gay and transgendered people are moral deviants, Nazis had a moral obligation to rid the German nation of its 'Jewish disease', and so on).

It is because moral beliefs and opinions can be misguided, misinformed and mistaken — and because people can make mistakes in their moral judgments — that those at the forefront of moral decision-making *must* provide strong 'warranties' (good reasons) for their decisions and actions. It is not acceptable for a person to claim that his/her point of view is more worthy and more moral than another's (is 'right') *just because* it is his/her point of view. For instance, I cannot claim that my point of view counts more or is more 'right' than your point of view *just* because it is my point of view. Much more is required, namely, there must be a *sound justification* for holding the point of view that is put forward. I must put forward good reasons why reasonable thinking and 'right' minded people should accept the point of view I am advancing. The question that arises here is: *What constitutes a 'sound justification'?*

In the discussion to follow, attention will be given to clarifying the nature and importance of justification to moral decision-making and the role of ethical theory (in particular, ethical principlism, moral rights theory and virtue ethics) in providing justification and warranties (moral reasons) for our moral decisions and actions in the workplace.

Moral justification

Moral conflict and disagreement occurs frequently in health care contexts. This is not surprising given the 'value ladeness' of the health care practices that occur in health care domains. And given the complexity of the values that operate in health care domains, sometimes the choices we make will be 'problematic' insofar as they may express moral values, beliefs and evaluations that are not shared by others or which others do not agree with.

When experiencing situations involving moral disagreement and conflict, it is tempting to rely on our own ordinary moral experience and personal preferences to sustain the point of view we are advocating. As mentioned previously, however, sometimes our own 'ordinary moral experience' and personal preferences may not be reliable or worthy action guides because, as Kopelman (1995, p. 117) warns us, these can result from 'prejudice, self-interest or ignorance'. In light of this, we need to look elsewhere to strengthen the warranties of (in short, to justify) our moral choices and actions. Moral theory (which has as its focus showing *why* something is moral in addition to showing *that* it is moral) is commonly regarded as the definitive source from which such warranties (justifications) can be reliably sought.

Justifying a moral decision or action involves providing the *strongest moral reasons* behind them. According to Beauchamp and Childress (1994, p. 13), 'the reasons that we finally accept, express the conditions under which we believe some course of action is morally justified'. This account is not, however, free of difficulties. As Beauchamp and Childress (2001, p. 385) later point out, 'Not all reasons are good reasons, and not all good reasons are sufficient for justification'. For instance, a majority public opinion supporting the legalisation of euthanasia may constitute a *good reason* for decriminalising euthanasia yet stop short of providing a *sufficient* reason for doing so. For example, other 'good and sufficient' reasons might be put forward demonstrating why public opinion is not relevant or adequate to justifying legalised euthanasia, such as: majority opinion tells us only that a certain class of people hold a point of view, not whether that point of view is morally right (euthanasia could still be morally wrong despite a majority view to the contrary); public opinion is notoriously fickle and hence unreliable as a moral action guide — what is deemed 'right' by the majority today, could equally be deemed 'wrong' tomorrow, violating the standards of consistency and coherency otherwise expected in the case of sound moral decision-making). Decision-makers thus need to not only provide 'strong reasons' for their decisions and actions, but to also distinguish:

> a reason's *relevance* to a moral judgment from its final *adequacy* for that judgment, [and also] to distinguish an *attempted* justification from a *successful* justification.

> (Beauchamp and Childress 2001, p. 385, emphasis original)

Here, *relevance* (from the Latin *relevāre* to lighten, to relieve) can be measured by the extent to which the reason (belief) has *direct bearing* on and makes a *material difference* to the evaluation made as part of the process aimed at making moral judgments and choices/decisions. *Adequacy* (from the Lain *adaequare* to equalise, from *ad-to* + *aequus* Equal) can, in turn, be measured by the extent to which it fulfils a need or requirement (in this instance to provide sufficient grounds for belief or action) without being outstanding or abundant. An *attempt* is simply to 'make an effort'; to *succeed* is 'to accomplish'.

The notion of moral justification is not, however, without difficulties. One reason for this is that there exist a number of different accounts of what constitutes a plausible model of moral justification, and even of how a given or 'agreed' model of justification might be interpreted and applied (Beauchamp and Childress 2001; Kopelman 1995; Bauman 1993; Dancy 1993; Nielsen 1989). Some even suggest, controversially, that there can be no adequate model of justification since there is always room to question the grounds that are put forward as 'good reasons' supporting a particular act or judgment (see, for example, Hughes 1995; Johnston 1989).

The problem of moral justification has long been recognised as a crucial one in moral philosophy. As Kai Nielsen reflects (1989, p. 53):

> In ordinary non-philosophical moments, we sometimes wonder how (if at all) a deeply felt moral conviction can be justified. And, in our philosophical moments, we sometimes wonder if *any* moral judgments *ever* are *in principle* justified. Surely, we can find all sorts of reasons for taking one course of action rather than another. We find reasons readily enough for the appraisal we make of types of action and attitudes. We frequently make judgments about the moral code of our own culture as well as those of other cultures. But how do we decide if the reasons we offer for these appraisals are good reasons? And, what is the *ground* for our decision that some reasons are good reasons and others are not? When (if at all) can we say that these grounds are sufficient for our moral decisions? (emphasis original)

Beauchamp and Childress (2001) suggest three possible answers to these questions, namely, that we can appeal to either: (1) moral rules, principles and theories; (2) lived experience and case examples of individual personal judgments; or (3) a synthesis of both these (theoretical and experiential) approaches. They conclude that of the three approaches, the one that is the most plausible and warranted is the *synthesised* (or a 'coherentist') approach. This approach, unlike the other approaches, involves a strong synergy between theory and practice, with each informing the other and neither being immune to revision. They explain that in everyday moral reasoning, 'we effortlessly blend appeals to principles, rules, rights, virtues, passions, analogies, paradigms, narratives and parables' and that 'we should be able to do the same' in bioethics (Beauchamp and Childress 2001, p. 408).

This issue will be explored more fully in Chapter 5, Moral problems and moral decision-making in nursing and health care contexts.

Theoretical perspectives informing ethical practice

Western moral philosophy has given rise to many different and sometimes competing theoretical perspectives or viewpoints on the nature and justification of moral conduct. Having some knowledge and understanding of these different perspectives is crucial not just to enhancing our understanding of the complex nature of moral problems and the controversies and perplexities to which they so often give rise, but also to enhancing our abilities to provide satisfactory solutions to the moral problems we encounter in our everyday lives. Unfortunately it is beyond the scope of this book to give an in-depth account of the many ethical theories that have been and remain influential in Western moral philosophical thought (see Chapter 4 of the previous edition of this work [Johnstone 1999a]). There are, however, three theoretical frameworks that warrant attention here, namely, those that involve respectively (and sometimes interdependently) an appeal to:

1. ethical principles (*ethical principlism*);
2. moral rights (*moral rights theory*);
3. moral virtues (*virtue ethics*).

These three approaches have emerged as having the most currency and credibility in contemporary health care contexts. Reasons for this include:

- they have largely emerged from and been refined by practice;
- they are able to be readily and meaningfully applied to and in practice; and
- they are amendable to being revised and refined in order to be more responsive to the lived realities of everyday practice.

Ethical principlism

One of the most popular theoretical perspectives used today when considering ethical issues in health care is the perspective called 'ethical principlism'. Ethical principlism is the view that ethical decision-making and problem solving is best undertaken by appealing to sound moral principles. The principles most commonly used are those of: autonomy, nonmaleficence, beneficence and justice. These principles are generally accepted as providing sound moral reasons for taking moral action.

Although not free of difficulties, ethical principlism has become increasingly accepted as a reliable and practical framework for identifying and resolving moral problems in health care contexts (Benjamin 2001; Little 2001). Since ethical principlism has gained much currency in contemporary discussions on ethical issues in health care (largely because of the influential work on the topic by Beauchamp and Childress [2001]), it is important that nurses have some knowledge and understanding of this approach.

What are ethical principles?

Ethical principles are general standards of conduct that make up an ethical system. To say that a principle is 'ethical' or 'moral' is merely to assert that it is a behaviour guide which 'entails particular imperatives' (Harrison 1954, p. 115). In this instance the imperatives involve specification (in the form of prescriptions and proscriptions) that some type of action or conduct is either prohibited, required, or permitted in certain circumstances (Solomon 1978, p. 408). By this view, an action or decision is generally considered morally right or good when it accords with a given relevant moral principle, and morally wrong or bad when it does not. To illustrate how this works, consider the action of making a measurement using a ruler. If the line you have drawn measures the desired length of, say, 12 cm — as measured against your ruler — you would judge the length as 'correct'. If, however, the line you have drawn is only 10 cm long — not the desired 12 cm — you would judge the length to be 'incorrect'. By analogy, principles also function like rulers, insofar as they provide a standard against which something (in this case, actions) can be measured. For example, if an action fails to 'measure up' to the ultimate standards set by a given principle, we would judge the action to be 'incorrect' or, more specifically, morally wrong. If, however, an action fully measures up to the ultimate standards set by a given principle, we would judge the action to be 'correct' or morally right. The next question is: what are these moral principles against which actions can be measured?

Moral principles commonly used in discussions on ethical issues in nursing and health care include the principles of autonomy, non-maleficence, beneficence, and justice. It is to examining the content, prescriptive force and application of these principles that this discussion now turns.

AUTONOMY

The term 'autonomy' comes from the Greek *autos* (meaning 'self') and *nomos* (meaning 'rule', 'governance' or 'law'). When autonomy is used as a *concept* in moral discourse, what is commonly being referred to is a person's ability to make or to exercise self-determining choice — literally, to be 'self-governing'. Included here is the additional notion of 'respect for persons'; that is, of treating or respecting persons as ends in themselves, as dignified and autonomous choosers, and not as the mere means (objects or tools) to the ends of others (Kant 1972; Benn 1971). The *principle* of autonomy, however, is a little different, and is eloquently formulated by Beauchamp and Walters (1982, p. 27) as follows:

> Insofar as an autonomous agent's actions *do not infringe on the autonomous actions of others*, that person should be free to perform whatever action he or she wishes (presumably even if it involves considerable risk to himself or herself and even if others consider the action to be foolish). (emphasis added)

What this basically means is that people should be free to choose and entitled to act on their preferences provided their decisions and actions do not stand to violate, or impinge on, the significant moral interests of others.

Both the concept and the principle of autonomy have important implications for nursing practice. For example, if autonomy is to be taken seriously by nurses, nursing practice must truly respect patients as dignified human beings capable of deciding what is to count as being in their own best interests — even if what they decide is considered by others (including nurses) to be 'foolish'. In short, nurses must allow patients to participate in decision-making concerning their care. Given this, it soon becomes clear that the whole practice of 'negotiated patient goals' and 'negotiated patient care' as advocated by contemporary nursing philosophy has its roots in the moral principle of autonomy, and the derived duty to respect persons as autonomous moral choosers. It is not derived merely from a concept of 'acceptable professional nursing practice'.

In application, the principle of autonomy would judge as being morally objectionable and wrong any act which unjustly prevents autonomous persons from deciding what is to count as being in their own best interests. The kinds of act which might come in for criticism here include, for example:

- treating patients without their consent;
- treating patients without giving them all the relevant information necessary for making an informed and intelligent choice;
- withholding information from patients when they have expressed a considered choice to receive it;

- forcing information upon patients when they have expressed a considered choice not to receive it; and
- forcing nurses to act against their reasoned moral judgments or conscience.

It should be noted, however, that while the moral principle of autonomy is very helpful in guiding ethically just practices in health care contexts, it is not entirely unproblematic. Indeed, its uncritical and culturally inappropriate application in some contexts may, in fact, inadvertently cause rather than prevent significant moral harms to patients, for reasons which are considered in Chapter 4).

NON-MALEFICENCE

The term 'non-maleficence' comes from the Latin *maleficent* — from *maleficus*, (meaning 'wicked', 'prone to evil'), from *malum* (meaning 'evil'), and *male* (meaning 'ill'). As a moral principle, *non-maleficence* (literally 'refuse evil'), prescribes 'above all, do no harm' which entails a stringent obligation not to injure or harm others. This principle is sometimes equated with the moral principle of 'beneficence' (considered below under a separate subheading) which prescribes 'above all, do good'. Trying to conflate these two obviously distinct principles under one principle is, however, misleading. As Beauchamp and Childress (2001, p. 114) explain, not only are these two principles obviously distinct (for instance, our obligation not to kill someone does seem qualitatively and quantitatively different from our obligation to rescue someone from a life-threatening situation), but it is important to distinguish between them so as not to obscure other important distinctions which might be made in ordinary moral discourse. One instance in which 'other important distinctions might need to be made' is in the case of where both principles might apply to a given situation, but where the strength of the respective moral imperatives of each may nevertheless differ significantly and thus might prescribe quite different courses of action. As Beauchamp and Childress point out:

> Obligations not to harm others are sometimes more stringent than obligations to help them, but obligations of beneficence are also sometimes more stringent than obligations of non-maleficence.

> (Beauchamp and Childress 2001, p. 114)

'Stringentness' thus stands as an important distinction that might be obscured if the principles of non-maleficence and beneficence were conflated into one single principle. Beauchamp and Childress (2001, p. 115) conclude, however, that generally 'obligations of non-maleficence are more stringent than obligations of beneficence', and, in some cases, may even override beneficence particularly in instances where beneficent acts, paradoxically, are not morally defensible (for example, depriving one's family of food for a week and failing to pay the rent [thereby increasing the risk of eviction] because of donating the household's weekly budget to charity).

Applied in nursing contexts, the principle of non-maleficence would provide justification for condemning any act which unjustly injures a person or causes them to suffer an otherwise avoidable harm (such as in the case scenarios presented in Chapter 1 of this book, involving nurses who mistreated elderly people in their care).

Before continuing, some commentary is warranted on the notion of 'harm' and how it might be interpreted (given that it is open to a variety of interpretations). For the purposes of this discussion, harm may be taken to involve the invasion, violation, thwarting, or 'setting back' of a person's significant welfare interests to the detriment of that person's wellbeing (Feinberg 1984, p. 34; Beauchamp and Childress 2001, pp. 116-17). Interests, in this instance, are taken to mean 'a miscellaneous collection, consist[ing] of all those things in which one has a stake' together with the 'harmonious advancement' of those interests (Feinberg 1984, p. 34). Interests are morally significant since they are fundamentally linked to human wellbeing; specifically, they stand as a *fundamental requisite* (although, granted, not the whole) of human wellbeing (Feinberg 1984, p. 37). Wellbeing, in turn, can include interests in:

> continuance for a foreseeable interval of one's life, and the interests in one's own physical health and vigour, the integrity and normal functioning of one's body, the absence of absorbing pain and suffering or grotesque disfigurement, minimal intellectual acuity, emotional stability, the absence of groundless anxieties and resentments, the capacity to engage normally in social intercourse and to enjoy and maintain friendships, at least minimal income and financial security, a tolerable social and physical environment, and a certain amount of freedom from interference and coercion.
>
> (Feinberg 1984, p. 37)

The test for whether a person's interests and wellbeing have been violated, 'set back', thwarted or invaded rests on 'whether that interest is in a worse condition than it would otherwise have been in had the invasion not occurred at all' (Feinberg 1984, p. 34). For instance, if a person (for example, a patient) is left psychogenically distressed (for example, emotionally distressed, anxious, depressed and even suicidal) or in a state of needless physical pain and/or disability as a result of his/her experiences (for example, as *a patient* in a given health care setting) our reflective commonsense tells us that this person's interests have been violated and the person him/herself 'harmed'. As the American philosopher Joel Feinberg (1984) further explains, the violation of a person's welfare interests renders that person 'very seriously harmed indeed' since 'their ultimate aspirations are defeated too'.

BENEFICENCE

The term 'beneficence' comes from the Latin *beneficus*, from *bene* (meaning 'well' or 'good') and *facere* (meaning 'to do'). The principle of beneficence prescribes 'above all, do good'; in practice, it entails a positive obligation to literally 'act for the benefit of others' *viz*. contribute to the welfare and wellbeing of others (Beauchamp and Childress 2001, p. 166). Acts of beneficence can include such virtuous actions as: care, compassion, empathy, sympathy, altruism, kindness, mercy, love, friendship and charity. It is recognised, however, that bestowing benefits on others is not always without cost to the benefactor. Thus there are some limits to the principle; that is, it is not 'free standing' and its application can be appropriately constrained by other moral (for example, utilitarian) considerations. To put this another way, we are not obliged to act beneficently towards others when doing so could result in our own significant moral interests being seriously harmed or compromised in some way.

Although the notion of 'obligatory beneficence' remains a controversial one in moral philosophy (for instance, it is popularly accepted that we are not 'morally required to benefit persons on all occasions, even if we are in a position to do so'), there are nevertheless a number of conditions under which a person can indeed be said to have an obligation of beneficence and that this obligation might, sometimes, be overriding. These conditions, devised by Beauchamp and Childress (2001, p. 171), are as follows:

a person X has a determinate obligation of beneficence toward person Y if and only if each of the following conditions is satisfied (assuming X is aware of the relevant facts):

1. Y is at risk of significant loss of or damage to life or health or some other major interest.
2. X's action is needed (singly or in concert with others) to prevent this loss or damage.
3. X's action (singly or in concert with others) has a high probability of preventing it.
4. X's action would not present significant risks, costs, or burdens to X.
5. The benefit that Y expected to gain outweighs any harms, costs, or burdens that X is likely to incur.

They go on to suggest that it is only when these conditions are satisfied that a person's 'general duty of beneficence' becomes a 'specific duty of beneficence' toward another given individual.

The principle stands to have an interesting and useful application in nursing practice. Consider the following case (personal communication; names have been changed).

Mrs Jones, a Jehovah's Witness, is admitted to an intensive care unit in a terminal condition, suffering from advanced hepatitis B and severe liver failure. She has a slow internal haemorrhage and is only semiconscious. Before her alteration in consciousness she had given her doctors a written statement specifically requesting that she not be given a blood transfusion under any circumstances. Upon her arrival in the unit, however, the attending doctor prescribes a unit of blood and requests that it be given immediately. Mrs Jones' husband and children are all present and, upon overhearing the doctor's request, become very upset. Mr Jones approaches the doctor and asks that his wife not be given the blood transfusion. He reminds the doctor that Mrs Jones has made explicit her wish not to have a blood transfusion under any circumstances. Nurse Smith, the registered nurse caring for Mrs Jones, hears the discussion and has to make a decision whether or not to intervene on her patient's behalf. In making her decision, Nurse Smith might appeal to the principle of beneficence in the following manner:

1. Mrs Jones, a terminally ill Jehovah's Witness, is at risk of suffering a significant loss (a violation of her spiritual values and beliefs) if she is given the prescribed blood transfusion;
2. action by Nurse Smith, the attending nurse, is needed to prevent Mrs Jones from experiencing the loss in question;
3. Nurse Smith's action of refusing to administer the prescribed transfusion would probably prevent Mrs Jones' loss;
4. Nurse Smith's action will not present a significant risk to her (for example, she will not lose her job);
5. the benefits gained by Mrs Jones outweigh any harms Nurse Smith is likely to suffer (given that Nurse Smith autonomously chooses to uphold Mrs Jones' interests, and does not stand to suffer any morally significant consequences of her actions).

In this particular case the nurse refused to give the transfusion which had been prescribed. When the doctor insisted that it be given, the nurse pointed out that the transfusion would probably be of no benefit to Mrs Jones, as she was clearly in the end stages of her disease — to put it bluntly, 'she was dying'. Nurse Smith then suggested to the doctor that perhaps he would prefer to administer the transfusion himself. Interestingly, the doctor declined this invitation, and the transfusion was not given. Mrs Jones died a short while later, without having to experience a needless violation of her expressed wishes, values and beliefs.

In summary, by this principle, any act which fails to address an imbalance of harms over benefits where this can be done without sacrificing a benefactor's own significant moral interests, warrants judgment as being morally unacceptable.

JUSTICE

The principle of justice (its nature and content), unlike the principles above, is not so amenable to definition or quantification. As a point of interest, questions concerning what justice is and what its origins are have occupied the minds of philosophers for nearly three thousand years, and to this day remain the subject of intensive philosophical debate (MacIntyre 1988; Solomon and Murphy 1990). Significantly, the end result of this great philosophical debate has not been the development of a singular and refined universal theory of justice, but the development of a range of rival theories of justice (MacIntyre 1988). Different conceptions of justice (from the Latin *justus* meaning 'righteous') have included: justice as revenge (retributive justice — for example, 'an eye for an eye'); justice as mercy (Christian ethics); justice as harmony in the soul and harmony in the state (Pythagorean ethics, 600 BC–1 AD); justice as equality ('equals must be treated equally, and unequals unequally'); justice as an equal distribution of benefits and burdens (distributive justice); justice as what is deserved ('each according to one's merit or worth'); and justice as love (Rawls 1971; Outka 1972; MacIntyre 1985, 1988; Waithe 1987; Solomon and Murphy 1990; Singer 1991; Beauchamp and Childress 2001).

Given these different conceptions of justice, the problem arises of what, if any, conception of justice nurses should adopt? While it is beyond the scope of this book to answer this question in depth, there is nevertheless room to advocate at least two senses of justice which nurses might find helpful: (1) justice as fairness; and (2) justice as the equal distribution of benefits and burdens. It is these two senses of justice which will now be considered.

Justice as fairness

Justice as fairness finds interpretation in terms of 'what is owed or due'. Here, it can be said that 'one acts justly toward a person when that person has given what is due or owed'; an injustice, by this view, would involve:

> a wrongful act or omission that denies people benefits to which they have a right or distribues benefits unfairly (Beauchmap and Childress 2001, p. 226).

If a person deserved something, justice is done when that person receives that particular something. Here, the 'something' may be either positive (a reward) or negative (a punishment). This view relies very heavily on an 'intuitive' sense of justice. For example, we may 'feel' it is unjust to punish or censure someone for a harm they did not cause, or not to punish someone for a harm they did deliberately cause. Likewise we may feel that it is unjust to reward someone for an accomplishment to which they contributed nothing, and yet not reward someone who contributed a great deal.

We do not need to look far in nursing practice to find sobering examples of where the principle of justice as fairness has been violated. Consider cases where nurses have been subjected to severe legal and professional censure on the basis of mistakes made by doctors (Johnstone 1994). The Somera case of 1929, referred to in Chapter 2, involving a nurse who was fined and sentenced to prison after following an incorrect medical order, stands as an important example here (Grennan 1930). While it may well have been 'fair' that Somera was censured for her part in the administration of an incorrectly prescribed drug, it was hardly 'fair' that the doctor — who prescribed the drug, checked it with Somera, and administered it — was acquitted.

Other less dramatic examples involve cases where nurses have gained promotion or have secured employment on the basis of their claiming credit for the work of either their peers or their subordinates; at the other end of the continuum, some nurses have been denied promotion or employment because their superior has ignored, or refused for whatever reasons to recognise significant professional achievements the nurse applicant has in fact made. The story of 'Sally Trihard', a registered nurse who had difficulty getting a job because of a past difference of professional opinion with a charge nurse, is a case in point (Johnstone 1987, p. 41; see also 'A costly misjudgment', *Australian Nurses Journal* 1988 p. 3).

How, then, might we make choices on this view of justice? One possible approach which has received widespread attention is that discussed by the contemporary American philosopher John Rawls, briefly mentioned earlier in this chapter. He argues, for example, that if parties are to exercise truly just or fair choices, they must choose from a hypothetically 'neutral' position, or from a position of what he describes as being 'behind the veil of ignorance' (Rawls 1971, p. 12). From such a position he argues (p. 12):

> no-one knows his [sic] place in society, his [sic] class position or social status, nor does anyone know his [sic] fortune in the distribution of natural assets and abilities, his [sic] intelligence, strength, and the like … [T]his ensures that no-one is advantaged or disadvantaged in the choice of principles by the outcome of natural chance or the contingency of social circumstances. Since all are similarly situated and no-one is able to design principles to favour his [sic] particular condition, the principles of justice are the result of a fair agreement or bargain.

While Rawls' view is problematic (for instance, it is open to serious question whether, in fact, all choosers are or could ever be 'similarly situated', as he assumes), it is nevertheless persuasive, particularly when considered in the light of broader philosophical demands which emphasise among other things that moral choice and judgment should be exercised from a position of impartiality and objectivity. However, whether in fact human beings are ever capable of exercising truly impartial and 'objective' choices — indeed, of choosing from behind that veil of ignorance — is a matter of great controversy. Despite its weaknesses, Rawls' justice theory helps us to come to terms with the notion of fairness and how it might be used in real life situations. It also alerts us to some of the potential difficulties of trying to determine and apply an uncontentious view of justice.

Justice as an equal distribution of benefits and burdens

A second sense in which justice can be used is that pertaining to 'distributive justice'; that is, an equal distribution of benefits and harms. By this view, all people are required to bear an equal share of their society's benefits and burdens. Such a view admits that all persons must have equal claims to liberty and opportunity, but in a way that is compatible with the claims of others. As well as this, there must be equal access (and opportunity to gain access) to positions of authority and power, and there must be an equal distribution of wealth and income. The only morally acceptable exception to this would be if an unequal distribution would work to everyone's advantage (Beauchamp and Childress 2001, p. 226); or where an unequal distribution of benefits would be necessary so as to 'maximise the minimum level of primary goods in order to protect vital interests in potentially damaging or disastrous contexts' (Beauchamp and Childress 2001, p. 226). Simply put, inequalities in distributing benefits and primary goods are 'just' as long as this results in the least well-off (that is, those who are already disadvantaged unfairly) achieving a decent minimum level of wellbeing (that is, being advantaged by the benefits which have been conferred unequally). Given this view, 'injustice' finds interpretation as 'simply inequalities that are not to the benefit of all' (Rawls 1971, pp. 60–1).

As with the fairness sense of justice discussed earlier, we do not need to look far to find sobering examples in nursing where the principle of distributive justice has been violated. In many cases, nurses have had to (and continue to) bear unequal and intolerable burdens on account of certain inequities in the distribution of scarce health care resources. For example, historically nurses have had to endure poor and unsafe working conditions with a maximum of responsibility and a minimum of financial or personal reward (Johnstone 1994, 2002).

In considering the fairness and the distributive senses of justice, it is instructive to note that both uphold two common minimal principles: formal equality ('equals must be treated equally, and unequals must be treated unequally'); and a mixture of autonomy and beneficence ('we all ought to bear certain burdens, usually of a minimal sort, for the common good') (Beauchamp and Childress 1989, pp. 256–306).

In calculating the balance or distribution of harms and benefits, notions of comparative and non-comparative justice are also used. Justice is 'comparative' when what a person deserves can be determined only by balancing the competing claims of others against the person's own claims (Beauchamp and Childress 2001, pp. 226–37). For example, whether a nurse qualifies for a job or a promotion will depend largely on the competing claims of the other applicants. If the other applicants are more qualified and more experienced, it seems reasonable to hold that they are more 'deserving' of the position being offered. Justice is 'non-comparative', on the other hand, when 'desert is judged by standards independent of the claims of others' (Beauchamp and Childress 2001, pp. 227–30). For example, a nurse who is guilty of breaching acceptable professional standards of conduct deserves to be censured, or even deregistered, if the breach of conduct warrants such an action; a nurse who is innocent of professional misconduct, however, does not deserve to be censured or deregistered.

Moral rules

Moral principles are not the only entities that make up an ethical system or ethical framework for guiding conduct. Moral rules also have a place in guiding and 'warranting' ethical conduct. Like moral principles, moral rules function by specifying that some type of action or conduct is either prohibited, required or permitted (Solomon 1978, pp. 408–9). What distinguishes a moral rule from a moral principle in certain contexts is its structure and nature. Moral principles, for instance, tend to be regarded as providing the content of morality, and the bases or the 'parent' forms from which general moral truths (insofar as these can be determined) are derived. In application, moral principles incline more toward a general focus. Consider, for example, the broad moral principle of 'autonomy'. In general, the principle demands that persons should be respected as autonomous choosers, capable of judging what is in their own best interests. As such, rational persons should be free to act as they wish provided their actions do not violate the moral interests of others.

Moral rules, on the other hand, stand as being merely derivative of moral principles and theories and, in application, are much more particular in their focus. Although it is difficult to draw a firm distinction between moral rules and moral principles, it is generally recognised that moral rules have different force, sanctioning power, conditions of existence, scope of application, and level of concreteness from moral principles (Solomon 1978). An example of a moral rule would be the demand, say, to 'always tell the truth' or 'never tell a lie'. Thus, if a patient asks an attending health care professional a question concerning a diagnosis and proposed treatment, the health care professional could be said to be obliged to give the information the patient has requested. The apparent 'obligation' here finds its force not just from the moral rule 'always tell the truth', but from the moral principle of autonomy which demands that rational people be respected as autonomous choosers, and be given the information required to make an informed and intelligent choice.

Another example can be found in a set of rules that prescribe such things as 'do not kill others', 'do not cause pain and suffering to others', 'do not affect detrimentally the physical and mental health of others', and so forth. The apparent obligations here find their force not just from the rules stated, but from the moral principle non-maleficence which prescribes 'do no harm'.

In order for a particular moral rule (or set of moral rules) to be justified, it must be fully derived from and reducible to established parent principles of morality.

In summary, moral rules derive from moral principles, and as such have only prima-facie force (i.e. they can be overridden by stronger moral claims). Given their prima-facie nature, moral rules cannot override the moral principles from which they have been derived. To accept that they could would be to suggest, somewhat paradoxically, that derived rules could meaningfully conflict with parent principles — which, of course, is absurd. The relationship between particular moral judgments, moral rules, moral prinicples and moral theories is shown in Figure 3.1.

Moral/Ethical theory
(e.g. Deontology/Teleology)
↑
Principles
(e.g. Autonomy – people ought to be respected as self-determining choosers)
↑
Rules
(e.g. Do not lie)
↑
Particular judgment
(e.g. Mr X has asked for and ought to be told the truth about his medical diagnosis)

Figure 3.1 Moral justification and direction of appeal

(adapted from Beauchamp, T. and Childress, J. [1994], *Principles of biomedical ethics*, 4th edn, Oxford University Press, New York, p. 15)

The question of moral rules is an important one for nurses, particularly as it relates to the broader issue of professional codes of conduct, an issue that will become clearer in the following chapters.

Problems with ethical principles

In considering ethical principlism it is important to be aware of a number of difficulties that can arise when appealing to the ethical principles described. For example, problems commonly associated with ethical principlism include:

- *deciding correctly which principles apply in a given situation* (e.g. 'Is it the principle of autonomy or beneficence that applies in this case, or both?');
- *interpreting correctly the imperatives of the principles chosen to guide ethical decision-making in a given situation* (e.g. 'What does the principle of autonomy require of me? Is it the case that the principle of autonomy ought always to be upheld?');
- *deciding correctly the relative weights of given principles* (e.g. 'Which principle has overriding consideration in this case — the principle of autonomy or the principle of nonmaleficence?');
- *balancing the demands of different principles in situations where their respective though equally weighted demands might conflict* (e.g. 'How can I uphold the principle of autonomy without, at the same time, violating the principle of justice which has an equal bearing in this case?');
- *deciding whether ethical principles apply at all* (e.g. 'This is a matter to be resolved by kindness and care — by being virtuous — not by appealing to ethical principles per se');
- *resolving disagreement with others regarding either of the above* (e.g. 'I feel strongly that respecting the patient's autonomy in this case means *withholding* the information about his diagnosis as he has requested, but others in the team do not agree and are going to tell him insisting he MUST be told so that he can make informed choices about his future treatment.').

The issue of moral uncertainty, moral dilemmas and moral disagreements in regard to the selection, interpretation and application of ethical principles will be explored further in the chapters to follow.

Moral rights theory

Of the moral theories that have been appealed to in the contemporary literature on ethics, a 'rights' view of ethics is probably the one that has the most currency among professional and lay communities alike. Certainly most people have a sense that they have 'rights' and that their rights, whatever these may be, 'ought to be respected'. Here important questions to ask are: What are moral rights? Who has them? and To what extent are others obliged to respect them?

Moral rights theory has emerged as an extremely influential theoretical perspective across the globe. Evidence of this can be found in the vast array of contexts in which moral rights discourse has been used. For example, we see moral rights discourse in: position statements and bills of clients'/patients' rights; professional codes of ethics and conduct (for example, the International Council of Nurses *Code for Nurses* and supporting position statements); statutory authorities (for example, the various Australian state and territory Human Rights and Equal Opportunity Commissions); government inquiries (for example, the *Report of the National Inquiry into the Human*

Rights of People with Mental Illness by Burdekin et al. 1993); and in global declarations (for example, the Universal Declaration of Human Rights in 1948 [United Nations 1978]). There is also an abundance of literature on the subject. If nurses are to participate effectively in discourses on moral rights, it is essential that they have some understanding of the theoretical underpinnings of a moral (and human) rights perspective on ethics. It is to providing a brief examination of moral rights theory that this section will now turn.

Moral rights

Moral rights (to be distinguished here from legal rights, institutional rights, civil rights, etc.) generally entail claims about some special entitlement or interest which ought, for moral reasons, to be protected. The kinds of interests for which protection might be sought include, for example, life, freedom, happiness, privacy, self-determination, fair treatment and bodily integrity. The language used in asserting rights typically involves expressions such as: 'I have a right to …', 'It's your right to …', 'They have a right to …', and so on. A rights claim is generally accepted as a sound moral reason for taking moral action.

There is no single thesis of moral rights. The following is a brief overview of better-known theories concerning the existence of moral rights and the conditions under which they can be validly claimed.

BASED ON NATURAL LAW AND DIVINE COMMAND

Natural rights theory argues that certain entitlements are simply 'built into' the universe like the laws of gravity, and as such are neither the products of human invention nor the constructs of other moral theories (Martin and Nickel 1980). A variation of this thesis is that natural rights have been divinely ordained for all human beings. From both these points of view, since the laws of nature and the ordinances of God apply equally to all human beings, it follows that all human beings, young and old, male, female, transgender and intergendered (e.g. haemophrodites), black, white and coloured unconditionally have natural rights.

Objections to this account of moral rights derive from those raised against a theological account of morality generally. For example, if it were shown that God did not exist, or that natural law did not exist, this account of moral rights would immediately collapse because its very foundation would be pulled out from underneath it. Another objection rests on the problem that natural rights essentially defy scientific verification.

BASED ON COMMON HUMANITY

Another popular natural rights thesis is that all human beings have rights simply by virtue of being 'human' and 'equal'. What is critical to this thesis is the notion that 'being human' is something over which we have no control; that is, we cannot choose to be either human or not human (Martin and Nickel 1980). In this sense, then, we can be said to enjoy a 'common humanity', a notion which Leah Curtin (1986) explores in her treatment of advocacy. This view of rights is vulnerable to the objection that not all human rights are *moral rights* per se. The human right to education, which is dependent on the availability of educational resources, is an example of a human right which is not a moral right per se.

Another more serious problem is that given the recent advancements made in the field of genetic engineering, 'being human' may indeed be something over which we have control in the near future. Human genes have already been cloned onto animals (for example, pigs); it is not far-fetched to imagine that scientists will succeed (if they have not already done so) in cloning animal genes onto humans. Persons with a genetic makeup comprising both human and non-human genes could be said to be not 'fully human', at least, not in a 'speciesist' sense, just as someone who is part Greek and part Chinese is not 'fully Greek' or 'fully Chinese' in a racial sense. Were someone to be not 'fully human', their claim to moral rights on the basis of a *common humanity* would be cast in doubt.

BASED ON RATIONALITY

A Kantian thesis (i.e. a thesis based on the philosophical views of the German philosopher Immanuel Kant) of natural rights holds rationality as being the sole basis upon which a right's claim can be made. In other words, only those people who are capable of rational, autonomous thought are entitled to claim moral rights. One disturbing consequence of this thesis is that any human being (or non-human being, for that matter) who is unable to reason is not regarded as having moral status. Such a view clearly excludes infants, brain-dead and intellectually disabled persons from having a just claim to moral rights. It might be tempting to dismiss this view as being merely an intellectual one, of interest only to moral philosophers. There is ample evidence, however, that this view is influential and enjoys considerable currency in the 'real world' of human affairs. (The most notable examples here can be found in the use of brain-dead persons as organ donors, and the suggestion that live-born anencephalic babies and fetuses should also be used as organ donors [Meinke 1989; Gillam 1989; Sanders and Moore 1991]).

BASED ON INTERESTS

The North American philosopher Joel Feinberg offers quite a different theory of moral rights. He argues that, in order for an entity to be able to claim rights meaningfully, that entity must have interests (Feinberg 1979). To have interests, the entity must be capable of being either benefited or harmed. In order to be either benefited or harmed, one must be able to experience pleasure and pain. In short, unless one has sentience one cannot have interests, and thus cannot be either benefited or harmed, and therefore cannot make claims. This theory of moral rights can be expressed diagrammatically as shown in Figure 3.2.

It can be seen that by this view it would be nonsense to assert, for example, that a rock has rights. Why? Because a rock does not have sentience and therefore cannot, strictly speaking, be benefited or harmed, and thus cannot meaningfully be said to have interests and hence rights. Those who value rocks (for example, conservationists, geologists, rock collectors) might be benefited or harmed by what happens to a rock, but it is not meaningful, philosophically speaking, to assert that a rock per se has rights. In contrast, any entity which can be shown to have sentience (that is, the capacity to experience pleasure or suffer pain) would, by this view, be entitled to be respected as having rights. Given this, it is clear that we can, for example, assert meaningfully that entities such as dolphins, puppies, kittens, horses, demented people and babies have moral rights.

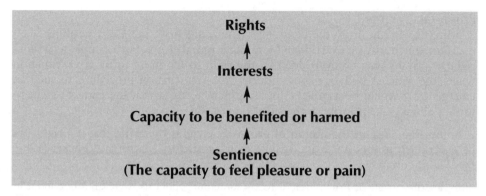

Figure 3.2 Feinberg's theory of moral rights

Like Bentham, the founding father of utilitarianism (to be discussed later in this chapter), Feinberg sees the *capacity to suffer*, not reason, as the ultimate basis upon which a person's interest claims become the focus of moral action.

One shortcoming of this view is that individuals must be able to represent their own interests. Feinberg (1979, p. 595) argues that, if individuals cannot represent their own interests, they have no more rights than 'redwood trees and rosebushes'. Unhappily, the 'human vegetable', it seems, is no better off under an interests-based thesis of moral rights than it is under a thesis based on reason.

Feinberg does not, however, offer an adequate account of why entities must be able to 'represent their own interests', and why others (who are quite capable of making sound judgments about the moral interests of vulnerable persons and acting in a way to protect those interests) could not speak for them when they are unable or incapable of speaking on their own behalf. On closer analysis, there is room to suggest that an interests-based thesis of moral rights could even justify such acts involving, as it were, 'surrogate' representation.

DIFFERENT TYPES OF RIGHTS

When speaking of moral rights, it is important to distinguish three different types which can be claimed: notably, inalienable, absolute and prima-facie rights.

Inalienable rights

An inalienable right is one which cannot be transferred under any circumstances. For example, if we accept the right to life as being an inalienable right, we are committed to accepting that it cannot be transferred to someone else or for some other cause under any circumstances. According to this view, sacrificing one's life either in suicide, martyrdom, or in an act of supreme altruism (for example, a mother sacrificing her life for her child) would be deemed as morally wrong. Of course, we may ask the question whether the right to life is an inalienable right.

Absolute rights

An absolute right, by contrast, is a right which cannot be overridden under any circumstances. For example, if we take the right to life as being absolute, we would be bound to respect it whatever the cost. By this view, any wilful taking of life, whether through war, self-defence, abortion, capital punishment, or any other act, would be morally wrong. Here the question arises whether the right to life really is an absolute right.

Prima-facie rights

A prima-facie right (from the Latin *primus*, meaning 'first', and *facies*, meaning 'face') is a right which may be overridden by stronger moral claims. For example, a patient's right to privacy may be overridden by the right to life in a cardiac arrest situation where the patient's body is exposed during the resuscitation procedure. In such an emergency, it would be a mistake for an ethicist to insist that the patient's right to privacy should take priority in the situation at hand.

Some argue against the notion of prima–facie rights by saying that if a right can be overridden it does not exist. Against such a criticism, Martin and Nickel (1980, pp. 172–4) comment:

> to describe a right as Prima Facie is to say something about its weight but not about its scope or conditions of possession ... Overridence depends on whether the case of conflict is central to the values that the right serves to protect or whether it is a marginal case and thus can be expected in all cases without great loss to those values.

MAKING RIGHTS CLAIMS

Having a right usually entails that another has a corresponding duty to respect that right. As Feinberg (1978, p. 1508) explains, when people assert their moral rights, they assert a kind of 'moral power' over us which we feel constrained to respect. Where claims have a special convincing force they have a coercive effect on our judgments, which in turn make us feel driven to both acknowledge and support the interest claims being made as being genuine rights claims.

Rights which entail a corresponding duty are typically referred to as 'claims rights'. These rights can be either positive or negative, and can entail either a positive or a negative rights claim. Positive rights claims generally entail a correlative duty to act or to do, in contrast with a negative rights claim which generally entails a correlative duty to omit or to refrain (Feinberg 1978, p. 1509). For example, if a patient claims a right not to be harmed, this claim imposes a negative duty on an attending nurse to refrain from acts which may cause harm. On the other hand, if a patient claims a right to be benefited in some way, such as by having an intolerable pain state relieved, this imposes a duty on an attending nurse to perform the positive act of promptly administering an effective analgesic. If a person's rights claims are not upheld, or are infringed or violated in some way, that person generally feels wronged or feels a serious injustice has been done. In a rights view of ethics, if someone claims a right this is generally regarded as providing a 'moral reason' (a warranty) for taking moral action.

Problems with rights claims

In discussing rights it is important to keep in mind at least five central problems that can arise when dealing with rights claims. First, rights and interests can seriously compete and conflict with one another. For example, a patient's right to life could seriously compete or conflict with another patient's right to life in a situation involving scarce medical resources; or a nurse's conscientious refusal to assist with an abortion procedure could conflict with a patient's right to have an abortion and to receive care following the procedure. In such instances there may be no easy solution to the conflict of interests at hand.

Second, it may be difficult to establish the extent to which a person's rights claim entails a correlative duty. For example, if someone claims a right to life, who or what has the corresponding duty to respond to that claim? Does it fall to the health professional, or to family, friends, the hospital, the state, or another body? There may be no satisfactory answer to this question.

Third, there may be disagreement about which entities have rights. For example, some might argue that brain-dead people, anencephalic babies, the intellectually impaired and babies do not have moral rights, while others might argue that they do. Again there may be no satisfactory solution to this type of disagreement.

Fourth, it may be very difficult to try and satisfy the rights claims of all people equally. For instance, if there is a genuine lack of resources, it may be impossible to satisfy all rights claims. Once again, we are left, unhappily, with an unresolved moral problem.

Fifth, and more seriously, is the controversial claim that moral rights theory is not a complete theory at all, but only 'a piece of a more general account of what makes a claim valid [and justified]' — a 'partial framework' as it were (Beauchamp and Childress 2001, p. 361). By this view, rather than being a comprehensive theory, a moral rights perspective is at best only an account of 'minimal and enforceable *rules* that communities and individuals must observe in their treatment of persons' (Beauchamp and Childress 1994, p. 76, emphasis added).

On account of these and other difficulties (not least, the inherent adversarial nature of rights claims and entitlements), some have sought to avoid a moral rights perspective altogether, or at least to 'replace the language of rights' (Beauchamp and Childress 2001, p. 362). (For example, when referring to people's moral entitlements, instead of using 'rights' language, some writers use such terms as 'interests', 'welfare', 'wellbeing', and so on.) Others, however, defend the use of rights language despite the theoretical weaknesses of a moral rights perspective. Beauchamp and Childress, for example, conclude (p. 362):

> No part of the moral vocabulary has done more to protect the legitimate interests of citizens in political states than the language of rights. Predictably, injustice and inhumane treatment occur most frequently in states that fail to recognise human rights in their political rhetoric and documents. As much as any part of moral discourse, rights language crosses international boundaries and enters into treaties, international law, and statements by international agencies and associations. Rights thereby become acknowledged as international standards for the treatment of persons.

The issue of moral rights is an important one for nurses — particularly as the issue relates to patients' rights and the patients' rights movement. As this is a substantial issue on its own, it is considered separately in Chapter 6 of this book.

Virtue ethics

In recent times there has been a resurgence of virtue theory in ethics and a re-examination of the importance of 'characterological excellence' as an ingredient of authentic moral conduct. Virtue ethics holds a particular relevance for nursing since virtuous conduct is intricately linked to therapeutic healing behaviours and the promotion of human wellbeing.

Virtue ethics (also known as character ethics) has an impressive history dating back to the ancient philosophical and theological texts of both Western and non-Western cultures (Beauchamp and Childress 2001; Pellegrino 1995; Kruschwitz and Roberts 1987). As Pellegrino (1995, p. 254) writes, 'Virtue is the most ancient, durable, and ubiquitous concept in the history of ethical theory'.

Despite its durability, virtue theory has experienced a significant decline particularly within the field of Western moral philosophy. This decline can be traced to the rise of scientism. By the late seventeenth and eighteenth centuries, for instance, the 'Enlightenment project of finding a rational justification for morality' saw moralists look away from the law of God 'to actual, observable human nature for a justification of traditional moral norms' (MacIntyre — cited in Krushwitz and Roberts 1987, pp. 12–13). Although virtue ethics has retained its currency in some fields, for example, the medical profession up until as late as the 1970s (Pellegrino 1995, p. 264), and the nursing profession up until the present time, its importance to and in moral philosophy has long been lost, having been seriously neglected by philosophers preoccupied with turning ethics into a science.

Significantly, over the past several decades, there has been a revival in virtue-based theories of ethics (Pellegrino 1995; Pence 1984). This revival (which has included both religious and non-religious approaches to virtue theory) has been driven by an increasing dissatisfaction and frustration among some philosophers with the otherwise narrow, abstract, impersonal and at times oversimplified approach of traditional theories of ethics, and the need to find an alternative approach that is more reflective of and responsive to the complexities of the moral life (Pellegrino 1995; Pence 1991). Of particular concern has been the questionable neglect within mainstream moral philosophy of considerations relating to the moral character of moral agents (persons who engage in moral actions). One aspect of this concern is expressed eloquently by Pence (1991, p. 256), who, commenting on what he sees as 'a common defect in non-virtue theories', points out:

> On the theories of duty or principle, it is theoretically possible that a person could, robot-like, obey every moral rule and lead the perfectly moral life. In this scenario, one would be like a perfectly programmed computer (perhaps such people do exist, and are products of perfect moral educations).

The idea that persons could function as 'moral robots' is both disturbing and unsatisfactory to virtue theorists, and, it might be added, to others who feel at least an intuitive unease about the prospect of morality being merely a matter of following a set of rules. We do seem to think, as Clouser (1995, p. 231) reminds us, that morality 'also encourages us to act in ways that go beyond what is required' — beyond a robot-like obedience to rules.

There does seem to be something 'missing' in the traditional picture of 'the moral life'. For virtue theorists, this 'something' is character. As Pence (1991, p. 256) writes:

> we need to know much more about the outer shell of behaviour to make such [moral] judgments, i.e. we need to know what kind of person is involved, how the person thinks of other people, how he or she thinks of his or her own character, how the person feels about past actions, and also how the person feels about actions not done.

Furthermore, there is a sense in which virtue theory is inevitable. As Pellegrino (1995, p. 254) points out:

> One cannot completely separate the character of a moral agent from his or her acts, the nature of those acts, the circumstances under which they are performed, or their consequences. Virtue theories focus on the agent; on his or her intentions, dispositions and motives; and on the kind of person the moral agent becomes, wishes to become, or ought to become as a result of his or her habitual disposition to act in certain ways.

Virtue theory raises some important questions, namely: (1) What is virtue? (2) What constitutes a virtuous person? and (3) Given virtue theory, does virtue ethics offer a plausible and viable alternative to traditional theories of ethics?

The notion of virtue

The term 'virtue' (from the Latin *virtus* meaning 'manliness', courage from vir meaning 'man') denotes the quality or practice of moral excellence. As an ingredient of moral theory, it can be defined as:

> a trait or character that disposes its possessor habitually to excellence of intent and performance with respect to the telos specific to a human activity. Virtue gives to reason the power to discern and to will the motivation asymptotically to accomplish a moral end with perfection.
>
> (Pellegrino 1995, p. 268)

Examples of the moral virtues include: care, compassion, kindness, empathy, sympathy, altruism, generosity, respectfulness, trustworthiness, personal integrity, forgiveness, friendship, love, wisdom, courage, fairness (justice), and so on (Beauchamp and Childress 2001; Blum 1994, 1980; Pellegrino 1995; Blustein 1991; Krushwitz and Roberts 1987; Walton 1986).

THE VIRTUOUS PERSON

The notions of 'virtue' and 'virtuous persons' are both universal constructs. As Pellegrino (1995, p. 255) points out:

> Every culture has a notion of the virtuous person — i.e., a paradigm person, real or idealised, who sets standards of noble conduct for a culture and whose character traits exemplify the kind of person others in that culture ought to be or to emulate.
>
> (Pellegrino 1995, p. 255)

Such paradigm persons include: Buddha, Confucius, Jesus Christ and, more recently, the Catholic nun, Mother Theresa (see Vardey 1995), hailed for her charitable works in India.

The question remains: what is a virtuous person? In a purely virtue-based theory of ethics, morally exemplary (virtuous) persons (including moral heroes and moral saints), are generally distinguished from other persons who 'do their duty' in a somewhat impersonal, impartial, universalistic rule-bound sense (Blum 1988). In a purely virtue-based ethic, a virtuous person is taken to be 'the good person, the person upon whom one can rely habitually to be good and to do the good under all circumstances' (Pellegrino 1995, p. 254).

Blum (1988) takes the notion of virtuous persons even further to include what he calls 'moral heroes' and 'moral saints'. A moral hero, by his view, is someone:

- who brings about a great good (or prevents a great evil);
- who acts to a great extent from morally worthy motives;
- whose moral-worthy motives are substantially embedded in his or her own personal psychology;
- who carries out his or her moral project in the face of risk or danger; and
- who is relatively 'faultless' or has an absence of unworthy desires, dispositions, sentiments, attitudes.

(adapted from Blum 1988, pp. 199, 203)

A moral saint, in contrast, is not altogether different from a moral hero, except for one feature. According to Blum (1988, p. 204), moral saints share three features in common with moral heroes:

> they are animated by morally-worthy motives, their morally-excellent qualities exist at a deep level of their personality or character, and they meet the standard of relative absence of unworthy desires.

The salient feature which distinguishes a moral saint from a moral hero, however, is that the moral saint exhibits 'a higher standard of faultlessness' viz. the absence of unworthy desires (Blum 1988, p. 204).

Virtue ethics and nursing

A virtue theory of ethics holds a particular pertinence for nursing ethics in terms of providing a justificatory framework for nursing moral decisions and actions.

The agreed end or *telos* of the profession and practice of nursing is the promotion of health, healing and wellbeing, together with the alleviation of suffering, in individuals, groups and communities for whom nurses care. This end is a moral end, and one that carries with it a strong moral action guiding force for nurses insofar as it requires nurses to engage in the behaviours necessary to promote health, healing and wellbeing in people, and, when manifest, to alleviate their suffering. In light of these ends, and the nature of the means necessary to achieve them (that is, 'good' nursing care), nursing thus stands fundamentally as a benevolent (virtuous) activity, or, more precisely, a 'moral practice' that aims to discover (through assessment), make explicit and accomplish (through cooperation and negotiation) whatever is 'good' for (read as 'conducive to the health, healing and wellbeing of') the individuals, groups and communities for whose care nurses share responsibility (Gastmans et al. 1998, p. 58).

In speaking of 'good' nursing care, it is important to clarify that something much more than merely 'competent' nursing care is being referred to. Rather, it is competent care integrated with a 'virtuous attitude' of caring. As Gastmans et al. explain (1998, pp. 45, 53, emphasis added):

> It is only by integrating a virtuous attitude of caring with the competent performance of care activities (*caring behaviour*) that *good care* can be achieved ... Morally virtuous attitudes are an integral part of nursing practice, since this practice takes place within a human relationship where the nurse and the patient are the main actors ...This is in essence what is meant by caring behaviour: *the integration of virtue and expert activity.*

'Virtuous caring' is integral to 'good' (moral) nursing practice (and, by implication, nursing ethics) in at least two important ways. First, virtuous caring or 'right attitudes' (which include the behavioural orientations of compassion, empathy, concern, genuineness, warmth, trust, kindness, gentleness, nurturence, enablement, respect, mutuality, 'giving presence' (being there), attentive responsiveness, providing comfort, providing a sense of safety and security, and others) have all been thoroughly implicated as effective nursing healing behaviours in the alleviation of human suffering (hence the notions in nursing of *caring as healing* and *nursing as informed caring for the wellbeing of others*) (Taylor 1995; Ching 1993; Larson and Ferketich 1993; Leftwich 1993; Swanson 1993; Connelly 1991; Geary and Hawkins 1991; Oliver 1990). Such behavioural orientations have been demonstrated as making a significant and positive difference not only to a patient's existential sense of — and actual — 'wellbeing', but to the effectiveness of drugs, to wound healing, and even to survival itself (it is well known, for example, that premature newborns will 'fail to thrive' in the absence of attentive, 'high touch' and informed nursing care and may even die; similarly, it is known that adults who are deprived of meaningful care will fail to heal and may even die prematurely from life-threatening diseases) (Ryffe and Singer 2001; Gastmans et al. 1998; Kanitsaki 1996; Dossey 1993, 1991; Moore and Komras 1993; Starck and McGovern 1992; Gaut and Leininger 1991; Peterson and Bossio 1991).

Second, 'virtuous caring' plays an important theoretical role in providing an account of moral motivation in nursing to act in beneficent ways. For instance, whereas in obligation-based theories the motivation to act morally is thought to be derived from a rationally appraised commitment to 'do one's duty', in the case of virtuous caring the motivation to be moral is derived from moral sentiment (for instance, caring about a thing in some way [Rachels 1988, p. 20]), specifically a nurse's affective involvement in (that is, *caring about*) the patient's wellbeing. The explanation of Gastmans et al. (1998, p. 54) is worth quoting at length. They write:

> In addition to the collection and availability of relevant information [to plan and implement patient care], the caring nurse needs to be affectively involved in the patient's wellbeing. The caring nurse needs to be emotionally touched by what happens to the patient, both in a positive and a negative sense. The cognitive and affective dimensions of the virtue of care are not rightly understood as merely two separate *components* — a cognition and a feeling-state — added together, rather they inform one another. The (altruistic) virtue of care is more than a passive feeling-state that has a person in a state of woe as their object. The (altruistic) virtue of care involves an active, motivational aspect as well, relating to the promotion of beneficent acts aimed at helping the other person. In other words, the caring nurse must be motivated to respond to the appeal of the patient. Common to the altruistic virtue of care is a desire for, or regard for, the good of the other (for his or her own sake). This desire prompts (intended) beneficent action when the nurse is in a position to engage in it.

The agreed ethical standards of nursing require nurses to promote the genuine welfare and wellbeing of people in need of help through nursing care, and to do so in a manner that is safe, competent, therapeutically effective, culturally relevant, and just. These standards also recognise that in the ultimate analysis nurses 'can never escape the reality that they literally hold human wellbeing in their hands' (Taylor 1998, p. 74), and accordingly must act responsively and responsibly to protect it. These requirements are demonstrably consistent with a virtue theory account of ethics.

Virtue ethics and nursing's ethic of care

Consistent with a virtue theory account of ethics is a nursing articulated 'ethic of care' regarded by many nurse theorists as the moral foundation, essence, ideal and imperative of nursing (Bowden 1994; Hodge 1993a, 1993b; Brown et al. 1992; Gaut 1992; Roach 1992, 1987; Cooper 1991; Gaut and Leininger 1991; Leininger 1991, 1990a, 1990b, 1988; Klimek 1990; Leininger and Watson 1990; Benner and Wrubel 1989; Fry 1989a, 1989b, 1988a, 1988b; Twomey 1989; Carper 1986; Watson 1985a, 1985b; Benner 1984). Despite this, there has been mounting criticism in recent years about the place of 'care' in nursing ethics. These criticisms have ranged from describing an ethic of care as being 'hopelessly vague' and as 'obscuring more than it promotes' (Allmark 1995), to rejecting that care is a virtue at all (Curzer 1993). Still others denigrate care as an untenable form of 'subjugation' of women on account of its apparent 'sexist service orientation' that could see women (nurses) carrying a disproportionate 'burden of care' in a society (or a system) that is, for the most part, *careless* (Puka 1989). A brief response to some of these criticisms is warranted here.

Firstly, as just demonstrated, a reflective articulation of an ethic of care in relation to the moral ends of nursing helps to clarify the precise behaviours expected of a 'good' nurse. It not only prescribes 'do good', but it describes *what* those 'goods' are (the promotion of health, healing and wellbeing, and the alleviation of suffering), and *how* to achieve them (through an integration of expert and virtuous caring comprising a range of 'healing promoting behaviours'). Second, given the mutually beneficial nature of 'virtuous caring' (it has demonstrable positive outcomes for *both* the receiver and the giver of authentic virtuous care), there is room to suggest that 'caring' that is unjustly burdensome is not only *not* 'virtuous caring' but not ethical. Arguments against 'virtuous caring' are thus not correctly aligned at the right target; they are, as it were, 'attacking a straw man'. Thirdly, the criticisms are not convincing. For instance, in the case of the criticism that an ethic of care could be unduly burdensome on women (nurses), it is not immediately clear why it would be any more burdensome than say an obligation-based theory of ethics. As the example of the Biblical story of Abraham demonstrates (Abraham came close to sacrificing his only son to fulfil his duty of obedience to God), 'doing one's duty' can, in some circumstances, be an extremely burdensome thing to do and further may not be able to be done without sacrificing something of moral importance. Further, to suggest that nurses might in someway become enslaved or 'subjugated' by an ethic of care, seems to imply erroneously that (and, it must be added, perpetuate the patriarchal myth that) nurses *qua* nurses lack the discretion and moral competence necessary to *decide for themselves* what moral standards they will adopt and uphold; in short, it seems to suggest, incorrectly in my view, that nurses will just 'follow slavishly' an ethic of care. Finally, these criticisms seem to overlook that an ethic of care is, paradoxically, protective of its practitioners in that it rejects symbiotic (over) emotional involvement with 'the other', emphasising instead moral virtue (characterological excellence) as its foundation (Gastmans et al. 1998, pp. 54–7).

Problems with virtue ethics

Virtue ethics, like other theories of ethics, is not free of difficulties. Key among these are: the 'circularity of justification' in virtue theory (virtuous persons do what is good, the good is what virtuous persons do); the inability of virtue theory to explain adequately its force as a moral action guide (that is, compared with other obligation-based theories that can rely on moral rules, principles and maxims to justify moral conduct); and the high expectations virtue theory imposes on people to be 'good' (while a good many of us can be conscientious in our actions, few of us can be 'exemplary' (Pellegrino 1995, pp. 262–3). These difficulties, however, may be more a product of the adversarial nature of philosophical inquiry and its use to critically examine and raise objections to virtue theory, than a problem with virtue ethics itself. For instance, given the distinctive non-rational quality of the moral virtues, it seems odd to suggest that virtuous actions require 'justification' (how does one 'justify' an inclination to be kind toward another, or to be fair? how does one 'justify' an act of saintliness or heroism?). Similarly, it seems odd to expect that virtue theory can be reduced to a set of justificatory rules, principles and maxims (noting that, what makes the virtues what they are is their spontaneous and unconditional expression *beyond* that otherwise required by rules, principles and maxims). There is room here to suggest that to 'justify' the virtues in a rational philosophical sense is to do violence to them and to all that they represent. Finally, it seems odd to suggest that expecting people to be 'decent' and 'morally excellent' human beings is 'too high an expectation'. Ethics is precisely about expecting people to strive to achieve the highest ideals of morality and to engage in morally excellent conduct. Virtue ethics is no different in this regard. That people may not achieve such an ideal is no reason to abandon ethics, and it is no reason to abandon virtue ethics either.

It is becoming increasingly accepted that while virtue cannot stand alone, it can be (and should be) 'related to other ethical theories in a more comprehensive moral philosophy than currently exists' (Pence 1984, p. 282; see also Pellegrino 1995, p. 254). As Beauchamp and Childress (1994, p. 66) conclude, the virtues have 'a special place in the moral life'. They are mostly compatible with traditional obligation-based theories (e.g. principles and rules) and where there exists a correspondence between them, even though 'rough and imperfect', they tend to be mutually reinforcing of each other. For example, respect for the principle of autonomy, requires the virtue of *respectfulness*; commitment to and upholding the principle of beneficence, requires the virtue of *benevolence*; and so on (Beauchamp and Childress 2001, p. 39).

Deontology and teleology

This discussion on moral theory would not be complete without reference being made to two main 'parent' theories of ethics, namely: *deontology* and *teleology* (also called consequentialism, of which utilitarian theory is a form).

Deontology

According to deontological ethics, duty is the basis of all moral action. Taken at its most basic, deontology asserts that some acts are obligatory (duty bound) regardless of their consequences. For example, a deontologist might assert that one has a duty to always tell the truth. By this view, the deontologist is duty bound to always tell the truth even when doing so might have horrible consequences. An important question to be asked here is: How do we know what our duty is?

One possible answer to this question can be found in classical deontological theory that derives from religious ethics. According to this view, it is God's command that determines our moral duties. If, for example, God commands 'thou shalt not kill', 'thou shalt not steal', and the like, then conduct that accords with (obeys) these commands is morally praiseworthy (right and justified). This is 'because and only because it is commanded by God' (Frankena 1973).

There are many examples of deontological ethics influencing decision-making in health care domains. For example, Jehovah's Witnesses are well known for their refusal of life-saving blood transfusions, on the grounds that to accept such treatment would be tantamount to violating God's command that, according to their beliefs, prohibits taking blood (Fry and Johnstone 2002, pp. 117–18). Another example can be found in a deontological adherence by some physicians and surgeons to the preservation of 'medically hopeless' human life whatever the costs (read consequences) resulting in the administration of 'futile' medical treatment to clients — sometimes even against their will (Schneiderman and Jecker 1995).

Another answer can be found in what is otherwise known as ethical rationalism. This view dates back to the work of the 18th century German philosopher Immanuel Kant who held that the supreme principle of morality was reason, whose ultimate end is good will. According to a 1972 translation, Kant stated that reason is free (autonomous) to formulate moral law and to determine just what is to count as being an overriding moral duty. Kant held duty to be that which is done for its own sake, and 'not for the results it attains or seeks to attain' (Kant 1972). Kant further believed that moral considerations (duties) were always overriding in nature — in other words, should take precedence over other (non-moral) considerations.

In terms of determining what one's actual duty is, Kant suggested that this can be done by appealing to some formal (reasoned) principle or maxim. In choosing such a maxim, however, Kant warned that we must take care not to choose something that would privilege our interests over the interests of others. Kant's solution to this problem was to establish a universally valid law called the 'categorical imperative'. This law states: 'Act only on that maxim through which you can at the same time will that it should become universal law' (Kant 1972). In other words, we should only act on maxims that we are prepared to accept as holding for everybody (including ourselves) throughout space and time. A variation of Kant's law can be found in what is popularly known as the Golden Rule: 'Do unto others as you would have them do unto you'.

Teleology

According to teleological theory (also known as consequentialism) actions can only be judged right and/or good on the basis of the consequences they produce. In this respect, teleological ethics denies everything that deontological ethics asserts.

The most popularly known teleological theory of ethics is *utilitarianism*, which has as its central concern the general welfare of people as a whole, rather than individuals. In short, utilitarianism views the world not in terms of certain individual rights which people may or may not claim, but in terms of people's collective and overall welfare and interests. The perspective of utilitarianism is persuasive in that it promotes a universal point of view; namely, that one person's interests cannot count as being superior to the interests of another, just because they are personal interests (Singer 1979; Smart and Williams 1973). To put this another way, I cannot claim that my interests are more deserving than your interests are, just because they are my interests.

Classical utilitarianism, first advanced by the English philosopher Jeremy Bentham (1748–1832) and later modified by the work of the British philosopher John Stuart Mill (1806–73), holds roughly that moral agents have a duty to 'maximise the greatest happiness/good for the greatest number' (Bentham 1962; Mill 1962). This view has resulted in classical utilitarianism being dubbed the 'greatest happiness principle'. Because of difficulties associated with calculating both individual and collective happiness and unhappiness, and the problem of individual interests being sacrificed for the collective whole, classical utilitarianism theory has been largely abandoned in favour of recent utilitarian theory. Of particular note is *preference utilitarianism*, which views the maximisation of autonomy and individual preferences as being of intrinsic value rather than the maximisation of happiness per se. This is because, as Beauchamp and Childress explain, what is intrinsically valuable is what individuals prefer to obtain, and utility is thus translated into maxmizing 'the overall satisfaction of the preferences of the greatest number of individuals' (Beauchamp and Childress 2001, p. 342).

Although not without difficulty, preference utilitarianism is also considered more plausible since it is relatively easy to calculate what people's preferences are: all we have to do is to ask people what it is they prefer. And where their preferences are at odds with ethical conduct, we have no obligation to respect them.

Moral duties and obligations

Common to all theoretical perspectives are the imperatives they impose for behaving in ways that respects the significant moral interests of others. It is generally accepted within moral philosophy that moral theories, moral principles, and moral rights all provide *sound moral reasons* for deciding and acting (behaving) in certain ways towards others and for explaining *why* we should act morally. For example, the *moral principle of autonomy* and the *moral right to informed consent* both seem to provide strong reasons ('moral warrants') for giving information to patients/clients and *why*; that is, to enable them to make prudent and intelligent choices about their care and treatment. More than this, they impose a *moral duty* on us to do so. To understand what this means and how *duties* (and their counterparts, *obligations*) 'bind' us to be moral it would be useful here to explain what duties and obligations are and how they work.

Moral duties

A moral duty (to be distinguished here from a legal duty, a civil duty, a professional duty, and so on) is an action which a person is bound, for moral reasons, to perform. Language used in identifying duties typically involves expressions such as: 'I have a duty to …', 'You have a duty to …', 'They have a duty to …', and so on.

Duties are primarily concerned with avoiding intolerable results; they are thought to provide the basic requirements that may be demanded of everybody (i.e. universally) in an effort to achieve a 'tolerable basis of social life' (Urmson 1958, in Feinberg 1969, p. 73). They also work 'to secure reliability, a state of affairs in which people can reasonably expect others to behave in some ways and not in others' (Williams 1985, p. 187). If a duty fails to avoid an intolerable result, there is room for questioning whether in fact it was a duty in the first place (Urmson 1958). It might also be argued that if a duty can be overridden (for example, where there appears to be a conflict of duties) it is not a duty at all; we have merely mistakenly thought that it was (Hare 1981, p. 26). On the other hand, it might be replied that just because a duty can be overridden this does not mean 'it was not a duty in the first place' but only that it was a 'prima-facie duty'. There is nothing philosophically wrong in holding that duties can be prima facie in nature (Ross 1930, p. 19).

As already stated, moral reasons binding people to act in certain ways can be provided from the following sources: a moral theory, a moral principle, or a moral right. For example, from a teleological perspective, duties generally derive from the consideration of some predicted moral consequence that ought to be furthered or upheld. It might be argued, for instance, that one has a stringent moral duty to prevent otherwise avoidable harmful consequences from occurring where this can be done without sacrificing other important moral interests. Given this 'teleological reason', if a person's action stands to prevent a particular harmful consequence from occurring, that person is duty-bound to perform that action, provided other important moral interests are not sacrificed in the process. An off-duty nurse, for example, could be said to be duty-bound to render life-saving care at the scene of a road accident, regardless of any inconvenience this might cause since mere inconvenience is not generally regarded as a morally significant consideration. If the life of the nurse were put at risk, however, the moral duty to render assistance would not be so clear-cut.

Similarly in the case of ethical principlism. For example, the ethical principles of autonomy, non-maleficence, beneficence, and justice all provide moral reasons binding people to act in certain ways toward others: the principle of autonomy, for instance, imposes on people a duty to respect the choices of others; the principle of nonmaleficence imposes on people a duty not to harm others; the principle of benefience imposes on people a duty to treat others well (beneficially), and the principle of justice imposes on people a duty to treat others fairly.

In a rights view of morality, and in contrast to the above approaches, a moral reason is supplied by a correlative *rights* claim. Thus if someone claims a right to be respected, this imposes on us a duty to respect that person; likewise, if someone claims a right to privacy, this imposes on us a duty not to disclose information of a private nature about that person, and so on.

The critical task for each of us is to decide just what our moral duties are. This, of course, is dependent on correctly determining what is to count as an overriding moral reason for doing something or, as in the case of rights, correctly determining whether a given rights claim is genuine, and, further, whether we, as moral agents, do in fact have a duty correlative to the claim in question.

Moral obligations

A notion that is strongly related to the notion of 'moral duty' is that of 'moral obligation'. The language of obligations is very similar to the language of duties, and typically involves expressions like: 'You have an obligation to …', 'I have an obligation to …', 'We have an obligation to …', 'They have an obligation to …', and so on. Although many philosophers treat the terms 'duties' and 'obligations' synonymously, an important and useful distinction can be drawn between them, which rests on the differing moral strengths each notion has, rather than on a difference in their essential moral nature. Duties are regarded as having a stronger force than obligations, or, to put this another way, duties are more morally compelling than are obligations. Dworkin (1977, pp. 48–9), an influential exponent of this distinction, gives the example that it is one thing to say a person has an obligation to give to a charity, but it is quite another to say that person has a duty to do so. While it would be 'good' if someone made a charitable donation, it would be a mistake to suggest a moral compulsion to do so. To a limited extent, Dworkin's thesis helps to alleviate the tension created by the problem of supposed conflicting duties.

The concept of obligation and its distinctiveness from duty has interesting and important implications for nurses, particularly in relation to the issue of following a doctor's or a supervisor's directives. For instance, it may well be that nurses have an *obligation* to follow a doctor's or a supervisor's orders, but it is far from clear that they always have a *duty* to do so, either morally or legally. In fact, if a doctor's or a supervisor's directives are 'dubious', a nurse has both a legal and a moral duty to question such directives. In some cases, the nurse may even have a duty to refuse to follow a given directive if, for instance, it is 'unreasonable', 'unlawful' or 'likely to cause otherwise avoidable harm'.

Clarifying the difference between rights and duties

Before concluding this discussion, the important task remains of clearing up some confusion which some nurses may have about their own rights and duties in relation to caring for patients. Consider, for example, a situation involving an abortion procedure. A nurse could reasonably claim either a *right* to refuse to participate in an abortion procedure or a *duty* to refuse to participate. What is important here is to distinguish the basis upon which each claim might rest and to remember that whereas *rights* basically concern claims about *one's own interests*, *duties* basically concern claims about the *interests of others*. Thus, in an abortion case, if a nurse claims the *right* to refuse, this is fundamentally a claim involving the protection of the *nurse's own interests* (as opposed to the interests of the patient). The nurse might, for instance, have a religious-based conscientious objection to abortion and assert an entitlement to practise the tenets of that faith. A refusal based on a *duty* claim is significantly different, however. In this instance, the refusal is based more on the consideration of *another's interests*; for example, the interests of the patient or the fetus. Here the duty to refuse would derive from the broader moral duty to, say, prevent harm or to preserve life.

By this brief account it can be seen that to use the terms 'rights' and 'duties' interchangeably is not only incorrect, but misleading. When nurses speak of their *right* to, say, care for a patient in a certain way, or to practise their code of ethics, it is quite possible they are really asserting that they have a *duty* to care for the patient in that way or a duty to uphold their code of ethics.

Limitations and weaknesses of ethical theory

Over the past several decades, there has been mounting dissatisfaction among some moral philosophers in regard to the ability of commonly accepted moral theories to provide an adequate account of moral conduct and the 'moral life', and to provide practical guidance on how to deal with concrete everyday ethical problems. There has also been a related dissatisfaction with bioethics and its apparent (in)ability to deal effectively with ethical issues in health care and related domains and to guide practical solutions to the many complex ethical problems encountered in those domains. Feminist moral philosophers have been among the most ardent critics arguing that moral theory (particularly traditional or mainstream moral theory):

- is too abstract to be able to deal effectively with the concrete circumstances of life;
- pays too much attention to upholding abstract rules and principles, rather than: (1) promoting quality relationships between people, and (2) upholding the genuine welfare and wellbeing of people;
- has tended to privilege dominant groups over marginalised groups (more specifically, they have tended to privilege the interests and concerns of white, middle-class, able-bodied, heterosexual, politically conservative males at the expense of those deemed 'other', and hence inferior — for example, women and children, people of non-English-speaking and culturally diverse backgrounds, the disabled, gay men and lesbians, the poor, the uneducated, and so on);
- emphasis on rational argument has tended to fuel rather than quell moral controversy, disagreement, and distress;
- has failed on account of its augmentative and adversarial approach tending to divide rather than unite and reconcile people in common bonds (see in particular Addelson 1994; Brabeck 1989; Braidotti 1986; Card 1991; Cole and Coultrap-McQuinn 1992; Gatens 1986; Gibson 1976; Gilligan 1987, 1982; Grimshaw 1986; Hoagland 1988; Hekman 1995; Holmes and Purdy 1992; Kittay and Meyers 1987; Little 1996; Morgan 1988; Moulton 1983; Mullet 1988; Noddings 1984; Parsons 1986; Porter 1991; Sherwin 1992; Tronto 1993; Walker 1998, 1992; Wolf 1996a, 1996b).

In several respects the criticisms leveled at both traditional and contemporary moral theory have been warranted, especially those criticisms that have been advanced from the perspectives of feminist ethics. There is ample evidence to suggest that ethical theory, as it has been traditionally taught and considered, has been too far removed from the realities of practice and has failed too often to provide practical guidance on how to respond effectively to the complex moral questions of day-to-day living and practice. It is evident therefore that what has been called 'spaceship ethics' (i.e. a conception of ethics that operates from 'the secluded comfort of the arm chair' or from 'abstract apriori principles from which it hopes to derive answers to complicated, real-life practical problems'), needs to change (Benjamin 2001, p. 29). Its opposite, however, 'subway ethics' – an approach 'that would have us focus on particular cases and contexts with little or no concern for theory' — is not the answer either (Benjamin 2001, p. 29). As Benjamin (2001) explains (p. 29):

> If spaceship ethics is too far removed from the concrete ethical problems that actually trouble us, subway ethics is too close to them.

Where then lies the solution? For all the criticisms and controversies generated in response to ethical theory, one thing is clear: the solution is not to abandon it, but to *enrich* it. As Little explains (2001, p. 33):

> ... whatever one thinks about them [the criticisms], they are clearly objections to *impoverished* moral theory, not to *moral theory* per se (emphasis added).

What is needed, therefore, is a richer moral theory (or, more to the point, moral theor*ies*) that are more responsive to the practical lived realities of everyday life. Whether we wish to admit it or not, ethical theory is 'essential to moral life' insofar as it provides useful generalisations that can be used to teach, persuade others to accept, and to justify morally worthy points of view (Little 2001, p. 39).

With or without 'grand theories' of ethics, the fact remains that we all theorise about and try to make sense of our moral experiences. As Little (2001) contends, it is not enough to know *that*, we also need to know *why*; and we cannot know *why* without some kind of theoretical abstraction. In other words, the moral landscape simply cannot be understood *without* theoretical reasoning. But neither can the moral landscape or our moral experiences be understood simply by adopting or applying one or two 'master' concepts or principles or theories of ethics (Little 2001, p.33). It is for this reason that we need to engage constantly in the positive project of constructing and developing alternative models, methods, procedures and discourses of ethics that are more responsive to the lived realities and experiences of people and the social–cultural contexts within which they live (Gross 1986). A key aim of this books is to assist practitioners to engage in such a project.

Moral justification and moral theory — some further thoughts

The discussion in this chapter has shown that moral theory not only has an important role to play, but is essential in terms of enabling people to give meaning and order to their everyday moral experiences. Moral/ethical theory does this by helping people to describe the moral world, devise meaningful moral standards and ideals, distinguish ethical issues from other sorts of issues, and to provide a systematic justification of the actual practice of morality. When well developed, a moral/ethical theory 'provides a framework within which agents can reflect on the acceptability of actions and can evaluate moral judgments and character' (Beauchamp and Childress 1994, p. 44). It should be added, however, that 'good' ethical practice also provides a framework for evaluating and reflecting on what constitutes a well developed ethical theory. In several respects, therefore, the relationship between moral theory and ethical practice is symbiotic; just as ethical practice cannot be evaluated independently of its theoretical underpinnings, neither can moral theory be evaluated independently of moral experience.

Ethical experience may, however, provide more than an evaluative framework for guiding theoretical reflections; in several respects it provides an important methodological starting point for developing moral theory (both 'ordinary' and 'formal'). Moreno (1995 p. 113), for example, defending what he calls 'ethical naturalism', persuasively argues that 'moral values emerge from *actual human experience* and are not superimposed on it by some transcendental reality' (emphasis added). Clouser (1995, p. 235), takes a similar position. He states:

> Ordinary moral experience is our starting point. After all, morality cannot be *invented*. 'Look, here's my idea for a new morality ... those with the most education get to say what happens to anyone with less education ...!' We must begin with the moral system that is actually used by thoughtful people in making decisions and judgments about what to do in particular cases. Ordinary morality is generally expressed in what can be regarded as moral rules — e.g. don't cheat, don't kill, don't lie — and moral ideals — e.g. relieve pain, promote freedom, help the needy. If one were just initiating a study of morality as it is practiced, these rules and ideals would constitute the demarcations of the moral realm; they are the earmarks of morality at work; they are the phenomena on which the study would focus. (emphasis original)

The importance of moral experience in nursing and its relationship to the development and refinement of nursing ethics will be explored further in the chapters to follow.

Conclusion

In this chapter, attention has been given to clarifying the relationship between moral theory and ethical nursing practice. Particular attention has been given to examining the nature and importance of moral justification to moral decision-making and how various ethical theories (for example, ethical principlism, moral rights theory and virtue ethics) work to provide 'good reasons' for deciding and acting morally toward others. The notions of 'duties' and 'obligations' and the distinction between 'rights' and 'duties' have also been clarified. Having now considered what ethics is, why nurses should be (i.e. have a *duty* to be) be ethical, and having examined a number of different ethical frameworks within which nurses can operate to guide their moral choices and conduct, there remains the task of exploring further some of the issues that nurses will encounter during the course of their work. Here it may be asked: What kinds of issues are nurses likely to encounter in health care contexts? What 'ethical competencies' do nurses need in order to address the issues they encounter? How should nurses respond to the ethical issues they encounter? It is to examining these and related questions that the following chapters will now turn.

CASE SCENARIO AND CRITICAL QUESTIONS

Case scenario

A registered nurse working in aged care was sacked by her employer of five years after she allegedly spoke out against the poor conditions at the nursing home where she worked. It had been previously reported in the media that residents at the home 'had been left lying wet in their beds for hours' and 'that there was broken plaster and exposed plumbing and that mice and rats had been known to climb through holes in the walls' at the home (Toy 2000, p. 5). The proprieters of the home reportedly denied the allegations and called a meeting of staff to discuss the allegations. At this meeting the nurse in question spoke freely about what she believed had been a decline in standards 'over the past two years because of staff cuts' and about her concern that this was 'jeopardising residents' safety' (Toy 2000, p. 5). After receiving a warning from her employer for allegedly behaving in an 'unacceptably aggressive' manner during the staff meeting and having a 'negative and disruptive attitude towards management' the nurse was dismissed (Toy 2000, p. 5). In support of the nurse, supervisors subsequently wrote to the employer indicating that she was 'an excellent nurse practitioner with excellent patient care skills' and requested her immediate reinstatement. The Australian Nursing Federation was reported as stating that this incident was 'a clear case of a nurse being punished for speaking out' and that, if left unchallenged, it could create 'a climate of fear and might prevent other nurses from speaking out on behalf of residents who often had no one else to advocate for them' (Toy 2000, p. 5).

Critical questions

1. Was the nurse's action of 'speaking out' in this case morally justified?
2. What moral reasons are there for either supporting or rejecting the position she took?
3. What would you have done in this situation?
4. How would you have decided what to do?

Chapter 4

Transcultural ethics and the ethical practice of nursing

LEARNING OBJECTIVES

Upon the completion of this chapter and with further self-directed learning you are expected to be able to:

- Explain what is meant by the notion of 'culture'.
- Discuss the critical relationship between culture and ethics.
- Examine critically the nature and implications of applying transcultural ethics in nursing and health care contexts.
- Discuss the ways in which ignoring cultural considerations in nursing and health care contexts could adversely affect the significant moral interests of patients and (their) families from diverse cultural and linguistic backgrounds.
- Outline at least four questions that nurses should ask in order to assess their own cultural–moral competency to make moral decisions when caring for people of diverse cultural backgrounds.

KEYWORDS

- Culture
- Ethics
- Moral diversity
- Moral imperialism
- Moral pluralism
- Nocebo phenomenon
- Placebo phenomenon
- Transcultural ethics

Introduction

One of the greatest challenges facing nurses and the health care teams in which they work is caring effectively, appropriately and ethically for people from diverse cultural and linguistic backgrounds. One reason why caring for people from diverse cultural backgrounds is challenging is that professional caregivers do not always know, understand or share the same cultural and moral values held by those for whom they care. This lack of knowledge and understanding of the different cultural life ways of different people can make it very difficult for professional caregivers to provide care that is culturally appropriate, therapeutically effective, and ethically just. This difficulty is compounded if professional caregivers also do not have appropriate knowledge and understanding of the complex relationship that exists between culture, health and healing (therapeutic) behaviours. A lack of knowledge and understanding about these things can result not only in disagreements between professional caregivers, and between professional caregivers and patients and families, but also in wrong judgments being made and 'wrong care' or what Kanitsaki calls 'toxic service' being provided (Kanitsaki 2003, 2000, 1996). This, in turn, can result in the undesirable moral consequences of patients' wellbeing and even their lives being placed in jeopardy, as examples to be given in this and the following chapters will show.

In order to respond effectively to the challenges posed by caring for people from diverse cultural backgrounds, it is vital that nurses and allied health care professionals understand the nature of culture and its relationship to ethics. What particularly needs to be understood is that *culture exists logically prior to ethics, not the other way around* as has been classically contended in moral philosophy. In other words, ethics and the various systems of ethics that exist are every bit the products of the cultures and the times from which they have emerged and which have shaped, developed, refined and sustained them. In short, ethics and its derivatives have been, and continue to be, 'culturally constructed' (Cortese 1990, p. 1; see also Anderson 1990; Moreno 1995). That is, they are *human inventions* and not, as some have asserted, naturally occurring material facts that are interwoven into the fabric of the observable world (McNaughton 1988; Brink 1989; Dancy 1993).

Transcultural nursing and ethics

Leininger (1990), an American leader in transcultural nursing, has made the important claim that 'culture has been the critical and conspicuously missing dimension in the study and practice of ethical and moral [sic] dimensions of human care' (p. 49). She has also criticised nurse ethicists for their failure to recognise the important and significant role that culture plays in guiding moral judgments and behaviour in human care contexts; and she contends further that some nurse ethicists have even 'deliberately avoided' the concept of culture altogether, preferring instead to assume the universality of the ethical principles, codes and standards of human conduct that have become so prevalent in mainstream nursing ethics discourse (Leininger 1990, p. 51). Leininger concludes that, if nurses are to provide appropriate ethical care to individuals, families and groups of different cultural backgrounds, they must have knowledge of and the ability to uphold sensitively and in an informed way the culturally based moral values and beliefs of the people for whom they care (Leininger 1990, p. 52). On this point, she states (pp. 52–3):

> most assuredly, the evolving discipline of nursing needs an epistemic ethical and moral [sic] knowledge base that takes into account cultural differences and similarities in order to

provide knowledgeable and accurate judgments that are congruent with clients' values and life-ways.

Without this knowledge base, Leininger contends, it is not possible for nurses to make the 'right' decisions or to provide the 'right' (ethical) human care when planning and implementing nursing care (Leininger 1990, p. 64).

Questions remain, however: What is culture? and, further, What is culture's relationship to and role in ethics generally, and nursing ethics in particular? It is to briefly answering these questions that this discussion now turns.

Culture and its relationship to ethics

Culture is an extremely complex concept, and one that has been defined, interpreted and analysed from a variety of disciplinary perspectives (see, for example, Kanitsaki 2000, 1994, 1993; Leininger 1991; Midgley 1991a; Helman 1990; Williams 1989; Fieldhouse 1986; Bullivant 1984, 1981; Wuthnow et al. 1984; Beals 1979; Spindler 1974; Kluckholn 1962; Sorokin 1957; Mead 1955). Not surprisingly, this has seen the emergence of a number of rival theories and viewpoints on what culture is, and on what its relationship to and role in human affairs is or should be (Kanitsaki 1992, p. 5). Even anthropologists do not agree about how culture should be defined, interpreted and analysed (Kanitsaki 1989a, p. 11). Nevertheless, there is some agreement among scholars that culture is a human invention and one which is critical for human survival and the development of human potential (Kanitsaki 1989a, p. 11).

What then is culture? As already stated, culture has been defined, interpreted and analysed in a variety of ways. Cohen, for example, argues that (1968, p. 1):

> culture is made up of the energy systems, the objective and specific artefacts, the organisations of social relations, the modes of thought, the ideologies, and the total range of customary behaviour that are transmitted from one generation to another by a social group and that enables it to maintain life in a particular habitat.

Bullivant argues along similar lines, adding to the description of culture that it is something which (1981, p. 19):

> can be thought of as the knowledge and conceptions embodied in symbolic and non-symbolic communication modes about the technology and skills, customary behaviours, values, beliefs, and attitudes a society has evolved from its historical past, and progressively modifies and augments to give meaning to and cope with the present and anticipated future problems of its existence.

A more accessible description of culture, however, and one which is very helpful to this discussion, comes from an Australian Professor of Transcultural Nursing, Olga Kanitsaki, AM (Member in the Order of Australia). Kanitsaki describes culture as follows (1994, p. 95):

> Culture includes a particular people's beliefs, value orientations and value systems, which give meaning, logic, worth and significance to their existence and experience in relation to both the universe and other human beings. These value orientations, value systems and beliefs in turn shape customs and traditions, prescribe and proscribe behaviour, determine the structure of social institutions and power relations, and identify and prescribe social relations, modes and rules of communication, *moral order*, and, indeed, the whole spirit and web of meaning and purpose of a given group in a particular place and time. Culture thus reflects the shared history, traditions, achievements, struggles for survival and lived

experiences of a particular people. Its influence extends over politics, economics, the development and use of technology, the boundaries and meaning of class, the determination of gender roles, and so on. (emphasis added)

Kanitsaki further explains that (2002, p. 22):

Culture can be seen as an inherited 'lens' through which individuals perceive and understand the world that they inhabit, and learn how to live within. Growing up within any society is a form of enculturation, formal and informal, whereby the individual slowly acquires the cultural 'lens' of that society. Without a common consciousness and shared perceptions of the world, both the cohesion and the continuity of any human group would be impossible.

Unfortunately, it is beyond the scope of this text to discuss the concept of culture at the level and depth it warrants, and its consideration must be left for another time. Nevertheless, there is room to emphasise the point that, regardless of the competing theories on what culture is, it is clear that it plays a fundamental and critical role in shaping people's values, beliefs, perceptions and knowledge about the world within which they live, that it influences people's behaviour and generally gives logic and meaning to a whole way of life in that world, and that it ultimately provides the 'blueprint' for their (human) survival in that world (Kanitsaki 1992, p. 5). It is also clear that culture's relationship to and role in ethics (including its relationship to the theoretical underpinnings and practical application of ethics) cannot be plausibly denied. One does not have to be a distinguished cultural anthropologist to recognise and accept the critical link between culture and people's moral values, beliefs, perceptions and knowledge of what constitutes morally right and wrong conduct. As Mary Midgley points out (1991a, p. 72), the 'communication explosion' has meant, among other things, that:

virtually everybody, even in quite remote corners of the world, now grows up with the background knowledge that there are many ways of life deeply different from their own — a kind of knowledge which once used to be quite rare.

Similarly, nearly all of us know that there are in the world many people whose moral values and beliefs are radically different from our own (Midgley 1991a, p. 72). And we also know that in any one society there is likely to be a diversity of valid moral viewpoints and approaches (moral pluralism), and that this has created the possibility for, and the actuality of, irreconcilable moral disagreements, examples of which are given throughout this text (Elliott 1992, p. 32). Questions arising here include: What, if any, is the best way to respond to moral pluralism? and, more specifically, How should nurses respond to the challenge of what can be appropriately referred to as transcultural ethics? It is to briefly answering these questions that this discussion now turns.

The nature and implications of a transcultural approach to ethics

It is not the purpose of this text to advance a substantive theory of transcultural ethics or cultural relativism, or to provide an in-depth study of the ethical concepts, theories and practices of different cultural groups. Such a task is beyond our present scope, and requires much more space than it is possible to provide here. (See, meanwhile, Fry and Johnstone 2002; Macklin 1998; Elliott 1992; Marshall 1992; Midgley 1991a; Singer 1991; Cortese 1990; Leininger 1990). Nevertheless, it is important to have some understanding of the nature and implications of transcultural ethics (a form of ethical pluralism), and of how nurses might respond better to the challenges it poses.

One crucial point requiring understanding is that, while all societies have some sort of moral system for guiding and evaluating the conduct of their members, the moral constructs of one culture (for example, North American or English culture) cannot always be applied appropriately or reliably to another culture — at least not without some modification (Silberbauer 1991, p. 15). Further, language usage alone, and the difficulties encountered in reaching accurate culturally thick (rich) translations of accepted moral terms and concepts, may even make meaningful moral discourse across cultures impossible (Stout 1988). These points have, however, been largely overlooked by mainstream (Anglo-American) moral philosophers, who have tended to support an imperialist model of morality — that is, that their way of moral knowing and thinking is not only superior but 'right', and is thus something to be applied (read imposed) universally on to others whose moral systems they have judged to be inferior — even 'savage' (Midgley 1991a, p. 78).

This is an inadequate and fraudulent approach to moral thinking and conduct, however, and one which should be questioned. Nevertheless, this does not mean that mainstream Anglo-American moral philosophy itself should be abandoned. To the contrary — its rich traditions offer us important insights into our own culture-specific moral values and beliefs about how to be moral beings. We must, however, pay much greater attention to the influences of the primary organising principle of morality, namely, culture. We also need to recognise that, while it is true that all cultures have some 'priority rules', or principles for arbitrating between conflicting obligations and duties, just what these rules and principles are, how they are defined and interpreted, when they will be applied, and who ultimately applies them (and to what end) will, contrary to an imperialist model of ethics, vary across — and even within — different cultures (Midgley 1991b, p. 11; see also Cheng-tek Tai and Chung Seng Lin 2001). In short, morality will be expressed differently cross-culturally and intra-culturally.

An interesting example of the different ways in which morality can be expressed cross-culturally or even intra-culturally can be found in the case of small-scale and large-scale societies. In small-scale or traditional societies, for example, morality tends to be viewed as a process — as a means to an end — and is expressed through the *quality of relationships* (characterised by upholding values such as friendship, loyalty to kin, empathy, altruism, familial trust, and so on), rather than a deontological adherence to abstract principles. Silberbauer explains (1991, p. 27):

> Morality is less of an end in itself but is seen more clearly as a set of orientations for establishing and maintaining the health of relationships. Morality, then, is a means to a desired, enjoyed end.

This view is in stark contrast to that upheld by large-scale (non-traditional or industrialised) societies, in which relationships are less proximate, less intense and less significant, both at the individual and the societal level. Here morality is viewed as an end in itself rather than as a means to an end, and is expressed by adherence to rules (*viz.* adjudicating the conduct between strangers) rather than by and in the quality of relationships per se. On this point, Silberbauer explains (1991, p. 27):

> Morality certainly provides a set of orientations and thus helps to create and maintain coherent expectations of behaviour, but operates *impersonally* in that there is not the same capacity for negotiation. Morality thus tends to be valued more as an end in itself and less as a means to an end. (emphasis added)

To illustrate the different ways in which small-scale and large-scale societies might each express their different moralities, Silberbauer (1991) uses the simple example of the relationship between a bus-conductor and a passenger. He suggests that, in large-scale societies, where relationships tend to be 'single-purpose and impersonal', the relationship between a bus-conductor and a passenger would be of limited importance, and would probably manifest itself quite differently than it would in a small-scale society, where relationships were more proximate, multi-purpose and personal. He points out (1991, p. 14):

> how different it would be if the conductor were also my sister-in-law, near neighbour and the daughter of my father's golfing partner — I would never dare to tender anything other than the correct fare. In a small-scale society every fellow member whom I encounter in my day is likely to be connected to me by a comparable, or even more complex web of strands, each of which must be maintained in its appropriate alignment and tension lest all the others become tangled. My father's missed putts or my inconsiderate use of a motor-mower at daybreak will necessitate very diplomatic behaviour on the bus, or a long walk to work and a dismal dinner on my return.

A more relevant example here can be found in the comparison of nurses working in large city-based university teaching hospitals with those who work in small, close-knit rural 'outback' country communities. It has been my experience that nurses working in small rural or remote ('outback') country communities (where 'everyone is known to everyone') are far more vulnerable to putting local community members 'off-side' by offending an individual member of that community than are nurses working in large city-based university teaching hospitals. In this instance, we could speculate that nurses working in small country-based community nursing care settings might put more weight on *preserving the quality of relationships* in that community than on *upholding abstract moral principles*. Conversely, nurses working in large and impersonal communities may put greater emphasis on upholding abstract principles of conduct than on preserving the quality of relationships with 'strangers' whom they are unlikely to encounter more than once during their working lives.

Bear in mind, however, that this is only an example, being used here to help clarify Silberbauer's point. In reality it is likely that nurses express morality both as a *process* (as a means to an end) and as *an end in itself*. Whether this is so, and the extent to which it is so (that is, where the balance lies), may depend ultimately on the nature of the context they are in — whether it is characterised by personal or impersonal relationships. When it is considered that it is not contradictory to view the maintenance of quality relationships as an important moral end in itself (not just a means to an end), there is room to suggest that the distinction Silberbauer makes may, in the final analysis, be overstated.

Despite this observation, Silberbauer is correct to point out that abstract moral principles do not always have currency in some cultural or social groups, and that, even if there do exist some commonly accepted standards of moral conduct, we cannot assume that these standards will be expressed or applied uniformly across, or even within, different cultural groups. A good example of this can be found in the wide and popular acceptance of the moral principles of autonomy, non-maleficence, beneficence and justice, which are considered in Chapter 3. These principles are referred to and used widely in mainstream bioethics discourse (see in particular Beauchamp and Childress 2001), and are viewed popularly as 'self-standing conceptual systems by which we can impose some sort of order upon ethical problems' (Elliott 1992, p. 29). But, as Elliott correctly points out, what proponents of this view tend to overlook is that in reality, ethics does not stand apart. It is one thread in the fabric of a society, and it is intertwined with others. Ethical concepts are tied to a society's customs, manners, traditions, institutions — all of the concepts that structure and inform the ways in which a member of that society deals with the world (Elliott 1992, p. 29). He goes on to warn that, if people forget this inextricable link between ethics and culture (p. 29):

> we are in danger of leaving the world of genuine moral experience for the world of moral fiction — a simplified, hypothetical creation suited less for practical difficulties than for intellectual convenience.

A poignant example of the inaccuracy and fraud of viewing moral principles as self-standing conceptual systems rather than as ethical concepts tied to a particular tradition (culture) can be seen in the way in which the principle of autonomy tends to be interpreted and applied in professional health care contexts. As stated in Chapter 3, the concept of autonomy refers to an individual's *independent* and *self-contained* ability to decide. As a principle, autonomy prescribes that an *individual's rational preferences* ought to be respected even if we do not agree with them — and even if others consider them foolish — provided they do not interfere with or harm prejudicially the significant moral interests of others.

At first glance, this articulation of the concept and principle of autonomy appears unproblematic. And it is probably true that most nurses familiarising themselves with the moral nature and application of the principle of autonomy value the 'right' to make their own self-determining choices, and would probably feel a strong sense of outrage if their considered wishes were overridden arbitrarily by another. They may also share a strong conviction that patients should always be informed about their diagnoses, and about the details of their proposed treatment and care, and that it would be a gross violation of patients' rights not to accept or facilitate patients' self-determining choices regarding their own care and treatment options. In most cases, this position would probably be a demonstrably justifiable one to take. It would, however, be a grave mistake to accept the concept and principle of autonomy (as articulated above) as holding *universally*; that is, without exception. Consider the following.

Earlier in this book, it was pointed out that definitions of ethical terms and concepts can be 'ethically loaded', and hence can themselves be an important influence on how a moral debate or analysis might be conducted and what the outcomes of a given debate or analysis might be. This is true even (or perhaps especially) in the case of moral principles — the moral principle of autonomy being a case in point. It will be noted, for example, that even the definition of the concept and principle of autonomy reflects the dominant cultural values of the highly individualised large-scale Western Anglo-American culture from which it has arisen (Cheng-tek Tai and Chung Seng Lin 2001; Marshall 1992). Of particular importance to this discussion are the italicised terms *individuals, independent, self-contained*. Here the ethical loading clearly rests on respecting individualism, independence, and isolation (insulation) from one's social 'connectedness'. (As a point of interest, in contemporary Italian culture the notion autonomy [*autonomia*] is often used synonymously for isolation [*isolamento*] [Surbone 1992, p. 1662].) For people who hold these values, this ethical loading is not a major problem. But for people who do not hold or share these values — who may, for instance, subscribe to the values of collectiveness, interdependence, and social connectedness (context) — it is open to serious question whether the concept and principle of autonomy as popularly defined and applied in mainstream bioethics discourse could, or indeed should, be given any currency in mediating the relationships, and the responsibilities within those relationships, of people who do not subscribe to the values embraced by autonomy as described.

To illustrate the kinds of moral problems that can arise as a result of applying the principle of autonomy in an abstract, universal and context-independent way rather than in a substantive, context-dependent, culture-specific way, consider the case of Mr G (taken from Johnstone and Kanitsaki 1991). Mr G, an elderly Greek who spoke no English, was admitted to hospital for investigations, and was later diagnosed as having cancer of the lung. Mr G had a number of other health problems, including a mildly debilitating hemiplegia — although he could move about with assistance. Before his admission into hospital, Mr G was totally dependent on and cared for by his family.

When radiological and laboratory tests confirmed the provisional medical diagnosis of a malignant lung tumour, Mr G's physician arranged for an interpreter to come to the ward and through him informed Mr G directly that he had cancer of the lung. In this instance, it was the physician's personal policy to be candid with his patients, and inform them according to what he judged to be 'their right to know and be informed', as prescribed by the moral principle of autonomy. Unfortunately, in this case, although well intended, the physician's approach was culturally inappropriate, and had the undesirable moral consequence of causing the patient and his family otherwise avoidable suffering (Johnstone and Kanitsaki 1991).

A mainstream ethical analysis of the physician's actions in this case would probably support the view that informing the patient of his cancer diagnosis was a 'morally right' thing to do. And, interestingly, when I present this case to students (nursing and medical students alike), most contend that the physician's actions were not only morally correct but *praiseworthy*, given the reluctance by some doctors to be candid with their patients about diagnostic, care and treatment matters of this nature.

From a cultural perspective, however, the physician's actions can be shown to be not only mistaken but morally harmful, for reasons that will now be explained. In this case it would have been more culturally appropriate and morally beneficial had the physician communicated the cancer diagnosis to the patient's *family* rather than to the patient himself (see also Kanitsaki 2000, 1994, 1993). This is because, as Johnstone and Kanitsaki point out (1991, p. 280), during a health crisis, patients like Mr G who are of a traditional (rural, small-scale societal) cultural background, tend to prefer:

> the close involvement of their family and value the supportive, protective and therapeutic role that the family can and does play when one of its members is ill or suffering … Indeed, the involvement of the patient's family is an essential and integral part of the therapeutic relationship and of the process required to uphold the patient's best interests.

By not recognising the protective authority of Mr G's family to decide '*if, when, how and by whom* the diagnoses should be disclosed to Mr G', the physician inadvertently 'pointed the bone' at his patient and thereby undermined rather than promoted Mr G's autonomy. The reasons for this are complicated, but important. Kanitsaki (1989a) explains that for many rurally based Greeks who emigrated to Australia during the 1950s and 1960s the very word 'cancer' carries a whole range of negative connotations and thus is something never to be mentioned, since to do so would be to risk stimulating the nocebo phenomenon. The *nocebo phenomenon* (from the Latinate *noceo*, 'I hurt', and the Greek *nosis*, 'disease') is defined by Helman (1990, p. 257) as 'the negative effect on health of beliefs and expectations — and therefore the exact reverse of the "placebo" phenomenon' (see also Dossey 1982, 1991; Weil 1983; Chopra 1989; Moyers 1993). Kanitsaki (1989a, p. 46) explains that during the 1950s and 1960s, rural

Greece had virtually no hospitals, and that if people required treatment for serious illness they would have to travel great distances to the nearest cities. She goes on to point out that, because of this, as well as because of a scepticism about scientific medicine's ability to treat diseases effectively, people from rural areas would seek hospital treatment only as a last resort. As Kanitsaki explains (p. 47):

> the reluctance to frequent doctors and hospitals was exacerbated by a general dislike of hospitals, rumours about the lack of nursing care and unkind nursing staff, and a fear of cities generally. Pressures of local work demands, a lack of economic resources, and the probability of having to travel alone and thus without the protection, support, and physical presence of the family, also militated against scientific medical services being used by rural community members.

As a result of this reluctance — and, indeed, inability — to access scientific medical services, many people suffering from cancer-related illness did not receive the optimal treatment available, and as a result frequently died painful and agonising deaths (Kanitsaki 1989a). And it is the memories of these kinds of cancer-related deaths that many rural Greek immigrants have brought with them to Australia. Kanitsaki explains (personal communication) that many Greek immigrants of this background simply do not have any experiential knowledge of, or even a conception of, the kind of treatment and care that is available in Australia today; thus, even mentioning the word 'cancer' is sufficient to trigger in ill persons an overwhelming sense of hopelessness which ultimately finds its expression in their losing their will to live. Under these circumstances, to tell such patients, 'You've got cancer' — no matter how benevolent the intention in doing so — would probably be sufficient to trigger the nocebo phenomenon, resulting ultimately in the ill person's premature death (Kanitsaki, personal communication).

The way to avoid this disastrous situation is for the patient to be spared the information likely to stimulate the nocebo phenomenon, and for the patient's family to be respected as having the authority to decide — in the moral interests of and for the wellbeing of their sick loved one — *whether, when, where, how and by whom* information about the diagnosis of a serious illness and poor prognosis will be given (Kanitsaki, personal communication). A major *moral* motivation for this, Kanitsaki explains (personal communication), is to avoid undermining the sick person's hope (about getting better and being able to go on living a meaningful life), and thereby to maximise the person's ability to continue making important life-interested choices; that is, to maximise the person's autonomy. In sum, maintaining hope is the linchpin to promoting autonomy. This is because, without hope there is simply *nothing left to choose for* (Kanitsaki, personal communication). Interestingly, research has shown that, even in contemporary Greek society, truth telling about a diagnosis of serious life-threatening illness (especially cancer-related illnesses) is still viewed by many Greeks (urban as well as rural) as being harmful and hence 'undesirable', on the grounds that it could undermine hope and the will to live (Georgaki et al. 2002; Mystakidou et al. 1996; Dalla-Vorgia et al. 1992).

It should be noted that this moral world-view is not held exclusively by Greeks of rural or traditional cultural backgrounds. People of other traditional cultural backgrounds also believe that in some circumstances patients should not be told that they have a serious life-threatening illness, and that to do so would be harmful (see, for example, Lee and Wu 2002; Karim 2002; Cheng-tek Tai and Chung Seng Lin 2001; Grassi et al. 2000; Macklin 1998; Surbone 1992; Pellegrino 1992). The following anecdote shows this. The case concerns an elderly non-English-speaking

Italian man who, like Mr G, had emigrated to Australia in the 1950s. He was admitted to hospital for tests which later confirmed a cancer diagnosis. Although the man's family explicitly requested that their father not be given any information about the test results if they were positive, an interpreter was called in their absence and the man was told of his cancer diagnosis and poor prognosis. This information caused the man to become extremely distressed and, as his son commented later, 'the life just went out of his eyes and we knew he would die very soon'. The son, who was Australian-born and a qualified pharmacist, decided in consultation with the rest of his family to remedy the situation. This he did by contacting Italian-Australian friends who worked as doctors at the hospital where his father was a patient and arranging for all his father's tests to be repeated. His friends agreed to explain to his father that the tests needed to be repeated because 'there had been a terrible mistake' and that 'his earlier tests results had got mixed up with someone else's'. They later returned to tell the man that his tests showed he in fact did *not* have cancer. The son explained that his father was told he still needed medical treatment, but that he would 'be all right'. Ultimately, the family took their father home and cared for him. He continued to live beyond the time limit suggested by his poor prognosis and, in fact, was still alive at the time the anecdote was being shared. The son attributed this to the fact that they were able to convince their father all was not hopeless, which in turn had the effect of restoring his will to live. In short, the son's actions reversed his father's sense of hopelessness, and thus promoted rather than undermined his father's autonomy.

Interestingly, when I have shared this anecdote with students, many are appalled at the blatant deception that was employed in this case. Others, however, notably those whose parents are from rural Greece or Italy, have expressed enormous relief at the insights this and other cases like it have given them. One postgraduate nursing student, for example, commented (personal communication):

> I've always felt that if either of my parents should get cancer they should be told their diagnosis. But when speaking of this issue, my mother — who is Italian — has always insisted, 'No! you must not allow that to happen'. My Australian side of me tells me it is wrong not to tell them. But now I can see it would be wrong *to tell* them, and that my mother is right. I can live with this now. It is such an enormous relief. I am no longer in a dilemma. Thank you.

The comments of this student are included here because, among other things, they demonstrate the very practical help that adopting a transcultural view of ethics can offer; of particular note, they help to support the view that, by tying ethical views to the cultural traditions that inform them, we will be in a much better position to embrace morality as an experience rather than as an abstraction (Marshall 1992, pp. 53–7). And that by embracing morality as an experience rather than an abstraction we can avoid falling prey to the unhelpful, idle fantasies of moral fiction which, as Elliott (1992, p. 2) suggests, are suited more to the purposes of intellectual convenience than to resolving genuine practical difficulties in the concrete circumstances of life. The student's comments and, indeed, the anecdotes themselves also show, to borrow from Cortese (1990, p. 157) that 'relationships … are the essence of life and morality', and that to view morality simply as conceptions of abstract reified rational principles is 'to remove us from the real world in which we live, and separate us from real people whom we love' (Cortese 1990, p. 157). The lesson to be learned here is that, unless we embrace morality as an experience rather than as an abstraction, what we will end up with is only a concept of morality and not morality itself. And, borrowing again from Cortese (1990, p. 158), unless we have a 'deep sense of relationship, we may have a conceptualisation of the highest level of justice, but we will not be moral'. The point being that without relationships, justice — morality — 'contains no system of checks and balances. It becomes primarily an end in itself without regard to the purpose of morality' (Cortese 1990, p. 158).

Although only the principle of autonomy has been considered here, the other principles considered in Chapter 3 (non-maleficence, beneficence and justice) could all be examined along similar lines. We could, for example, ask in regard to each of these principles: From whose perspective are these principles to be meaningfully and appropriately defined, interpreted, analysed and applied? In the case of non-maleficence, for instance, meaningful questions can be asked about what constitutes a 'harm' in a given culturally-constructed clinical context? By whose standards and cultural perspectives is the notion of harm to be measured and evaluated? Likewise for the principles of beneficence and justice.

Where then does this leave the role of moral principles and culturally different moral viewpoints and approaches in our nursing ethics discourse? In answering this question, it might be useful at this point to consider the nature and implications of diversity or pluralism in moral values and moral world views.

Moral diversity and the challenge of moral pluralism

The world in which we now live is characteristically multicultural in its nature and outlook. This situation, in turn, has brought with it a diversity or pluralism of moral values and beliefs. Some fear that this diversity or pluralism of values may be 'the barrier to agreement' (Elliott 1992, p. 32), and, hence, the catalyst to producing a world hopelessly divided by radical and destructive moral disagreement. Others reject moral pluralism outright on the grounds that, in their view, it is 'just another name for confusion' (Stout 1988, p. 1). Moral diversity need not lead to destructive disagreement, however, nor to blinding confusion. Indeed, as is well recognised within the discipline of moral philosophy, moral disagreement has historically been the beginning and has seen the development of moral thinking, not its end or disintegration (see also Stout 1988; Benhabib and Dallmayr 1990). Further, as Mary Midgley correctly points out, 'nobody is infallible; and for that reason many different points of view are needed' (Midgley 1991a, p. 83).

What must also be recognised and understood here is that a diversity of values and beliefs is the key to morality's survival; it prompts critical reflection, rather than uncritical acceptance, and in so doing invites constant revision and creative refinement. Moral diversity also helps to ensure that no one moral point of view dominates; in short, it helps to prevent what might otherwise be termed 'moral fascism'. Meanwhile, its emphasis on *understanding difference* rather than *striving for uniformity* will help to ensure that the moral systems we end up embracing will be of a nature that is truly responsive to the lived realities and experiences of all human beings, not merely those of a select few whose positions of power have enabled them to manipulate morality into a tool for repressing unwanted truths and legitimating further the authority of moral imperialists who would impose their values on others as a means of maintaining rather than challenging their cultural hegemony.

Adopting a transcultural approach to ethics can be beneficial in a range of ways. Among other things, at a global level, it can enable cross-cultural interactions that 'build bridges of understanding between persons and cultures that make cooperation possible and conquest unnecessary' (Fasching 1993, p. 6). It can also help to avoid the perils of 'moral suprematism' such as those which have been amply exemplified during wartime (see, for example, Fasching 1993). For instance, during the second world war, the world bore witness to Nazis believing in 'their own moral superiority (supported by ultimate justification)' and the consequential rendering as mute 'all opposing views' (Gergen 1994, p. 113). As Gergen points out in relation to this historical period (p. 113):

> Had the means been available much earlier for an unobstructed interpretation of meaning systems — Nazi, Jewish, Christian, Marxist, feminist, and the like — one must imagine that the consequences would have been far less disastrous.

We thus stand warned that what is sometimes presented as *the* 'superior morality' might well prove to be little more than 'the morality of the superior' (meaning the extremely powerful and the dominant), with little to recommend itself to 'the other', rendered by it (the 'superior morality') as having only inferior moral status, or worse, as having no moral status at all (as indeed happened in the case of Nazi characterisations of the Jews) (Bauman 1993, p. 228).

At a more local level, a transcultural approach to ethics can enrich greatly our moral view of the world and the various relationships (including nurse–patient relationships) we experience within it. In the case of the nurse–patient relationship, however, a transcultural approach to ethics may not only enhance the moral quality but also the therapeutic effectiveness of that relationship (most notably through avoiding the harmful consequences of the nocebo phenomena [Kanitsaki 1996]), and hence the moral ends of nursing itself (referred to in the previous chapter).

An important lesson for nurses here is, I believe, that moral diversity is not something to be feared, but something to be embraced as a means of challenging our complacent thinking about the moral world we live in, and of improving our understanding of and ability to experience both ourselves and others as moral beings who have a mutual interest in living a worthwhile and meaningful life. Further, whether we wish to admit it or not, as Elliott points out (1992, p. 35):

> Moral disagreement will be with us as long as there is disagreement about what way of life is best for human beings. It is not at all obvious that this is a question that is answerable, even in principle. There may be no best life, only better and worse lives. And if morality is tied to a form of life, then it is a mistake to think that we can eliminate moral differences without eliminating the differences in cultures, and in individuals, to which morality is tied.

Elliott goes on to make the additional point that (p. 35):

> Though the biological characteristics humans share will mean that some lives, and some features of lives, are necessarily good or bad for human beings, there is no compelling reason, universally applicable, for adopting any one particular sort of life over all others — even if we had the choice, which we do not. For this reason, we should expect diversity in the sort of lives that people live, as well as the moral differences that inevitably follow.

Dealing with problems associated with a transcultural approach to ethics in health care

Before concluding this discussion, it is important to acknowledge that upholding a transcultural view of ethics can sometimes be extremely difficult, and may give rise to serious ethical dilemmas for health care professionals — nurses included. For instance, it is not uncommon for nurses to encounter a situation in which a patient requests one thing and his or her family requests another. A typical scenario is as follows.

A patient from a traditional cultural background (for example, Greek or Italian) discloses to an attending nurse: 'If my test results come back positive and I have cancer, *I* want to be told. I know my family has told you not to tell me, but I must ask you not to take notice of them. I want to know. And that is the end of the matter'. The family, meanwhile, may request: 'If our father's test results come back positive and he has cancer, under no circumstances is he to be told. We know him. Such news will kill him. You must give *us* the information and we will deal with it. This is family business and that is the end of the matter'. Usually, the attendant nurses in these kinds of situations are desperate to do what is best for all concerned, but are troubled about how to decide what, in fact, *is best* for all concerned. Typically, the questions they ask include: 'Who do I listen to — the patient, or the family? How best can I serve the patient's interests given that the family just might be right — that is, the information might "kill him"? What should I do?'. Just what attending nurses ought to do, all things considered, might not be as problematic as at first it appears to be. Consider the following.

In responding to the kind of scenario just outlined, it is vitally important that nurses do not *stereotype* people of different cultural backgrounds and assume that 'all immigrants' *ipso facto* practice traditional life-ways, or that 'all immigrants' *ipso facto* practice a family-centred (versus an individualistic) model of informed decision-making in health care contexts. Many immigrants to a host country assimilate to the mainstream culture of their new country, and have internalised very effectively the core cultural values of the (new) mainstream culture. Immigrants to Australia are no exception in this regard. Thus, when a 'new Australian' (as immigrants to Australia have been known in the past) makes an explicit request to the effect 'If my test results come back positive and I have cancer, I want to be told', it is highly probable that not only does he or she mean it, but will also be able to deal with it in a culturally adapted way. In such instances, there is no question that the nurse's primary responsibility is to initiate steps to ensure that the patient's request for information is honoured. Where then does this leave the family's request?

Giving primacy to the patient's request for information does not mean that the family's request has no bearing on the matter or should be ignored altogether (see, for example, Kuczewski 1996) (this issue will be considered in more depth in Chapter 6, page 140). To the contrary. The family's request is just as deserving of consideration as is the patient's — not least because *they too* are experiencing the health crisis of their loved one. What differs, however, is the way in which nursing and medical staff might respond to a family's requests. Kanitsaki, for example, advises (personal communication) that after securing consent from the patient, the following actions might alleviate the situation considerably:

- Inform the family that the patient has explicitly requested to be told the details of a diagnosis, and that the doctors and nurses have a legal and moral obligation to honour this request.
- Express understanding of the pain of the situation, and acknowledge that the family is only trying to do what is 'good and right' for their loved one.
- Invite the family to be present when the information is to be given to their loved one.
- Negotiate a plan of care that, in the event of a 'bad' diagnosis, all parties can be mutually supported; for example,

- it might be necessary to arrange for the family to meet with the attending physician on a regular basis in order to obtain and discuss details of their loved one's health status and progress;
- it might be necessary to organise culturally relevant help (for example, counselling — noting, however, that it might be necessary not to call it 'counselling' for cultural reasons) to assist family members and their sick loved one to re-establish communication patterns that the 'telling, not telling' scenario has possibly disrupted, and consequently left each family member feeling alienated from each other.

In most instances, a 'commonsense' approach to managing individuals and families experiencing grief crises will result in satisfactory outcomes and a 'therapeutic partnership' between lay and professional (nursing) carers.

Another kind of problem that is not uncommon in nursing care domains involves extended-family members visiting in contravention of hospital visiting rules; for example, visiting outside of a hospital's regulated visiting hours and/or in numbers in excess of two-visitors-per-patient visiting rule. In regard to the latter, this is seen as problematic by nurses since it sometimes compromises the privacy and other entitlements of other patients — especially when the presence of a large number of extended-family members creates undue conversational 'noise'. It is also seen as problematic by nurses since it is not uncommon, over the duration of their visit and/or the patient's hospital stay, for different family members to ask the same nurse the same question about the health condition of their loved one. Nurses not infrequently cite being frustrated at repeatedly being asked the same question by different family members as, among other things, this is commonly seen by nurses to stretch even further their already strained 'time resources' to attend other patients. All things considered, however, this problem is also not as problematic as at first it might appear to be and is amenable to remedy.

In addressing this kind of problem it is important for nurses to understand that 'presencing' by extended-family members is a crucial component of the lay–therapeutic relationship (Kanitsaki 2003, 2000, 1994, 1993, 1989a, 1989b). By being 'present', family members believe they are contributing to the healing process by 'giving strength' to their loved one. Significantly, it is not uncommon, especially in the case of seriously ill patients, to see family members strategically placed around the bed of a sick person, for example, with one family member touching the head, another the left hand, another the right hand, another the left foot, and another the right foot of the ill person. This 'touching' (often manifest as massage of a given part of the body or the sprinkling of healing waters over the part) is an important component of the process of giving 'healing energy' to the ill person and to assist them to 'get well'. The loved one, meanwhile, generally regards the presence of his or her family member as an indication of their 'caring'. To ask family members to leave under these circumstances thus stands as a major violation of the lay–therapeutic relationship, and it is understandable that extended-family members might react 'badly' to a nurse's directives to 'be considerate' of other patients and to observe a 'two-visitors-per-patient' rule. The question to arise here is: How can nurses best manage the situation?

Key to the effective management of extended-family visiting is for nurses themselves to understand the lay–therapeutic (healing) nature of this visiting, as well as the crucial role it also plays as a 'quality assurance' check of the care a loved one might be receiving. For instance, the repeated questioning of nursing staff by family members is an attempt to secure as much information as possible about the care of their loved one, which can subsequently be interrogated by family members for its consistency, accuracy and hence reliability (Kanitsaki 2003, 2000, 1996, 1994, 1993, 1989a, 1989b). Obviously, if six family members ask the same nurse the same question, yet receive six different answers, they would have grounds to be suspicious about whether their loved one was, in fact, receiving optimal care. Similarly, if their repeated requests for information are met with annoyance or hostility by nurses, this could be construed as meaning that the nurses 'do not care' and, again, that their loved one is not receiving optimal care. This, in turn, could result in the family removing the loved one from a given location of care and taking them elsewhere for care — even overseas (Kanitsaki 2003, 2000, 1996, 1994, 1993, 1989a, 1989b).

There are a number of strategies which nurses might use to help remedy a situation such as this. These include:

- asking the family to nominate a spokesperson for the family and for a primary nurse to agree to meet with this person, as required, to answer any questions the family might have;
- advise the family (in non-serious cases) of the constraints under which nurses are forced to operate and explain the need for considering the interests of other patients;
- in the case of seriously ill patients, move the patient to a single room so that the lay–therapeutic relationship can be expressed as fully as is possible under the circumstances (adapted from Kanitsaki 2000, 1996, 1994, 1993, 1989a, 1989b).

Feedback from nurses over the years has indicated that the implementation of these and related kinds of strategies have been very effective in maximising the quality of care experienced by patients (and their chosen carers) of culturally diverse backgrounds, and improving nurses' job satisfaction when involved in the care of such patients.

The third and final kind of problem to be considered here, and which nurses not infrequently have to deal with, concerns the codified demand on nurses to respect certain religious and traditional practices of patients. The nature of the problem is as follows.

The International Council of Nurses (2000) *Code for Nurses* prescribes that 'in providing care, the nurse promotes an environment in which the human rights, values, customs and spiritual beliefs of the individual, family and community are respected'. The *Code of Ethics for Nurses in Australia* (2002) likewise prescribes that 'Nurses respect individuals' needs, values, culture and vulnerability in the provision of nursing care'. The nursing ethics codes of other countries carry similar provisions. The problem for nurses, however, is that some religious and traditional practices either pose a threat or are actually harmful to patients — the case of female genital mutilation being an obvious example here. In such instances, nurses are troubled by what appears to be two conflicting demands: on the one hand, to respect the patient's cultural values and beliefs; and yet, on the other hand, to protect the patient from harm. This dilemma is compounded by postmodernist requirements to explain: 'harm' by *whose standards*? 'harm' by *whose world view*?, and to demonstrate that the apparent moral dilemma at issue is not merely a creation of 'moral ethnocentrism' or 'cultural (moral) imperialism' (James 1994).

This kind of problem is enormously complex, and requires a much deeper examination than is possible here. Further, addressing this kind of problem requires a deep understanding of the cultural complexities and dynamics informing the practices at issue. Nevertheless, at the risk of oversimplifying the issue, I offer the following comments.

Most nurses would agree, I believe, that they have at least a prima facie obligation to respect the cultural practices of their patients. More specifically, they would probably accept that:

> Intolerance of another's religious or traditional practices that pose no threat of harm is, at least, discourteous and at worst, a prejudicial attitude. And it does fail to show respect for persons and their diverse religious and cultural practices.
>
> (Macklin 1998, p. 7)

This does not mean, however, that nurses are obliged — either on the basis of the above view or of the nursing profession's formally adopted code of ethics — to tolerate, *without reflective judgment*, all religious and cultural practices of their patients. There are a number of reasons for this. Firstly, to borrow from Macklin (1998, p. 17), we can 'be respectful of cultural difference *and at the same time acknowledge that there are limits*' (emphasis added). Second, the 'limits' to our obligation of respect can be discerned by a critical examination of: (1) the internal cultural justifications and considerations raised in support of a given 'harmful' religious or traditional practice; and (2) external viewpoints (that is, from other cultural groups) about the 'harmfulness' of the practice (recognising here that culture is not static and can change in positive ways when exposed to relevant influences). Thirdly, we are not obliged to be respectful of practices which, when examined comparatively from an intra-cultural and cross-cultural perspective, are themselves disrespectful and oppressive of persons.

The question remains, however, of how these considerations might apply to the case of requests being imposed on nurses to assist with medical procedures that are culturally prescribed, but nevertheless judged by nurses to be 'harmful' to persons? Let us consider a possible answer to this question in relation to the practice of female genital mutilation, taken here as referring to a traditional procedure (as opposed to a medically therapeutic procedure, say for cancer) that may involve 'only' a clitoridectomy, or may include (as well as the removal of the clitoris) the excision of parts of the labia minoria or the removal of virtually all of the external female genitalia (James 1994, pp. 6–7).

Transcultural ethics and the case of female genital mutilation

It is estimated that the practice of female genital mutilation (usually performed on girls between the ages of 7 days and 15 years [Robson 1994, p. 15], and traditionally carried out by mothers, grandmothers and family friends) has affected between 100 to 136 million girls and women in more than 45 countries (Gilmore nd; Walker and Parmar 1993; World Health Organisation 1998; Affara 2000). In 1998, an information letter distributed by Amnesty International Australia estimated that during any one 24 hour period, 6000 young girls will undergo 'the knife' believing that 'they will become more feminine, clean and obedient' (Gilmore nd). It has been further estimated that an additional 2 million girls are at risk annually of having their genitals mutilated (World Health Organisation 1998; Affara 2000).

There are a number of internal cultural justifications offered for the brutal practice of female genital mutilation; these include 'appeals to custom, religion, family honour, cleanliness, esthetics, initiation, assurance of virginity, promotion of social and political cohesion, enhancement of fertility, improvement in male sexual pleasure, and prevention of female promiscuity' (Sherwin 1992, p. 62). Significantly, most of these justifications do not stand up when considered from an internal cultural perspective.

Firstly, although practised by Muslims, Christians, Jews and animists alike, female genital mutilation as such is not supported by any formal doctrine of religion. Rather, its support 'can be attributed, at least partly, to the manipulations of knowledgeable, male religious elites' who continue to this day to perpetuate 'false understandings among their followers' that the procedure is a religious requirement rather than an inherited custom (James 1994, p. 10). Perhaps an important lesson for nurses here is to ascertain whether a given questionable 'cultural' practice does in fact have the legitimacy being claimed.

Secondly, there is ample evidence to show that the practice of female genital mutilation fails to achieve a large number of the outcomes for which it is thought to be internally justified, namely: the promotion of family honour, cleanliness, aesthetics, assurance of virginity, promotion of social and political cohesion, enhancement of fertility, and the prevention of female promiscuity. Research has shown that the negative health effects of the procedure far outweigh the supposed benefits. As James explains (1994, pp. 8–9):

> Typically, for those undergoing the process, the operation results in severe pain, shock, infection, difficulty urinating and menstruating, malformation and scarring of the genitalia, physical and psychological trauma with sexual intercourse, bleeding, increased vulnerability to the AIDS virus, difficulty with childbirth, increased risk of sterility and infant mortality. There is also the risk of death to the female from the direct effects of the operation ... Fear, anxiety, pain, scarring and emotional trauma from circumcision combine to produce severe psychological disturbance and sexual dysfunction in many women subject to the procedure.

It is also known that the procedure does not 'assure virginity' or prevent 'female promiscuity'.

Thirdly, it is wrong to assume that female genital mutilation is unanimously supported in the countries and cultures where it is practised. For instance, many internal sub-cultural groups of the cultures believed to support female genital mutilation are actively working for the eradication of the practice (James 1994; Walker and Parmar 1993). The workings of these groups have included the development of local community health education programs, the production of film documentaries, and political lobbying (James 1994; Walker and Parmar 1993). There is also an increasing religious tolerance in some countries for supporting an international human rights approach to help eradicate the practice. James (1994, p. 24) writes, for example, that there is some suggestion 'Islam would be favourable to international human rights protection based on the equality of women and the moral wrongness of discrimination on the basis of sex' since in Islam, 'piety alone was to be the final test of a person's worth — woman or man'.

Another important consideration is that many cultural groups and countries condemn the practice of female genital mutilation (and the cultures that support it) on grounds of human rights violations; in some instances, countries have even outlawed the practice (for example, the United Kingdon) (James 1994; Robson 1994). In Australia, girls facing 'female circumcision' have been regarded as 'at risk' by child protection agencies and placed under supervised care (see, for example, the 1994 case of an 18 month supervision order granted by a Victorian court for the protection of two children aged 21 months and 3 years [Saunders 1994, p. 2]). Amnesty International, among other organisations, has also been at the forefront of campaigning against female genital mutilation, and the contravention of children's rights and the rights of women 'to equality, integrity and health' that the procedure constitutes. In 1994, the Australian Medical Association called on the federal government to outlaw female genital mutilation in Australia (Robson 1994). These and other groups have presented substantive evidence supporting the harmful nature of the practice and the need for its eradication.

To some, the activities of powerful Western lobby groups like medical associations or international human rights organisations might seem little more than 'Western cultural imperialism' or an instance of the 'morality of the superior' being imposed as *the* 'superior morality'. There is room to suggest, however, that to characterise the moral activism of these and like groups as 'moral ethnocentrism' or 'cultural (moral) imperialism' is rather hollow. The millions of females who have suffered as a result of this practice might have quite a different view. And I wonder what the answer would be if these women were asked the question: 'If there was another way — a way that would enable you to function fully as respected members of your society without the need to undergo genital mutilation — would you still submit to such a procedure?'. But then, for many women, this question would be redundant, since being mutilated was never a matter of 'real' choice for them. And currently, for 6000 girls per day, it still is not — notwithstanding the powerful enculturation process that occurs in young girls from the day they are born to accept the practice as 'normal' and to submit to it else risk the shame, stigma and social ostracism that would inevitably follow should they refuse. As Boulware-Miller (1985, p. 167) explains:

> The stigma associated with not being circumcised attaches early, virtually compelling a choice to undergo the operation.
> An un-excised, non-infibulated girl is often despised, ridiculed and referred to as el *beydourha meno* ('who wants her?') and el *beyaresha meno* ('who marries her?').

The activism of a range of groups (not just one cultural group) aimed at eradicating female genital mutilation at the very least draws attention to the need to question and to call into question things as they are. It reminds us that while culture can provide a group with a 'blue print for life', it can also be imprisoning, oppressive, cruel, and provide a 'blue print for death'. In such instances, 'minding our own cultural business' (viz. 'looking the other way' and allowing mutilating traditions to arbitrarily supplant moral considerations of human wellbeing) can be just as 'imperialistic' (viz. exercising supreme authority) as 'making other people's cultures our business'.

The activism of external cultural groups reminds us of both the possibility and the importance of making *critical discretionary judgments* about the kinds of religious and traditional practices which we, as health care professionals, ought and ought not to respect. This critical discretionary judgment may, however, rest less on questions of 'tolerance' (including the problematic questions of intolerance and over-tolerance), than on questions of culturally informed critical reflection grounded in the lived experiences of those who suffer demonstrably and intolerably on account of cultural practices that no longer serve the survival and prosperity interests of the group if, indeed, they ever did. By engaging in such critical reflection we should be able to discern the practices against which our conscientious objection, at least, is warranted if not our fully committed collective activism aimed at their eradication.

When discerning and focusing on 'harmful' traditional and religious practices, however, it is important that we do not become distracted from our original project of improving understanding and informed tolerance of cultural diversity, or the merits of a transcultural approach to ethics. Every culture has its 'down side' in regard to upholding questionable and possibly harmful traditional values, beliefs and practices. Furthermore, just because a certain behaviour is seen to be characteristic of a given culture, it does not follow that the behaviour in question is either accepted or regarded as being acceptable by all members of that culture. For instance, child abuse and domestic violence are characteristics of Australian society and culture. Aside from the perpetrators of such abuse and violence (religious elites among them), the Australian people would, I suggest, firmly reject any notion that such abuse and violence is culturally accepted and acceptable.

The above considerations are all important and need to be taken into account when 'reading the cultural world' and drawing upon it for cues to guide our moral actions both as individuals and as professionals. But most important of all, they remind us of the need to remain committed to acquiring and maintaining a deep understanding of the cultural complexities and dynamics that inform the range of practices which people from different cultural groups may observe, and the potential for disagreement (both from within and outside of those cultural groups) about the moral acceptability of those practices.

Conclusion

Transcultural ethics, like feminist ethics, recognises the inherent difficulties associated with genuine moral problems in human life being 'confronted as abstraction rather than experiential realities' (Marshall 1992, p. 52), and affirms that, if moral abstractions are to count for anything, they must be brought 'back to earth' (Stout 1988, p. 8). It also recognises the inability of abstract and decontextualised moral thinking to provide concrete answers to complex questions concerning a range of human experiences. Key among these experiences are: human pain and suffering, intense and sometimes conflicting human emotions, ambivalent and ambiguous human relationships, and, not least, differing cultural world views about the value and meaning of life — all of which often (too often) have to be dealt with in the face of overwhelming uncertainty, the unpredictability of probable outcomes (positive and negative), fallible modes of communication, and the fallibilities of decision-makers (Elliott 1992; Marshall 1992; Cortese 1990; Stout 1988).

Unlike other moral critiques, however, transcultural ethics offers an optimistic outlook. Its suggestion that acceptance of — and achieving a harmony of — moral diversity offers the key to sustaining the existence and purpose of morality provides an important basis upon which we can all develop, not just our moral thinking and sensibilities, but our ability to actually *be* moral in a world characterised by diverse and competing valid world views. This is not merely compromise, as some might believe, or even tolerance — the blinded eye of an indiscriminate mind (see Midgley 1991a; Wolff et al. 1969). Nor is it confusion. Rather, it is celebration. In particular, it is the celebration of the 'other' as different, but not inferior or fallacious or superstitious — as having something worthwhile to share, not as being something worthless to be marginalised, trivialised and ignored. If we accept this, we will all be in a much better position to judge what is really unethical as opposed to being merely disliked; what is truly wrong, as opposed to being merely unfamiliar and strange; and what is really confusion as opposed to simple misunderstanding of another's moral language with which we are not familiar (Stout 1988). This insight is, among other things, what we stand to gain by embracing a diversity of moral values and beliefs as being the beginning of morality and not its end.

In conclusion, I should like to list a number of questions nurses ought to ask when making moral decisions about the nursing care of people from diverse cultural backgrounds. Borrowing from Kanitsaki (1989b, p. 70):

- Is my understanding of this person's values and value systems such that it entitles me to override her or his family's requests or instructions?
- Can I by way of a third party (such as an interpreter) really ensure that my interventions will result in benefits not harms to that person?
- Are my values and frame of reference the only ones which warrant overriding consideration in this relationship?
- How do I know my judgments in this relationship are morally and culturally appropriate? In short, how do I know I am right?

By asking these and similar questions, and by seeking the 'right' answers to them, nurses will demonstrate successfully that they are able to embrace morality as something more than a set of abstract self-standing principles. They will also demonstrate that, in the ultimate analysis, it is people and relationships that count — not a blind deference to rules, which, when stripped of their cultural content and context, become little more than intellectual curiosities empowered by arbitrary will, incapable of responding to the lived realities and needs of human beings who have been born into circumstances which are very often beyond their control. Embracing this approach will also remind us that:

> any theory of ethics is, in the end, only as plausible as the complete picture of the world of which it forms a part.
>
> (McNaughton 1988, p. 41)

CASE SCENARIO AND CRITICAL QUESTIONS

Case scenario

A 69-year-old Greek-born man, who had grown up in a village and who spoke little English, was admitted to a major metropolitan hospital in Melbourne for follow-up assessment and tests for a cancer-related illness that had been diagnosed and treated some years earlier. Initially, when first diagnosed and treated, the man's prognosis was thought to be 'good' and his disease 'under control'. Unfortunately, his condition changed unexpectedly and his test results revealed that his cancer had spread and that only palliative care could now be offered for his condition. He was in no pain, however, and although tired was eager to return home. Meanwhile, his treating doctor decided that before being discharged the man had a right to be told the change in his prognosis and of what lay ahead. The man's Australian-born daughter, however, took a different view and insisted that 'under no circumstances was her father to be told his poor prognosis' since this would 'destroy his hope' and affect his quality of life (confidential source, personal communication 2003). When the doctor objected to her request, the daughter explained that, in their (Greek) culture, it was wrong to tell someone they had terminal cancer; she then begged the doctor not to tell her father his test results or that 'they [the doctors] were not going to do anything [medically] for him, other than to provide palliative care' (confidential source, personal communication 2003). The doctor again objected to the daughter's request, arguing that the matter was 'not about culture, but about ethics' and that her father 'had a right to know' (confidential source, personal communication 2003).

Critical questions

1. If you were a nurse assigned to the care of this elderly Greek-born man and you came across the doctor and the man's daughter arguing about his 'right to know', how would you respond to the situation?
2. What values and beliefs would you draw on to inform your decisions and actions?
3. What assistance would the ICN *Code of ethics for nurses* provide in helping you to decide what to do?
4. What might be the consequences to the man and his family if the doctor ignores the daughter's requests, calls an interpreter and tells the patient that his prognosis is poor and that only palliative care can now be offered to him?

5. Upon what basis, if at all, is imposing unwanted information (e.g. a poor prognosis) on a patient morally justified?

Chapter 5

Moral problems and moral decision-making in nursing and health care contexts

LEARNING OBJECTIVES

Upon the completion of this chapter and with further self-directed learning you are expected to be able to:
- Discuss the three distinguishing features of a moral problem.
- Explain why moral problems are different from other kinds of (non-moral) problems.
- Discuss the nature of the moral problems listed below and their possible implications in regard to the ethical practice of nursing:
  - moral unpreparedness
  - moral blindness
  - moral indifference
  - amoralism
  - immoralism
  - moral complacency
  - moral fanaticism
  - moral disagreement
  - moral dilemmas
  - moral stress, moral distress, and moral perplexity.
- Define moral decision-making.
- Discuss critically the role that reason, emotion, intuition and life experience might play in moral decision-making.
- Discuss processes for dealing effectively with moral disputes.
- Explore a range of 'everyday' ethical issues that nurses might face in the course of providing nursing care to patients.

KEYWORDS

- Everyday moral problems/ethical issues
- Moral consensus
- Moral decision-making
- Moral disputes
- Moral differences
- Moral problems
- Quantum morality

Introduction

A *problem* (from Late Latin *problēma*, meaning something that has been put forward or thrown forward) may be defined as 'any thing, matter, person, etc., that is difficult to deal with, solve or overcome' and as a puzzle or question that stands in need of a solution (*Collins English Dictionary*, 2003). A moral problem may be similarly defined, that is, as a moral matter or issue that is difficult to deal with, solve or overcome and which stands in need of a (moral) solution.

Nurses at all levels and in all areas of practice encounter moral problems during the course of their everyday professional practice. These problems range from the relatively 'simple' to the extraordinarily complex, and can cause varying degrees of perplexity and distress in those who encounter them. Whereas some moral problems may be relatively easy to resolve and may cause little if any distress to those involved; other problems may be extremely difficult or even impossible to resolve, and may cause a great deal of moral stress and distress for those encountering them.

Nurses, like other health professionals, have a stringent moral responsibility to be able to identify and respond effectively to the moral problems they encounter (whether 'simple' or 'complex'), and, where able, to employ strategies to prevent them from occurring in the first place. In order to be able to do this, however, nurses must first be able to distinguish moral problems from other sorts of (non-moral) problems (for example, legal and clinical problems), and to be able to distinguish different types of moral problems from each other. It is to advancing knowledge and understanding of the different kinds of moral problems that nurses might encounter in the course of their day-to-day practice — and how best to deal with them— that provides the focus for this chapter.

Distinguishing moral problems from other sorts of problems

All health professionals encounter a variety of problems in the course of their everyday practice, and nurses are no exception. Significantly, most of these problems probably have a moral dimension to them. It is important to clarify, however, that not all problems that have a moral dimension are *moral problems* per se. This raises the question of how are we to distinguish a bona fide moral problem from other kinds of (non-moral) problems. One clue to answering this question lies in the degree to which the moral dimension of a given problem might be deemed 'weightier' and thus *prima facie* as 'overriding' of the other dimensions of the problem, and the kinds of solutions that might be fruitfully employed to resolve the problem. Consider the following example.

A patient is in severe and intolerable pain due to not receiving pain medication. Nevertheless, while this is a problem and one which clearly has a moral dimension, it is not immediately evident that the problem is a 'full-blown' moral problem per se requiring moral analysis, debate and possibly the intervention of an 'ethics expert' or clinical ethics committee. Further analysis is required. It might be, for instance, that the patient's pain management has, for some reason, been neglected. What is required in this instance is a competent and compassionate clinical assessment of the patient and the swift administration of needed analgesia. The problem may thus be correctly characterised as a 'technical or practical problem' requiring, and resolvable by, a 'clinical solution'. It might also be, however, that the patient is in pain due to her refusing pain relief on religious grounds. In such an instance even the most competent and compassionate of clinical assessments will not necessarily result in the identification of a satisfactory solution to the problem of the patient's pain since the obvious 'clinical solution' (that is, of giving analgesia) is precluded by the moral demand to respect the patient's autonomous wishes. The problem may thus be correctly characterised as a moral problem (not merely a clinical problem) since:

- the patient's moral interest and wellbeing are at risk (if her autonomous wishes are respected, she will suffer the harm of intolerable pain; conversely, if her pain is alleviated by the administration of analgesia, she will suffer the harm of having her autonomous wishes violated);
- the nurses' moral interests and wellbeing are at risk on account of the moral distress they experience at their genuine inability to maximise the patient's moral interests in not suffering unnecessarily; and, finally,
- assistance is required to help attendant nurses to answer the question: *What should we do?*

To help clarify the basis upon which the above distinction has been made, the following framework is offered. It is generally accepted that something involves a (human) moral/ethical problem where it has as its central concern:

- the promotion and protection of people's genuine wellbeing and welfare (including their interests in not suffering unnecessarily);
- responding justly to the genuine needs and significant interests of different people; and
- determining and justifying what constitutes right and wrong conduct in a given situation (Beauchamp and Childress 2001; Bond 1996; Blum 1994, 1980; Singer 1993; Amato 1990; McNaughton 1988; Frankena 1973).

The nursing profession is fundamentally concerned with the promotion and protection of people's genuine wellbeing and welfare, and in achieving these ends, responding justly to the genuine needs and significant moral interests of different people. The nursing profession is, therefore, fundamentally concerned with 'moral problems' as well as other kinds of problems (for example, technical, clinical, legal, and so forth).

In order to deal with moral problems appropriately and effectively it is evident that nurses need to know, first, what form a moral problem might take and how to recognise it; and, second, how best to decide when dealing with them. It is to answering these questions that this discussion now turns.

Identifying different kinds of moral problems

The nursing literature has, to date, tended to focus predominantly on one type of moral problem; namely, the moral dilemma (also referred to as an *ethical dilemma*). While it is true that the moral/ethical dilemma is an important moral problem in nursing and health care domains, it needs to be clarified that it is by no means the *only* moral problem nurses (or others) will encounter when planning and implementing care. Indeed, there are at least ten different kinds of moral problems that can and do arise in nursing and health care contexts; these are:

1. moral unpreparedness
2. moral blindness
3. moral indifference

4. amoralism
5. immoralism
6. moral complacency
7. moral fanaticism
8. moral disagreements and conflicts
9. moral dilemmas
10. moral stress, moral distress, and moral perplexity.

If nurses are to respond effectively to the moral problems encountered in nursing and health care contexts, it is important that they understand the nature and implications of the different kinds of moral problems that can arise. It is to examining this issue further that the following discussion now turns.

Moral unpreparedness

The first type of moral problem to be considered here is that of general 'unpreparedness' to deal appropriately and effectively with morally troubling situations. What invariably happens here is that a nurse (or other health professional) enters into a situation without being sufficiently prepared to deal with the moral complexities of that situation specifically. The nurse (or other health professional) may lack the requisite moral knowledge, moral imagination, moral experience and moral wisdom otherwise necessary to be able to deal with the moral complexities of the situation at hand (this could also count as *moral incompetence* or *moral impairment* [Johnstone 1998]). When eventually faced with a particular moral problem, the nurse acts in bad faith by pretending that the situation at hand is one which can be handled 'with one's given moral apparatus' (Lemmon 1987, p. 112). The room for moral error here is considerable.

To illustrate the seriousness of moral unpreparedness, consider the analogous situation of clinical unpreparedness. A nurse who is not educated in the complexities of, say, intensive care nursing, but who is nevertheless sent to 'help out' and care for a ventilated patient in intensive care, would not only be inadequate in this role, but could even be dangerous. Such a nurse might not have the learned skills necessary to detect the subtle changes in a sedated patient's condition — changes indicating, for example, the need for more sedation, or the need to perform tracheal suctioning, or the need to increase the tidal volume of air flow or oxygen administration. Neither might this nurse be able to distinguish the many different alarms that can go off on the high-tech equipment being used to give full life support to the patient, or to detect any malfunctioning of this sophisticated equipment. Without these skills, a nurse working in intensive care would be likely to place the life and wellbeing of the patient at serious risk.

The argument of the seriousness of unpreparedness also applies to the complexities of sound ethical reasoning and ethical health care practice generally. Such a nurse, left to deal with a morally troubling situation, would not only be inadequate in that role but, as the intensive care example shows, his or her practice could be potentially hazardous. Without the learned moral skills necessary to detect moral problems and to resolve them in a sound, reliable and defensible manner, an unprepared nurse, no matter how well intentioned, could fail to correctly detect moral hazards in the workplace, and therefore fail to act or respond in a way that would prevent a moral catastrophe from occurring.

The kinds of moral catastrophes or near catastrophes that can occur as a result of nurses' (and other allied health professionals') moral unpreparedness to deal appropriately and effectively with moral problems in health care contexts are well documented in the nursing, bioethical, legal and other related literature. To give just one example, consider the notorious case of the Chelmsford Private Hospital in Sydney, Australia. In this case, many people were left permanently damaged and scarred — some even died — as a result of receiving deep sleep therapy (DST) prescribed by Dr Harry Bailey, a consultant psychiatrist, who later suicided in connection with the scandal that was eventually uncovered (Bromberger and Fife-Yeomans 1991; Rice 1988). It is now known that approximately one thousand patients were 'treated' with DST at this hospital. It is also known, as revealed as early as 1977 by the current affairs television program '60 Minutes', that many of these patients did not receive the standard of care and treatment they were entitled to receive. Among other things — including the deaths of seven people between 1974 and 1977 — the '60 Minutes' program revealed that 'recognised standard precautions for the safety of patients were not taken; and that patients received the treatment without their consent' (Bromberger and Fife-Yeomans 1991, p. 142). In the Chelmsford Royal Commission that was eventually established in 1988 to 'examine the provision of Deep Sleep Therapy and the administration of Chelmsford Private Hospital', it was confirmed that:

> The signature of some [consent] forms were obtained by fraud and deceit. Some were signed by people whose judgment was compromised by drugs. Some patients were even woken up from their DST [Deep Sleep Therapy] treatment to complete their authorisation. Other patients were treated contrary to their express wishes and some were treated despite the fact they had specifically refused the treatment.
>
> (Commissioner Slattery, cited in Bromberger and Fife-Yeomans 1991, p. 171)

Nursing care was also seriously substandard. In one notable case, the nursing care had been so negligent that a patient developed severe decubitus ulcers between her knees, which became 'glued' together as though they had been skin-grafted. The former patient recalled:

> I was having hallucinations about a lot of coloured ribbons and trying to climb out through them finding the world again. I woke up in a bath tub and two nurses were bathing me. I felt really dirty. One of the nurses said, 'My God, look at her knees.' I looked down and they were joined together. The nurses gently pulled them apart.
>
> (Bromberger and Fife-Yeomans 1991, p. 94)

Bromberger and Fife-Yeomans (1991, p. 94) comment that the patient 'still retains the scars on the inside of her knees'.

Another example of the substandard nursing care that was provided (or more to the point, not provided) can be found in the experiences of another patient, Barry Hart, outlined in the following statement read to the New South Wales Parliament in 1984:

> Basic, commonsense nursing practice was ignored. Patients were sedated for ten days and given no exercise during this period. They were incontinent of faeces and urine most of the time and were left lying incontinent of faeces until they woke up.
>
> There was no attempt to maintain a fluid balance. Patients wet the bed and remained lying in the urine until the sheets were changed. The staff made an approximation of whether the patients were actually passing urine (i.e. a fluid output) by seeing how wet the bed was.
>
> (cited in Rice 1988, p. 47)

One of the troubling things about the whole Chelmsford scandal is that rumours about Dr Bailey's unscrupulous practices had been circulating for years, yet nothing was done about it (Bromberger and Fife-Yeomans 1991, p. 176). Equally disturbing is the fact that it was not until 1988 — 24 years after the investigated death of the first 'deep sleep' patient, and only after 'treatment' had led to the deaths of 24 patients — that a Royal Commission was set up to investigate the allegations concerning the patient abuse that was subsequently proved to have occurred at Chelmsford Private Hospital (Bromberger and Fife-Yeomans 1991, p. 162). Significantly, in the Royal Commission of Inquiry that was conducted, and in the report on its findings, it was revealed that between 1963 and 1979 only *two* nurses took action in an attempt to expose the unscrupulous practices they had observed (*Report of the Royal Commission into Deep Sleep Therapy* 1990, p. 127). There is room to speculate here that had nursing personnel been better prepared to recognise and respond effectively to violations of professional ethical standards, the trauma and suffering experienced by the patients at Chelmsford could have been reduced considerably, if not avoided altogether.

Not all moral catastrophes occurring in health care contexts are as ethically dramatic as those that occurred in the Chelmsford Private Hospital case, however. Moral catastrophes can and do occur on a much more commonplace level in the health care arena, as examples to be given in the following chapters of this book will show.

Moral blindness

A second type of problem that nurses often encounter is that of what I shall call 'moral blindness'. A morally blind nurse (or other health professional) is someone who, upon encountering a moral problem, simply does not see it as a *moral* problem. Instead, they may perceive it as either a clinical or a technical problem. Carlton (1978, p. 10) argues, on the basis of her field research, that there is a tendency by many health professionals (particularly doctors) 'to translate ethical issues into technical problems which have clinical solutions'.

Moral blindness can be likened, in an analogous way, to colour-blindness. Just as a colour-blind person fails to distinguish certain colours in the world, a morally blind person fails to distinguish certain 'moral properties' in the world. Perhaps a better example can be found by appealing to a set of imageries commonly associated with Gestalt psychology and theories on the nature of perception. What I particularly have in mind here are the two drawings which are popularly presented in psychology texts to demonstrate certain perceptual phenomena, including perceptual organisation and the influence of context on the way in which an object is perceived.

The first of these drawings (Figure 5.1) depicts what initially appears to be a white vase or goblet against a black background; after a more sustained glance, the drawing changes (or rather, one's perception 'shifts') and what is perceived instead are two black facial profiles separated by a white space. Some people see the alternating vase–face images relatively quickly and easily, while others struggle to shake off what for them remains the dominant image (i.e. *either* the vase *or* the faces).

The second ambiguous drawing (Figure 5.2) depicts what can be seen as either an unsophisticated-looking old woman or a very sophisticated-looking young woman. As with the vase–face drawing, some people see the alternating old woman–young woman images relatively easily, while others literally get 'stuck' with a dominant perception of *either* the young woman *or* the old woman.

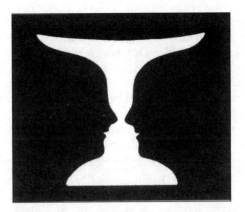

Figure 5.1 Reversible figure and background

(reproduced with permission from R. L. Atkinson, R. C. Atkinson and E. R. Hilgard (1983) *Introduction to psychology* (8th edn). Harcourt Brace Jovanovich, New York, p. 139)

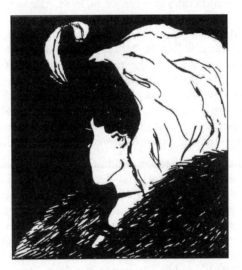

Figure 5.2 Ambiguous stimulus

(reproduced with permission from R. L. Atkinson, R. C. Atkinson and E. R. Hilgard (1983) *Introduction to psychology* (8th edn). Harcourt Brace Jovanovich, New York, p. 139)

Psychologists claim, however, that people's perceptions can be altered by context — in this instance, by showing photographs before the ambiguous drawings are viewed. They claim that, on an initial viewing of this drawing, 65 per cent report seeing the young woman first. If subjects are shown photographs of an old woman before seeing the drawing, however, almost all see the old woman first. The same 'reversals' can be achieved by conditioning subjects with photographs to see the young woman first (Atkinson et al. 1983, p. 147).

I am not here attempting to present an elaborate theory of moral perception but rather trying to illustrate what I believe is a common and potentially morally risky phenomenon in health care contexts: that of impaired moral perception. There is, I think, room to suggest that health professionals (including nurses) are sometimes so conditioned by the 'clinical imagery' (context) around them that, when they do encounter a bona fide moral problem, it tends to be perceived not as a *moral* problem, but as a *clinical* or a *technical* problem and, as such, one requiring a clinical solution, not a moral solution. Some health professionals have a healthy perception of the alternating moral–clinical images depicted by a given scenario; others, however, remain stuck with a dominant *clinical image* and do not see the alternative *moral image*, which for them is less discernible. One unfortunate consequence of this, is that *technically correct* decisions are sometimes made at the expense of *morally correct* decisions.

The extent to which clinical perceptions and judgments can dominate over moral perceptions and judgments can be illustrated by the once common practice of defending 'Do Not Resuscitate' (DNR) directives (also called 'Not For Resuscitation' or NFR directives) on hopelessly or chronically ill patients on medical grounds ('medical indications') *alone*. In the past many doctors and nurses perceived DNR directives as involving a *clinical issue*, not a *moral issue*, and, as such, one to be decided by doctors, not ethicists. The clinical–moral Gestalt problem became particularly clear to me at a nursing law and ethics conference in 1988. After presenting a paper on the nature and moral implications of DNR/NFR directives, I was approached by several registered nurses with what became a familiar and distressing comment: 'My God! I had never thought about it [DNR/NFR] as a *moral* issue before … What have I done?'. The issue was taken up by the media (see Miller 1988, 1989; Schumpeter 1988; Craig 1989; *Upfront* 1988); other nurses wanted to challenge or attack the view that DNR/NFR directives involved moral considerations and moral decisions. The then State President (in Victoria) of the Australian Medical Association, Dr Bill McCubbery, was prompted to respond to the issue, and is reported as saying that 'NFR decisions had to depend on professional judgment' (Schumpeter 1988, p. 21).

Today there is a much greater recognition of the moral dimensions of DNR/NFR directives and the degree to which such directives are informed by moral considerations (see the discussion on DNR in Chapter 12 of this book). The once common view that DNR/NFR decisions are based 'simply' on medical concerns/indications (not ethical concerns) and are more a matter of 'good medical judgment' (rather than — or as well as — sound moral judgment) is rarely advanced in contemporary debate, at least not credibly. Nevertheless, this kind of thinking persists in regard to other issues. For example, in 2001, in a highly publicised surgery ban imposed on smokers by doctors in the Australian State of Victoria, surgeons were reported as defending their stance by arguing that, '*Medical concerns*, not moral judgments, were the bottom line in banning smokers from a range of life-saving treatments' [emphasis added] (Chandler 2001, p. 9; Taylor 2001, p. 4). The specific treatments banned, in this instance, were reported to include: artery by-passes, coronary artery grafts, lung reduction surgery and lung and heart transplants (Taylor 2001, p. 4).

The issue of 'moral blindness' among nurses is an important one, since, as with the problem of moral unpreparedness, it could result in otherwise avoidable moral harms occurring. This problem is not insurmountable, however. Just as people can be 'conditioned' to see the old woman rather than the young woman in the ambiguous drawing shown in Figure 5.2, so too can nurses and allied health professionals be 'conditioned' (or rather educated) to see the moral dimension of an ambiguous scenario which can be perceived as involving either a moral problem or a clinical or technical problem. Arguably, the best way to achieve such a Gestalt moral shift in perception is by appropriate ethics education and reflective ethical practice.

Moral indifference

A third type of problem which nurses may encounter is that of 'moral indifference'. Moral indifference is characterised by an unconcerned or uninterested attitude toward demands to be moral; in short, it assumes the attitude of 'why bother to be moral?'. The morally indifferent person is someone who typically refrains from expressing any desire that certain acts should or should not be done in all comparable circumstances (Hare 1981, p. 185). An example of a morally indifferent nurse would be a nurse who is both unconcerned about and uninterested in alleviating a patient's pain, or is unconcerned about or uninterested in the fact that a DNR ('Do Not Resuscitate') directive or a directive to perform ECT (electroconvulsive therapy) has been given on an unconsenting patient, or is unconcerned about and uninterested in any form of violation of patients' rights, for that matter. As well as this, a morally indifferent nurse would probably refrain from expressing a desire that anything should be done about such situations.

The problem of moral indifference in nursing is well captured by Mila Aroskar (1986) in her classic article 'Are nurses' mind sets compatible with ethical practice?'. Aroskar (1986, p. 72) cites the findings of a study undertaken in the late 1970s which showed that nurses tended to defer to institutional norms 'even when patients' rights were being violated'. She also points out that, despite the North American nursing profession's formal commitment to ethical practice (as manifested, among other things, by its formal adoption of various codes and standards of practice), arguments were still widely heard among nurses that 'ethical practice is too risky and requires a certain amount of heroism on the part of nurses' (Aroskar 1986, p. 69). Although written almost two decades ago, Aroskar's words still apply today. As Jill Iliffe of the Australian Nursing Federation reflects (2002, p. 1):

> What do you do when something happens that you know to be wrong, unethical or inappropriate? [...] A colleague behaves unprofessionally; health care is provided that you know to be inappropriate; a decision is made that is ethically questionable; there is an adverse outcome that could have been avoided, as was perhaps even the result of negligence. What do you do? It is often a difficult decision to make, particularly when the other person or persons are more senior to you and in a position of power and authority.

The retreat by nurses into moral indifference, while not condonable, is understandable. There are many examples that demonstrate the kinds of difficulties nurses might find themselves in when attempting to conduct morally responsible, professional practice, and the ultimate price that can be paid for taking a moral stand on a matter. One such example concerns the highly publicised United Kingdom case of a registered nurse by the name of Graham Pink. Pink was found guilty of 'gross misconduct' by his employing health authority after he publicly exposed unacceptable standards of care (including poor staff–patient ratios) in the hospital at which he worked (Turner 1992, 1990; Tadd 1991). Pink's ordeal began in 1989 when he wrote to the local health authority detailing his concerns about the substandard care that was being given to elderly residents at the hospital where he worked. The health authority followed up the complaint and agreed that 'something must be done' and instructed the hospital 'to look at' staffing levels (Turner 1992, p. 28). When these instructions were not actioned, Pink communicated his concerns in writing to the chief executive of the National Health Service, the health secretary and the prime minister Mrs Thatcher. He received a written reply from the latter two 'thanking him' for the information but pointing out that it was 'a local matter' (Turner 1992, p. 28).

Subsequently Pink was persuaded by a member of parliament to allow a selection of his letters to be published in the *Guardian* newspaper. This action resulted in enormous public support. Pink, meanwhile, was warned 'not to speak out further' (Turner 1992, p28). Even though his actions ('to take appropriate action') were supported by the United Kingdom Central Council's *Code of Professional Conduct* (1984) and advisory document *Exercising Accountability* (1989), they nevertheless placed him at odds with his employer. Pink was suspended from duty, and the hospital management initiated disciplinary procedures against him. After one year of hearings and appeals, Pink was found guilty of gross misconduct and offered a transfer to a community setting. Pink refused this offer, however, and was dismissed by his employer. Summing up the implications of this case, one nurse is reported as commenting: 'It is difficult to imagine anybody ever speaking out again — they just wanted to get him and they did' (Turner 1990, p. 19). Another commentator concludes succinctly: 'Graham Pink's experience show[s] that once nurses raise their heads above the parapet they may not be far from disciplinary action' (Turner 1990, p. 19).

Although this case occurred several years ago, the lessons it provides remain current and are indicative of the difficulties nurses worldwide often face when trying to deliver ethically responsible care (see also Chapter 13 of this book). We all know (and have possibly personally experienced) the forces that can be brought to bear upon a nurse who takes a moral position which conflicts with established hospital norms and etiquette. It is then perhaps understandable (even though not excusable) that nurses become morally indifferent to the violations of patients' rights and other unjust practices in health care domains. Compounding this situation, institutional and legal constraints may make it very difficult for nurses to act morally (Johnstone 2002a, 1994). The price paid for acting morally or for taking a moral stand can be intolerably high, as other examples to be given in the chapters to follow will show. What this signifies, however, is not that nurses should abandon the demands of morality; rather, they should seek ways in which morality's demands can be upheld safely and effectively.

Amoralism

A fourth type of moral problem which nurses might encounter, and which is similar to moral indifference, is that of 'amoralism', which is characterised by an absence of moral concern and a rejection of morality altogether (a position significantly different from *immoralism*, [discussed below] which accepts morality, but violates its demands). An amoral person is someone who refrains from making moral judgments and who typically rejects being bound by any of morality's behavioural prescriptions and proscriptions. If an amoralist were to ask: 'why should I be moral?', it is likely that no answer would be satisfactory. (For a helpful response to the question 'Why should I be moral?', see Nielsen 1989.)

A nurse who is an amoralist would reject any imperative to behave morally as a professional. For example, the amoral nurse might reject that he or she has a moral duty to uphold a patient's rights. The amoral nurse would also probably claim that it does not make any sense even to speak of things like a patients' 'rights' since moral language itself has no meaning. The amoralist's position in this respect is analogous to the atheist's rejection of certain religious terms. The extreme atheist, for example, would argue against uttering the word 'God', since it refers to nothing and therefore has no meaning. Such an atheist might also claim that there is no point in engaging in a religious debate on the existence of God, since there is just nothing there to debate. To try and debate the existence of God would be like trying to debate the existence of 'a black cat in a darkened room when there isn't one'. The amoralist may argue in a similar way in relation to the issue of morality.

It can be seen that the amoralist's position is an extreme one, and one which is very difficult to sustain. (Even thieves, who may appear amoral, act on the 'moral' assumption that it is 'good/right' to steal.) Perhaps the most approximate example that can be given here is that of psychopaths or frontal lobe damaged persons who simply lack all capacity to be moral (see Damasio 1994). If amoralism is encountered in health care contexts, it is likely that very little can be done, morally speaking, to deal with it. The only recourse in dealing with the amoral health professional would be to appeal to non-moral censuring mechanisms such as legal and/or professional disciplinary measures (see, for example, Johnstone 1998).

Immoralism[1]

At its most basic, immoral conduct (also known as moral turpitude and moral delinquency) can be defined as any act involving a deliberate violation of accepted or agreed ethical standards. Moral turpitude (a notion which has received more stringent attention in the United States of America than in Australia) has been defined specifically as:

> anything done knowingly contrary to justice, honesty, principle, or good morals ... [or] an act of baseness, vileness or depravity in the private or social duties which a man [sic] owes to his fellow man [sic] or to society in general. The term implies something immoral in itself.
>
> (*Seary v State Bar of Texas* — cited in Freckelton 1996, p 142)

Moral delinquency, in turn, is taken here as referring to any act involving moral negligence or a dereliction of moral duty. As in the above definitions, moral delinquency in professional contexts entails a deliberate or careless violation of agreed standards of ethical professional conduct.

Accepting the above account, an immoral nurse can thus be described as someone who knowingly and wilfully violates the agreed norms of ethical professional conduct or general ethical standards of conduct towards others. Judging immoral conduct, by this view, would require a demonstration that the accepted ethical standards of the profession were (1) known by an offending nurse, and (2) deliberately and recklessly violated by that nurse. There are many 'obvious' examples of immoral conduct by nurses. These include: the deliberate theft of patients/clients money for personal use; the sexual, verbal and physical abuse of patients/clients; xenophobic behaviours (including racism, sexism, ageism, homophobia and a range of other unjust discriminatory behaviours); participation in unscrupulous research practices; and other morally unacceptable behaviours, examples of which are given throughout this book.

It should be noted that regardless of whether an act involving the violation of agreed professional or general ethical standards results in a significant moral harm to another, it would still stand as an instance of immoral conduct. For example, a nurse who knowingly and recklessly breaches a patient's/client's confidentiality would have committed an unethical act even if the breach in question did not result in any significant moral harm to the patient/client.

Moral complacency

A sixth type of moral problem nurses can encounter is that of 'moral complacency', defined by Unwin (1985, p. 205) as 'a general unwillingness to accept that one's moral opinions may be mistaken'. It could also be described as a general unwillingness to 'let go' the primacy of one's own point of view or to regard one's own point of view as *just one of many to be compared, contrasted and considered*. Again, we do not need to look far to find examples of moral complacency in health care contexts.

I recall, several years ago, once being approached by a then gerontology clinical nurse specialist lamenting the 'short-sightedness' of some of her students, who were of the view that elderly people in residential care homes should be resuscitated in the event of cardiac arrest, and that the blanket DNR ('Do Not Resuscitate') status that was automatically given to all elderly residents upon entering a residential care home was both immoral and illegal. The nurse specialist was insistent that the students were morally wrong, and was clearly disturbed and outraged by their position.

In my response to her, I enquired concerning the discussion she had with her students whether anyone had thought to ask the elderly residents what their preferences were — whether, in the event of cardiac arrest, *they* wished to be resuscitated or not? It should be noted that, at that time, elderly people entering a residential care agency were invariably asked whether upon their death they wished to be cremated, or where they wished to be buried; they were not always asked, however, whether they wished to be resuscitated in the event of a cardiac arrest. The nurse specialist became obviously agitated by my question, and exclaimed: 'surely it is ludicrous to ask all elderly residents whether they wish to be resuscitated!'. After I had expressed my disagreement and pointed out the minimal requirements of the moral principle of autonomy, the nurse specialist retorted: 'would you really expect us to ask each and every resident whether they wish to be resuscitated? It's ludicrous! It's silly! It's unnecessary …'. To this retort, I reminded the nurse specialist that elderly residents are already asked whether they wish to be cremated or where they wish to be buried upon their death so what was so difficult about asking them whether they wish to be resuscitated? The nurse specialist was still unconvinced, and persisted in rejecting the view I was putting to her. She further maintained that it was right and proper that all elderly residents should be uniformly designated DNR upon admission to a residential nursing care home. The attitude of the nurse specialist in this anecdote is an example of moral complacency.

Like moral unpreparedness and moral blindness, moral complacency is something which can be rectified by moral education and moral consciousness raising. The objective of taking this action would be, of course, to produce in the morally complacent person the attitude that nobody can afford to be complacent in the way they ordinarily view the world — least of all the moral world. This is particularly so in instances where *other* people's moral interests are at stake. It is a grave mistake to assume that our moral opinions are 'right' *just because* they are our own opinions. As ethical professionals, our stringent moral responsibility is to *question* our taken-for-granted assumptions about the world, and not to presume that they are always well founded and unable to be challenged.

Moral fanaticism

A seventh type of moral problem which may be encountered by nurses, and which is similar in many respects to moral complacency, is that of 'moral fanaticism'. The moral fanatic is someone who is thoroughly 'wedded to certain ideals' and uncritically and unreflectingly makes moral judgments according to them (Hare 1981, p. 170). Richard Hare's celebrated case of the fanatical Nazi is a good example here (Hare 1963, Chapter 9). The fanatical Nazi in this case stringently clings to the ideal of a pure Aryan German race and the need to exterminate all Jews as a means of purging the German race of its impurities. The Nazi falls into the category of being a 'fanatic' when he/she insists that, if any Nazis discover themselves to be of Jewish descent, then they too should be exterminated along with all the rest of the Jews (Hare 1963, pp. 161–2).

Examples of moral fanaticism exist in health care contexts. The surgeon who repeatedly performs 'futile' surgery in an attempt to prolong the life of a terminally ill patient, regardless of the dying patient's wishes to the contrary and the suffering it causes, is an important example here. Morally fanatical doctors in this instance might defend their position by claiming that it is not only medically indicated but strongly warranted from a moral point of view. The maintenance of absolute confidentiality, even though harm might be caused as a result, is another good example. So, too, is the example of a doctor or a nurse forcing unwanted information on a patient in the fanatical belief that all patients must be told the truth - even if the patient in question has specifically requested not to receive the information, and the imposition of the unwanted information on the patient can be shown to be a 'gratuitous and harmful misinterpretation of the moral foundations for respect for autonomy' (Pellegrino 1992, p. 1735).

In the case of moral fanatics, an appeal to overriding considerations or principles of conduct would not be helpful (Hare 1981, p. 178). As with the amoralist, the problem of the moral fanatic in health care contexts is likely to have disappointing outcomes. In the final analysis, it may be that other (non-moral) mechanisms will have to be appealed to in order to resolve the moral problems caused by moral fanaticism; for example, it may be necessary to seek the involvement of a public advocate, a court of law or a disciplinary body to arbitrate the matter.

Moral disagreements and conflicts

An eighth type of moral problem nurses will very often encounter is that involving 'moral disagreement' — concerning, for example, the selection, interpretation, application and evaluation of moral standards. In his classic article 'Moral deadlock', Milo (1986) identifies two fundamental types of moral disagreement: internal moral disagreement and radical moral disagreement.

INTERNAL MORAL DISAGREEMENT

Three forms of internal moral disagreement can occur. The first of these involves a fundamental conflict about the force or priority of accepted moral standards. For example, two people may agree to common moral standards but disagree about what to do when these standards come into conflict. Milo (1986, p. 455) argues that the disagreement here is not necessarily attributable to 'any disagreement in factual beliefs or to bad reasoning', but to a disagreement in *attitude* (see also McNaughton 1988, pp. 17, 29). Consider the following hypothetical example to illustrate Milo's point.

Two nurses might both accept a moral standard which generally requires truth-telling, but may disagree on when this standard should apply. Nurse A, for instance, might favour (that is, have a 'pro-attitude' towards) telling the truth to patient X about a pessimistic medical diagnosis. Nurse B, on the other hand, might not favour (i.e. might have a 'con–attitude' towards) telling the truth to patient X about this diagnosis and prefer a pro–attitude to avoiding unnecessary suffering (e.g. as a result of a nocebo effect that might be inadvertently stimulated upon learning about the diagnosis). It is not that these two nurses have different criteria of relevance, as such, but rather have *different principles of priority* (Milo 1986, p. 457).

A second type of internal disagreement centres on what are to count as acceptable exceptions and limitations to otherwise mutually agreed moral standards. As Milo explains, we generally accept that moral standards are limited by other moral standards, as well as by the competing claims of self-interest. (Morality does not usually expect us to risk our own lives or our own important moral interest in morally troubling situations.) People might agree that as a general rule we ought all to make certain modest sacrifices in terms of our own interests (a minimal requirement of justice), but may disagree 'about what constitutes a modest sacrifice' (Milo 1986, p. 459). In many respects this type of disagreement could be loosely described as a disagreement in interpretation of an accepted moral standard. Consider another example.

Two nurses might agree that patients' rights should not be violated. Nurse A might further hold that, in situations involving violations of patients' rights, a nurse should act — even if this means threatening the nurse's job security (which nurse A views as a modest sacrifice). Nurse B, on the other hand, might agree that nurses should in principle act to prevent a patient's rights from being violated, but disagree that nurses should do so if they stand to lose their jobs as a result (something which nurse B views as an unacceptable and extreme sacrifice). What these two nurses are essentially disagreeing about is not the moral standard per se (that nurses should act to prevent violations of patients' rights), but about when morally relevant considerations can be and cannot be overridden by self-interest. In disagreements like this, and where the disagreement is based on preferences rather than attitude, there may well be no happy solution, a situation which Milo calls a 'moral deadlock' (1986, p. 461).

A third and final type of internal moral disagreement centres on the selection and applicability of accepted ethical standards. This kind of disagreement has nothing to do with whether a standard can be overridden by other considerations, but concerns whether it should have been selected or appealed to in the first place.

For example, two nurses may agree that killing an innocent human being is wrong. They may disagree, however, that abortion is wrong. Nurse A, for example, might argue that, since the fetus is not a human being, abortion does not entail the killing of an innocent human being and therefore is not wrong. Appealing to a moral standard prohibiting the killing of innocent human life would then, for nurse A, be quite irrelevant. Nurse B, on the other hand, may argue that the fetus is a human being, and therefore abortion, since it entails killing an innocent human being, is absolutely morally wrong. Appealing to a moral standard prohibiting the killing of innocent human life would then, for nurse B, be supremely relevant. The disagreement between these two nurses hinges very much on a disagreement about the moral relevance of the facts on what constitutes a human being.

RADICAL MORAL DISAGREEMENT

Milo (1986) identifies two types of radical moral disagreement: the first type he calls 'partial radical moral disagreement', and the second type 'total radical moral disagreement'.

In cases of *partial radical moral disagreement*, dissenting parties might agree on some criteria of relevance but not all. For example, a nurse might argue that directly killing terminally and chronically ill patients with a lethal injection is morally wrong, whereas merely 'letting nature take its course' or 'letting patients die' is not morally wrong. Another nurse might agree that directly killing terminally and chronically ill patients is wrong, but thoroughly disagree that merely 'letting patients die' is less morally offensive. Here there may be no court of appeal to reconcile the distinction between direct 'killing' and merely 'letting die'. In this case, partial radical disagreement is very similar to internal moral disagreement. It may be very difficult to distinguish between the two, a point which Milo reluctantly concedes.

In cases of *total radical moral disagreement*, disputants do not agree on any criteria of relevance, and do not share any basic moral principles. For Milo (1986, p. 469), this is 'the most extreme kind of moral disagreement that one can imagine'.

An example of total radical moral disagreement would be where two theatre nurses radically disagree with each other about the moral acceptability of organ transplantations. Nurse A argues that retrieving or harvesting organs from so-called 'cadavers' is an unmitigated act of murder, since the person whose organs are being retrieved is not yet fully dead. (Nurse A, in this instance, rejects brain–death criteria as indicative of death.) Nurse A also argues that, even if the potential cadaver is restored to nothing more than a persistent vegetative state, and even if another person may die as a result of not getting a life-saving organ transplant operation, this does not justify violating the sanctity of life of the potential organ donor. The death of another person through not receiving a new organ, while 'unfortunate', cannot be helped. Such are the tragic twists of life.

Nurse B, on the other hand, argues that retrieving organs is nothing like murder since, among other things, the person is already dead. (Nurse B, in this instance, totally accepts brain–death criteria as indicative of death.) Nurse B also totally rejects a 'sanctity of life' view, arguing that it has no substance; only quality of life considerations have ethical meaning. Nurse B further argues that, even conceding the unreliability of brain–death criteria as indicative of death, retrieving the organs is still morally permissible, since the donating person can at best look forward only to a 'vegetative existence' and one devoid of any 'quality of life' (which is cruel and immoral), whereas an organ recipient could look forward to a renewed quality of life.

In the dispute between nurse A and nurse B, resolution is unlikely. As Milo points out, in total radical disagreement the disputants reach a total and irreconcilable impasse. The possibility of this situation occurring in health care contexts is, I believe, something which needs to be taken very seriously, and which has important implications for conscientious objection claims (an issue that is given separate consideration in Chapter 13 of this book).

It should be clarified here that, while moral disagreements can certainly be problematic (particularly if a person's life and wellbeing are hanging in the balance, and an immediate decision is needed about what should be done), these need not be taken as constituting grounds upon which morality as such should be viewed with scepticism or, worse, rejected altogether. As Stout (1988, p. 14) argues persuasively, the facts of moral disagreement 'don't *compel* us to become nihilists or sceptics, to abandon the notions of moral truth and justified moral belief'. One reason for this, he explains, is that moral disagreement is, in essence, just a kind of moral diversity or, as he calls it, 'conceptual diversity' (Stout 1988, pp. 15, 61). While moral disagreement may rightly challenge us to 'meticulously disentangle' diverse and conflicting moral points of view, it does not preclude or threaten the possibility of moral judgment per se, either within a particular culture or across many cultures (Stout 1988, p. 15).

As argued previously, moral disagreement has historically been the beginning of critical moral thinking, not its end. Given this, there is room to suggest that we should be very cautious in accepting Milo's pessimistic conclusions about the irreconcilability of radical moral disagreement. Instead, we should look towards a more optimistic solution, and view such disagreements as an important and necessary opportunity for 'enriching [our] conceptions of morality through comparative inquiry' (Stout 1988, p. 70), and thereby augment our collective wisdom about what morality is, and what it really means to *be* moral in a world characterised by individual and collective (cultural) diversity. In the ultimate analysis, the solution to the problematic of moral disagreement may not be to engage in adversarial dialogue (fight/litigate), or even to negotiate a happy medium between conflicting views (compromise). Rather, the solution may be, to borrow from Edward de Bono (1985), to engage in 'triangular thinking'; to engage in moral disagreement, not as a judge or as a negotiator, but as a 'creative designer' who is able to escape the imprisonment of the positivist logic and language that is so characteristic of mainstream Western moral discourse, and to engage in moral disagreement as someone who is able ultimately to resolve the conflicts and disagreements which others have long since abandoned as hopeless and irreconcilable impasses. Such an approach, however, requires not just an ability to think about new things, but, as Catharine MacKinnon (1987, p. 9) puts it, to engage in 'a new way of thinking'. Possible approaches to dealing effectively with moral disagreements and disputes will be considered shortly in this chapter under the subheading 'Dealing with moral disagreements and disputes'.

Moral dilemmas

Another significant moral problem to be considered here (and one which has been widely discussed in both nursing and bioethical literature) is that of the proverbial 'moral dilemma' (also called 'ethical dilemma'). Broadly speaking, a dilemma may be defined as a situation requiring choice between what seem to be two equally desirable or undesirable alternatives; it may also be described as an 'awful feeling of being stuck'. A moral dilemma, however, is a little different, and can occur in one of several forms.

First, a moral dilemma can occur in the form of *logical incompatibility* between two different moral principles. For example, two different moral principles might apply equally in a given situation, and neither principle can be chosen without violating the other. Even so, a choice has to be made. Consider the case of a nurse who accepts a moral principle which demands respect for the sanctity of life, and who also accepts another moral principle (non-maleficence) which demands that persons should be spared intolerable suffering. Now, imagine this nurse in the situation of caring for a terminally ill patient who is suffering intolerable and intractable pain. In this situation, if the nurse accepts the sanctity of life principle, the administration of the large and potentially lethal doses of narcotics that might be required to relieve the patient's intolerable pain would probably be prohibited. On the other hand, if the principle of non-maleficence were followed, the nurse might be required to administer the potentially lethal doses of narcotics, even though this could hasten the patient's death. In this situation, the nurse is unavoidably confronted with the profound and troubling dilemma that to uphold the sanctity of life principle could violate the principle of non-maleficence, and to uphold the principle of non-maleficence could violate the sanctity of life principle. The ultimate question posed for the nurse in this situation is: which principle ought I to choose?

The options open to the nurse are:

- to modify the principles in question so that they do not conflict (i.e. by adding 'riders' to them);
- to abandon one principle in favour of the other;
- to abandon both principles in favour of a third (for example, autonomy and respect for the patient's rational wishes, or the virtue of compassion).

It should be noted that none of these options is free of moral risk.

A second type of moral dilemma is that involving *competing moral duties*. Consider the following case. A nurse working in a specialised unit is assigned a patient with a known history of drug addiction, and is instructed to chaperone the patient when there are visitors to make sure that illicit drugs are not 'slipped in'. The nurse, however, believes that the duty to protect this patient from harm (such as might occur from receiving illicit drugs) competes with the duty to respect the patient's privacy. The question for the nurse in this scenario is: which duty ought I to fulfil?

In another case, a nurse is assigned a patient of traditional Greek background who has recently been diagnosed with metastatic cancer. The doctor has ordered that the patient not be told his diagnosis. The patient, however, keeps asking the nurse and his family for information about his diagnosis. The family knows the diagnosis, but wants the doctor to tell the patient. Here the nurse is caught between a duty to tell the truth to the patient, and a duty to respect the wishes of the family. The nurse is also bound to follow the doctor's directives (although the question of whether there is a *duty* to follow them is another matter). The question for the nurse in this scenario is, again: which duty ought I to fulfil — my duty to the patient or to the family, or to the doctor, or to whom?

Philosophical answers to questions raised by a conflict of duty are varied and controversial. In the classic work *The right and the good*, W. D. Ross (1930) argues that duties are prima facie or 'conditional' in nature. Thus, when two duties conflict, we must 'study the situation' as fully as we can until we are able to reach a 'considered opinion (it is never more) that in the circumstances one of them [the duties] is more incumbent than any other' (Ross 1930, p. 19). Once we have worked out which of the conflicting duties is the more 'incumbent' on us, we are bound to consider it our prima facie duty in that situation. Richard Hare (1981, p. 26), however, takes quite a different view. He argues that, if we find ourselves caught between what appear to be two conflicting duties, we need to look again. For it is likely that, in the case of an apparent conflict in duties, one of our so-called 'duties' is not our duty at all; we have only mistakenly thought that it was. In other words, what happens here is that one of the two apparently conflicting duties is eventually 'cancelled out', so to speak.

Williams (1973) disagrees. While he believes that one of the conflicting *oughts* has to be rejected (but only in the sense that both conflicting duties/oughts cannot be acted upon), he does not agree that this means that the duties or oughts in question do not apply equally in the situation at hand, or that one of the conflicting duties must inevitably be 'cancelled out'. To the contrary: our reasoning may assist us to deal with a conflict of duty and may assist us to find a 'best' way to act, but this does not mean that we abandon one or other of the duties in question. How do we know?

Even after making a choice between two conflicting duties, we are still left with a lingering feeling of 'regret'. And it is this very feeling of regret which tells us that we have not altogether abandoned or 'cancelled out' the duty we decided could not, in that situation, be also acted upon.

In the drug addict case, we might well side with Richard Hare and unanimously agree that the nurse is mistaken in a belief that there is an overriding duty to respect the patient's privacy, and that clearly the primary duty is to prevent the patient from suffering the harms likely to be incurred by the administration of illicit drugs. But here the question arises: Is it really a nurse's duty to act as a kind of police warden? What if the patient is not receiving any form of therapy for the immediate drug addiction problem, and is at risk of developing severe and life-threatening withdrawal symptoms? How is the nurse's duty to 'prevent harm' to be regarded in this instance? Does cancelling out one of the conflicting duties here relieve the moral tension created in this scenario? Or is there more to be achieved by exploring ways in which they can be reconciled with each other?

In the cancer diagnosis case, we might unanimously agree that the nurse's primary duty is to the patient, and that any apparent duty owed to the family is not a bona fide one (after all, does not the moral principle of autonomy demand respect for the patient's rational wishes in this scenario?). Placed in a cultural context, however, the scenario takes on a whole new dimension. As was considered in Chapter 4 of this book, families from a traditional cultural background often play a fundamental and highly protective role in mediating the flow of information to a sick loved one. To ignore a family's request in such a situation could be to risk terrible violence to the wellbeing of the patient. Where this is likely, it is imperative that the nurse works closely with the family and ensures that the transfer of information to the patient is handled in a *culturally appropriate manner*. While the family may be perceived as 'interfering', in reality it may be providing an important and key link in ensuring that the patient's wellbeing and moral interests are fully upheld (an issue that will be explored further in Chapter 6, page 140). Cancelling out one of the duties in this scenario is unlikely to relieve the moral tension generated by the patient's request for and the doctor's refusal to give the medical information on the patient's diagnosis. Had the only criterion for action been what superficially appeared to be a primary duty to the patient, the nurse may have unwittingly facilitated the flow of information in a culturally *inappropriate* and thus harmful manner. By reconciling the apparent conflict in duties, and by working closely with the family, however, the nurse is able to facilitate the flow of information to the patient in a culturally appropriate and thus less harmful manner. In this instance, by fulfilling the duty owed to the family, the nurse could also succeed in fulfilling the duty owed to the patient.

It might be objected that the examples given here do not involve difficult cases, and that the required choices are relatively easy to make. But even if we admit 'hard cases', Hare's position is somehow unsatisfactory, as is his argument that when there is an apparent conflict in duties, it is likely that one of the duties involved is not our duty at all. There is always room to question how we can ever be really sure that a 'cancelled' duty was not our duty in the first place. The cancer diagnosis case, I think, illustrates this point well. Ross's and Williams's positions, on the other hand, remind us that matters of moral duty are never clear-cut; and, further, that we always have to be very careful in our appraisal of given situations and in the choices we make regarding to whom our moral duties are owed and what our moral duties actually are.

A third kind of moral dilemma, and one closely related to a dilemma concerning competing duties, is that entailing *competing and conflicting interests*. Here the question raised for the moral observer is: whose interests ought I to uphold?

Consider the following case. A clinical teacher on clinical placement at a residential care home was informed by a student that an elderly demented resident had been physically and verbally abused by one of the ward's permanent staff members, as witnessed by the student. The clinical teacher was temporarily undecided about what to do. It was a very serious matter — and, indeed, a very serious accusation — but it would be very difficult to prove. If the incident was not reported to the home's nursing administrator, the staff member concerned would probably continue to abuse the home's residents. If the incident was reported, there was a risk that the interests of both students and the school of nursing could be threatened. (The home's administrator might, for example, refuse to continue allowing students to be placed at the home for the purposes of gaining clinical experience.) The dilemma for the clinical teacher was whether or not to report the matter and thereby protect both the students' and the school's interests in having continued clinical placements, or to report the matter fully, whatever the consequences to the school and the students, and thereby protect the residents' interests.

The teacher and the student mutually agreed that the matter was too serious to ignore and decided they would risk the consequences of reporting the incident. The exercise, as feared, proved extremely distressing and painful for both the student concerned and the clinical teacher. The accused staff member denied having abused the elderly resident, and in turn accused the student of lying and of being the one who had really committed the abuses. The opinion of the patient could not be sought, as the elderly resident concerned was demented. Fortunately, the matter was eventually resolved to everyone's satisfaction. The administrator took the allegation seriously and, later, took the initiative to emphasise to *all* staff the importance of protecting and upholding residents' rights. The student was reassured that she had done the 'right thing', and that she had fulfilled her professional and moral obligations both (i) in *reporting* the incident, and (ii) in the *manner* in which she had reported it (i.e. she had followed proper processes). The clinical supervisor and administrator reached an agreement that any matters of concern discussed during clinical teaching placements be referred directly and immediately to the administrator for action. The staff member who was the subject of the unsubstantiated allegation was counselled in confidence by the administrator.

A fourth type of dilemma is taken from a feminist moral perspective, and is described by Gilligan (1982, 1987) in terms of being caught between attachments to people and trying to decide upon ways that will avoid 'hurting' each of these 'attached people'. Gilligan uses the example of a woman contemplating an abortion; she argues that generally a woman faced with having to make a choice in this situation 'contemplates a decision that affects both self and others and engages directly the critical moral issue of hurting' (Gilligan 1982, p. 71). Here the question to be raised in contemplating a difficult choice is: how can I avoid hurting the people to whom I am attached?

It might be objected here that Gilligan's sense of 'hurt' and 'avoiding hurt' is not very different from the general moral principle of non-maleficence and its demand to avoid or prevent 'harm'. While I concede that 'hurt' is a type of harm, there is a subtle distinction between 'hurt' in the sense that I think Gilligan is using it and 'harm' in an abstract sense as used by philosophers. It is important to draw a distinction between these two notions so as not to obscure other important distinctions which can be drawn in our moral discourse. Let us examine this point a little more fully.

The sense in which 'hurt' is being used here is not simply 'physical', but rather existential, spiritual, and even 'soulful' or 'soul-felt'. There is even room to make the radical claim that the notion of 'avoiding hurt' is not being asserted as a *principle* as such, but more as an *attitude*, and one which reminds us that we need to take very special care in our selection, interpretation and application of general moral principles in our everyday personal and professional lives. In short, it is an attitude which serves to *mediate* the use of more general moral principles. Consider, for example, the demand to 'avoid hurt' in a situation involving a patient who has yet to be told an unfavourable medical diagnosis. The demand to 'avoid hurt' reminds us that it is not enough just to *give* the patient the diagnosis (as may otherwise be required by the moral principle of autonomy), but that it must also be given in a caring, compassionate and culturally appropriate manner. Furthermore, it is not clear to me that the principle of non-maleficence fully captures the demand to be caring, compassionate and culturally appropriate in manner when performing such an unpleasant task as giving someone an unfavourable medical diagnosis. And in some instances, taken to its extreme, the principle of non-maleficence might even instruct that the diagnosis should not be given at all. 'Avoiding hurt', on the other hand, recognises that the information that needs to be given could be 'harmful' and is probably 'hurtful', but that there is a way of *lessening* if not *avoiding* this harm and hurt. To illustrate this point, consider the following case (told to me by a nursing colleague).

A young doctor walked into a patient's room, stood at the end of the bed, and in full view and hearing distance of other patients in the room, and without greeting the patient or smiling, stated abruptly: 'We've looked at your throat and the lump you have there is cancer'. Without another word, the doctor then briskly walked off. The patient had previously expressed a desire to know the diagnosis when it was available, so in many respects we could conclude that the doctor acted 'ethically' in that the patient's wishes had been respected and the requested information had been relayed to the patient. What is evident in this case is that the doctor had not considered ways to give the information less 'hurtfully' — or, if such ways had been considered, they were not heeded. For example, the doctor might have at least greeted the patient, used a compassionate tone of voice, drawn the curtains around the patient before speaking, sat down on a chair to be at the same level as the patient, and stayed long enough to allow the patient to ask questions, which the patient stated later would have been desirable. If the doctor felt inadequate to deal with this situation, it might have been advisable to wait until a colleague or a nurse was available to accompany him. Or, more simply, the doctor should have passed the task over to someone else who was more experienced and better prepared to deal with the situation. By using such an abrupt manner, the doctor not only failed to 'avoid hurt', but exacerbated it. To make matters worse, the diagnosis given to the patient later turned out to be incorrect. At the time of learning that in fact there was no cancer, the patient was still in a state of psychological shock. This could have been avoided had the situation been handled more compassionately and caringly, and with an attitude intent on 'lessening hurt'. Within the same week, two other patients confided in my colleague that they had undergone similar experiences with the same doctor.

Of course, doctors are not the only ones who have exhibited hurtful attitudes towards others. I have seen many instances where nurses have likewise failed to avoid or to lessen the hurt of a given situation. I recall the tragic case of a middle-aged man who was dying from advanced cancer. A close friend and members of his family were greatly distressed about his deteriorating condition, and even accused the nursing staff of 'trying to kill' their loved one by giving him morphine for his pain. On one occasion the nursing staff observed the family friend clutching his friend and pleading with him not to accept the morphine injections, telling him: 'don't you see, they are killing you! They are killing you! You don't have to have them …'. The nursing staff tried to get the friend to leave, but he refused to go. When he became abusive, the nursing staff contacted a hospital security officer, and he was forcibly removed. There is, I believe, room to speculate about this case: had the friend's grief been properly addressed by the nursing staff, and the dynamics and benefits of effective pain management fully explained to him, both he, and the patient, the patient's family and attending nursing staff would have been spared the 'hurt' that this tragic situation caused.

These two cases demonstrate that 'avoiding hurt' is not something that can be fully directed or achieved by an abstract moral principle. Rather, it requires that we draw heavily on our past experience, knowledge, intuition, feelings, and interpersonal skills, as well as on a thorough and systematic analysis of the facts of the situation at hand.

Moral stress, moral distress and moral perplexity[2]

It has long been recognised that nurses experience moral stress, moral distress and moral outrage during the course of their work (see, for example, Severinsson 2003; Sundin-Huard and Fahy 1999; Tiedje 2000; Corley and Raines 1993; Andersen 1990; Cahn 1989; Wilkinson 1987/88; Andrews and Fargotstein 1986; Jameton 1984). Defined as 'the psychological disequilibrium and negative feeling state experienced when a person makes a moral decision but does not follow through by performing the moral behaviour indicated by that decision' (Wilkinson 1987/88, p. 16), moral stress/distress can arise in a number of situations. Jameton (1984, p. 6) points out, for example, that nurses experience moral distress when they know the right thing to do, 'but institutional constraints make it nearly impossible to pursue the right course of action'. In such instance, unchecked moral stress and distress can turn into moral outrage which can, in turn, compound the original distress. Andersen explains (1990, p. 9):

> Moral outrage is a product of the emotional turbulence, pain, incredulity, indignation, and rage that … occurs when a logical attempt to solve a moral problem results in denial of the problem and an assault on the nurse's integrity by those who have sacrificed their integrity and the welfare of patients to preserve the status quo of submarginal performance. The psychobiological remnants of moral distress are then compounded by the experience of moral outrage.

Moral distress can also follow from moral perplexity, taken here to be a state of moral confusion or bewilderment that arises when a person is faced with a morally problematic situation, recognises it (the situation) as being morally problematic, has the resources for dealing with it, but genuinely does not know what is the right thing to do. Nurses can and do suffer moral perplexity when confronted with a range of moral problems (examples of which are given in this book). Perhaps among the most perplexing of moral problems faced by nurses are those otherwise known as moral dilemmas and moral disagreements (just discussed above). These problems can be particularly perplexing in instances where it becomes apparent that, due to a variety of reasons, they may not be or indeed are not amenable to resolution.

Making moral decisions

When encountering a moral problem, there comes a point at which we have to decide what to do about it and how best to go about doing what we have decided; that is, how best to address the problem (or problems) we have encountered. Invariably, when encountering a moral problem, the question arises of: 'How do I decide what to do?' and 'How, if at all, should I act on what I have decided?'. Before considering these questions, it would be useful to first clarify what a moral decision is and the various processes that might be used for making moral decisions. Following this, attention will then be given to examining briefly how to deal with moral disagreements and disputes in workplace contexts.

Moral decision-making — a working definition

The word 'decision' (from the Latin *dēcisiō*, literally a 'cutting off') may be defined as 'a judgment, conclusion or resolution reached or given'; it may also be defined as 'the act of making up one's mind' (*Collins English Dictionary*, 2003). A moral decision may be similarly defined, that is, as a moral judgment, moral conclusion or moral resolution reached or given, notably, about what constitutes 'right' and 'wrong' conduct. Moral decision-making may be further defined as that which is fundamentally concerned with reconciling moral disagreements between disputing parties, each of whom may hold equally valid moral viewpoints and may reach different yet reasonable conclusions on what constitutes 'right' and 'wrong' conduct in a given context (Wong 1992). These two different yet related aspects of moral decision-making are depicted in Figure 5.3.

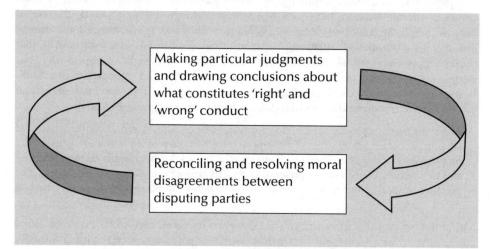

Making particular judgments and drawing conclusions about what constitutes 'right' and 'wrong' conduct

Reconciling and resolving moral disagreements between disputing parties

Figure 5.3 Two aspects of moral decision-making

An essential and distinguishing feature of moral decisions is that they are based on and informed by *moral considerations*, which are regarded as paramount to the moral decision-making process. Another distinguishing feature of moral decisions is that they provide a definitive starting point from which moral action can be taken in order to prevent moral harms from occurring and to promote morally desirable or at least tolerable outcomes (see Figure 5.4).

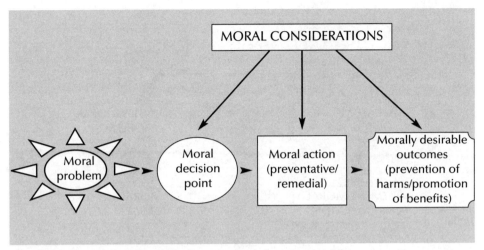

Figure 5.4 Distinguishing features of moral decision-making

Processes for making moral decisions

Moral decisions can be made either by an individual (e.g. a nurse, doctor, and so on) or by a collective entity (e.g. a health care team, a stakeholder group, or a committee). In either case, the decision-making process needs to be approached with the utmost diligence and vigilance. Decision makers need to take particular care in ensuring that a careful appraisal is made of the relevant *facts* of the matter as well as of the *values* that are operating in the given context at hand. One reason for this is that facts/values can each exert considerable influence on the other and, as a consequence, may even lead to profound changes in our conceptions of them and hence the moral decision we ultimately make. This is because, as Benjamin (2001, p. 25) explains:

> What counts as relevant factual considerations may change as explorations of an ethical issue progresses. In some cases, facts considered important at the outset fade into the background as others, barely noticed at first, come to the fore. In others [...] we not merely replace one set of factual considerations with another, but the facts either alter our ethical values and principles or we revise factual consideration in the light of values and principles.

One way of ensuring that moral decision-making is approached in a diligent and vigilant way is to use a systematic step-by-step decision-making process, much like the five-step decision-making process that has become universally associated with the nursing process. Such a five-step process requires moral decision-makers to:

1. assess the situation (including making a diligent appraisal of the relevant facts of the matter and operating values in the situation at issue);
2. diagnose or identify the moral problem(s) at hand;
3. set moral goals and plan an appropriate moral course of action to address the moral problems identified;
4. implement the plan of moral action;
5. evaluate the moral outcomes of the action implemented.

(Note: in the event that a morally desirable outcome has not been achieved, this process will need to be repeated.)

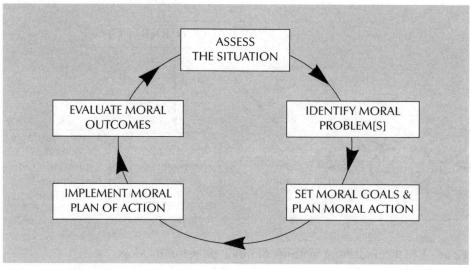

Figure 5.5 Moral decision-making model

This model may be expressed diagrammatically as shown in Figure 5.5.

It needs to be clarified at this point that when using a systematic moral decision-making process, deliberations during each of the steps identified involve appeals to reason, emotion and intuition, with each of these, in turn, being informed or 'fine tuned' by life experience (see Figure 5.6, page 117). Moral decision-making also requires moral imagination — that is, an ability to reflect and imagine possible moral 'futures' (options) and solutions to problems, and possible ways of progressing these even in situations that are hostile to moral considerations and which may also involve a 'moral deadlock' (see also Johnson 1993; Tuan 1989). Since the role of reason, emotion, intuition, and life experience in moral decision-making is not always understood and, ironically, has itself been the subject of moral dispute, some further discussion of it is warranted here. Consider the following.

Reason and moral decision-making

Throughout history dating back to the days of the Ancient Greek philosophers, it has been popularly assumed (and argued) by moral philosophers that, in order for a moral decision to be 'sound', it must be based on rational or 'reasoned' (abstract) moral principles of conduct. The thinking behind this view (which dates back to the works of the ancient Greek philosophers) is that, unlike *feelings* (e.g. emotion and intuition which are, by their nature, value-laden and subjective), *reason* is value-neutral and objective, and therefore more reliable and hence supreme as an enlightened authority on how best to conduct one's behaviour in the world of competing self-interest. By this view, *to be rational is to be moral* since, by upholding rationality as the supreme principle of morality, decision-makers will be able to avoid the 'corrupting influences of the passions' and thereby avoid falling prey to deciding in favour of their own self-interests.

An influential advocate of this view was the German philosopher, Immanuel Kant (1724–1804).

Kant contended that what distinguished human beings from other (non-human) beings was their capacity to reason. His reasoning behind this view was that *reason is free* (i.e. *autonomous*) to *formulate moral law* (something that animals, for example, cannot do) and to determine just what is to count as being an overriding moral duty — the basis of all moral actions. A duty, according to Kant, is that which is *done for its own sake* — for its own intrinsic moral worth — and 'not for the results it attains or seeks to attain' (Kant 1972, p. 20). What is to count as one's duty, in turn, is determined by appealing to some formal (reasoned) principle or 'maxim'. In choosing such a principle or maxim, however, decision-makers must take care not to choose something which serves merely to uphold their own individual interests or to satisfy their own unruly desires. Indeed, Kant went on to assert that it is precisely because of our human weaknesses (especially our inclinations towards satisfying our own desires and interests) that the maxim we adopt must have the characteristics of being a universally valid 'law' — that is, something which 'commands or compels obedience' and which is binding on all persons equally (Kant 1972, p. 21).

Kant believed that moral considerations are always overriding ones. Thus, in situations where a number of considerations are competing (for instance, between practical, economic, political, moral and cultural considerations), it is always the moral considerations which should 'win out'. For example, if a nurse is in the position of having to decide whether to risk losing his or her job (a practical consideration) by exposing the unethical conduct of a supervisor (a moral consideration), it is the moral consideration which is, according to Kant's view, the weightier of the two; the nurse, by this analysis, should expose the supervisor.

As well as holding that moral considerations should always override non-moral considerations, Kant maintained that moral imperatives (as based on universal moral law) are by their very nature unconditional, absolute and inescapable. This means that moral imperatives, or duties in this instance, are both overriding and binding regardless of their consequences. Therefore we, as rational autonomous moral choosers, cannot escape the demands which a moral imperative may place upon us; the bottom line, according to Kant, is that we are absolutely required and therefore compelled to fulfil our moral duties. By this view, morally decent persons are those who fulfil their duties and who are not distracted by self-interested or practical considerations; morally indecent persons, on the other hand, are those who shirk or abandon their moral duties — probably in favour of other considerations such as the pursuit of material self-interest and pleasure. How do we know this? According to Kant, because reason tells us it is so. This viewpoint remains influential today.

Emotion and moral decision-making

Not everyone agrees that reason is the supreme principle of morality or that reason provides a more reliable guide to moral decision-making and action than other human faculties such as emotion or intuition. The Scottish philosopher David Hume (1711–76), for example, maintained that 'reason is, and ought only to be, the slave of the passions and can never pretend to any other office than to serve and obey them' (Hume 1888, p. 415).

Hume rejected reason or science as having ultimate moral authority, arguing that these things are nothing more than the 'comparing of ideas and the discovery of their relations' (Hume 1888, p. 466). He regarded reason as 'utterly impotent' (p. 457) in moral domains and said that it is 'perfectly inert, and can never either prevent or produce any action or affection' (p. 458). The only power reason has, in Hume's conceptual framework, is to shape beliefs — and, even then, beliefs cannot be relied upon to move one to action, unless they are relevant to the satisfaction of some passion, desire or need (Harmon 1977, p. 5).

The question remains, how do Hume's views capture the making of moral judgments and decisions? In essence, Hume's morality is something to be 'properly felt' rather than 'rationally judged', with goods and evils being known simply by particular sensations of pleasure and pain (Hume 1888, p. 470). He argued (p. 469):

> Nothing can be more real, or concern us more, than our own sentiments of pleasure and uneasiness; and if these be favourable to virtue, and unfavourable to vice, no more can be requisite to the regulation of our conduct and behaviour.

In summary, Hume's account of morality sees the sensations of pleasure (moral sentiments) as distinguishing that which is virtuous, and the sensations of pain or uneasiness as distinguishing that which is vicious. If something appears either virtuous or vicious, there is no reason to doubt that appearance or to resist an inclination to act in response to them. On this point, Hume argued famously that 'Tis not contrary to reason to prefer the destruction of the whole world to the scratching of my finger' (Hume 1888, p. 416). In other words, it is perfectly 'reasonable', paradoxically, to respond to and act upon a sentiment or sensation.

Hume has not been alone in his critique of reason as a moral action guide. The supremacy and role of rationality and 'pure practical reason' in moral decision-making has also been challenged more recently both by moral philosophers (particularly feminist philosophers) and by biomedical scientists. The contemporary British philosopher, Alasdair MacIntyre, for example, raises the provocative question: 'What is it about rational argument which is so important that it is the nearly universal appearance assumed by those who engage in moral conflict?' (MacIntyre 1985, p. 9). His short answer to this is that there is nothing compelling or important about it at all. If anything, the rational paradigm of moral argument is uncomfortably aligned with a 'disquieting private arbitrariness' (MacIntyre 1985, p. 8). What appears to be a 'rational' approach is not a rational approach at all, at least not in the genuine 'critically reflective' sense. Philosophical opponents enter into moral debates with their minds already firmly made up. Their lack of irrefutable criteria to convince their opponents inevitably sees what should be an instructive and enlightening debate reduced to nothing more than a battleground characterised by dogmatic assertions and counter-assertions (MacIntyre 1985, p. 8). Small wonder, MacIntyre ponders, that 'we become defensive and therefore shrill' in our public arguments.

Feminist moral philosophers have also been extremely critical of reason being regarded as the supreme principle of morality. In their critiques of this assertion, they have resoundedly rejected the view that reason (1) is 'value-neutral' (they assert that reason is no more objective than the subjectivity that prefers and values it [Gatens 1986, p. 25]), and (2) is a reliable guide to sound moral decision-making and action (Walker 1998; Addelson 1994; Tronto 1993; Cole and Coultrap-McQuin 1992; Frazer et al. 1992; Holmes and Purdy 1992; Sherwin 1992; Card 1991; Porter 1991; Brabeck 1989; Code et al. 1988; Hoagland 1988; Andolsen et al. 1987; Kittay and Meyers 1987; Braidotti 1986; Gatens 1986; Grimshaw 1986; Noddings 1984; Harding and Hintikka 1983). They have also raised serious questions as to why reason should be regarded as having any more authority in moral thinking and decision-making than the moral sentiments of, for example, empathy, compassion, sympathy, kindness, friendliness or caring. The short answer to this question is, that it does not and any assertion to the contrary is utterly baseless and contrary to life experience.

Biomedical scientists have also argued persuasively that sound and effective moral decision-making requires an appeal to emotion and intuition as well as to reason. In a popular work on the subject, entitled *Descartes error: emotion, reason, and the human brain*, the renowned neurologist Antonio Damasio (1994) presents a persuasive account of the crucial role of emotion in moral decision-making. In this book, Damasio examines a number of case studies involving people who have suffered serious brain injuries. Significantly, his research has found that, under certain circumstances, just as *too much* emotion can disrupt reason, so too can *too little* emotion. Calling into question traditional accounts of the relationship between reason and emotion, Damasio (1994, p. 53) suggests that a reduction in emotion may, paradoxically, 'constitute an equally important source of irrational behaviour'. It can also give rise to annihilistic decision-making. On the basis of observations made of people with 'defective emotional modulation' (in particular, those who could be described as being 'flat' in emotion and feeling), Damasio concludes that there is a significant 'interaction of the systems underlying the normal processes of emotion, feeling, reason, and decision-making'; where the emotion centres of the brain are affected adversely, so too is a person's capacity to make important life-sustaining (moral) judgments (Damasio 1994, pp. 40, 54). Significantly, this is so even in the case of where a brain-injured person's basic intellect, language ability, attention, perception, memory and language remain intact. In sum, to borrow from Damasio, a decline in the emotions can and do result in serious 'decision-making failures'.

Drawing on his scientific findings, Damasio (1994) goes on to warn of the inherent dangers to personal and interpersonal human relationships, and to human survival, of adopting a purely rationalistic and rule-bound approach to moral decision-making. He writes (p. 171):

> The 'high-reason' view, which is none other than the commonsense view, assumes that when we are at our decision-making best, we are the pride and joy of Plato, Descarte and Kant. Formal logic will, by itself, get us to the best available solution for any problem. An important aspect of the rationalist conception is that to obtain the best results, emotions must be kept *out*. Rational processing must be unencumbered by passion.

After outlining a step-by-step approach to 'pure' rational decision-making, Damasio continues (p. 72):

> Now, let me submit that if this strategy is the *only* one you have available, rationality, as described above, is not going to work. At best, your decision will take an inordinately long time, far more than acceptable if you are to get anything done that day. At worst, you may not even end up with a decision at all because you will get lost in the byways of your calculations. [...] You will lose track. Attention and working memory have a limited capacity. In the end, if purely rational calculations is how your mind normally operates, you might choose incorrectly and live to regret the error, or simply give up trying, in frustration.

He concludes that experience with brain-damaged patients such as those considered in his book suggest that 'the cool strategy advocated by Kant, among others, has far more to do with the way patients with prefrontal damage go about deciding than with how normals usually operate' (Damasio 1994, p. 172).

In contrast, 'integrated' decision-makers will fare much better. This is because somatic markers ('gut feelings'/emotions) help improve both the accuracy and efficiency of the decision-making process. Damasio explains (p. 173):

> [The somatic marker] focuses attention on the negative outcome to which a given action may lead, and functions as an automated alarm signal which says: Beware of danger ahead

if you choose the option which leads to this outcome. The signal may lead you to reject, *immediately*, the negative course of action and thus make you choose among other alternatives. The automated signal protects you against future losses, without further ado, and then allows you to choose from among fewer alternatives. There is still room for using a cost/benefit analysis and proper deductive competence, but only *after* the automated step drastically reduces the number of options.

Given the findings of Damasio's research, there is considerable room to suggest, contrary to the rationality thesis, that sound moral decision-making requires a collaboration between *reason* and *emotion*. Anything less could risk the practice of a defeatist and life-destructive ethic — that is, an ethical perspective that justifies annihilation rather than survival, such as is already evident in debates about 'just wars', and about euthanasia and assisted suicide.

Intuition and moral decision-making

Like emotion, intuition also has an important role to play in guiding moral judgments and moral decision-making. Like those who support the role of emotion in moral decision-making, supporters of *moral intuitionism* — the theory that moral principles and moral judgments are known to be true simply by intuition — reject outright the view that reason has ultimate moral authority (Frankena 1973, pp. 102–5) and claim, instead, that it is *intuition* that stands as the 'prime avenue to truth' (Goldberg 1983, p. 17).

The question remains, how does intuitionism actually determine the moral rightness or wrongness of a particular act? The short answer is that it determines the intrinsic good or bad nature of a given act, which in turn derives from the properties of that act — whether they are intrinsically good or bad. For example, an intuitionist might claim that the wilful act of leaving a child road-accident victim to die needlessly has the self-evident property of wrongness, whereas the thoughtful act of assisting and resuscitating a child road-accident victim and thereby preventing a needless and untimely death has the self-evident property of goodness.

The process of knowing by intuition the rightness or wrongness of an action goes something like this: first, properties making the act in question right or wrong must be determined. These properties in turn are classified as being either 'prima-facie right' (i.e. the 'rightness' of the properties may be overridden by stronger moral properties) or 'wrong, all things considered' (i.e. in light of other morally significant considerations, and when these considerations have been weighed up against each other, the act is wrong) (Baier 1978a, p. 415). For example, resuscitating a child road-accident victim may be regarded as 'prima-facie right' where other stronger moral considerations do not impinge (for example, the rescuer may risk her or his own life in the attempt to resuscitate or save the victim); whereas leaving the child road-accident victim to die needlessly might be regarded as 'wrong all things considered' (for example, when the rescuer is regarded as well qualified to instigate life-saving measures, and would be likely to succeed in the attempt, but is in too much of a hurry to stop, having promised to meet friends for a social dinner).

The second step involves determining the relative weight of given properties and deciding which imposes the more stringent of duties on a person to act. Once it has been decided which of the duties in question is the more stringent, the 'final duty', or 'duty, all things considered', can be established (Baier 1978a, p. 415). For example, once it is determined that the duty to save a child road-accident victim's life is more stringent than the duty to fulfil one's promise to friends to share a social meal with them, so too is it established that saving the life of the child road–accident victim is the 'final duty' or 'duty, all things considered'. How do we know this is our final duty, it might be asked? The answer: we 'just know', it is 'self-evident', and that is all there is to say on the matter.

Moral intuitionism is considered by many philosophers to be implausible. They have severely criticised intuitionism on the grounds that it is misleading; that it fails to answer important moral questions; that it is unable to define and analyse the properties to which ethical terms refer; that it lacks objectivity; that it fails to provide a theory of moral motivation (i.e. what motivates people to do morally good acts); that it fails to provide a convincing theory of moral justification; and, more seriously, that it cannot be relied upon to resolve moral conflict (Swanton 1987; Baier 1978a; Frankena 1973; Rawls 1971; Warnock 1967).

While these criticisms are serious, they should not be taken as implying that intuition has no role to play in moral or other forms of decision-making. Such a conclusion would be at odds with recent scientific and scholarly research demonstrating the nature of intuition and its practical importance to and in a range of activities characteristic of human living (see, for example, Davis-Floyd and Arvidson 1997). Furthermore, it is important to note that not all moral philosophers agree that intuition has no place in our moral schemes. For example, in his classic book *Moral Thinking: its levels, method and point*, Richard Hare (1981) concedes the role of intuition in moral thinking.

Although Hare completely rejects intuition as the basis of moral thinking, and rejects its independent ability to resolve moral conflict, he nevertheless accepts that (1981, p. 210):

> the intuitive level of moral thinking certainly exists and is (humanly speaking) an essential part of the whole structure.

Hare basically argues that neither intuition nor reason is adequate on its own to deal effectively with moral problems. A sounder or more complete approach to moral thinking and decision-making, he suggests, would be to admit a kind of 'collaborative relationship' between these two faculties and to cease viewing them as being necessary opponents (p. 44):

> Let us be clear, first of all, that critical and intuitive moral thinking are not rival procedures, as much of the dispute between utilitarians and intuitionists seem to suppose. They are elements in a common structure, each with its parts to play.

Admittedly, Hare views intuition in somewhat rationalistic terms. He regards intuition essentially as being comprised of prima-facie moral principles which have been selected by critical thinking or reason (Hare 1981, pp. 49–50). This might lead intuitionists to be somewhat suspicious of his account of moral thinking. However, it should not detract from the worth of Hare's thesis or the significant contribution it can make to the development of a more progressive and flexible moral theory.

Psychologists also stress the importance of intuition in our everyday practical and working lives, and the need to enhance it if we are to make better rational decisions. Goldberg (1983, p. 33) argues that intuition is very much a part of reason, and in fact plays a crucial role in aiding the reasoning process itself. Intuition does this by feeding and stimulating rational thought and then by evaluating its products. If a reason or a thought does not 'feel' right, the reasoner or thinker simply switches tracks. Goldberg even makes the radical suggestion that 'reason is merely slow intuition' (p. 37), and that intuition has a particularly important role to play when dealing with problems which are too complex to be solved by rational analysis (p. 23). Goldberg's thesis, again, is not incompatible with Hare's views, but his prescriptions are more fruitful. What is needed, concludes Goldberg (p. 28), is:

> a balance and a recognition of the intricate, mutually enhancing relationship between intuition and rationality. We need not just more intuition but better intuition. We need not only to trust it but to make it more trustworthy. And at the same time we need sharp, discriminating rationality.

Regardless of the classic objections raised against intuition, it has its place both in our moral thinking and in our everyday lives (see also Davis-Floyd and Arvidson 1997; Vaughan 1979). As Urmson (1975, p. 119) correctly points out, intuition is needed to weigh up the 'plurality of primary moral reasons for action', something which, in his view, is no cause for either surprise or distress. Why is this? The answer is that the need for an intuitive weighing up of a plurality of moral reasons is 'not an irrational anomaly but our ordinary predicament with regard to reasons in most fields' (Urmson 1975, p. 119).

Life experience and moral decision-making

It is becoming increasingly accepted that *life experience* is critical to the process of moral decision-making on account of its practical effects (both positive and negative) on the capacity of people to make sound moral choices in their daily lives and to take appropriate action based on those choices (Beauchamp and Childress 2001; Benjamin 2001; Little 2001; Moreno 1995; Walker 1998). It is also becoming increasingly recognised that moral viewpoints and the theoretical stances underpinning them are not set in stone, and that they can and do change (and sometimes ought to change) in the light of life experience and the new knowledge(s) gained in the process. As Anderson (1990, p. 258) points out, many have come to accept 'morality, and moral discourse, as a living and central element in human existence'. He explains (pp. 258–9):

> We see our interpersonal relationships as collaborative efforts in constructing values. We see education as, among other things, a training in the skills of moral reasoning — morality not merely handed down but learned and created and re-created out of experience. And when there is conflict about that, as there inevitably will be, we accept the conflict also as an arena for expressing and creating values ... Morals are not being handed down from the mountaintop on graven tablets; they are being created by people out of the challenges of the times. The morals of today are not the morals of yesterday, and they will not be the morals of tomorrow.

It is this possibility for creating and re-creating (changing) our moral viewpoints and refining the moral values that inform them that makes the project of reconciling disputes about moral matters possible, feasible, viable, hopeful and sustainable. Consider the following.

As discussed in Chapter 3 of this book, we seem to recognise and accept that some moral choices and actions are better than others (e.g. acts of kindness are better, morally speaking, than acts of cruelty). It is also evident that when some moral beliefs are shown to be 'wrong' or 'mistaken', people can and do change them. For instance, as Benjamin (2001, p. 26) explains:

> Some of us may have been raised to believe that black people, gay people, poor people, or rich people don't have the same basic hopes, fears, wishes, and values as we do, or that there

can be no morality without God, but what we read and experience for ourselves makes these [beliefs] seem doubtful.

Benjamin goes on to explain that when our beliefs are found to be at 'odds' with our life experiences we subsequently revise our beliefs to ensure a better (more coherent) 'fit' between them and our lived experiences. In instances where our background beliefs seem 'wrong' and lacking 'fit' with the world, Benjamin writes (p. 26):

> we revise our overall outlook to achieve a better overall fit among its elements. None of them is basic or sacrosanct. Each may be modified in the interests of the outlook's achieving greater overall breadth and coherence. Sometimes we'll revise an increasingly dubious particular judgment in the interests of coherence with some more secure values or principles or background beliefs and theories. At other times, we'll revise an obsolete value or principle to fit with a particular moral judgment and background belief and theory. In some cases ... we'll even revise a background belief or theory — our understanding of what the world is like — to square with particular judgments and values and principles.

Benjamin further contends that if we are to succeed in our quest to develop a practical and plausible approach to ethics — and one that will be successful in improving, if not resolving 'concrete practical problems' — then sometimes our moral viewpoints *have* to change; he contends (p. 25):

> Values and principles, in the light of experience, sometimes *have to* be revised, modified, or replaced. Moreover, in some cases, a commitment to certain ethical values and principles will *require* that we revise our understanding of the world, the facts. (emphasis added)

Reason, emotion, intuition and life experience — some further thoughts

Reason, emotion, intuition and life experience all have an important role to play in guiding our moral judgments and moral decision-making. Acting in 'collaboration', these processes can work effectively as 'mutually correcting resources in moral reflection' (Callahan 1988) and tutor, test and fine-tune our perceptions of and responses to moral problems in the workplace and elsewhere. This collaboration is expressed diagrammatically in Figure 5.6.

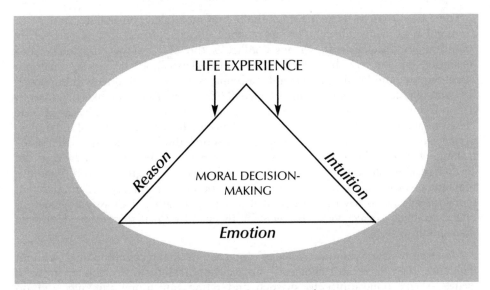

Figure 5.6 Processes influencing moral decision-making

Dealing with moral disagreements and disputes

As pointed out in Chapter One, moral problems and disagreements constitute an inevitable and unavoidable aspect of both our personal and professional lives. Wong (1992, p. 763) suggests that we might even expect serious conflict to feature *regularly* in our ethical lives, 'involving people with whom continuing relationships are both necessary and desirable'. One reason for this is that 'informed, thoughtful individuals will not always agree about complex moral and political issues' and 'a number of important conflicts will have no clear resolution' (Benjamin 2001, p.27). This is because (as already alluded to in this chapter, in the discussion on moral disagreement):

- different individuals can interpret the same evidence differently and draw quite different yet reasonable conclusions from that evidence;
- the evidence itself may be contradictory, leading reasonable people to draw reasonably different conclusions;
- even when individuals agree about what the relevant facts or considerations of a given matter are, they may nevertheless reasonably disagree about the weightings that should be given to the facts and considerations, and arrive at quite different conclusions (e.g. the debate about the moral permissibility of abortion and euthanasia rests more on disagreement about the *weightings* of relevant moral principles, than about the applicability of the moral principles per se);
- moral concepts are often ambiguous and open to a variety of interpretations; individuals may make different reasonable interpretations of these which, in turn, may lead to different though reasonable conclusions (adapted from Benjamin 2001 — citing Rawls 1971, 1993).

Compounding the problem of moral disagreements is that there are 'no neutral criteria for determining that one reasonable world view and way of life is in all respects superior to the others' (Benjamin 2001, p. 28).

The question that arises here is: How are we to respond to disagreements about moral matters and the conflicts that they sometimes give rise to? It is to briefly answering this question that the remainder of this chapter now turns.

There is a variety of ways in which the task of moral decision-making in the face of moral disagreement might be approached. One approach that is particularly promising for dealing with serious conflict is the little known approach called 'quantum morality' (Zohar 1991; Zohar and Marshall 1993, 2000). Quantum morality uses a model of thinking and reasoning associated with quantum physics or the 'new physics' as it is sometimes called (Heisenberg 1990). Unlike the *either/or* divisionary way of thinking commonly associated with the classical physics of Isaac Newton (and from which Western moral philosophy has borrowed heavily), this new perspective rests on a *both/and* approach to moral thinking and moral decision-making. Whereas the classical model of Western moral thinking advocates an adversarial approach to interrogating ideas and discovering 'the moral truth', quantum morality advocates a cooperative and creative approach that accepts many different moral viewpoints as having the potential to be right, rather than assuming there is only one single correct view that *must* be defended even if this means destroying other points of view.

Underpinning a 'quantum morality' approach is the recognition that without difference, there is no real choice — no real opportunity to develop, to grow, to evolve — no opportunity to sharpen and refine our moral thinking, and no opportunity to learn to understand another's point of view and to discover the 'creative unity in our differences' (Zohar and Marshall 1993, p. 273). Here, quantum morality takes as its starting point the view that being open to different viewpoints expands the potential of a situation, allows for more questions to be asked and more to be learnt, and ultimately allows for common ground to be found.

Moral decision-making, by this view, is seen as involving a shared and cooperative venture, where people have time and *can take time* to dialogue, to *really listen* to other people's points of view (and thereby give recognition to others by listening), and to negotiate choices that strike 'a creative balance between more fixed attitudes of control at the one extreme or total receptiveness at the other' (Zohar and Marshall 1993, p. 102). For this approach to work, however, participants must come to the moral deliberating process with a willingness to: (1) 'let go' their own point of view as the *only* point of view, and (2) to put their own views alongside others 'as one of many to be compared, contrasted and considered' (Zohar and Marshall 1993, p. 235). Through cooperative and creative dialogue, the differing viewpoints of all participants can evolve into a new 'synthesised' complex whole. In so far as evaluating whether the 'correct' choices have been made, the following applies: if the values and meanings of the choices break down 'and the moral equivalent of physical chaos sets in', the participants may conclude that 'everything has fallen apart' and that a morally good outcome has not been achieved (Zohar 1991, p.182). Conversely, if the values and meanings of the choices made do not break down, and the moral equivalent of physical order and unity sets in, the participants may conclude that everything has stayed together as a harmonious whole evolving toward a viable and sustainable future, and that a morally good outcome has been achieved.

Benjamin (2001), Moreno (1995), Wong (1992) and Jennings (1991), among others, argue along similar lines. These authors contend that, at the very least, moral decision-making in the face of moral disagreement must be approached in a consensual rather than a conflictive (adversarial) manner; democratically rather than dictatorially; with a genuine interest in and commitment to learning about moral differences and bridging the gap between them, instead of denigrating and dismissing differences as 'other' and hence deviant and wrong; and with a willingness to reciprocate rather than reproach attempts to create (new) common ground even — and, perhaps, especially — in instances where it may appear that none exists. In defence of a consensual and democratic approach to moral problem-solving, Benjamin argues (2001, p. 28):

> Balancing personal conviction with respect for reasonable differences, the democratic temperament combines the standpoints of agent and spectator. The trick – and part of being human – is being able to retain both standpoints while judiciously tacking between them.

Wong (1992), however, contends that in the case of serious moral conflict much more than 'democratic discussion' is required. He explains (p. 780):

> An openness to be influenced by others, to bridge differences, may also take the form of a preparedness to expand one's conception of the good and the right upon further understanding and appreciation of other ways of life. This sort of preparedness goes beyond what could be required by the ideal of fair and democratic discussion – beyond, for example, the passive virtue of being prepared to change one's views in the face of undermining evidence. Learning from others often requires instead an *active willingness* to gain a more vivid and detailed appreciation of what it is like to live their ways of life, an appreciation that can only be achieved through significant interaction with them [emphasis added].

Unfortunately, not all are willing to engage in a quantum moral approach to moral disagreements or to cultivate an 'active willingness to gain a more vivid and detailed appreciation of what it is like to live [others] ways of life'. Tragically, this unwillingness to consider other points of view has sometimes lead to moral disputes being expressed via extraordinary acts of violence, resulting in serious injuries to and even the deaths of people whose viewpoints moral dissidents do not share. For example, in 1993, Dr David Gunn, a medical practitioner engaged in abortion work at the Pensacola Women's Medical Services clinic in the Unites States, was fatally wounded by an anti-abortion demonstrator engaged in a pro-life protest outside of the clinic (Rohter 1993, p.7). Described by authorities as the first slaying of its kind in the United States, the incident exemplified the increasing violence against abortion clinics and workers across the nation. In regard to the death of Dr Gunn, Rescue America (a pro-life group) was reported as commenting that 'while Gunn's death is unfortunate, it's also true that quite a number of babies' lives will be saved' (Rohter 1993, p. 3).

Just over a year later, again in the Unites States, a second doctor was killed outside an abortion clinic by a pro-life protester (Sharkey 1994, p. 3). At the time, a British commentator on anti-abortion protests in the United States was reported as saying that the slaying was 'the start of the new Pro-Life movement, the new activism' (Sharkey 1994, p. 3). This new 'pro-life activism' has involved bombing and arson attacks against clinics, and the murder and injury of health workers. It has been reported that 'one hundred per cent of the bombers, arsonists and now murderers are Christian fundamentalists' (Sharkey 1994, p. 4).

The United States of America is not, of course, the only country troubled by the increasingly public and sometimes violent manifestations of radical moral disagreements about bioethical issues. Australia has encountered its own problems. For example, in 1995 the Brisbane *Courier-Mail* reported that a member of the group called Christians Speaking Out stated that 'it is a Christian's duty to stop abortionists by any means' (13 May, 1995). The member is also reported as condoning the killing of abortionists arguing that it was 'justifiable homicide' (*Courier-Mail* 13 May, 1995).

In light of these and other examples, perhaps one of the greatest challenges ahead may not be how to devise new ways of thinking about ethics or about developing better models of moral decision-making for dealing with moral conflict. Rather, the challenge may be to find new ways of *motivating* moral behaviour and to foster among those who hold differing moral values and beliefs a genuine interest in approaching moral disagreement in a consensual rather than a conflictive manner, and in a manner that seeks first to understand before seeking to be understood.

'Everyday' moral problems in nursing[3]

Before concluding this chapter, some comment is required on the less 'exotic' issue of 'everyday' moral problems in nursing practice. As already stated, nurses have to deal with ethical issues *everyday*. The nursing ethics literature does not, however, always represent or reflect the reality of the kinds of 'everyday' problems that nurses face. Instead, this literature has borrowed heavily from mainstream bioethics to shape nursing ethics discourse and in a way that has sometimes been at the expense of nurses' own experiential wisdom.

In Chapter 2 of this book, under the discussion on nursing ethics, it was suggested that the actual lived experiences of nurses and the lived realities of nursing practice provide a more reliable methodological starting point to nursing ethics inquiry than do the 'top down' theories of Western moral philosophy and the field of bioethics which is derivative of it. This is because an examination of nurses' lived experiences and lived realities of practice would yield important knowledge about and insights into the actual everyday ethical issues and moral problems that nurses have to deal with. Examples include problems concerning the:

- *moral boundaries of nursing* (e.g. nurses as carers being 'in relationship' with others, as opposed to being what the North American philosopher, John Rawls, advocates, the 'detached observers choosing from behind a veil of ignorance' [Rawls 1971]);
- *catalysts to moral action in nursing* (e.g. 'experiential triggers' such as 'the look of suffering in a patients eyes', as opposed to abstract moral rules and principles);
- *operating moral values in nursing* (e.g. sympathy, empathy, compassion, human understanding, and a desire 'to do the best we can', rather than an obsession to 'do one's duty');
- *ethical decision-making processes in nursing* (e.g. which tend to be collaborative, communicative, communal and contextualised, rather than independent, private, individual, solo, and decontextualised);
- *barriers to ethical practice in nursing* (e.g. which tend to be structural rather than knowledge based; that is, the power and authority of doctors to determine patient care, organisational norms forcing compliance with the status quo, and negative attitudes and a lack of support from co-workers and managers);
- *need for cathartic moral talking in nursing care domains* (e.g. 'talking through' moral concerns in a safe and supportive environment to help relieve the moral distress that so often arises as a result of trying to be moral in a world that appears to becoming increasingly amoral).

What talking with nurses so often reveals is that it is *not* the so-called paramount ('exotic') bioethical issues (for example, abortion and euthanasia) that trouble them, but the more fundamental issues of:

- how to help a patient in distress in the 'here and now';
- how to stop 'things going bad for a patient';
- how to best support a relative or chosen carer during times of distress and when the 'system' appears to be against them;
- how to make things 'less traumatic' for someone who is suffering;
- how to reduce the anxiety and vulnerability of the people being cared for;
- where to get help with their (the nurses') own moral distress; and
- how to make a difference in contexts which have become manifestly indifferent to the moral interests of others;

The above and other related concerns are all issues worthy of attention and consideration both within and outside of the nursing profession. They are also issues that deserve to be recognised as 'moral problems in nursing' just as the other 'paramount' issues of bioethics are.

Conclusion

Nurses will encounter many complex moral problems in the course of their work. To be effective in dealing with these problems and preventing the kinds of moral harms that can follow as a consequence of them, it is imperative that nurses have an informed knowledge and understanding of the nature of moral problems, the various forms in which they can manifest, and the kinds of processes that can be used for dealing with them effectively. This chapter has sought to provide such knowledge and understanding. Consideration of other processes, for example, conscientious objection, seeking the advice of a clinical ethics committee, or whistleblowing will be considered further in Chapter 13 of this book.

In the past, when confronted by the moral problems of life, it has been 'too easy to reach solutions that fail to do justice to the difficulty of the problem' (Nagel 1991, p. xi). We do not have to look far to see that many of the answers gained and the solutions reached in contemporary bioethics have been found seriously deficient and inadequate when applied to and in the concrete circumstances of life. Arguably, what is required to help remedy this situation is a mind set that not only seeks to ask questions, but seeks to *call into question* things as they are (Freire 1970, 1972). There also needs to be a recognition that when faced with morally perplexing issues:

- we need to think better and harder about the issues in question (Boyle 1994);
- we need to remember that moral ambiguity, uncertainty, controversy and disagreement can and do have many causes, both practical and theoretical (McCullough 1995); and
- we need to accept that addressing moral problems in a sound and effective manner requires an appeal to a moral approach that recognises a *multiplicity of possible solutions* to a given problem, and that a moral approach which insists on there being just one single correct answer (a 'final solution') to a given moral problem may compound rather than remedy that problem (Fasching 1993).

CASE SCENARIO AND CRITICAL QUESTIONS

Case scenario[4]

An intensive care nurse of several years experience was assigned the care of man who had been estranged from his identical twin brother for several years. The man's condition was serious and it was evident that he was dying. Despite being aware of his deteriorating condition, the man was adamant that 'he did not want any contact with his twin brother' and that 'his twin brother was not to be contacted and told about his condition'. Having had personal experience of the relationship dynamics between twins in her own family, and having an 'intuition' that the man was not making the 'right choice' in the circumstances at hand, the nurse decided to 'respectfully disagree' with her patient's request and to go against his expressed wishes.

Recognising that time was running out (the man was not expected to live very long), she immediately set in motion a chain of events that resulted in the estranged brothers being reunited and reconciled before the ill brother died. Prior to the ill twin's death, both brothers were adamant that the nurse had 'done the right thing' and expressed their deep appreciation for her insights, sensitivity and actions — especially her decision to 'go against the ill-twin's expressed wishes'. Other staff in the unit, however, had reservations about the way in which the nurse had handled the situation. They were especially concerned about her decision to go against the patient's expressed wishes, which they perceived as a violation of his right to decide.

Critical questions

1. What are the moral problems the nurse encountered in this case?
2. What decision-making processes do you think the nurse used to address the moral problems that emerged?
3. Should the nurse have sought advice from others before taking the action she did?
4. In your view, did the nurse make the right moral decisions in this case?
5. If you were the nurse who had been assigned to care for this patient, what would you have done in this situation?
6. What processes would you have used in order to address the moral problems identified?
7. Do you think your 'ordinary' moral values, beliefs, knowledge and experiences (e.g., such as those acquired before you entered into nursing or studied ethics) would have been adequate to guide you on how to act in this case?

---

1   Adapted from Johnstone, M-J (1998). Determining and responding effectively to ethical professional misconduct in nursing: a report to the Nurses Board of Victoria. Melbourne. Section 6: Responding effectively to breaches of ethical standards of conduct in nursing, pp. 71–96.

2   Adapted from Johnstone, M-J (1998). Determining and responding effectively to ethical professional misconduct in nursing: a report to the Nurses Board of Victoria. Melbourne. Section 3: 'Defining ethical professional misconduct in nursing', pp. 17–28.

3   An earlier version of this chapter was first published in the *INEN Bulletin* 5(1), pp. 1–4 (1997)(the Newsletter of the International Nursing Ethics [& Midwifery] Network, Maastricht, The Netherlands). It has been revised for inclusion in this present work.

4   Taken from Johnstone, M. (2003) *Effective writing for health professionals: a practical guide to getting published.* Allen & Unwin, Sydney, pp. 3–4.

Chapter 6

Patients' rights to and in health care

LEARNING OBJECTIVES

Upon the completion of this chapter and with further self-directed learning you are expected to be able to:

- Discuss the relationship between patients'/clients' rights and moral rights.
- Consider the right to health care and:
  - discuss at least three senses in which the right to health care can be claimed;
  - outline some controversial arguments raised both for and against the right to health care;
  - explain why an economic framework is morally inadequate for deciding issues of health care justice.
- Consider the right to make informed choices and:
  - outline the doctrine of informed consent;
  - explore the notion of the 'sovereignty of the individual' and its implications for informed consent practices;
  - examine critically the five analytical components of informed consent;
  - discuss critically at least five common objections raised against the right to give an informed consent;
- Examine the notion of competency and its implications for patients with impaired decision-making capacity.
- Discuss critically the notion of 'surrogate decision-making' in the case of rational incompetence.
- Discuss the nature and moral implications of paternalism in nursing and health care.
- Consider the right to confidentiality and:
  - state the International Council of Nurses' position on confidentiality;
  - outline the moral basis and requirements of the principle of confidentiality;
  - discuss briefly the conditions under which demands to keep information confidential may be justly overridden;
- Discuss critically the right to dignity and dying with dignity.
- Discuss critically the right to be treated with respect.

KEYWORDS
- Competency
- Confidentiality
- Dignity
- Discrimination
- Health care
- Human rights
- Informed consent
- Informed decision–making
- Patients'/clients' rights
- Privacy
- Respect
- Stigma

Introduction

In 1996, in what has been described by media commentators as 'the first case of its kind' in North America, a patient sued his treating physician for 'keeping him alive' against his expressed wishes and for not offering him an 'elective demise' (Reed 1996, p. 14). The patient in this case was a 66-year-old man who had been diagnosed with amyotrophic lateral sclerosis, a degenerative nerve disorder. Despite having made a 'living will' that clearly stated his wishes 'not to be attached to a respirator' should his condition deteriorate, the patient was nevertheless placed on an artificial life support machine when he began experiencing breathing difficulties. As a result of this paternalistic medical decision, he was left totally dependent on 24-hour nursing care, depleted of his life-savings, and deprived of what he regarded as a 'dignified death' (Reed 1996, p. 14). The patient's life expectancy was estimated at the time of the report to be between five to ten years.

A little over one year later, in New Zealand, a case of a very different kind unfolded. In this case, a man suffering from an end-stage illness, was denied kidney dialysis treatment on 'economic grounds' (Field 1997, p. 10). Outraged by the hospital's decision not to treat their father, and in a desperate bid to secure life-saving treatment for him, the man's family applied to the New Zealand Court of Appeal to intervene. The court is reported as ruling, however, that the hospital managers 'did not need to resume kidney dialysis treatment' (Field 1997, p. 10). In response to the case, the then associate Health Minister was reported to have said that 'health rationing was now a fact of life'. It was subsequently observed that (p. 10):

> Although formal rationing has not previously been acknowledged here [New Zealand], from July every New Zealander referred for surgery in the public health system will be scored for points on clinical and social criteria to determine when they will be treated.

In 2002, a major Australian newspaper reported on the assault and substandard care of a 87-year-old woman in a State Government-run aged care facility (Miller 2002). The report stated that the woman was allegedly assaulted (by another resident) on at least four occasions, found smeared with faeces a number of times, and had had at least six falls resulting in injuries. The woman's daughter is reported as also alleging that 'some of the ward emergency buzzers were broken, the toilets were often found in a disgraceful condition' and that she had seen 'rats and mice on the ground floor of the aged care center' (Miller 2002, p. 3). The daughter is also reported as stating that 'for months she complied with the hospital's internal complaints procedures but abandoned it "when it proved itself to be a futile process" ' (Miller 2002, p.3).

These reports on treating patients against their will, denying patients life-saving treatment for economic reasons, and the provision of substandard care are just some among many examples of patients' rights violations that can and do occur in health care contexts. Other examples of patients' rights violations include: breaches of confidentiality, inadequate consent practices, not being treated with respect, and being stigmatised and discriminated against in health injurious and harmful ways. It is to examining patients' rights and their implications for members of the nursing profession that this and the following chapters now turn.

The issue of patients' rights

People requiring or receiving health care are not, and never have been, obliged to be the passive recipients of unnegotiated care. Yet the more we examine the realities of health care practice and the way our health care institutions and services operate, the more apparent it becomes that the rhetoric surrounding the idealism of people's rights to and in health care does not always match the reality. As the bioethics, legal, professional and lay literature, and our own everyday experience, make plain, people continue to be denied equitable access to the quality and quantity of health care they need; they continue to be denied the opportunity to make informed choices about their care and treatment options; and they continue to be harmed physically, psychologically, spiritually and morally as a result of morally questionable practices in our health care services and institutions.

Over the past two decades, the issue of patients' rights has received considerable attention both in Australia and overseas. There exists a vast body of literature on the subject (too numerous to list here), and there has been a proliferation of dramatised accounts of people's 'life stories' on the matter both in books and films. There have also been significant policy and law reforms in the area of patients' rights, for instance, in relation to:

- clarifying people's common law right to refuse orthodox medical treatment;
- the lawful appointment of 'surrogate decision-makers' (e.g. persons with medical power of attorney) in the case of patients who become incompetent to decide their own medical treatment options;
- formulating 'living wills';
- the right to an 'assisted death';
- the establishment of clinical ethics committees (CECs) and 'client support' persons;
- the establishment of statutory health services complaints mechanisms;
- the role of a public advocate in the case of disagreement about treatment decisions;
- the development of public consumer advocacy groups;
- the establishment of national ethics committees and commissions.

Despite these important innovations, however, the area of patients' rights remains problematic.

There is no denying that enormous progress has been made over the past two decades in regard to patients' rights: violations are monitored more carefully; redress of violations is more substantial; and more effort is now being put into preventing patients' rights violations from occurring (notably under the rubric of corporate/ clinical risk management). Nevertheless it is evident that we still have a long way to go in order to ensure that the rights of patients are properly respected and protected in health care domains — dispute remains about who has rights to and in health care; there are disagreements about what rights patients can meaningfully and reasonably claim in certain contexts; there is a lack of certainty about who has corresponding duties to patients' rights claims; and there is no consensus on how best to resolve disputes in cases where patients' rights claims compete and conflict. Important questions remain of: How and what can we learn about the disputes and disagreements that remain concerning patients' rights? How might we prevent patients' rights from being violated in the domains in which we work? and How do those who have violated patients' rights, and the patients whose rights have been violated, come to terms with the aftermath of those violations?

In 1990, the Consumers' Health Forum (CHF) pointed out that the Australian legal system has not been responsive to protecting the needs of health care consumers. In its report on the *Legal Recognition and Protection of the Rights of Health Consumers*, CHF states (pp. 1–2):

> For some consumers the diversity of the Australian legal system has provided some benefits. Unfortunately, for the majority it has been far more effective in creating an inequitable and unresponsive legal maze. As it currently stands:
>
> – there is no comprehensive, consistent, consumer-orientated health law that recognises individual consumers' and the community's health and wellbeing as a fundamental objective;
> – there is no clear direction for consumers as to how they should act, how others should act, and what redress they have if things go wrong (their rights depend upon which State consumers live in or even whether they attend a public or private health facility); and
> – the interests of bureaucrats and professional groups are better reflected in existing law than the interests of consumers and the community in such matters as information, participation, accountability and openness.

At the time of writing, this situation has not changed significantly and there are no indications that it will change significantly in the immediate future. It can be seen then that the issue of patients' (clients') rights is of obvious importance to the nursing profession. If nurses are to respond effectively to this issue, however, they need to have knowledge and understanding of, first, what patients' rights are, and second, how these rights can best be upheld. It is to advancing an understanding of these matters that this discussion will now turn.

What are patients' rights?

To put it simply, patients' or clients' rights are a subcategory of human rights. Statements of patients' or clients' rights are merely statements about particular moral interests that a person might have in health care contexts and that require special protection when a person assumes the role of a patient or client. Referring to this particular set of interests in terms of 'patients' rights' or 'clients' rights' serves more the purposes of manageability than those of philosophy. For example, when the notion patients' rights or clients' rights is used, we know immediately what kind of context and what kind of rights claims are likely to be encountered. The notion of patients' rights or clients' rights in this instance immediately 'sets the scene', or identifies the domain of concern. In the case of human rights language, the scene that is set is much broader. Some might consider human rights language in health care contexts to be somewhat cumbersome to manage. This is not to say that it would be inappropriate to use the notion of human rights in health care contexts; quite the reverse. In many respects, using human rights language might be more compelling and more effective in drawing attention to and demanding respect of the deserving moral interests of people in health care domains.

It is perhaps important to clarify that patients' rights statements tend to include a mixture of civil rights, legal rights and moral rights. Popular examples of patients' rights include: a right to health care, a right to be informed, a right to participate in decision-making concerning treatment and care, a right to give an informed consent, a right to refuse consent, a right to have access to a trained health interpreter, a right to know the name, status and practice experience of attending health professionals, a right to a second opinion, a right to be treated with respect, a right to confidentiality, a right to bodily integrity, a right to the maintenance of dignity, and many others. Many of these rights statements derive from the broader moral principles of autonomy, non-maleficence, beneficence and justice, already discussed in this book. Unfortunately there is insufficient space here to discuss every type of patients' right that has been formulated at some time or another. For the purposes of this discussion, attention is given to only five broad categories of rights, under which many other narrower rights claims fall. These category claims include the rights to health care, to make self-determining choices (informed consent), to confidentiality, dignity, (including the right to die with dignity), and to be treated with respect.

The right to health care

The right to health care (taken here in its broadest sense, and not to be confused with *medical* care) is complex and controversial. As well as being a sensitive moral issue, it is also a highly charged political issue, as ongoing debates on health care resource allocation make plain.

Bioethicists have yet to find a happy medium between the many competing and conflicting views on the subject. Some philosophers argue that health care is something all people are equally entitled to receive, regardless of the cost. Where human life is at stake, they contend, decisions should not be constrained by economic considerations (Brody 1986). If more money is required, the solution is relatively simple: redirect society's resources (for example, away from gross expenditures on arsenals of arms and other life-threatening instruments of war). Others argue that it is implausible and impossible to provide a high standard of health care to all persons equally. At best, all that people can reasonably claim is a 'decent minimum' of health care, as measured in terms of the amount necessary to secure a minimally decent or 'tolerable' life (Engelhardt 1986, p. 336; Buchanan 1984; Fried 1982). Still others argue that there is no such thing as a right to health care. One philosopher even claims that it is *immoral* to speak of health care as a 'right' (Sade 1983), and another that the expression 'a right to health care' is nothing but a 'dangerous slogan' (Fried 1982).

Charles Fried (1982, p. 400) makes the interesting and, if taken from the perspective of medical treatment, I think correct claim that the 'impossible dilemma posed by the promise of a right to health care' is really nothing more than a product of 'our culture's inability to face and cope with the persistent facts of illness, old age, and death'. He goes on to assert controversially that (p. 400):

> Because we are little able to come to terms with the hazards which illness proposes, because the old are a burden and an embarrassment, because we pretend that death does not exist, we employ elaborate ruses to put these things out of the ambit of our ordinary lives.

Whether the right to health care is a bogus claim or a dangerous slogan or cultural quirk will, however, depend very much on how the notion of 'health care' is interpreted. I suspect that many philosophers' criticisms derive from their erroneously equating 'health care' with 'medical care'. Since medical care makes up only a small proportion of overall health care, it is obviously not synonymous with health care. Once the notion of 'health care' is understood in more holistic terms, the right to such care may not seem so outrageous or fraudulent or even culturally odd as a claim. Every culture has its way of dealing with sickness, illness, pain and suffering, and of caring for the sick. Not every culture embraces Western scientific medicine as the most effective way of dealing with sickness and related illness experiences, however. And thus not every culture is posed with the dilemma of economic restrictions on resource allocation; this, I suspect, is what lies at the root of the debate about whether people have a right to health (that is, medical) care. Once health care, in its more holistic sense, is seen as an important means of promoting a person's *total* (and not merely physical) wellbeing, it becomes increasingly difficult to deny that claims to it are valid and morally justified. What makes a claim to health care compelling is precisely that, once it is accepted, it has the moral power to prescribe actions to relieve the distressing symptoms caused by disease and illness, to promote human wellbeing (a moral end) and, indeed, to promote human life itself (also a moral end). If we deny entitlements to health care, we must also deny entitlements to a range of other interests, including those of life, happiness and even the exercise of self-determining choices.

It is beyond the scope of this text to deal with the many arguments and counter-arguments raised in response to the question of whether people have a right to health care. What is of concern here is to clarify the *nature* of the claim to a *right to health care*, and what might be meant by such a claim.

People's entitlement to receive health care first received global recognition with the signing of the United Nations Declaration of Human Rights on 10 December 1948. Article 25 states:

> Everyone has the right to a standard of living adequate for the health and wellbeing of himself [sic] and his [sic] family, including food, clothing, housing and medical care and necessary social services, and the right to security in the event of unemployment, sickness, disability, widowhood, old age or other lack of livelihood in circumstances beyond his [sic] control.
>
> (United Nations 1978, p. 8)

It is worth noting here that the right to health care embodied by this statement extends far beyond a claim of mere *medical* care, and embraces a more holistic interpretation of health care.

Since the signing of this declaration the question of the right to health care has taken on a new meaning, and has emerged largely as a result of what people perceive to be an 'unjust or unfair state of affairs' involving present structures of health care, which are seen as diminishing and even eliminating possibilities for the enhancement of the quality of human life and for human life itself (Teays and Purdy 2001; McCullough 1983).

In speaking of the right to health care, it is important to distinguish at least three different senses in which it can be claimed: that is, the right to equal access to health care; the right to have access to appropriate care; and the right to quality of care.

THE RIGHT TO EQUAL ACCESS TO HEALTH CARE

Access to health care refers to 'whether people who are — or should be — entitled to health care services receive them' (Emanuel 2000, p. 8). The right to equal access to health care raises questions of distributive justice and of how the benefits and burdens associated with health care service delivery ought to be distributed. It also raises questions of whether people or institutions can be found morally negligent for failing to provide equal access to health care for persons requiring it. Responses refuting this sense of a right to health care typically centre on such arguments as: 'there is not a "bottomless pit" of health care resources, and somebody has to do without'.

Specifically, the 'scarce resources, but unlimited wants' argument tends to be constructed as follows:

1. the demand for health care has outstripped supply;
2. this is fundamentally because health care resources are limited;
3. different people have different health needs, and different views on how existing resources should be used to meet these needs;
4. it is true that existing health care resources can be used in alternative ways; and
5. nevertheless, health care resources are limited, so it is not possible to satisfy everybody's needs and wants (Johnstone 1990, p. 3; see also Teays and Purdy 2001; Beauchamp and Steinbock 1999; Fuchs 1983).

The ultimate conclusion drawn from these premises — the 'bottom line', so to speak — is that, inevitably, choices will have to be made. In particular, borrowing from Sheehan and Wells (1985, p. 59), choices will have to be made about:

1. the conditions for which scarce resources should be made available; and
2. the priority with which given conditions should be treated.

It remains an open question, however, whether we have to accept the premises of this 'scarce resources, but unlimited wants' argument, and, further, whether we have to accept its apparent 'inevitable' conclusions. As I have argued elsewhere (Johnstone 1990), it is far from clear that we do have to accept them — particularly when the politics of health care resource allocation is considered fully, including the vested and powerful interests that the whole health care economics debate is serving. Further, it is also open to serious question whether we are obliged to accept that economic principles ought to supplant morality as the ultimate test of conduct, as an economic rationalisation approach to health care dictates. Human life is not something that can be reduced, like an object, to mere economic worth, and as moral beings we ought to resist attempts to do so; if we do not resist, we risk seeing 'worthless' human beings denied the health care entitlements they would otherwise be entitled morally to receive.

It is important to recognise that the issue of resource allocation goes far beyond the simple question of merely how to allocate dollars and cents. It involves much broader questions of how to measure quality of life, efficacy of health care and medical treatment, and quality of care, and of how to calculate cost-effectiveness, as well as complex socio-cultural questions pertaining to power, politics, and profit (Johnstone 1990; see also David Lindorff's controversial and provocative text *Marketplace medicine: the rise of the for-profit hospital chains* [1992]). Fundamentally, it also involves questions of how best to promote health, not merely access to health care services in 'bricks and mortar' hospitals (Johnstone 2002b; Teays and Purdy 2001; Emanuel 2000).

Unless nurses address these other broader questions — both academically and professionally — they will never be in a position to offer a convincing account of why *health care* (whatever form this may take), not merely medical care, needs to be better recognised and why it must be more appropriately funded. A strong stand must be taken on the need to recognise and to fund the promotion of *health* better (not just health care services), and there is considerable scope to suggest that it would be appropriate for the nursing profession to lead such a stand (see also Christensen et al. 2001). More than this, the nursing profession has a moral obligation to lobby effectively for the community as a whole, and the individuals who comprise it, to have better access to the processes that promote health, not merely to medical or hospital care and related services (Johnstone 2002b; Christensen et al. 2001).

THE RIGHT TO HAVE ACCESS TO APPROPRIATE CARE

The right to have access to appropriate care is a second sense in which a right to health care can be claimed. This sense raises important questions concerning the cultural relativity or ethno-specificity of care and its ability to accommodate people's personal preferences, health beliefs, health values and health practices. As examples given in Chapter 4 of this book have already shown, failing to provide health care in an appropriate manner can have harmful consequences (clinically, legally and morally).

Many other examples can be given here. The complementary therapy movement, for instance, has posed all sorts of new dilemmas for the scientific health professional, particularly in instances where patients prefer to try scientifically 'unproven' vitamin or herbal remedies, meditation, and other 'alternative' therapeutic agents for serious diseases, rather than risk the known and unpleasant side effects of more orthodox medical treatments. To some extent this type of problem has been overcome on account of alternative therapies being better researched, and more widely accepted by health professionals. Today, it is not uncommon for patients to receive a combination of orthodox and unorthodox treatments (for example, performing surgery as well as administering vitamin and herbal therapies, or administering orthodox drugs as well as performing spinal manipulation, acupuncture and acupressure, facilitating meditation, and the like).

Another aspect of 'appropriate care' entails patients having access to people (lay, folk and professional) of their own choosing. It also includes patients' entitlements to seek a second medical opinion, to refuse a recommended medical therapy or folk therapy, to choose an alternative health therapy, to be surrounded by family and friends, to have unrestricted visiting rights, and to decline to be 'ordered' to do anything they do not wish to do (including getting out of bed, having a shower every day, and taking prescribed medication). As the Australian Consumers' Association (1988, p. 16) pointed out long ago, patients do not need a doctor's or nurse's 'permission' (to be distinguished here from *advice*) for anything!

If nurses are to respond to this sense of a right to health care, they need to gain knowledge and understanding of their patients' health beliefs and health practices and to negotiate ways in which these can be accommodated and met appropriately.

THE RIGHT TO QUALITY OF CARE

A right to quality of care is the third and final sense in which the right to health care can be claimed. This sense raises questions concerning the accountability, responsibility and competency of health professionals and health care providers, and about the standard of care that is actually delivered. Not only are practical and technical skills at issue here, but also attitudinal factors such as a health care provider's attitude towards patients as human beings with needs and interests, who are entitled to participate in decision-making concerning their care. A claim to receive quality care also raises questions concerning what should be done in the case of the 'impaired professional'— that is, someone who functions below an otherwise acceptable professional standard (Johnstone 1998).

Quality health care as a right is an ambiguous and complex notion. Nevertheless, an attempt must be made to understand and use it in a meaningful way. This can be achieved by appealing to the agreed standards of the profession, experience, commonsense (for example, concerning the distinctions that can be readily made between 'quality care' and 'substandard care'), formal quality assurance processes, formal measures of patient outcomes, and the like. The task for the nursing profession is to ensure that health care delivery never falls to a level that compromises patient safety and wellbeing; nurses in many parts of the world have already demonstrated their willingness to 'blow the whistle' or to take strike action when patient safety is compromised by substandard conditions and resources.

Challenges posed by the right to health care

It can be seen that all three senses of the right to health care pose a significant challenge to the nursing profession. As far as the right to equal access is concerned, nurses have much to contribute. Nurses know very well the areas in which access to health care has effectively been denied to people, and why (for example, lack of appropriate resource allocation, inappropriate structuring of health care delivery, obstructive institutional policies and legal laws, language and cultural barriers). Despite their knowledge and experience in relation to these matters, however, nurses are not always included in the processes for deciding important policy or health resource allocation matters.

Nurses must directly participate in high-level decision-making concerning health care matters, an imperative already well argued for by Paul Gross (1985) two decades ago. If nurses fail to influence policy and decision-making, the prospects for patients' rights, not to mention the nursing profession's ability to promote and protect these, will remain limited.

The right to health care, in the senses pertaining to both appropriate health care and quality health care, also poses significant challenges to the nursing profession, in terms not only of its own standards, but also of those applied in health care contexts generally. If the nursing profession is to succeed in providing appropriate nursing care (a subcategory of health care), it needs to pay careful and continuous attention to developing its curricula and to ensuring that its members are educationally prepared to meet and to respond to the needs of society, and in particular the needs of the culturally and individually diverse people comprising it. As well as this, the nursing profession must pay careful attention to developing reliable mechanisms for guiding its members in their attempts to deliver safe, therapeutically effective, culturally appropriate and morally accountable care, and for censuring those of its members who fail to do so (Johnstone 1998).

Nurses, individually and collectively, have a moral responsibility to respond to the serious threats mounting against a person's right to health care; they must therefore develop a well organised and effective lobby to champion a more balanced approach to resource allocation and a more balanced approach to the structuring of health care facilities generally. Nurses also have a moral responsibility to inform the community at large of its entitlements to, in and against health care, and to educate the community that the 'technologically big' is not necessarily the 'health care best'.

The right to make informed decisions

Of all the patients' rights which might be claimed in a given health care context, none is perhaps more challenging to the power, authority and sometimes the integrity of attending health professionals than the patient's right to make informed choices about his or her care and treatment. This might help to explain why, despite the apparent success of the patients' rights movement over the past two decades, the right of patients to give an informed consent to care and treatment continues to be problematic in some areas. For example, over the past ten years I have conducted a number of workshops and seminars addressing ethical issues in nursing. Disturbingly, nurses attending these educational activities have consistently identified the following problems in relation to consent to treatment practices:

- patients signing consent forms without having any comprehension of what it is they are consenting to (see Figure 6.1 for an example of a typical consent form);
- nurses assuming incorrectly that treating doctors have explained a recommended medical procedure or treatment to a patient/relatives before obtaining the patient's consent;
- relatives/chosen carers being upset at discovering that a recommended medical procedure had not been properly explained to a loved one before being performed;
- signed consent forms being treated as generic, that is, as signifying a consent to 'anything deemed necessary' during the period of hospitalisation;
- patients giving consent to a particular procedure being performed, only to discover later that a different procedure was performed without any 'real choice' being given (for example, the patient may have consented to having a biopsy *only*; upon recovery, however, he or she finds that radical surgery has been performed);
- verbal consents being obtained from relatives/chosen carers over the telephone in situations which are not of a true 'emergency' nature (for example, where there has been a last minute cancellation from a private list and a bed has become vacant for a new elective surgery patient);
- consents being obtained from people of non-English-speaking backgrounds without the assistance of qualified health interpreters;
- patients consenting to a procedure, knowing what the procedure involves, but having no knowledge of associated risks or potential adverse side effects of the procedure in question;
- consent being obtained from patients after they have received a pre-medication or when they are under the influence of alcohol or other mind-altering drugs; and
- procedures performed without consent being obtained from the patient at all.

CONSENT FOR OPERATION AND ANAESTHETICS

I, ... of ....

.... hereby consent to undergo

the submission of my (child) (ward) .... to undergo

the operation of ....

the nature and purpose of which have been explained to me by

Dr/Mr ....

I also consent to such further or alternative operative measures as may be found appropriate during the course of the abovementioned operation, and to the administration of general, local or other anaesthetics for any of these purposes.

No assurance has been given to me that the operation will be performed by any particular practitioner.

Date .... Signed ....

*Patient/Parent/Guardian

I confirm that I have explained the nature and purpose of this operation to the *patient/parent/guardian.

Date .... Signed ....

*Medical/Dental Practitioner

*Delete as appropriate

Figure 6.1 Typical consent form for operation and anaesthetics procedure

(from J. Fordham (1988) *Doctor's orders or patient choice*. Leo Cussen Institute, Melbourne, p. 68)

In disclosing these problems, the nurses have also expressed considerable distress at what they see as their inability 'to do anything about the problem'.

The issue of informed consent has obvious implications for nurses, not least on account of them being at the forefront of receiving requests from patients and relatives for 'information'. As well, nurses are at the forefront of being expected to take appropriate action when patients' information needs are not being met and/or when their (the patients') entitlements in regard to consent practices are unjustly violated. It is therefore important that nurses have a thorough understanding of the nature and function of informed consent, as well as their responsibilities as nurses in relation to facilitating a patient making informed choices about recommended care and treatment options. It is to exploring these two issues that this discussion will now turn.

WHAT IS INFORMED CONSENT?

The doctrine of informed consent, although having a profound ethical dimension, is essentially a legal doctrine developed partially out of recognition of the patient's right to self-determination and partially out of the doctor's duty to give the patient 'information about proposed treatment so as to provide him or her with the opportunity of making an "informed" or "rational" choice as to whether to undergo the treatment' (Robertson 1981, p. 102; see also Gert et al. 1997; Beauchamp and Childress 2001).

In distinguishing the differences between a legal and a moral approach to informed consent, Faden and Beauchamp (1986) explain that the legal law's approach to informed consent 'springs from pragmatic theory', which focuses more on a doctor's duty to disclose information to patients and not to injure them. By contrast, moral philosophy's approach to informed consent 'springs from a principle of respect for autonomy that focuses on the patient or subject, who has a right to make an autonomous choice' (Faden and Beauchamp 1986, p. 4).

Whether such a clear-cut distinction can be drawn between a legal and a moral approach to informed consent is a matter of some controversy, however. The moral demand to respect autonomy is clearly the prime motivator of the doctor's duty to disclose information, and the moral principle of non-maleficence is the prime motivator of the doctor's duty not to injure or harm patients. It seems that, while the moral and legal approaches to informed consent can be loosely distinguished, they are nevertheless inextricably linked. It is this linkage which highlights the other important functions, besides the promotion of patient autonomy, that the application of the doctrine of informed consent also serves, namely those of protecting patients, avoiding fraud and duress (i.e. as occurs when information is not disclosed), of encouraging self-scrutiny by health professionals, of promoting 'rational' and systematic moral decision-making, and of involving the public 'in promoting autonomy as a general social value and in controlling biomedical research' (Capron 1974; Gert et al. 1997; Beauchamp and Childress 2001).

There is no question that consent practices have improved considerably over recent years. Health professionals have increasingly recognised the benefits of ensuring that patients (and their proxies) are informed appropriately about their care and treatment options, and patients (and their proxies) are more willing to question the information that they have been provided in order to inform their choices and consent to treatment (Tweeddale 2002; Chaboyer 2000). Nevertheless nurses continue to witness instances in which consent practices have been questionable and where patients' rights to make informed choices have been violated. For example, I have been told of several instances in which nurses have been 'ordered' by an operating surgeon to obtain the written consent of a patient who has already been given a pre-medication and who is drowsy and awaiting transfer to the operating theatre. In each instance, the fact that consent given under the influence of sedating or narcotic drugs is legally invalid seems to have been ignored by the surgeons in question. In one case, the gynaecologist 'ordered' a registered nurse to obtain the signature of a non-English-speaking and already pre-medicated woman on whom he was about to perform a dilatation and curettage (D&C) of the uterus. However, there was some suggestion that the gynaecologist also intended to sterilise this woman, and the nurse involved in the case was deeply concerned that the matter of surgical sterilisation had not been properly discussed with the woman. Further, the patient was in no state to give a valid consent, since she was very drowsy from the effects of her pre-medication. As well, no interpreter was immediately available to transmit to the woman the information she needed in order to give an informed consent. On the basis of her assessment of the situation the registered nurse refused to comply with the gynaecologist's order. Upon hearing her refusal the gynaecologist became abusive and was overheard to yell at her. Fortunately, other nurses on the ward came to her defence and supported her decision not to seek the woman's signature. Needless to say, the woman did not go to theatre that day.

Another example concerns the case of a 66-year-old Greek woman ('Mrs G') who had been admitted to hospital for elective surgery to treat a kidney disorder (Kanitsaki 1992). As in the previous cases, informed consent was not obtained. Describing the circumstances surrounding the failure to obtain an informed consent from this woman, Kanitsaki writes (1992, pp. 2–3):

> The morning of Mrs G's operation arrived, and it was observed by the nurse who was to prepare her for theatre, that Mrs G's consent form was not signed. The nurse reported this to the charge nurse who rang the relevant doctor to come and obtain Mrs G's signature on the consent form. The surgical registrar arrived, and in an irritable tone asked 'why this was not done the day before'. The nurse remarked that Mrs G only spoke a few words of English, and would need an interpreter to explain to her what she was signing and why. The doctor replied 'I know. But I have no time to wait. It will be alright'. He then proceeded to instruct Mrs G how to sign the consent form. Mrs G sat up in bed, however, and looking puzzled, uttered 'Me no understand. Me no understand'. The doctor then proceeded to pick up Mrs G's hand, placed a pen into it, and by holding and directing her hand, made a cross on the consent form. Once this was achieved, the doctor gently touched Mrs G's hand and said 'Good. Good'. He then left the ward.

One reason why consent practices in Australia and New Zealand are problematic relates to the model they are based on. Unlike the United States and Canada, which use a *reasonable patient standard* model of consent (emphasising trespass and battery), Australia and New Zealand use a *reasonable doctor standard* model (emphasising negligence and malpractice). Understanding the difference between these two models is important to any debate on informed consent, and I will briefly outline them here. (For a more detailed discussion on the legal aspects of informed consent to medical treatment, see Forrester and Griffiths 2001; Kirby 1995; Wallace 1991; Law Reform Commission of Victoria et al. 1987; Faden and Beauchamp 1986; Andrews 1985.)

In the *reasonable doctor standard* model of consent, a consensus of reasonable and established medical opinion provides the 'objective' measure. On the basis of this model, a doctor has the duty to use reasonable skill and may *withhold* information if, in the doctor's opinion, its disclosure would be injurious to the patient. If patients are to successfully sue for damages on account of a failure to disclose information relevant to the consent process, they have to show, first, that the doctor failed to provide information and advice to a patient that accords with the 'practice existing in the medical profession' (Law Reform Commission of Victoria et al. 1987, p. 8), and, second, that injury was suffered as a (causally) *direct result* of this negligence. In establishing whether the doctor did in fact use 'reasonable skill', the law would appeal to the *reasonable doctor standard* model and would ask what most or many reasonable and competent doctors in a given particular branch of medicine would do and say in such circumstances; that is, what would be considered 'accepted medical practice' in this situation? If there were conflict, the answer to this question would be sought from an expert medical witness, or witnesses, who would testify what they, as reasonable and competent doctors in a particular branch of medicine, would probably do or say in the circumstances under question. For example, the question of whether a doctor should have disclosed to a patient a 0.1–0.2 per cent risk of quadriplegia in cases involving cervical spinal surgery would ultimately be decided on the basis of whether *other* reasonable and competent doctors in the field usually disclose this information. If it could be established that other reasonable doctors do not disclose to their patients a 0.1–0.2 per cent risk of quadriplegia in cases involving cervical spinal surgery, it is likely that a doctor who failed to disclose such information to a patient would not be found negligent or causally responsible for the patient's injuries in the case of a material risk manifesting itself (such as quadriplegia).

In the *reasonable patient standard* model, on the other hand, the standard is set 'by reference to hypothetical behaviour of adult, competent people in the sorts of situations which are presented to courts and other tribunals for decision' (Law Reform Commission of Victoria et al. 1987, p. 8). On the basis of this model, a doctor has the duty to *disclose* to the patient all the information necessary to making an intelligent and 'rational' choice (including information pertaining to small material risks). For example, consider the hypothetical case of a patient who has suffered the complication of quadriplegia following a cervical spinal fusion. Consider further that the patient claims that, had information been given about the associated risk of quadriplegia, the operation would never have been consented to in the first place. The famous *Sidaway case* provides a good and thought-provoking example of this kind of situation (Law Reform Commission of Victoria et al. 1987, pp. 3–4, 37–9; Andrews 1985, p. 14). In the hypothetical case, the question of whether a doctor should have disclosed to the patient a 0.1–0.2 per cent risk of quadriplegia in cases involving cervical spinal surgery would ultimately be decided on the basis of whether:

1. the information that was withheld was critical to the patient's making an intelligent choice;
2. the information would have caused the patient to make a different choice had she or he been informed of the associated risks before giving consent;
3. the patient's desire to know of the given associated material risks was consistent with the desires of a hypothetical reasonable and competent adult;
4. the risk was considered to be severe (i.e. the injury, were it to occur, would be of a serious nature; quadriplegia in this instance is clearly 'severe' viz. 'of a serious nature'); and
5. the probability of the risk occurring was high.

If it could be established, in this instance, that the patient would not have consented to the procedure, and that the patient's declining to give consent would have been consistent with what a hypothetical reasonable and competent adult would do in a similar situation, then the patient's original consent would be vitiated and the doctor would be found guilty of trespass and battery.

Both models depend on the further consideration of a patient's rational or legal *competence* — a matter that, rightly or wrongly, only the courts can decide (the question of patient competency will be considered later in this discussion).

The issue facing us is whether we should totally abandon the reasonable doctor standard model in favour of the reasonable patient standard model, or whether we should opt for some middle ground between the two. There is some suggestion that this middle position has already been opted for in one or two Australian court cases (Russell 1987, p. 18); however, further legal opinion would be necessary to explore the issue in more depth.

Whatever the legal considerations and arguments for or against these models, from a moral point of view (and, indeed, a pragmatic point of view) neither is free of difficulties. It takes little imagination to see how the reasonable doctor standard can be unreliable. As books, articles, anecdotal case studies and media commentaries make plain, doctors are often reluctant to testify against their colleagues. Commenting on Australia's medical defence unions, Stephen Rice writes (1988, p. 124):

> the medical defence unions operating in Australia claim they do not object to their members testifying against colleagues. But they stress to members in newsletters: — 'Avoid unnecessary criticism of the work or conduct of other practitioners.'

Rice also cites the experience of a Sydney solicitor (and former legal secretary of the Australian Medical Association) who, when addressing a medico–legal seminar organised by the AMA, was unable to find one doctor in the audience who was prepared to give evidence against another doctor at a court hearing. Rice comments further: 'Even with his impeccable contacts in the medical community, he [the solicitor] has discovered it is not easy to find willing witnesses' (p. 124). This traditional situation has changed little in the intervening years.

The reasonable patient standard, however, can also be unreliable. For example, who is to say what is to count as a 'reasonable' patient, hypothetical or otherwise? Are we really expected to believe and accept that an abstract 'hypothetical reasonable and competent adult' — divorced from any cultural, social, historical and spiritual context of living — is able to represent reliably and truthfully what an actual person whose 'reasonableness' is at issue would ultimately desire? What one patient might consider *reasonable*, another might equally reject; and vice versa. The case of Jehovah's Witnesses and their well recognised refusal to accept life-saving blood transfusions is a point in question. It is not difficult to imagine a 'reasonable patient' of the Jehovah's Witness faith refusing a blood transfusion against an overwhelming body of public opinion that such a refusal was 'unreasonable' and even 'mad' or 'idiotic'. The case of children (mature minors) reasonably refusing burdensome medical treatment against adult opinion is another example. A particular example of this can be found in the controversial English case involving a 15 year old girl who underwent a heart transplant by order of a British High Court. The girl did not want the transplant explaining 'I would feel different with someone else's heart — that is a good enough reason not to have a heart transplant, even if it saved my life' (Boseley and Dyer 1999, p. 19). Treating doctors and the Court disagreed, however, and the girl's wishes were overridden on the 'reasonable' grounds that the heart transplant would save her life.

In dealing with these and other difficulties, as well as with other more general objections which may be raised against the doctrine of informed consent, it is important not to lose sight of the various theoretical perspectives underpinning and justifying the right of people to make informed choices about their care and treatment. For instance, key to both the legal doctrine and moral right of informed consent is (1) the liberal democratic notion of the *sovereignty of the individual*, and (2) ethical principlism, considered under separate subheadings below.

INFORMED CONSENT AND THE SOVEREIGNTY OF THE INDIVIDUAL

Informed consent rests heavily on the view that the individual is sovereign alias the *sovereignty of the individual*. This highly individualistic notion characterises the person (patient) as a solitary competent individual who possesses 'a sphere of protected activity or privacy free from unwanted interference'; by this view, although 'influence is acceptable', coercion in any form is not (Kuczewski 1996, p. 30). Kuczewski explains that (p. 30):

> Within this zone of privacy, one is able to exercise his or her liberty and discretion. Within this protected sphere take place disclosure, comprehension, and choice, which express the patient's right of self-determination ... The person is opaque to others and therefore the best judge and guardian of his or her own interests. Although the physician may be the expert on the medical 'facts', the patient is the only individual with genuine insight into his [sic] private sphere of 'values'. Because treatment plans should reflect personal values as well as medical realities, the patient must be the ultimate decision-maker.

One serious and significant implication of this view is that the patient's family, friends and/or chosen carers (acknowledging here that not all patients have families or, if they do, desire the involvement of their families) are conceived 'as comprising competing interests'; they are also seen as having no entitlements whatsoever in regard to any consent to medical treatment processes that the 'sovereign individual' might otherwise engage in (Kuczewski 1996). This may help to explain some of the tensions examined previously in Chapter 4 (pages 77–80) in regard to family members of traditional cultural backgrounds seeking active participation in consent to medical treatment processes and the reluctance by some doctors and nurses to involve these family members in such processes.

Bioethicists and clinicians (particularly palliative care physicians) are, however, rethinking their traditional opposition to the involvement of family or chosen carers in consent to treatment practices (Chaboyer 2000; see also Chapter 4, pages 77–80 of this book). There is increasing recognition that illness can seriously undermine the patient's capacity to make prudent self-determined choices (autonomy) and to be an effective judge and guardian of his or her own self-interests. This has been matched by an increasing questioning of the traditional legalistic approach to informed consent that, among other things, presupposes that the values of the 'sovereign individual' are well-developed, fixed and adequate to the task of choosing between difficult treatment options, and that all the chooser needs in order to make an informed choice is 'information' (Gert 2002; Kuczewski 1996).

Increasingly, family members and chosen carers are recognised as having a vital role to play in consent processes. By being intimately acquainted with ('knowing well') the patient, family members or chosen carers are able to provide appropriate and meaningful feedback to their loved ones, and to generally assist in 'reality checking' their loved one's choices and the values, beliefs (new and old), and deliberations influencing these choices. In sum, the involvement of family members and/or chosen carers in consent to treatment processes can play a vital role in restoring the otherwise diminished autonomy of their sick loved ones (Kuczewski 1996). Furthermore, by fulfilling this role, they are also able to strengthen the bonds of their relationship with the patient and with each other — in short, to express their care of and for each other.

The ultimate conclusion of this new approach is this: we need to reconceptualise informed consent as a *shared* rather than as an *individual* decision-making process (Kuczewski 1996).

INFORMED CONSENT AND ETHICAL PRINCIPLISM

Informed consent also rests heavily on ethical principlism (discussed in Chapter 3 of this book), both for its content and justification as an action guide. The principles of particular importance here include those of:

- *autonomy* — which demands respect for patients as self-determining choosers, and justifies allowing them the option of accepting risks;
- *non-maleficence* — which demands the protection of patients from battery, assault, trespass, exploitation, and other harms that may result from inadequate or inappropriate consent processes (including the inadequate or inappropriate disclosure of information);
- *beneficence* — which demands the maximisation of patient wellbeing via consent processes;
- *justice* — which demands fairness and that patients not be unduly or intolerably burdened by consent processes.

It should be noted that while autonomy is *a* value underlying the doctrine of informed consent it is not the value, nor an *absolute* value. As Faden and Beauchamp (1986, p. 18) point out, at best autonomy is only a prima facie value, and to regard it as having overriding value would be both historically and culturally 'odd'. This is not to say that autonomy does not have a significant place in a moral approach to informed consent. It merely means that it does not have a sole place, and can be justly restricted by other competing moral principles, such as those already mentioned.

Having now reviewed the function and theoretical underpinnings of informed consent, let us proceed critically to examine the constituents and nature of informed consent.

THE ELEMENTS OF AN INFORMED AND VALID CONSENT

It is generally recognised within bioethics that disclosure, comprehension, voluntariness, competence and consent itself form the analytical components of the concept of informed consent (Faden and Beauchamp 1986, p. 274).

Morally speaking, for a consent to be regarded as informed, it must satisfy a number of criteria, including those relating to the *informational* aspect of the consent and those relating to the *giving of consent* itself. Beauchamp and Childress (2001, pp. 77–98) argue that for consent to be informed: there must be a *disclosure* of all the relevant information (including both benefits and risks); the patient *must fully understand* (comprehend) both the information which has been given and the implications of giving consent; the consent must be voluntarily given (i.e. the patient must be free of coercion or manipulation); and, lastly, the patient must be competent to consent (i.e. be both 'rational' and prudent). Faden and Beauchamp (1986, p. 54) argue along similar lines, and recommend what they believe are less 'overdemanding' and plausible criteria, notably:

(1) a patient or subject must agree to an intervention based on an *understanding* of (usually disclosed) relevant *information*, (2) consent must not be controlled by influences that would engineer the outcome, and (3) the consent must involve the intentional giving of *permission* for an intervention.

It needs to be noted that patients frequently do not realise that in giving consent they are not merely acknowledging the receipt of information concerning a recommended medical treatment or procedure, but are also actually *giving permission* to an attending health professional to go ahead and perform the treatment or procedure in question.

Faden and Beauchamp's foundational work and theory of informed consent is probably one of the most comprehensive to date, and one which, although written from the cultural perspective of the United States, deserves to be given serious attention by those furthering the informed consent debate in Australia, New Zealand and other common law countries. As well as advancing their ethical theory, these authors also make a number of useful practical suggestions on how informed consent practices could be made more 'workable'.

It should be noted that the doctrine of informed consent has been the subject of much controversy, most notably amongst health professionals. Common objections include:

- obtaining an informed consent is unacceptably time-consuming;
- when patients are told the information they need to know, they forget it;
- most patients do not want to know all the details of the risks and benefits associated with a recommended medical treatment or procedure, and forcing information on them would be just as paternalistic as withholding it;
- most patients would not understand the information required to make an informed choice;
- giving information to patients can be harmful (for example, they might refuse a life-saving procedure or drug because of a negligible risk); and
- informed consent is impractical and thus unworkable.

These and similar objections are, however, difficult to sustain in the face of research findings, anecdotes and professional experience. For example, it is well recognised that people in stressful and unfamiliar situations are vulnerable both to information overload and short-term memory loss. The stress of being admitted to hospital; of coping with feelings of pain, fear and anxiety; of being separated from the familiarity of one's home, family and friends; the general disruption of one's life, not to mention the effort required to adapt to a new (hospital) environment characterised by strange smells, sights, noises, tastes, routines, faces, procedures and sensations — all contribute, predictably, to lessening an individual's capacity to pay attention to and to recall information that has been disclosed. It is small wonder that patients forget. Information overload and stress-induced short-term memory impairment in turn compromise the individual's actual understanding of information received.

To complicate matters, health professionals seeking consent or giving information do not always manage their encounters with patients very well. Some use a hurried, uninterested and sometimes positively intimidating approach when seeking a patient's consent. When seeking consent from a patient, health professionals too often give little attention to controlling their tone of voice, choosing a suitable time and place to approach the patient, ensuring privacy, using the appropriate body language and facial expressions, choosing the right words, avoiding complicated jargon, sitting at the patient's level, and so on. When dealing with non-English-speaking patients, these problems are considerably worse. For example, health professionals may shout unnecessarily (a problem which also sometimes occurs when they are dealing with blind or physically handicapped people who nevertheless have perfect hearing), or they may use inappropriate body language and facial expressions, use the wrong intonations in speech, or use terms which cannot be readily interpreted into the patient's spoken language.

As far as patients who do not want to know the details of an impending medical procedure are concerned, there are few who seem to fit into this category. In some instances patients have declined information (on the basis of personal and cultural health beliefs and practices), but even then only certain select pieces of information have been declined; in these instances, patients have not voiced a blanket and unconditional rejection of all relevant information. In many instances, what has superficially appeared to be a 'refusal' was in fact more a demand that the information be given in a culturally appropriate manner (see discussion in Chapter 4 of this book). If, however, patients do make an informed and authentic choice not to receive certain relevant pieces of information, and on reflection are not open to changing their minds about receiving the information in question, then to give this information to the patients would certainly count as a paternalistic act (the subject of 'paternalism' will be considered shortly below).

The objection that patients would not be able to understand the necessary information in order to make an intelligent and informed choice is also difficult to sustain. It is sometimes difficult to avoid the impression that the claim that a patient cannot understand is more an assumption than a matter of sound deliberation and determination. Buchanan (1978, p. 386), for example, argues that to assume a patient would not understand given information is to make a 'dubious and extremely broad psychological generalisation', which, of course, ordinary doctors and nurses are not particularly qualified to make. Faden and Beauchamp (1986) also argue that most patients are able to understand the information given to them, and, what is more, that a patient's level of understanding can be ascertained and measured.

Even if patients do not fully understand the information given, this does not always imply that it is the fault of the patient. A patient's inability to understand may be directly related to a doctor's or a nurse's inappropriate behaviour and communication (Roth et al. 1983, p. 176). The onus then is on those seeking to obtain consent to improve their approach to patients, and to presume a patient's *ability* to understand information rather than an inability to understand. On this point Muyskens (1982, p. 119) argues:

> as in a court of law in which one's innocence is presumed until proven otherwise, the client's ability to comprehend and understand what is going on and to be able to make judgments based on the data must be presumed until firm evidence establishes the contrary.

Just as there is no compelling evidence to suggest that patients would not understand information disclosed to them about a proposed medical procedure, there is no compelling evidence to suggest that patients would be unduly injured or harmed by disclosures. Bok (1980) has long contended that very few patients withdraw their consent when informed of material risks or other so-called 'harmful' pieces of information concerning a proposed medical procedure. She further contends that in fact 'it is what patients do not know but vaguely suspect that causes them corrosive worry' (Bok 1980, p. 234).

Buchanan (1978) is even more critical of the view that the disclosure of information material to a treatment decision may cause harm to patients, arguing that such a view reeks of nothing more than wide and unfounded 'psychiatric generalisations', which ordinary doctors and nurses are not qualified to make. He argues further that even qualified psychiatric specialists would probably find it very difficult to judge correctly whether a patient would be significantly harmed by disclosure.

The 'information causing harm' objection, of course, also ignores the moral point that, even if a patient refused to undergo a recommended medical procedure on the basis of information received about certain material risks, this is, after all, something which any competent patient is morally entitled to do — whatever the risks involved and regardless of what others might think of their refusal (see also Tweeddale 2002). At best, all attending health professionals can morally do is to persuade patients *non-coercively* about the known benefits of undergoing a given medical procedure; but they are not entitled to interfere with the patient's choice if such persuasion fails (Faden and Beauchamp 1986).

Even if critics concede that these objections cannot be sustained, the objection still remains that informed consent procedures are impractical because they are unrealistically and unacceptably time-consuming. It is quite true that obtaining a voluntary consent (i.e. one free of coercive or manipulative influences) and a truly informed consent from a patient will take more time than the type of consent that is likely to be obtained in an 'assembly line' approach. But, then, so it *should* take more time. Health professionals should take more time (and as much as is required) to interact and communicate with their patients in a way that facilitates making informed choices and realising morally acceptable outcomes. If health professionals really do care about the wellbeing of their patients, there can be no excuse whatsoever for denying patients the time needed to deal with an anxiety, to answer a worrisome question, or to be reassured. Patients must have sufficient time to make an adequate decision and must have sufficient time to contemplate viable and real alternatives; anything less will result in information overload and will undermine their ability to make voluntary and informed choices (Faden and Beauchamp 1986, p. 326).

In a culture so heavily dominated and constrained by considerations of 'time', it is easy to accept 'time constraint' as a valid reason for abrogating one's moral responsibilities. This, however, is not acceptable morally. There are ways around the difficulties posed by time constraints, and these must always be fully explored. In the case of informed consent, the one possible solution is to involve others in the processes of information transfer to and sharing with patients. As considered above, these 'others' could include lawful proxies, family and/or chosen carers.

While it is obviously and properly the responsibility of treating doctors to obtain informed consents to treatment from the patients they are treating, there is nevertheless considerable room to suggest that a collaborative approach to meeting patients' information needs would contribute substantially to maximising the patients' moral interests. Rightly or wrongly, nurses already play a major, although unacknowledged, role in meeting patients' information needs. This situation has arisen for many reasons, including the reality that treating doctors sometimes fail to meet the information needs of their patients — even when specifically requested to do so, either by patients themselves, or by nurses, or even by other doctors. In situations like this, an attending nurse is often the only immediately available person patients have to turn to in order to obtain the information they want. Indeed, nurses are very often the ones whom patients ask directly about what to expect of a given or pending medical procedure or treatment. In such instances, nurses can find themselves in a very difficult situation — particularly if an attending doctor will not respond appropriately to a patient's request for information. The nurses' dilemma is compounded by the fact that they know they can contribute a great deal to allaying patient anxiety related to knowledge deficits concerning proposed and rendered medical care and treatment options, but do not have the legitimated authority to undertake this role. Thus, if and when they are giving information to patients about medical treatments, nurses know they are 'taking a risk', since this could be construed as 'interfering with the physician–patient relationship' — as, indeed, has happened in a number of high profile legal cases (see Johnstone 1994).

Studies have long shown that nurses can greatly assist patients in coming to understand their illness experience and physician directives given during medical consultations (Uyer 1986). One study also shows that the task of giving information to patients and satisfying patients' information needs is '*impossible* without systematic collaboration between medical and nursing staff' (Engstrom 1986, emphasis added). It is clear that this is a matter which requires much greater attention than it has been given up until now with a view toward legitimating the role of nurses in meeting patients' information needs.

A second obvious strategy which could be used to help resolve the time constraint problem is to restructure the time frame itself during which consents are usually sought. In elective admissions, consents are usually sought on the day before or evening before a scheduled medical or surgical procedure. The moral disadvantages of this are obvious. As Faden and Beauchamp ask (1986, p. 325):

> who would want, on the eve of surgery after having disrupted one's life, gathered one's courage, and entered the hospital, to change one's mind? And thus who would want to pay attention to information that challenges the wisdom of the decision?

Such a short time frame is hardly conducive to patients exercising voluntary and informed consent. One possible solution — and one that is routinely practised in some areas — would be to give patients all the 'usual' information during a pre-admission clinic a week or so before the procedure. In this way, patients have time to go home, contemplate the information received, discuss it with family and friends, formulate any further questions they would like to ask, or even change their minds and decline the recommended therapy or procedure if they so desired. If patients are allowed time to reflect on the information given to them, not only would their consents to treatment be of better quality, but so too would their decisions to enter hospital.

The time factor involved in obtaining consent is crucial to the realisation of morally just outcomes. If sufficient time is not allocated for the purposes of gaining a patient's consent, a very real risk exists that the voluntary and informed nature of the consent will be seriously compromised, thus having the domino effect of violating underlying moral principles such as autonomy, non-maleficence, beneficence, and justice. In other words, a complete moral collapse of the situation could occur. In emergency or life-threatening situations, of course, it is not always possible to seek an informed consent and it could be hazardous to try and do so. The law recognises that in emergency or life-threatening situations consent can be 'waived'; morality likewise recognises situations in which consent can be justly waived.

The challenge to doctors and nurses and other health professionals is to restructure their thinking on informed consent, and to view it as something which 'should help overcome the inclination that many people have to yield compliantly to proposals from powerful authority figures' (Faden and Beauchamp 1986, p. 372). Faden and Beauchamp (1986, p. 305) argue that the questions that all health professionals and policy and law makers should be asking are not what patients should be told or even who should tell them, but 'What can professionals do to facilitate obtaining informed consents based on substantial understanding?', or 'How can professionals enable patients and subjects to make informed autonomous choices?'.

If informed consent procedures are to work and to achieve their desired ends, a number of other practical considerations need to be attended to. First, consent forms should be made available in the patient's own language and obtaining consent facilitated by the involvement of trained health interpreters. It was once the practice to ask cleaners or orderlies or kitchen hands who speak languages other than English to interpret for a non-English-speaking patient (see also Stone 1991, p. 4). This situation still arises on occasion despite being unacceptable. First, orderlies and cleaners and kitchen hands are not trained as interpreters and thus may seriously misinterpret the information being relayed, or may give their own assessment of and interpretation of a question being asked. For example, Olga Kanitsaki (who is Greek-speaking) describes a case involving a Greek-speaking patient. In this case, a cleaner called in to interpret for the doctor exclaimed to the patient, in Greek, 'Well, if you only have a headache why don't you take an aspirin? What did you come into hospital for? Why are you bothering the doctor?' (personal communication).

Another problem here, and one often overlooked by health professionals, is that orderlies and cleaners and kitchen hands do not have a professional relationship with the patient; thus, involving them as interpreters is tantamount to breaching confidentiality. Who is to know whether these 'informal' interpreters will keep confidential the information disclosed during an interpreting session? Since they are not bound by any professional code of ethics, they may not fully appreciate their moral responsibilities not to disclose the confidential information they have become privy to while acting as interpreters.

A second practical consideration is that patients' consent must be continuously *re-evaluated* so as to check whether their original consent still holds. This is particularly crucial in situations involving 'Not For Resuscitation' directives (also called 'Do Not Resuscitate' directives) or refusal to consent to given life-saving therapies. In some instances, the terms of a patient's original consent may need to be modified. It has been asserted informally by those working in the area that the term 'informed consent' should be abandoned in favour of the term 'informed decision-making'. The rationale given is that the notion of *informed consent* has an air of finality about it — that is, once consent has been obtained that is the end of the process. With the notion of *informed decision-making*, however, the connotations are quite different. In contrast, it has an air of 'open-endedness' about it — of a process that is *ongoing*. Given this, it is thought, the notion of informed decision-making, unlike the notion of informed consent, seems to invite the continuous re-evaluation of any decisions made about care and treatment options. This change in thinking, however, has yet to be reflected fully in literature on the subject.

A third consideration is that patients must be informed of their entitlement to *refuse* a recommended medical or nursing procedure, and the opportunity to refuse must always be present without prejudice to the patients. Fourth, patients must be kept up to date on the relevant details pertaining to their cases. Details which are not readily understood should be explained (in understandable language), and reinforced through planned patient health education programs (something that nurses are educationally prepared to undertake).

Lastly, health professionals need to remind themselves constantly that many factors can deter patients from exercising informed and voluntary choices, including, but not limited to, *fear of victimisation*. For example, patients may fear that if they refuse to give consent to some aspect of the proposed procedure they may be victimised by being denied other forms of treatment or by being verbally and emotionally abused. Other factors include: feelings of guilt where patients might feel, for example, that somehow they ought to give consent for the sake of their families (see Roberts 1987; Hyun 2002); fear of unknown outcomes; frank disagreement and value conflict, where patients might refuse simply because they do not agree with a given recommended medical therapy and would prefer to try an alternative health modality; pain or grief states which can cloud patients' prudence; 'rational incompetence', and an associated inability to exercise self-determining choices; and incompetent or impaired health professionals who may, for instance, be poor communicators, have poor interpersonal skills, be rushed or hurried, or lack the relevant information to give to the patient.

Before concluding this discussion two further issues remain to be addressed — the problem of the so-called 'rationally incompetent' patient and medical paternalism.

THE PROBLEM OF RATIONAL COMPETENCY

Critical to satisfying the requirements of informed consent is competency to decide. The issue of competency is, however, controversial and complicated. This is because there is no substantial agreement on the characteristics of a 'competent person' or on how 'competency' should be measured. Nor is there any legal test of competency that 'commands general acceptance' (Gert et al. 1997, p. 131). To complicate this matter further, there is also no substantial agreement on what constitutes *rationality* which, as has been argued elsewhere, is very much a matter of subjective interpretation (Johnstone 1999a, 122). As Gibson (1976) points out in an early article on the subject, rationality cannot escape the influences of the social patterns and institutions around it and, for this reason, any value-neutral account of rationality is quite inadequate. She further suggests that at most rationality should be regarded as a value, rather than a property that all 'normal' people have (Gibson 1967, p. 193). In summary, the notion of 'rational competency' is problematic because there is no precise definition of, or agreement on, what it is.

Even if there was agreement on what constitutes rational competency, there remains the problem of 'whereby the definition of competence changes in different clinical situations' (Gert et al. 1997, p. 135). For example, an elderly demented resident may be deemed competent to eat his/her evening meal alone, but deemed not to be competent to refuse treatment (e.g. suturing) of a deep and bloody laceration to his/her arm. As Gert et al. (1997, p. 132) go on to explain, we need to appreciate that persons as such are 'not globally "competent" but rather "competent to do X", where X is some specific physical or mental task'. In other words, competence is always 'task-specific' and determining or measuring competence is thus always 'context-dependent' (see also Mukherjee and Shah 2001).

Significantly the issue of competency rarely arises in contexts where the patient agrees with and consents to a doctor's recommended or prescribed treatment. Gert et al. (1997, p. 142) suggest controversially that this is because 'doctors almost always recommend treatments that it would be rational for patients to choose'. They go on to argue that it is mostly in 'cases of treatment refusals, especially those that appear to be irrational, that the question of a patient's competence most frequently and appropriately arises' (Gert el al. 1997, p. 142). A good example of this can be found in the much publicised Australian case of John McKewan that occurred in the mid-1980s and which sparked an unprecedented public inquiry into the so-called 'right to die with dignity' (Social Development Committee 1987).

John McKewan, a former Australian water skiing champion, was left a ventilator-dependent quadriplegic after a diving accident at Echuca, Victoria. Throughout his hospitalisation, he repeatedly asked to be allowed to die. At one point, desperate to achieve his wish, he went on a hunger strike and instructed his solicitor to draw up a 'living will', which stated 'that he did not wish to be revived if and when he fell into a coma' (*Bioethics News* 1985, p. 2). According to media reports, this act led to a psychiatrist certifying him as rationally incompetent, thereby enabling John McEwan to be treated (fed) against his will. The psychiatrist's judgment was revoked a few days later, however, when John McEwan 'agreed to end his hunger strike and accept a course of antidepressants' (*Bioethics News* 1985, p. 2).

A little over a year after his accident, and despite still being ventilator-dependent, John McEwan was discharged home. The round-the-clock day care he required was given by family members and friends who had received special training in how to care for him. In the weeks following his discharge from hospital, John McEwan continued to express his wish to be allowed to die (Social Development Committee 1987, pp. 310–11). This prompted the general practitioner who was medically responsible for him to inform the senior nursing assistant that:

> John McEwan at his own request could come off the ventilator from time to time but had to be reconnected if he became distressed *even if it was against his own wishes*.
> (Social Development Committee 1987, p. 312, emphasis added)

During one incident, while at home, John McEwan was observed to be angry at having been reconnected to the ventilator against his wishes. And in another incident shortly before his death, he talked openly with his general practitioner about 'hiring someone to blow his [John McEwan's] brains out or kill him as he felt his wish to die was being frustrated' (Social Development Committee 1987, p. 316). There was no reason to suspect that John McEwan's wishes were irrational. Before his accident he had been a committed sportsman and for him the life of a helpless quadriplegic was intolerable.

At four o'clock in the morning on 3 April 1986, John McEwan was found dead by his nursing attendant. At the time of discovery he was disconnected from his ventilator.

It is perhaps easy to think of competency in cases such as this in purely medical or psychiatric terms. In their classic and still frequently cited work, Roth et al. (1983) argue, however, that the concept of competency is not merely a psychiatric or medical concept, as some might assume, but is also fundamentally social and legal in nature. They go on to warn that there is no magical definition of competency, and that the problems posed by so-called 'incompetent' persons are very often problems of personal prejudices and social biases, or of other difficulties associated with trying to find the 'right' words.

The critical issue in developing tests of competency is how to strike a happy balance between serving a rationally incompetent person's autonomy and also serving that person's health care, nursing care and medical treatment needs. Also of critical concern is finding a competency test which is comprehensive enough to deal with diverse situations, which can be applied reliably, and which is mutually acceptable to health care professionals, lawyers, judges and the community at large.

Roth et al. suggest (1983, p. 173) that competency tests proposed in the literature basically fall into five categories:

1. evidencing a choice;
2. 'reasonable' outcome of choice;
3. choice based on 'rational' reasons;
4. ability to understand;
5. actual understanding.

The test of *evidencing a choice* is as it sounds, and is concerned only with whether a patient's choice is 'evident'; that is, whether it is *present or absent*. For example, a fully comatose patient would be unable to evidence a choice, unlike a semi-comatose patient or a brain-injured person, who could evidence a choice by opening and shutting their eyes or by squeezing someone's hand to indicate 'yes' or 'no'. The *quality* of the patient's choice in this instance is quite irrelevant. One problem with this test, however, is whether, say, the blinking of a patient's eyes can be relied upon as evidencing a choice; in a life and death situation one would need to be very sure that a patient's so-called 'evidencing a choice' is more than just a reflex.

The test of *reasonable outcome of a choice* is again as it sounds, and focuses on the *outcome* of a given choice, as opposed to the mere presence or absence of a choice. The objective test here is similar to that employed in law, and involves asking the question: What would a reasonable person in like circumstances consider to be a reasonable outcome? The reliability of this measure is, of course, open to serious question — as previously objected, what one person might accept as reasonable another might equally reject.

The test of *choice based on rational reasons* is a little more difficult to apply. Basically, it asks whether a given choice is the product of 'mental illness' or whether it is the product of prudent and critically reflective deliberation. A number of objections can be raised here. For example, contrary to popular medical opinion, there is nothing to suggest that a person's decision to suicide is always the product of mental disease or depression. A patient could without contradiction 'rationally' choose to suicide as a means of escaping an intolerable life characterised by suffering intractable and intolerable pain. Alternatively, a depressed and so-called 'irrational' person might refuse a particular psychiatric treatment, such as psychotropic drugs, electroconvulsive therapy, or psychosurgery, out of a very 'rational' and well-founded fear of what undesirable effects these treatments might ultimately have.

The test of *ability to understand*, on the other hand, asks whether the patient is able to comprehend the risks, benefits and alternatives to a proposed medical procedure, as well as the implications of giving consent. Here objections can be raised concerning just how sophisticated a patient's understanding needs to be. The problem also may arise of patients perceiving a risk as a benefit. Roth et al. (1983, p. 175), for example, cite the case of a 49-year-old woman psychiatric patient who was informed that there was a one in three thousand chance of dying from ECT. When told of this risk she replied, happily: 'I hope I am the one!'.

The fifth and final competency test is that of *actual understanding*. This test asks how well the patient has actually understood information which has been disclosed. This can be established by asking patients probing questions and inviting them to reiterate the information they have received. On the basis of educated skill and past experience, the health professional is usually able to ascertain the level at which the patient has understood the information received and what data gaps or misunderstandings remain.

A variation of this test is advanced by Grisso and Appelbaum (1998, p. 31), and includes assessing patients' for their abilities to:

1. express a choice;
2. understand information relevant to treatment decision making;
3. appreciate the significance of that information for [their] own situation, especially concerning [their own] illness and the probable consequences of [their] treatment options; and
4. reason with relevant information so as to engage in a logical process of weighing treatment options [emphasis original]

Issues raised by this test criteria are much the same as those already considered above in relation to Roth et al's competency test (Gert et al. 1997).

Whatever the patients' competency to decide and quality of their autonomous choice may be, any duty of respect owed would still ultimately depend on the demands of other competing moral considerations, as already discussed. Thus, what may appear to be a dilemma involving whether to respect a patient's autonomy may not in fact be a dilemma at all. For example, if an elderly demented patient keeps wandering aimlessly from his bed, and is at risk of falling and fracturing his hip, overriding considerations do exist which would justify interfering with the choice to wander. If, after careful analysis of all available alternatives, the only way to stop this elderly patient from sustaining a fractured hip is to restrain him, it may well be that the use of a comfortable restraining device is the morally compelling option in this case. If, however, the elderly person is not at risk of falling and sustaining a fractured hip, and his wandering is merely an 'inconvenience' to staff, the solution might be better found in securing door locks so as to prevent the patient from wandering out onto the street where there is a very real risk of injury — say, of being hit by a car. This solution is already employed in a number of residential care homes which have installed combination locks on all their doors; only those residents who know the combination of the locks on the doors can freely come and go. Either way, entitlements and corresponding duties in the case of 'rational incompetence' must ultimately be determined by critical reflection and not, as can happen, by misguided or unfounded assumption.

It should be noted that competency is a key issue not just in aged care or psychiatric nursing, but in any health care context where judgments of competency are critical to deciding: (1) whether a patient can or should decide and/or be permitted to decide for herself or himself, and (2) the point at which another or others will need to or should decide for the patient — that is, become what Buchanan and Brock (1989) term *surrogate decision-makers* and what others call 'proxies' (Chaboyer 2000). The question remains, however, of how these things can be decided in a morally sound and just way. This question becomes even more problematic when it is considered that patients deemed 'rationally incompetent' (or at least, cognitively impaired) can still be quite capable of making 'reasonable' self-interested choices, and, further, that the choices they make — even if 'irrational' — are not always harmful (Williams 2002).

Commenting on the moral standards which should be met when deciding whether to respect or override the expressed preferences of a patient deemed 'incompetent', Buchanan and Brock (1989) argue that it is important to be clear about what statements of competence refer to. Like Gert et al. (1997), cited earlier, they argue that statements of competence (i.e. in clinical contexts) usually refer to a person's competence to *do something*, in this instance, to *choose and make decisions*; by this view, competence is, therefore, 'choice and decision-relative'. Given this, determining competence in health care contexts fundamentally involves determining a person's ability to make particular choices and decisions under particular conditions (Buchanan and Brock 1989, pp. 311–65; see also Mukherjee and Shah 2001).

An important problem particularly in psychiatric contexts is that severe mental illness can significantly affect the capacities needed for competent decision-making (for instance, understanding, reasoning, and applying values), and hence the ability generally of severely mentally ill persons to make sound decisions about their own wellbeing — including the need for care and treatment (Buchanan and Brock 1989). For example, as Buchanan and Brock comment (1989, p. 318):

> a person may persist in a fixed delusional belief that proffered medications are poison or are being used to control his or her mind. Such delusions or fixed false beliefs obviously may also impair a person's capacity to reason about whether hospitalisation and treatment will on balance serve his or her wellbeing. Severe mental illness can also affect and seriously distort a person's underlying and enduring aims and values, his or her conception of his or her own good, that one must use in evaluating hospitalisation and treatment for an illness.

It is precisely in situations such as these that attending health care professionals need a reliable framework within which to decide how best to act — notably: (1) whether to respect a patient's preferences even though the patient is deemed 'incompetent', or (2) whether to override patients' preferences in the interests of protecting or upholding what has been deemed by *others* to be in the patient's overall 'best interests'. Just what such a framework would — or indeed should — look like, is, however, a matter of some controversy. Nevertheless, as Buchanan and Brock's substantive work *Deciding for others: the ethics of surrogate decision-making* (1989) has shown, it is possible to devise at least a prima facie working framework to guide professional ethical decision-making in this sensitive, complex and problematic area. Specifically, Buchanan and Brock (1989) suggest that the whole issue hinges on:

1. setting and applying accurately standards of competency to choose and decide; and
2. achieving a balance between (i) protecting and promoting the patients' wellbeing (human welfare), (ii) protecting and promoting the patients' entitlement to and interest in exercising self-determining choices, and (iii) protecting others who could be harmed by patients exercising harm-causing choices.

In regard to setting and applying accurately standards of competency to choose and decide, Buchanan and Brock suggest that, among other things, ethical professional decision-making in this problematic area should be guided by the following considerations (p. 85):

> No single standard of competence is adequate for all decisions. The standard depends in large part on the risk involved, and varies along a range from low/minimal to high/maximal. The more serious the expected harm to the patient from acting on a choice, the higher should be the standard of decision-making capacity, and the greater should be the certainty that the standard is satisfied.

In other words, the extent to which an attending health care professional is bound morally to respect the choices of a person deemed 'rationally incompetent' depends primarily on the severity of the risks involved to the patient if her or his choices are permitted. The higher and more severe the risks involved, the higher and more rigorous should be the standards for determining the patient's decision-making capacity, and the more certain attending health care professionals should be that the patient has met these standards. This framework is expressed diagrammatically in Figure 6.2.

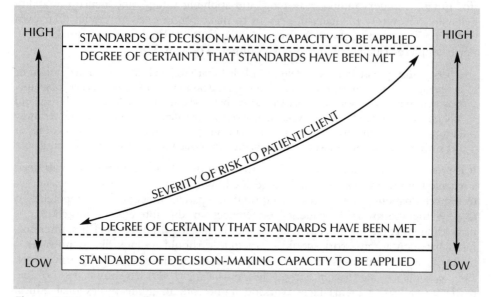

Figure 6.2 Assessing risks and permitting choices of patients deemed 'rationally incompetent'

For example, if a patient with severe mental illness chooses to refuse hospitalisation, the extent to which an attending health professional is obliged morally to respect this choice will depend on how severe the risks to the patient are of not being hospitalised — for instance, whether a failure to hospitalise the patient will result in her or him suiciding, or will result only in her or him being left in a state of moderate, although not life-threatening, depression. In the case of suicide risk, the grounds for not honouring a patient's choices do seem at least prima facie stronger than possible grounds for overriding the choices of a patient who is only moderately depressed. (Whether or not the risk of suicide does provide strong grounds for overriding a patient's choices to refuse hospitalisation and treatment is another question, however, and one which is considered separately in Chapter 10 of this book.)

While Buchanan and Brock's (1989) 'sliding scale' framework is useful, it is not free of difficulties. For instance, there remains the problem of how to determine what is a harm, what is a low/minimal and high/maximal risk of harm, and who properly should decide these things — the answers to which involve complex value judgments. Consider, for example, the following case (personal communication).

An involuntary psychiatric patient refuses to take the psychotropic medication he has been prescribed. In defence of his refusal, the patient argues 'reasonably' that the adverse side effects of the drugs he is being expected to take are intolerable, and that he would prefer the pain of his mental illness to the intolerable side effects of the drugs that have been prescribed to treat his mental illness. Staff on the ward in which he is an involuntary patient are divided about what they should do. The more experienced staff in this case insist that the patient should be given his medication forcibly by intramuscular injection. They argue in defence of this decision that the patient's condition is deteriorating rapidly, and that if he does not receive the medication prescribed he will 'spiral down into a psychiatric crisis' (in other words a total exacerbation of his condition), which would be even more intolerable and harmful than the unpleasant side effects he has been experiencing as a result of taking the psychotropic drugs in question. They make the additional value judgment that it would be 'better' for the patient if his psychiatric condition was prevented from deteriorating, and that their decision to administer his prescribed medication forcibly against his will is justified on these grounds.

The less experienced staff on the ward disagree with this reasoning, however, and argue that, even though the patient's psychiatric condition is deteriorating, and this is a preventable harm, the patient is nevertheless able to make an informed choice about this and therefore his wishes should be respected. In defence of their position, they argue that the patient's complaints are justified — the adverse side effects of his psychotropic drugs have indeed been 'awful', and are commonly experienced by other patients as well; and that he has experienced a decline in his psychiatric condition before, and hence knows what to expect. Further, they argue, if he is given the medication against his will, an even greater harm will follow: specifically, he will trust the nursing staff even less than he does already, and will be even less willing to comply with his oral medication prescription than he is now.

In this case, the more experienced staff outnumbered the less experienced staff, and the patient was held down and forcibly given an intramuscular injection of the medication he had refused. Later, after recovering from this incident, the patient was, as predicted by the less experienced nursing staff, grossly mistrustful of the nursing staff on the ward, and even less willing to comply with his oral medication prescription. His requests for different and less drugs, and more counselling, went unheeded.

This case scenario demonstrates the difficulties that can be encountered when accepting/rejecting a patient's ability to choose and decide care and treatment options, and deciding when and how to override a patient's preferences. Not only is there the problem of how to determine accurately what a harm is and how a given harm should be weighted morally when evaluating whether a patient's choices should be respected or overridden; there is the additional problem that attending health care professionals may disagree radically among themselves about how these things should be determined — to a point that may even cause rather than prevent harm to the patient, as happened in this case. What else then should health care professionals do?

One response is to insist on the development of reliable (research-based) criteria for deciding these sorts of problematic issues. The need to do this becomes even more acute when the problem of determining and weighting harms is considered in relation to the broader demand to achieve a balance between protecting and promoting the patient's wellbeing, protecting and promoting the patient's autonomy, and protecting others who could be harmed if a mentally ill person is left free to exercise harm-causing choices (as happened in the *Tarasoff case*, to be considered later in this chapter).

Just what these criteria should be, however, and how they should be applied, is an extremely complex matter, and one that requires much greater attention than it is possible to give here. Nevertheless, Buchanan and Brock (1989) provide an important starting point by identifying the following three factors which should be (and are already being) taken into consideration when deciding whether to override a mentally ill person's choices, namely (1) whether the person is a danger to herself or himself; (2) whether the person is in need of care and treatment; and (3) whether the person is a danger to others. In regard to the consideration of being a danger to self, Buchanan and Brock (1989, pp. 317–31) correctly argue that what is needed are stringent criteria of what constitutes a danger to self; in the case of the need for care and treatment, that what is needed are stringent criteria for ascertaining deterioration and distress; and in the case of harm to others, that what is needed are stringent criteria of what constitutes a danger to others. And while applying the criteria developed may inevitably result in a health care professional assuming the essentially paternalistic role of being a surrogate decision-maker for a given patient, this need not be problematic provided the model of surrogate decision-making used is *patient centred* — that is, committed to upholding the patient's interests and concerns insofar as these can be ascertained (something which was not done in the case given above).

A patient-centred model of surrogate decision-making, in this instance, would have as its rationale *preventing harm to patients*, and would embrace an ethical framework which is structured 'for deciding *for* patients for *their benefit*' (Buchanan and Brock 1989, pp. 327, 331). This is in contrast with a non-patient or 'other'-centred decision-making model, which would have as its rationale *preventing harm to others*, and which embraces an ethical framework 'for deciding *about* others for *others' benefits*' (Buchanan and Brock 1989, pp. 327, 331). It should be noted, however, that these two models are not necessarily mutually exclusive and indeed could, in some instances, be mutually supporting (a man contemplating a violent suicide involving others is not only a danger to himself but to the innocent others he plans to 'take with him'). Just which model or models are appropriate, and under what circumstances they should be used, will, however, depend ultimately on the people involved (and the relationships between them), the moral interests at stake, the context in which these moral interests are at stake, the resources available (human and otherwise) to protect and promote the moral interests that are at risk of being harmed, and, finally, the accurate prediction of possibilities and probabilities in regard to the achievement of desirable and acceptable moral outcomes. This, in turn, will depend on the competence, experience, wisdom and moral integrity of the decision-makers, and the degree of commitment they have to: (1) ensuring the realisation of morally just outcomes, and (2) protecting and promoting the wellbeing and moral interests of those made vulnerable not just by their mental illnesses, but by the inability of their caregivers to respond to the manifestation of their illnesses in morally sensitive, humane, therapeutically effective and culturally appropriate ways.

PATERNALISM AND INFORMED CONSENT

The word *paternalism* comes from the Latin *pater* meaning 'father', and literally means 'in the manner of a father, especially in usurping individual responsibility and the liberty of choice' (*Collins English Dictionary* 1995). In the bioethics literature, paternalism has been defined in a variety of ways. Literature published in the early 1970s, for example, defined paternalism (construed as a principle viz. the *Paternalistic Principle* [Beauchamp 1980, p. 98]) as:

the interference with a person's liberty of action justified by reasons referring exclusively to the welfare, good, happiness, needs, interests or value of the person being coerced.

(Dworkin 1972, p. 65)

Subsequently, paternalism was defined more specifically as:

interference with a person's freedom of action or freedom of information, or the deliberate dissemination of misinformation, where the alleged justification of interfering or misinforming is that it is for the good of the person who is interfered with or misinformed.

(Buchanan 1978, p. 372)

A further modification in definition resulted in the suggestion that for an act to be paternalistic:

There must be a violation of a person's autonomy ...There must be a [sic] usurpation of decision-making, either by preventing people from doing what they have decided or by interfering with the way in which they arrive at their decision.

(Dworkin 1988, p. 123)

A more recent definition of paternalism holds it to be:

the intentional overriding of one person's known preferences or actions by another person, where the person who overrides justifies the action by the goal of benefiting or avoiding harm to the person whose preferences or actions are overridden.

(Beauchamp and Childress 2001, p. 178)

Early literature on the subject distinguished between two types of paternalism: (1) harm paternalism, and (2) benefit paternalism (Beauchamp 1978; Beauchamp and Childress 1994). *Harm paternalism* (underpinned by the principle of non-maleficence) was thought to be justified where it had as its objective protecting individuals from self-inflicted harm. In contrast, *benefit paternalism* (underpinned by the principle of beneficence) was thought to be justified where it had as its objective securing a good or a beneficence that an individual would not otherwise get — for example, because their liberty is limited. These two forms of paternalism were, in turn, categorised still further, with the following distinctions being made: (1) strong paternalism and (2) weak paternalism, considered below.

In the case of *strong paternalism*, it was thought to be 'proper to protect or benefit a person by liberty-limiting measures *even when his [or her] contrary choices are informed and voluntary* (Beauchamp 1978, p. 1197). An example of 'strong paternalism' would be where a consultant physician refuses to release a competent although seriously ill patient from hospital even though the patient has requested discharge and knows the potentially fatal consequences of his/her request.

Strong paternalism is in contradistinction to *weak paternalism* where interference with an individual's conduct is only justified in cases where that person's conduct is 'substantially nonvoluntary or when temporary intervention is necessary to establish whether it is voluntary or not' (Feinberg 1971, pp. 113, 116). In short, where a person's autonomy has been compromised in some way (e.g. as a result of pain, drug ingestion, psychogenic distress, physical trauma to the head that interferes with memory, and the like), it is acceptable to paternalistically override a person's choices or restrain their liberty of conduct. This form of paternalism has been widely accepted in law, medicine and moral philosophy (Beauchamp 1995, p. 1915). An example of 'weak paternalism' would be where an attending health care professional attends the scene of a motor vehicle accident and picks up an injured, partially coherent victim and takes him/her to hospital even though the victim has refused an ambulance (Beauchamp 1995, p. 1915).

As a point of clarification, it should be noted that harm paternalism is thought to be easier to justify and uphold than benefit paternalism. One reason for this is that it was (and is) generally thought, controversially, that we have a greater duty to avoid harm than to promote good — which may not always be within our capacity in given contexts and thus not something for which we could be held morally responsible for not doing. If it was our duty to do or promote good — even where we lacked the resources to do so — this would risk us being condemned as 'unethical' for not doing something that we could not do anyway, which would be untenable.

However defined or conceptualised, it should be noted that *paternalism* remains morally controversial since it always entails the *choices or actions of one person being overridden by another without consent*. Even if a person's stated preferences do not originate from a substantially autonomous and authentic choice, 'overriding his or her preference can still be paternalistic' (Beauchamp 1995, p. 1915). This is because, even in the case of 'diminished autonomy', persons (for example, young children, the intellectually disabled and the mentally ill) can still be capable of exercising self-interested choices. It is against this backdrop then that a key question arises, namely: Is paternalism ever justified? and if so, under what conditions?

IS PATERNALISM JUSTIFIED?

The literature reveals at least three possible answers to the question of whether paternalism is justified:

1. pro-paternalism (always justified);
2. anti-paternalism (never justified); and
3. prima-facie paternalism (sometimes justified).

These three possible answers are discussed below.

Pro-paternalism (always justified)

Pro-paternalism positions hold that paternalism is always justified to 'protect individuals against themselves' (Hart 1963, p. 31). This position is supported by an appeal to either of the principles of human welfare, beneficence (e.g. as in the case of overriding the harmful choices of children) and/or 'rational consent' (meaning consent that 'would otherwise have been given'; in this instance, paternalism is thought to be justified as a kind of 'social insurance policy' for our own protection (Beauchamp 1995, p. 1916). Further, it is held that sometimes an immediate act of paternalism may, paradoxically, protect a person's 'deeper autonomy', for example, such as in the case of someone who is depressed and suicidal (Beauchamp 1980, 1995). Justificatory considerations for strong paternalism, include the following conditions:

- no acceptable alternative to the paternalistic action exists;
- risks to the person that are introduced by the paternalistic action itself are not substantial;
- projected benefits to the person outweigh risks to the person;
- any infringement of the principle of respect for autonomy is minimal.

(Beauchamp 1995, p. 1917)

Anti-paternalism (never justified)

Anti-paternalism positions hold that paternalism is never justified. This is because paternalism always involves a violation of moral rules, for example, that we ought to respect people's choices even if we do not agree with them, provided they do not harm others; the individual is sovereign and any coercion or interference with their self-determining choices is morally unacceptable. Acts of paternalism also violate a person's privacy and fail to treat them as the moral equals of others (Childress 1982, cited in Beauchamp 1995, p. 1916).

Prima-facie paternalism (sometimes justified)

Prima-facie paternalism (also known as ambivalent-paternalism) holds the position that paternalism is sometimes justified, though severely limited. Any action of coercion against or interference with another's conduct carries a heavy burden of justification. Paternalism is only justified where:

1. the evils prevented from occurring to the person are greater than the evils (if any) caused by violating the moral rule;
2. it is universally justified under relevantly similar circumstances always to treat persons in this way

(Gert and Culver 1976)

These three positions may be expressed diagrammatically as shown in Figure 6.3.

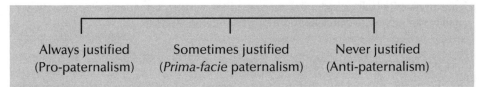

Always justified   Sometimes justified   Never justified
(Pro-paternalism)   (*Prima-facie* paternalism)   (Anti-paternalism)

Figure 6.3 Three positions on paternalism

Despite the apparent differences between these three positions, however, there is some agreement between the positions of 'weak paternalism' and 'anti-paternalism'. These are (Beauchamp 1995, p. 1917):

(i) it is justifiable to interfere in order to protect persons against harm from their own substantially non-autonomous decisions; and
(ii) it is unjustifiable to interfere in order to protect persons against harm from their own substantially autonomous decisions.

One reason for this closeness in position is that, as some contend, 'weak paternalism' is not really paternalism at all since it cannot be substantively distinguished from anti-paternalism. In the ultimate analysis both rest on the principles of beneficence and non-maleficence, and both reject strong paternalism (which justifies overriding strongly autonomous choices). However, when it is considered that even strong paternalism rests on the principles of beneficence and non-maleficence, the differences between all three positions may, in the end, be overstated.

APPLYING THE 'PATERNALISTIC PRINCIPLE' IN HEALTH CARE

Applying the 'Paternalistic Principle' in health care contexts is not clear-cut and indeed raises a number of important questions, such as: How are we to justify overriding another's choices? What constitutes beneficial and harmful outcomes for the patient? What constitutes a patient's 'best interests'? How are we to measure the quality of another's autonomy and autonomous choices? Do people have the right to refuse life-saving/enhancing treatment? What if treatments are 'harmful'?

The abuses of paternalistic decision-making and the rise of individualism and 'patients' rights' in the 1970s and 1980s saw a backlash against paternalism in health care. The past three decades have, however, seen a tempering of this rejection (see also Gert et al. 1997; Beauchamp and Childress 2001). As Beauchamp concludes (1995, p. 1920):

> Paternalism seems likely to continue to be a viewpoint that will gain or lose adherents as the issues and larger social context shift. We may never again see the concentrated flurry of scholarly interest in this subject that was exhibited from the mid-1970s to the mid-1980s, but paternalism is not likely to be an issue that will soon disappear.

One author has argued controversially that medical paternalism in health care contexts (which he states is often practised 'covertly') is not only here to stay, but is 'essential' to ethical practice and the promotion of patient autonomy; he writes:

> Although patient autonomy is dominant in current ethical discussions, medical paternalism is not extinct. Indeed it cannot become so, for the exercise of paternalism is essential to the practice of medicine. After all, we are the medical experts, and we are required to recommend what is medically best for the patient. It is therefore arguable that some measure of paternalism is involved in most treatment decisions. This covert paternalism is not necessarily bad, provided it is recognised for what it is, and is used appropriately to guide and support patient autonomy rather than to override it.
>
> (Tweeddale 2002, p. 236)

INFORMED CONSENT AND NURSES

The discussion given here on informed consent (and its counterparts, competency and paternalism) is less than complete; much more can be said on the matter. Nevertheless, in the light of what has been discussed it is evident that nurses have much to contribute to the informed consent debate. Further, it is evident that the nursing profession needs to pay much greater attention to the doctrine of informed consent and its moral implications for nurses — not least the duties it imposes on nurses to obtain patients' informed consent to *nursing* care and procedures, and the issues it raises concerning 'nursing paternalism.' It is perhaps important to emphasise that, although the doctrine of informed consent has traditionally been discussed primarily in regard to medical treatment and care, the underlying moral values, moral principles and moral requirements of this doctrine apply equally to other kinds of health care practices and procedures, including nursing care and procedures. This is because nurses are no less exempt than are any other health care professionals from the moral standards governing consent procedures, including the demands to:

- disclose all relevant information necessary for making an informed choice about proposed nursing cares and procedures;
- ensure that the patient understands the information received and the implications of giving consent;
- ensure that the consent is given voluntarily (that is, that nurses do not coerce or manipulate the patient into giving consent); and
- ensure that the patient has the capacity to make an informed choice, and, if not, that any surrogate decision-making on the patient's behalf is in accordance with rigorous moral standards.

Likewise the issue of paternalism. Although paternalism has primarily been discussed in regard to the profession of medicine (medical paternalism), the issues raised apply just as well to nursing (nursing paternalism). These issues both stand as fertile ground for further debate, research and scholarship.

The right to confidentiality

The principle of confidentiality has long been recognised as an important and fundamental guide to action in health professional–client relationships. This principle is recognised in law as well as in ethics. In so far as the law is concerned, Wallace (1991, p. 146) explains:

> It is unlawful for any person to disclose any information relating to patients, except with their consent, when required by law, or to lessen a serious threat to the life and health of the individual.

From an ethical perspective, the requirement to uphold the principle of confidentiality is similar to the legal position, as will now be shown.

There are widely divergent views among health professionals and patients/clients about the nature and 'bindingness' of confidentiality (Winslade 1995, p. 454). For example, the International Council of Nurses (ICN) *Code for Nurses* (2000) takes a prima facie (discretionary) position, stating: 'the nurse holds in confidence personal information and *uses judgment in sharing this information*' [emphasis added]. By contrast, the *International Code of Medical Ethics* (1983) takes an absolutist position, stating: 'A physician shall preserve *absolute confidentiality on all he [sic] knows about his [sic] patient even after the patient has died*' [emphasis added] (p. 6). It should be noted, however, that the position of the *International Code of Medical Ethics* has not been adopted universally by local medical associations. The Australian Medical Association's *Code of Ethics*, for example, recognises that information may be divulged with the patient's permission' and that 'exceptions may arise where the health of others is at risk or you [the doctor] are required by order of a court to breach patient confidentiality'.

Historically, the principle of confidentiality has been interpreted as an absolute principle. In application it was (and still is in some contexts, e.g. the priest confessional) taken as demanding that information gained in a professional–client relationship must be kept secret, even when its disclosure might serve a greater public good. An example of the extent to which confidentiality was once regarded by professionals (especially doctors) as being absolute can be found in a 1904 case in which a physician refused to warn a prospective victim that her fiancé was a syphilitic, thereby risking both her and her offspring being exposed to the disease (Bok 1980). Commenting on the case, the physician wrote (p. 147):

> A single word […] would save her from this terrible fate, yet the physician is fettered hand and foot by his cast-iron code, his tongue is silenced, he cannot lift a finger or utter a word to prevent this catastrophe.

Over the past two-three decades, however, both real and hypothetical cases have exposed the inappropriateness and moral unacceptability of holding confidentiality as being an *absolute* principle (i.e. cannot be breached under any circumstances).

It is now widely recognised that in cases where innocent victims stand to be significantly harmed by a failure to disclose, the demand to breach confidentiality becomes morally compelling. This was the view taken in the noted United States legal case *Tarasoff v Regents of the University of California* (1974). The case involved a university student, Prosenjit Poddar, who had met and fallen in love with a young woman, Tatiana Tarasoff. Unfortunately, Tarasoff did not share Poddar's feelings, and told him so. Consequently, Poddar became very depressed and sought psychiatric help on a voluntary outpatient basis at the Cowell Memorial Hospital at the University. During a consultation with his psychologist, Dr Lawrence Moore, Poddar revealed that he seriously intended to kill Tarasoff. After receiving this information the psychologist wrote to the campus police and informed them that Poddar was 'at this point a danger to the welfare of other people and himself', also pointing out that Poddar had been threatening to kill an unnamed girl who he felt had 'betrayed him' and had 'violated his honour' (Daley 1983, p. 243). The psychologist then went on to ask the police for assistance in detaining Poddar for psychiatric assessment. Daley writes that the campus police detained Poddar 'but released him when he appeared rational and promised to stay away from Tarasoff' (p. 235).

Following this, Poddar's psychologist was directed by a superior to take no further action and to destroy his client's records (a practice which is sometimes followed by psychologists, psychotherapists and psychiatrists in order to ensure confidentiality). Two months later, as he had threatened to his psychologist, Poddar carried out his intention and killed Tarasoff with a butcher's knife.

Daley (1983) notes that neither the girl nor her parents were warned of Poddar's threat. It seems that none of the psychotherapists involved considered it part of their professional morality to warn the victim. Even the California Supreme Court acknowledged recognition of the general rule that 'there is ordinarily no duty to control the conduct of another or to warn those endangered by such conduct' (Daley 1983, p. 235). However, the Supreme Court also recognised certain exceptions to the general rule, and its final decision in the *Tarasoff* case imposed a new duty to warn upon doctors and psychiatrists under its jurisdiction. The psychiatric profession 'reacted with alarm' to the California Supreme Court's ruling, claiming that it would 'cripple the use of psychotherapy by destroying the confidentiality vital to the psychiatrist–patient relationship' (Daley 1983, p. 234).

In a more recent Australian case, the duty to warn an intended victim at risk of harm by another became the subject of media commentary and controversy after a Sydney woman, who contracted HIV from her husband, 'successfully sued the medical practice where the couple had received premarriage testing for sexually transmitted diseases' (Lamont 2003, p. 1). The woman (who was in her late twenties) sued the practice for failing to tell her of her husband's HIV-positive status. Damages of $727,000 were awarded to the woman on the grounds that 'the doctors had not adequately counselled either partner about their results' (*The Age* – Editorial 2003, p. 14). The woman only learned about her husband's HIV-positive status 15 months after they had both been tested when she found a laboratory report showing that her husband was HIV-positive; previously, the husband had shown her a falsified report declaring him to be HIV-negative. Although the court upheld the principle of doctor–patient confidentiality and affirmed that 'doctors cannot be sued for damages by maintaining the confidential relationship', it also affirmed that doctors 'must safeguard patients through proper counselling protocols and, if necessary, notify the Director of General Health, who has the power to breach confidentiality and directly warn someone they are at risk of infection' (Lamont 2003, p. 1). An editorial appearing in *The Age*, concluded (2003, p. 14):

> Doctor-patient confidentiality is an important principle and policy-makers are right to do their utmost to uphold it. But human life is even more precious and doctors have a duty to do all they can to protect those whom they believe are at risk.

The *Tarasoff case* and others like it (such as the Sydney case, cited above) raise interesting and thought-provoking questions about the nature and force of the principle of confidentiality and the extent to which health professionals are obliged morally to uphold it.

In general the demand to keep secret information disclosed in a professional–client relationship is thought to derive from the broader moral principles of autonomy, non-maleficence, justice and the obligation to keep one's promises. In the case of autonomy, it is held that individuals are entitled to choose who should have access to information about themselves, as well as what information should be disclosed, if any. Non-maleficence, on the other hand, demands that people are entitled to be protected from the harms that might flow from disclosure (which, as we know, can be both considerable and intolerable). And justice demands that a person, about whom 'private' information is known, deserves to be treated fairly. Promise-keeping, simply put, demands that 'added respect is due for that which one has promised to keep secret' (Bok 1980, p. 149), although it is generally recognised that a promise to do morally evil things is either not binding at all or 'deficient in its binding power' (Freedman 1978, p. 12).

In health care contexts, the supremacy of the principle of confidentiality is thought to be particularly justified on grounds that it is crucial to preserving the fiduciary (trust) nature of the health professional–patient relationship (Beauchamp and Childress 2001; Gert et al. 1997). If patients/clients can trust their attending health professionals to keep secret certain information disclosed in the professional relationship, it is thought that patients/clients will be more likely to reveal information crucial for making a correct assessment/diagnosis, and thus a correct prescription of care and treatment.

Understandably, if it were common practice to breach confidentiality, patients/clients would probably lose their trust and confidence in their attending health care professionals, and would probably refrain from divulging critical information to them. Worse, they might not seek professional help at all — something which might have the undesirable consequence of individuals, groups and indeed the community at large, suffering a health status inferior to that which might otherwise be enjoyed.

The question remains, however, of whether the principle of confidentiality really is as binding as professionals seem to think it is. Where does it come from? And, as Bok (1980, p. 154) correctly asks: 'Was it ever meant to stretch so far as to require lying?'; 'Why is it so binding that it can protect those who have no right to impose their incompetence, their disease, their malevolence on ignorant and innocent victims?'.

In answering these questions, it is important to understand the nature of the principle of confidentiality. One reason why I think it has been so problematic and has caused so many controversies in health professional practice is that people have mistakenly viewed it as an *absolute* principle — that is, one which cannot be overridden under any circumstance, as the *International Code of Medical Ethics* seems to demand. If we examine its parent principles, that is, the broader moral principles from which it has been derived, we can soon see that this absolutist view is questionable.

CONFIDENTIALITY AS A PRIMA-FACIE PRINCIPLE

On close analysis it can be seen that, at best, the principle of confidentiality is, and can only ever be, a prima-facie principle. Confidentiality has a special link to a person's *right to privacy*, which may be loosely defined as the right to 'have control over information about ourselves' or 'control over who can sense us' (Parker 1974; McCloskey 1980; Thomson 1975). This in turn is connected with the principle of autonomy, which demands that people should be respected as autonomous choosers, and have the right to act on their choices provided these do not seriously impinge on the moral interests of others. Given this, it seems reasonable to hold that, where the maintenance of confidentiality results in the moral interests of others being violated, the principle can and must be overridden. This conclusion is also partially supported by the principles of non-maleficence and justice. Thus, in instances where keeping a confidence or a secret has the unhappy consequence of causing or failing to prevent an otherwise avoidable harm, and/or indeed results in an unequal distribution of harms over benefits, there is a very strong case supporting disclosure of the information being kept secret.

When subjected to the scrutiny of broader moral principles, it can be seen, first, that there are serious limits to the duty of secrecy and of maintaining confidentiality. Second, it is clear that, while in some instances the norm of confidentiality might justifiably extend to include lying, this does not hold unconditionally in all cases. (Given a consequentialist analysis, lying can only ever be justified on the grounds that it is necessary to prevent an otherwise avoidable harm from occurring, and that there is no other alternative action which can be taken to prevent the foreseen harm in question.) Third, it can be seen, given the competing demands of the moral principles of non-maleficence and justice, that the principle of confidentiality can never be used morally to protect those who would impose their incompetence, their diseases and their malevolence on to innocent and uninformed victims.

Unfortunately, the moral principle of confidentiality has sometimes been (ab)used to prevent the disclosure of unscrupulous practices. A poignant example of this can be found in the Chelmsford case referred to in Chapter 5. Of particular relevance to this discussion is the point that, after the '60 Minutes' program in 1977, when some advice was sought by medical authorities on how to deal with the Chelmsford case, the principle of confidentiality was used to impose a duty of silence on the matter, or at least to delay its exposure. When, for example, an eminent professor of psychiatry at Cambridge University was approached about the matter, he advised:

> The inhumanity and cruelty to which the patients appear to have been subjected is quite unique in my experience, and the Scientologists and other organisations will have obtained ammunition for decades to come. There is therefore a pressing need for maintaining strict confidentiality at this stage until one can set these unique barbarities in the context of contemporary practice in psychiatry in a carefully prepared statement that comes from colleges and other bodies concerned.
> (Sir Martin Roth, cited in Bromberger and Fife-Yeomans 1991, p. 143)

This appeal to the principle of confidentiality is questionable, and stands as an example of how conventional ethical principles of conduct can be (ab)used to maintain and reinforce the status quo rather than to challenge it. Further, when more parochial interpretations and applications of the principle of confidentiality are considered, what emerges is not a respect for ethical conduct, but rather what Bok (1980) describes as 'primeval tribal emotions: the loyalty to self, kin, clansmen, guild members as against ... the unrelated, the outsiders, the barbarians' (p. 149). Bok (1980, p. 149) concludes by warning that the principle of confidentiality can sometimes serve little more than the drive for 'self-preservation' and 'collective survival in an hostile environment' (see also Forrester and Griffiths 2001, p. 75). The Chelmsford case is an example of this.

It is not being argued here that the principle of confidentiality ought not to be respected. On the contrary: confidentiality is an important moral requirement of any health care professional–patient/client relationship, and one that is crucial to ensuring the protection of a patient's/client's wellbeing and moral interests. Indiscriminate breaches of confidentiality can have morally undesirable and catastrophic consequences for patients/clients. For example, careless breaches of confidentiality concerning persons who are HIV positive can result — and have resulted — in people being dismissed from their jobs, being evicted from their rented accommodation, and being subjected generally to a wide range of negative discrimination and abuse. Similarly, careless breaches of confidentiality concerning a person's mental health status (including mild depression and grieving states) can also result — and have resulted — in harmful consequences, including persons losing their jobs or having their career prospects hampered (see also Johnstone 2001). It is crucial, therefore, that every effort is made to ensure that information disclosed in the professional–client relationship is kept secret. This is not to say, however, that there is not a need for the principle of confidentiality to be interpreted better and applied more justly than it has been in the past. Points of clarification which need to be particularly addressed are summarised as follows:

- confidentiality is at best only a prima-facie principle, not an absolute one, and thus is one which may be overridden by stronger moral considerations;
- confidentiality should not be upheld in instances where doing so would result in otherwise avoidable harms occurring to innocent others; and
- while patients/clients as a general rule have an entitlement to have certain information about themselves kept secret, the entitlement is forfeited where it stands seriously to impinge on the moral interests of innocent others.

If these points of clarification are accepted, it must also be accepted that patients (or anybody else, for that matter) might not always be entitled to have certain information about themselves kept secret; and that disclosure, in some instances, might even be an overriding moral duty, particularly in cases where non-disclosure entails the probability of innocent others suffering unnecessary and avoidable harms (for example, children as in the case of child abuse). This second demand is also enshrined in legal law, which requires health professionals to report certain infectious diseases (commonly referred to as 'notifiable diseases'), suspected cases of child abuse (to be examined in depth in Chapter 8 of this work), and other activities 'which [are] potentially or actually dangerous to the health of others' (Wallace 1991, p. 303; see also Forrester and Griffiths 2001, pp. 75-81).

Whatever the situation at hand, nurses' decisions to keep secret or to disclose certain information gained in a professional–client or other type of relationship (for example, an employee–employer relationship) must always be based firmly on sound moral justifications and moral decision-making procedures. Nurses also need to remember that arbitrary disclosure is just as morally capricious as arbitrary non-disclosure, and may have just as many devastating consequences. As in any morally troubling situation, dilemmas posed by a controversial application of the principle of confidentiality must be resolved in a way which ensures the realisation of morally just outcomes.

The right to dignity and dying with dignity¹

The right to dignity, and, in particular, the *right to die with dignity*, have both been widely considered in the bioethics and nursing literature (too voluminous to list here).

The terms dignity and dying with dignity have gained popular usage in contemporary debates concerning the invasive and sometimes encroaching nature of technological scientific medical care. They have also featured as key words in debates concerning the moral rights and wrongs of euthanasia and assisted suicide. Yet, while the terms 'dignity' and 'dying with dignity' have been and are freely used, there is room to question whether those who use them have a clear understanding of what precisely they mean.

Another concern is that these terms have come to be used in a rather clichéd sense, and thus could have the undesirable consequence of a blanket definition of dignity being applied uncritically in all situations, regardless of their ethically significant differences, and in a way which could result in a serious distraction from (rather than a focus on) the moral issues at stake. For example, some speak of the removal of a life-support system, or the withdrawal of some other orthodox medical therapies, as tantamount to 'letting a person die with dignity' (Social Development Committee, Victoria 1986, 1987). What such views presume, however, is that the terms 'dignity' and 'dying with dignity' in these contexts have a clear-cut, commonsense meaning and use, and, furthermore, implicitly justify the acts or omissions in relation to which they have been expressed.

Two central questions invariably arise here: How should the notions 'dignity' and 'dying with dignity' be defined? What might be the implications of given definitions of these terms for nursing practice?

CAN DIGNITY BE DEFINED?

The word dignity comes from the Latin *dignitas*, meaning 'merit', and *dignus*, meaning 'worthy'. Needless to say, there are as many definitions of 'dignity' as there are dictionaries. *Collins English dictionary*, for example, defines dignity as:

[1]..a formal, stately, or grave bearing ... [2]. the state or quality of being worthy of honour ... [3]. relative importance; rank ... [4]. sense of self importance ...

According to the *Oxford English dictionary*, dignity is:

[1]. the quality of being worthy or honourable; worthiness, worth, nobleness, excellence ... [2]. Honourable or high estate, position, or estimation ... [4]. Nobility or befitting elevation of aspect, manner, or style ...

Webster's dictionary says dignity is:

[1]:.the quality or state of being worthy: intrinsic worth: EXCELLENCE ... [2]:.the quality or state of being honoured or esteemed: degree of esteem ... [5]:.formal reserve of manner, appearance, behaviour, or language: behaviour that accords with self-respect or with regard for the seriousness of occasion or purpose ...

Interestingly, the unabridged international edition of *Webster's dictionary* also gives consideration of the word 'decent' (i.e. of the mind and character) as a definition of dignity. It is perhaps worth noting here that the term 'decent' comes from the Latin *decens*, meaning 'suitable', and from *decere*, meaning 'to be fitting'.

The question of dignity has also been a topic of significant philosophical debate. For example, in 1651 the English philosopher Thomas Hobbes defined it as (1968, p. 52):

> (T)he publique worth of a man [sic], which is the Value set on him [sic] by the Common-Wealth ... And this Value of him [sic] by the commonwealth, is understood, by offices of Command, Judicature, public Employment; or by Names and Titles, introduced for distinction of such Value.

Later philosophers, however, rejected this 'social worth' view and sought to define dignity in more sophisticated moral terms. The German philosopher Immanuel Kant, for instance, defines dignity in quite different terms as 'an intrinsic, unconditioned, incomparable worth or worthiness' (1972, p. 35). Rejecting the 'market value' or 'social worth' interpretations of dignity, he goes on to assert that (p. 35):

> Morality or virtue — and humanity so far as it is capable of morality — alone has dignity. In this respect it cannot be compared with things that have economic value (a market price) or even with things that have an aesthetic value (a fancy price). The incomparable worth of a good man [sic] springs from his [sic] being a [moral] law making member in a kingdom of ends.

More recent definitions and interpretations have tended to capture the essence of Kant's views. One philosopher, for example, argues that dignity is akin to 'justified happiness' (a happiness which is 'interpenetrated with a sense of meaning, reason, and worth') and the attainment of 'just goals'; that is, morally valuable ends (Swenson 1981). The behaviourist B. F. Skinner (1973, pp. 48–62) sees dignity and what he calls the 'struggle for dignity' as having many features in common with freedom and the 'struggle for freedom'.

Some of the most revealing and instructive definitions of dignity and dying with dignity, however, come from a group of first year undergraduate nursing students from the former Phillip Institute of Technology (now RMIT University). Comments were sought from the students after their clinical placement at a residential care home for the elderly. The results are summarised as follows.

- 'Dying with dignity is dying the way you want to die.'
- 'Dignity is a feeling of pride ... of feeling good about yourself.'
- 'Dignity and dying with dignity is maintaining self-value, self-respect, and self-image ...'
- 'I don't know, but I think, as it is used today, it all boils down to having to look good for other people.'
- 'Dignity is having pride without shame.'
- 'Dignity and dying with dignity is being happy with oneself, and what one has achieved in life.'
- 'Dying with dignity is having no pain, no fear. Feeling valued, and having your opinions valued. Yes. That's it! It involves having control and being valued.'
- 'Dying with dignity is putting yourself above whatever is going on around you.'
- 'Dignity is concerned with self-respect, and how this is related to society — your social worth.'
- 'Dignity is being accepting of one's self, and of what's to come ... the problem is, however, that a lot of people base their self-worth on what other people think of them.'

As the last student voiced her comments, another student interjected with frustration, exclaiming: 'Oh! How can you die with dignity if you have no say about it?'.

In considering all these definitions, it soon becomes apparent that the notions 'dignity', and 'dying with dignity', essentially defy precise definition. What this inevitably warns, of course, is that nurses — and indeed health care professionals generally — must never take the notion of dignity (and its usage) for granted. They must also be cautious in treating these terms as if they had clear-cut, commonsense interpretations. What one person might consider 'dignity', another person might equally reject —and this has important implications for nursing care delivery in particular, and health care management generally.

How, then, should dignity be defined? And what might be the implications of a given definition for nursing practice?

Despite the variety of definitions and interpretations of the notions 'dignity' and 'dying with dignity', there are a number of common elements. In summary, these include:

- that persons have intrinsic moral worth, and thus ought to be treated with respect (see below);
- that persons should be respected as autonomous choosers, and thus as beings capable of exercising self-determining choice;
- that persons should be facilitated and supported in the course of exercising their autonomous choices;
- that persons should be facilitated and supported in their attempts to maintain their self-respect and self-esteem.

IMPLICATIONS FOR NURSES

Whatever nurses or allied health workers take dignity and/or dying with dignity to mean, it is important that they do not unfairly impose their interpretations on their patients. It is morally imperative that patients' preferences (which might include them abdicating their autonomy to a surrogate decision-maker) are respected, even if others do not agree with these. This means that, where possible, and in a manner that is culturally appropriate, patients are morally entitled to participate in decision-making concerning their care, and are morally entitled to give a fully informed consent to the use and withdrawal of recommended medical or other therapies. If patients are not able to participate in decision-making concerning their care and treatment, every effort must be made to establish what their considered preferences might be. Either way, in the final analysis, what is to count as dignity and dying with dignity must be decided from the patients' (or their advocates') point of view, not that of the health professionals.

Given this, nurses should not be asking 'What is dignity?' or 'What does it mean to die with dignity?'; rather, they should be asking: 'What is dignity for *this* or *that* person?' and 'What is dying with dignity *for them*?'.

The challenge to nursing is not just to allow patients the right to the maintenance of dignity, but actually to find out what the patient considers as being dignity and/or a dignified death, and ensuring that this is permitted and upheld on terms of what the patient wants, and not on what the *nurse thinks* the patient wants.

The right to be treated with respect

People (regardless of their age, sexuality, cultural backgrounds and social position) have a special interest in being treated with respect. Furthermore, there are significant moral reasons why this interest ought to be protected. Thus, the claim that people have a *right* to be treated with respect is a meaningful one.

Underpinning most moral claims (rights claims included) is the principle that *people ought to be treated with respect*. Otherwise referred to in moral philosophy as 'respect for persons', this principle is generally regarded as being of paramount importance to the establishment, development and maintenance of moral relationships between people, and to moral practice generally (Tadd 1998, pp. 1–3).

The notion of 'respect for persons' is widely used, often without qualification, in the bioethics literature (its meaning more or less taken for granted), and, of significance to this discussion, it is widely used in codes of professional ethics. For instance, common to most nursing codes of ethics is a prescribed demand to 'respect patients' in the provision of nursing care. This demand tends to be interpreted in varying ways as including an obligation to treat with respect a patient's needs, values, beliefs, and culture. As well, nursing codes of ethics prescribe respect for patients' rights. Consider the following examples.

The International Council of Nurses (2000) *Code for Nurses* states:

Inherent in nursing is respect for human rights, including the right to life, to and to be treated with respect. [...] In providing care, the nurse promotes an environment in which the human rights, values, customs and spiritual beliefs of the individual, family and community are respected.

The Australian Nursing Council's (2002) *Code of Ethics for Nurses in Australia* takes a similar position. It states:

- Nurses respect individuals' needs, values, culture and vulnerability in the provision of nursing care (Value statement 1).

The Nursing Council of New Zealand's *Code of Conduct for Nurses and Midwives* (2001) also emphasises the respect for patients' rights. Principle three of the Code states:

The nurse or midwife respects the rights of patients/clients.

Despite the term's common use in the ethics literature and in codes of ethics, however, just what constitutes 'respect' and 'respect for persons' has received surprisingly little attention by authors. In the remainder of this chapter an attempt will be made to remedy this oversight. Specifically, brief attention will be given to exploring the nature and moral implications of 'respect' and 'respect for persons' — particularly as these pertain to the ethical practice of nursing and the promotion of patients' rights generally.

Every culture has its own conception of respect and 'its own norms of behaviour and ways of being that are considered respectful' (Sugirtharjah 1994). Asian cultures, for example, tend to treat respect as a moral *duty* expressed through such concepts (tautologically) as: *duty, respect* and *honour* (Sugirtharjah 1994). Western cultures, however, tend to give greater primacy to respect as an individual moral *right* (Sugirtharjah 1994, p. 740).

Western conceptions of *respect* and, specifically, the *principle of respect for persons* has borrowed heavily from the work of the 18th Century German philosopher, Immanuel Kant. In his celebrated work the *Fundamental principles of the metaphysics of ethics*, Kant (1959, p. 56) prescribes the (now famous) practical imperative: 'So act as to treat humanity, whether in thine own person or in that of any other, in every case as an end withal, never as means only'. This practical imperative has been variously translated to mean that *people should always be treated as ends in themselves, and never as mere means (for instance, as objects) to the ends of others.* Although commonly accepted, this conception of 'respect for persons' is, however, miserably inadequate and requires expansion to enhance its usefulness as a guiding principle in health care domains. There is, for instance, considerable scope to suggest that respecting persons entails something far more than fulfilling the negative duty of not treating individuals as 'mere means' to the ends of others. It also involves the positive duty of treating people in a manner that is affirming of their *personal identity* as dignified human beings, that is, affirming of *who they are.*

In clarifying the nature and moral implications of rights claims involving respect in health care contexts, it is important first to draw a distinction between respecting *persons* per se, and respecting *the rights* of persons. While the latter is obviously a critical ingredient of the former, the two are nevertheless distinct. In regard to the latter, respecting *the rights* of persons means honouring a range of special interests (moral entitlements) that people might have, say, upon entering a health care domain; for example, the right to health care, to make informed choices, to have information about themselves treated as confidential, to be treated with dignity, and to be treated with respect itself. Moral demands to treat *persons* with respect, in contrast, is fundamentally tied to enhancing the self-identity of persons and involves, in complex ways, acknowledging persons for who they are and responding to them in a manner that *prima facie* preserves the integrity of their self-identity and the promotion of moral goods that this preservation will facilitate. Let us explore this claim further.

Respect (from the Latin *respicere*, meaning 'to look back, pay attention to', from *specere*, meaning 'to look') is essentially a moral attitude that when translated into action is manifest as the showing of admiration, regard, esteem, and/or kindly consideration for another. In short, *respect* manifests as the 'good' treatment of people, and invariably results in their being 'humanised' (that is, enabled to experience their 'beingness' both as human persons and as moral entities, and/or characterised as having moral worth). Disrespect, in contrast, manifests as the 'bad' (or ill) treatment of people, and invariably results in them being 'dehumanised' (deprived of qualities that otherwise enables them — and others — to feel they are 'human beings' of moral worth). Or, to borrow from Asian thought, disrespecting another is to 'take away' that other's 'face'; to 'lose face', in turn, is to diminish that person's very identity and dignity, and consequently to 'pollute the web of relationship' (Rivers 1996, pp. 54–5). Respect, in contrast, keeps the door of relationship' open (Rivers 1996, p. 55).

An important example of the manifestation of disrespect in health care can be found in the case of the stigmatisation, prejudicial treatment of, marginalisation and (negative) discrimination of certain groups of people (for instance: the mentally ill; people of different cultural backgrounds and whose first language is not English; the aged; the disabled; people living with blood borne pathogens [for example, HIV]; the homeless and the poor; gay men, lesbians, transgendered and intergendered [viz. hermaphrodite] people). Consider the following.

Stigma (from Latin via Greek meaning 'brand' or 'bodily sign') is literally a distinguishing mark of social disgrace. It presupposes the acquisition of an attribute or attributes that others (usually those who are dominant members of a mainstream culture or group) find or regard as deeply discrediting (personally, socially and morally) (Goffman 1963). What is regarded as a 'distinguishing mark of social disgrace' will, however, depend on the culture from which it has originated.

The process of stigmatisation evolves into a situation in which an individual is disqualified from full social and cultural acceptance on the basis of his or her carrying a given 'distinguishing mark of social disgrace' (for example, being old, immigrant, disabled, homosexual, mentally ill etc.) (Goffman 1963). Inevitably this means that stigma almost always carries with it commensurate processes of discrimination; that is, the unfair treatment of persons on the basis of their 'distinguishing mark(s)'. This treatment is unfair since judgments are made on the somewhat arbitrary basis of morally irrelevant *distinguishing marks*, rather than on *moral considerations per se*; hence the notion that stigma and stigmatisation are unjustly discriminatory. This outcome is unethical since, by focusing on one (or more) arbitrary characteristic(s) of a person (that is, the marks that may 'distinguish them'), stigma and discrimination undermine the moral worth of a person (results in them 'losing face', if you will) and thus dehumanises them. The stigmatising and (negative) discriminatory treatment of persons thus stands in contradistinction to the respectful treatment of persons. In the case of respectful treatment, responses to persons are guided by profoundly moral considerations, not merely arbitrary ones. (For a comprehensive study of stigma and discrimination in the case of caring for people living with HIV/AIDS, see Crock 2001).

What then are the ingredients of respectful health-professional (nurse–patient) interactions? In conclusion to this discussion on the right to be treated with respect, I would like to suggest that minimally a nurse's respectful interactions with patients, chosen carers and significant others must contain the following:

- acknowledgment of the moral worth and dignity of human beings;
- an unconditional positive regard and valuing of persons for *who they are* as moral beings;
- focused attention on persons (that is, being 'fully present' and being *fully alert to another's presence*, viz. not treating persons in a dismissive, belittling or marginalising manner);
- empathically attuned listening (taking seriously what another says and knows);
- supportive actions aimed at promoting another's moral interests and wellbeing; and
- strategies aimed at 'saving face' and preserving the web of relationship.

Conclusion

The issue of patients' rights to and in health care is an important one for members of the nursing profession. Although a patients' rights approach to ethics in health care is not free of difficulties (as examples throughout this book show), it nevertheless serves a number of important functions. Among other things, discourse on patients' rights helps to remind both health professionals and the laity alike: firstly, that upon entering health care domains for care and treatment, people have special interests and entitlements which ought to be recognised and protected; secondly, and related to this first claim, people (patients) are not — and never have been — obliged to be the passive recipients of unnegotiated care. Thirdly, patients' rights discourse helps to remind health professionals (nurses included) that their relationships with patients and their chosen carers are constrained by morally relevant considerations. Fourthly, patients' rights discourse highlights the vulnerability of people in health care contexts and the 'special' actions that are required by others (including nurses) to help reduce this vulnerability and to promote generally the significant moral interests of patients and their chosen carers. Finally, patients' rights discourse helps to remind us that moral decision-making in health care is not just a matter of 'working through normative hierarchies of values', but is also 'a matter of personal extension into the lives and values of other human beings' which deserve respect (Thomasma 1990, p. 250).

Despite the enormous progress that has been made in recent years in regard to the whole issue of patients' rights to and in health care, it is nevertheless evident that serious violations of patients' rights continue to occur unacceptably across the continuum of care. In light of this, it is evident that the nursing profession has a fundamental role to play in advocating the promotion and protection of patients' rights — not just 'at the bedside', but in the broader socio–political sphere as well. Specifically, the nursing profession has an important and justifiable role to play in actively lobbying for such things as:

- the formulation and global recognition of a comprehensive list of principles, together with a set of interpretive statements, which can be appealed to for both identifying patients' rights and guiding their protection (in short, a universal declaration of patients' rights);
- the establishment and maintenance of accessible, just, reliable and enforceable health complaints mechanisms;
- the improvement of health professional education programs aimed at preparing health professionals better to recognise and respond appropriately to patients' rights claims;
- the introduction of broadly-based community information programs aimed at better informing its community members of their rights to, in and against health care; and
- the staging of regular state, national and international multidisciplinary and transcultural symposiums on patients' rights, with a commitment by all concerned (including health care professional groups and governments) to act upon these symposiums' findings.

If such aims can be achieved, we will be able to rest assured that the rights of patients (and their surrogates/advocates) will be truly promoted and protected in health care domains.

CASE SCENARIOS AND CRITICAL QUESTIONS

Case scenario 1

A 20-year-old Jehovah's Witness woman has given birth to her first child. Unfortunately, following the delivery of her child, she starts to bleed badly. Her attending doctors offer the woman and her husband a stark choice: 'one hour to decide between a blood transfusion and a hysterectomy', or else death (Magazanik 1998, p.1). If the woman has a hysterectomy, this means that her first child will be her last. The blood transfusion, however, is not an option since it is against her religion. Her refusal to have a blood transfusion is expressed clearly and frequently (both verbally and in writing), has been formerly documented, and is widely known by hospital staff. The woman is observed by her husband to be very 'strong, confident and calm about the whole matter' (Magazanik 1998, p. 2).

A hysterectomy is performed, but the woman continues to bleed and she is transferred to the intensive care unit of a major hospital for further care. She starts to drift in and out of consciousness, and her condition becomes poor. Worried that the woman could die, her attending doctors seek legal advice. The advice received is recorded as follows: 'Continue supportive measures. Not for blood unless at direction of court' (Magazanik 1998, p. 2).

The woman's condition continues to deteriorate and it is probable that, within an hour, she will suffer irreversible brain damage. Distraught at the prospect of his wife dying, the husband changes his mind about a blood transfusion and, upon seeking advice from hospital authorities, successfully obtains a court order giving him legal guardianship over his wife and hence the lawful authority to consent to a blood transfusion being given. The husband provides his consent to hospital authorities immediately and his wife is given a blood transfusion. The woman recovers quickly and is well enough to leave hospital one week later.

According to media reports, however, the husband feels 'guilty' about the transfusion and the woman is 'furious' that the blood was given to her against her wishes. According to a Supreme Court document, the woman stated:

> I view the blood transfusion that was forced upon me at the [name of hospital deleted] as equivalent to rape. To me, it feels as if someone has forced an abortion on me while I was under sedation. I am angry about what has happened and I have cried about it a number of times (quoted in Magazanik 1998, p. 2).

The woman is also reported as stating that she 'would have "screamed" and "fought" against the transfusion had she not been sedated' and that she is 'considering suing the hospital, doctors, nurses and lawyers involved in giving her blood' (Magazanik 1998, p.2). The Jehovah's Witness organisation is reported to be deeply involved in the legal action that is being pursued, stressing its position that 'We want to be certain that if people say "I do not want blood", then that is respected' (Magazanik 1998, p. 2).

Case scenario 2

A man who was HIV-positive was admitted to hospital after being knocked unconscious in a car accident. Upon regaining consciousness, his first thoughts were 'to inform staff of his HIV status because he was bleeding heavily from a head wound' and he noticed that attending staff were not using 'universal precautions' (Crock 2001, p. 218 – citing Herdman and Kippax 1995). Disclosing his HIV status, however, resulted in him being treated in a stigmatised and discriminatory manner. In regard to his experience, the man recounts:

> During the time I was there it was the worst experience I've ever had. They [the staff] were horrendous. I had every doctor, nurse, orderly, kitchen staff, whatever come through and look at me and [...] the doctors all wanted to know how I had the HIV [...] and I said I'm here because I've got a broken nose, my head's cut open, I've got gravel rash all over my face [...] the HIV isn't the issue except wear a pair of gloves (Crock 2001, p. 218; Herdman and Kippax 1995).

The man went on to add that an attending doctor declared that his nose was not broken even though he had not examined it, and that the lacerations on his head did not require suturing even though the blood loss indicated that suturing would probably be beneficial. Despite being covered in blood, a nurse advised him that he could go home. Crock (2001, p. 218) writes that when the man asked for his wounds to be cleaned up, the nurse 'handed him a washer held between the tips of her thumb and forefinger' (Herdman and Kippax 1995, p. 56). And when the man asked where the toilet was so that he could use a mirror to clean himself up, 'the nurse took him to look at his reflection in a stainless steel cabinet, leading him to suspect that she did not want him to use the toilets' (Crock 2001, p. 218 – citing Herdman and Kippax 1995).

Critical questions

1. What patients' rights have been violated in these two cases?
2. What were the moral duties of the nurses in these scenarios in regard to upholding and protecting the rights of the patients concerned?
3. How might the violations that occurred in these cases have been prevented?
4. What might be done to assist the patients whose rights have been violated in the cases to come to terms with the aftermath of their experiences?

---

1 Section 4, 'The right to dignity and dying with dignity', is revised from M.-J. Johnstone (1989) 'Dying with dignity', *New Zealand Nursing Journal* 81(12), pp. 34, 37.

Chapter 7

Human rights and the mentally ill

LEARNING OBJECTIVES

Upon the completion of this chapter and with further self-directed learning you are expected to be able to:

- Discuss critically the nursing implications of human rights to and in mental health.
- Examine critically the ways in which a human rights approach to mental health might not always benefit the mentally ill.
- Explore ways in which members of the nursing profession might improve its advocacy of people with mental health problems and severe mental illnesses.
- Discuss critically the use of psychiatric advance directives ('Ulysses contracts') in mental health.

KEYWORDS

- Advocacy
- Discrimination
- Ethics
- Human rights
- Mental health
- Mental health ethics
- Mental illness
- Psychiatric advance directives
- Stigma
- 'Ulysses contracts'

Introduction

Discussions on patients' rights to and in health care have tended to have as their focus persons with 'physical health' problems. While important, this focus has nevertheless been at the expense of attention being given to the moral entitlements of people with 'mental health' problems. Indeed, the subject of moral rights and the mentally ill has been relatively neglected in mainstream bioethics discourse (Johnstone 2001, 1995; Christensen 1997). In light of the past neglect of mental health care ethics in both the mainstream bioethics and nursing literature, 'special' attention to the moral plight of the mentally ill is warranted. In this chapter, a brief overview will be provided of some of the disproportionate and hence unjust burdens that the mentally ill have to carry in the cultural context of Australia. While drawing on the Australian experience, however, this discussion has relevance for other countries.

Discrimination against the mentally ill

It is accepted internationally that people suffering from mental health disorders, mental illness and other mental health-related problems are among the most stigmatised, discriminated against, marginalised, disadvantaged and hence vulnerable individuals in society (World Health Organization 2001; Guimón 2001; Johnstone 2001).[1]

Furthermore, it is widely accepted that despite the advances made in mental health over the past several decades, the status quo remains relatively unchanged. In Australia, for example, a 1993 national inquiry into the human rights of people with mental illness found that people affected by mental illness suffered from 'widespread, systematic discrimination and are consistently denied the rights and services to which they are entitled' (Burdekin et al. 1993, p. 870). The inquiry also found that discrimination was particularly widespread in mainstream society, with the mentally ill experiencing 'stigma and discrimination in almost every aspect of their lives', ranging from restrictions on eligibility for insurance and superannuation schemes, to employment, education and training (Burdekin et al. 1993, p. 925). Equally disturbing was the inquiry's additional finding that underpinning this discrimination were deeply ingrained (and often structurally reinforced) societal attitudes of fear, ignorance and intolerance of mental illness and mental health disorders. A decade later, a nation-wide review of the experiences of users and providers of community-based mental health services in Australia has found that the human rights of mentally ill persons (including their right of access to appropriate mental health services) continue to be violated (Groom and Hickie 2003; Groom et al. 2003; see also Armstrong 2003, 2000; Muir-Cochrane et al. 2002). Tragically, this situation is not confined to the cultural context of Australia. According to the World Health Organization (2001, p.3), mental ill-health and the burden of suffering associated with it (including that imposed by stigma and discrimination) has been largely ignored or neglected in most parts of the world. The World Health Organization (WHO) estimates that currently over '450 million people suffer from a mental or behaviour disorder, yet only a small minority of them receive even the most basic treatment' (WHO 2001, p.3). Most individuals with mental illness, WHO asserts, 'are left to cope as best they can with their private burdens such as depression, dementia, schizophrenia, and substance dependence' (WHO 2001, p. 3; see also James Glass's classic 1989 study, *Private terror/public life: psychosis and the politics of community*).

Although human rights violations have occurred repeatedly in the mental health care sector since the inception of contemporary bioethics, the issue of the human rights of people with mental health problems has received relatively little attention in the mainstream bioethics and related literature. Just why this is so, is a matter for speculation. One explanation might be that the issue of human rights in mental health care simply lacks the kudos that, say, other more popular bioethical issues (such as euthanasia, abortion, reproductive technology, organ transplantation, and the like) have. Or, it might be that, the issue itself carries some degree of stigma from which authors writing in the field of health care ethics (bioethics) would prefer to obtain some distance.

In recent years significant efforts have been made in Australia (and elsewhere) to redress the problem of human rights violations in mental health care settings, and to provide a framework for assuring the protection of the moral entitlements of people suffering from mental health problems.[2] However, it is evident that a great deal more needs to be done to improve the status quo. Certainly, initiatives aimed at educating the public, promoting mental health through mainstream health promotion activities, establishing preventative mental health programs as an essential component of care provision to people at risk of mental health problems, and promoting research, are all essential to promoting better 'mental health outcomes'. If, however, there is to be a genuine promotion and realisation of 'social justice, equity, access and a compassionate society with mental health as a primary goal' (Raphael 1995), what is also required is the development, promotion and practice of a substantive mental health care ethic which recognises, among other things, that mental health is a 'multi-dimensional, dynamic and interactive phenomenon' (Tippett et al. 1994, p. xii).

The moral responsibilities of nurses in mental health care

The *Code of Ethics for Nurses in Australia* (Australian Nursing Council 2002) makes explicit the moral responsibility of nurses to care for human beings in a manner that gives just and due consideration to — and is not prejudicially comprised by — an individual's or a group's 'ethnicity, culture, aboriginality, gender, spiritual values, sexuality, disability, age, economics, social or health status, or any other grounds' (p. 1). Underpinning this stated moral responsibility of nurses is a recognition of nursing care as being a profoundly moral activity that 'is based on the development of a therapeutic relationship and the implementation and evaluation of therapeutic processes' (Australian Nursing Council 2002, p. 1). Therapeutic processes, in this instance, are interpreted to include 'health promotion and education, counselling, nursing interventions and empowerment of individuals, families or groups to exercise maximum choice in relation to their health care' (Australian Nursing Council 2002, p. 1). The moral imperatives arising from this interpretation have an obvious significance and poignancy for those working in the area of mental health care.

It has been acknowledged that nurses are at the forefront of providing care to people suffering from mental illness, mental health disorders and other mental health-related problems (Burdekin et al. 1993, pp. 175–8). By virtue of this primary position in mental health care, nurses have a fundamental role to play in promoting social justice, equity, access, compassion and destigmatisation in mental health domains. While many nurses may already be well intentioned in this regard, much more than 'good intention' is required. Specifically, nurses need to be well informed about the ethical issues confronting them, and the kinds of strategies required in order to address these issues in ways that are responsive to and reflective of the lived experiences of the people for whose mental health care they share responsibility. Many of the topics covered in this text will assist nurses to develop a requisite understanding of the ethical issues they face when caring for people with mental health problems. However, it is also important that they have a 'special' understanding of the now widely accepted 'human rights' approach to and in mental health, a brief overview of which will now be given.

A human rights approach to and in mental health care domains

In Australia, as in other countries, it has become increasingly recognised at a social, cultural and political level that people suffering from mental illnesses, mental health disorders and other mental health–related problems need to be protected from abuse and neglect, something which for a variety of reasons they are especially vulnerable to experiencing. This need of protection has also been recognised at an international level as evident by the United Nations General Assembly's adoption in 1991 of the principles for 'The Protection of Persons with Mental Illness and for the Improvement of Mental Health Care' and, more recently, by the World Health Organization's release of its *World Health Report 2001. Mental Health: New Understanding, New Hope (WHO 2001)*.

In attempting to secure protection of the mentally ill and disordered from abuse and neglect, a human rights model of mental health care ethics has been adopted. Underpinning the selection of this model is the view that 'all people have fundamental human rights' and that people with mental health problems or disorders should not be precluded from having or exercising these rights *just because* of their mental health difficulties. As the Mental Health Consumer Outcomes Task Force puts it (1995, p. ix):

> The diagnosis of mental health problems or mental disorder is not an excuse for inappropriately limiting their [people with mental health problems or disorders] rights.

In March 1991, the Australian Health Ministers acknowledged and accepted the above viewpoint, and adopted, as part of Australia's national mental health strategy, the final report of the Mental Health Consumer Outcomes Task Force, titled *Mental Health Statement of Rights and Responsibilities*. This report has been reprinted twice since its initial publication (latest edition 1995), and stands as an influential guiding force behind other public policy initiatives and statements such as the *National Mental Health Policy* (Australian Health Ministers 1995) as well as health care professional practice in mental health care settings.

The *Mental Health Statement of Rights and Responsibilities* makes explicit and seeks to inform a range of stakeholders of a number of key rights (in fact, a mixture of moral, civil and legal rights) affecting 'individuals seeking promotion or enhancement of mental health or care and protection when suffering mental health problems or mental disorders' (Mental Health Consumer Outcomes Task Force 1995, p. 1). Included in its list are consumers' rights to:

- access adequate, high quality and culturally appropriate mental health care services;
- make informed choices about care and treatment;
- privacy, dignity and respect;
- be treated fairly;
- mechanisms of complaint and redress;

- advocacy;
- have legislation affirm their fundamental rights;
- have mental health legislation reviewed and updated as necessary;
- have access to relatives and friends;
- rehabilitation; and
- 'the right equal to other citizens to health care, income maintenance, education, employment, housing, transport, legal services, equitable health and other insurance and leisure appropriate to one's age' (Mental Health Consumer Outcomes Task Force 1995, p. 1).

As well as specifying a number of key rights, the statement also lists key responsibilities; included here are mental health consumers' responsibilities to 'respect the human worth and dignity of other people; and to participate as far as possible in reasonable treatment and rehabilitation processes' (Mental Health Consumer Outcomes Task Force 1995, p. 2). The rights and responsibilities of service providers, carers and advocates are also listed.

At first glance, the content and intent of the *Mental Health Statement of Rights and Responsibilities* seems to provide an important step forward toward the protection of the human rights of people made vulnerable by mental health problems. On closer examination, however, there is room to suggest that the statement may, in reality, offer those working in the field little guidance on what to do when faced with morally problematic situations involving people who are mentally ill, mentally unwell, mentally disordered or whatever other description may be appropriate of someone experiencing a mental health problem. One reason for this relates to the problematic nature of a human rights approach to ethics itself (discussed earlier in Chapter 3 of this book). Let us consider this claim further.

Human rights claims entail a range of 'special interests' deserving protection for a variety of reasons. Human rights include moral rights, legal rights, civil rights and so forth, and thus do not exclusively concern moral rights. Of pertinence to this discussion is the *moral rights* aspect of human rights.

As previously explained, a moral right can be defined as a special interest or entitlement which a person has and which ought to be protected for moral reasons. Having a moral right usually entails that another has a corresponding duty to respect that right. Fulfilling a corresponding duty can involve either doing something 'positive' to benefit a person claiming a particular right or, alternatively, refraining from doing something 'negative' which could harm a person claiming a particular right. For example, if a patient claims the right to make an informed choice concerning prescribed psychotropic medication or electroconvulsive therapy (ECT), this imposes on an attending health care professional a corresponding duty to ensure that the patient is fully informed about the therapeutic effects and the adverse side effects of the treatments in question *as well as* to respect the patient's choice to either accept or refuse the treatment, even where the health professional may not agree with the ultimate choice made. The moral force of the right's claim in this instance is such that if an attending health care professional does not uphold or violates the patient's choice in regard to the treatment options considered, that patient would probably feel wronged or that a serious injustice had been done. The health care professional in turn could be judged, criticised and possibly even censured on grounds of having infringed the patient's rights.

As already explained in this text, a human rights approach to ethics is widely used. It is not, however, without difficulties. For example, the *Mental Health Statement of Rights and Responsibilities* (cited throughout this discussion) itself acknowledges that the freedom of people to exercise their human rights (and responsibilities) is 'inherently linked to the mental health functioning of individuals and communities' (Mental Health Consumer Outcomes Task Force 1995, p. ix). Here serious questions arise concerning the status and usefulness of a human rights approach for people who are so mentally ill that they are unable to exercise their own rights. While it might be responded that in such instances an advocate could and indeed should (that is, has a *duty* to) act on behalf of the person in question, this merely begs the question of who can and should undertake this role, as well as when, where and how?

For example, should the role of, and the duty to act as, an advocate fall to an attending health care professional (who may or may not have intimate knowledge of the mentally ill person)? Or a family member (who, while having intimate knowledge of the mentally ill person, may for some reason be estranged from him or her)? Or a friend (who has no legal relationship with the person, but nevertheless has the person's best interests at heart). Or a lawyer or some other legal representative (who, despite having the legal authority to act on behalf of the person, may be a complete stranger and not really be in a position to advocate the person's 'best interests' at all)? How is a matter of this nature to be decided and by whom? There may be no easy answers to the questions posed. An additional problem concerns the philosophical issue of whether human rights are of a nature that allows another to validly act as a 'surrogate decision-maker' and make rights claims 'by proxy' on behalf of another. To put this another way, is the freedom to exercise a human right something that can be 'abdicated' to another? Or does this defeat the whole purpose of having individual human rights in the first place?

Another difficulty is that rights can conflict and compete with one another. For example, the patient's stated right to have 'access to family and friends' could seriously conflict with the family's and friend's moral interests and entitlements to be spared the certain harms that might flow from contact; for example, in the case of a patient who is physically violent and has demonstrable homicidal tendencies. In a case such as this, the patient's right to privacy and confidentiality might also stand in serious conflict with the moral interests of family and friends to be warned of a possible threat to their safety and wellbeing; for example, in instances where the client has disclosed a serious intention to kill a given person, as tragically happened in the 1974 American legal case *Tarasoff v Regents of the University of California* (discussed in Chapter 6). While a human rights approach to ethics may tell us what rights people have, it offers very little guidance in regard to what should be done when stated rights conflict and compete with one another.

Related to the above is the additional difficulty of establishing the extent to which a patient's rights claim entails a correlative duty. Consider, for example, a person's right to access appropriate and quality mental health care services. Consider also that such a claim may be extremely difficult to uphold in instances where services are either seriously under-resourced or simply do not exist (such as in remote areas). Here difficult questions arise concerning who or what has a corresponding duty to respond to a mentally ill person's rights in this instance: is it an individual nurse? another mental health worker? a mental health service? a general hospital? family? friends? the state? a philanthropist? or some other entity? Compounding this difficulty is the problem of competing rights claims. For example, a number of persons might make equally deserving claims to mental health care services (as they do) but, because of a shortage of resources, it is genuinely difficult to satisfy the rights claims of all persons equally. Compounding these difficulties still further is the additional question of whether it makes sense to even claim a right to something that does not exist, in this instance, a particular type of health care service in a particular region? Further, is it reasonable to condemn someone for not providing a service where no such service exists or where existing services have been totally exhausted? There may be no satisfactory answers to these questions.

Finally there is the paradoxical problem of a human rights approach to mental health care ethics being abused to advance dominant political interests. For instance, trends over the past three decades favouring the deinstitutionalisation of the mentally ill might be cynically appraised as having been motivated not by humane concern for people with mental health problems confined to institutional care, but by blatant political interest in reducing the cost (both financial and political) of institutionalised mental health care services around the country — some of which were shown to be seriously substandard (see, for example, the publicly documented cases of the *Chelmsford Hospital in New South Wales* [Bromberger and Fife-Yeomans 1991], *Ward 10B of Townsville Hospital in Queensland* [Carter 1991], and the *Lakeside Hospital in Victoria* [Burdekin et al. 1993, p. 870]). Consider the following.

In his controversial text *Nowhere to go*, Torrey (1988), an American psychiatrist, persuasively argues that sometimes rights (for example, civil and legal rights) designed to protect the mentally ill often protect their 'right' to *remain* mentally ill. In illustrating this, Torrey (1988) cites an American case of a man suffering from schizophrenia and who was the subject of a committal hearing. The man had been refusing food, but was said to have been ingesting his own faeces. Although in a state of neglect and in need of institutional care and treatment, the man could not be institutionalised against his will without a court order. Significantly, while the court acknowledged that the man was eating his own faeces, it did not regard this as constituting a 'danger to self' (or to others, for that matter). The court subsequently upheld the man's 'civil liberty' not to be institutionalised against his will. An important point to be drawn from this case is that while that man's civil liberties (rights) were protected by the court in this instance, his genuine human welfare and wellbeing was not. As one observer cited by Torrey (1988, p. 31) phrased it, 'we are protecting the civil liberties [of the mentally ill] much more adequately than we are protecting their minds and their lives'.

Problems associated with a human rights approach to mental health care ethics

From the brief discussion above, it can be seen that a human rights approach to mental health care ethics can be very problematic. One reason for this can be found in the nature of a rights approach to ethics itself and the difficulties which can be experienced in determining who has rights, who has corresponding duties to these rights, and how best to try and satisfy all valid rights claims of all people equally. Another difficulty is that what are sometimes put forward as moral rights are not, technically speaking, moral rights at all, but rather a mixture of civil rights (special interests and entitlements people have by virtue of being civilians), legal rights (special interests or entitlements bestowed by law and which ought to be protected for legal reasons) or institutional rights (special interests or entitlements bestowed by an institution in which one is participating in some way) — all of which have differing moral force. This mixture can confuse judgments on what is a morally correct course of action to take and can compound many of the problems outlined above.

An important question to arise here is: If statements on human rights and responsibilities in mental health care are so problematic, is there any point in having them? The short answer to this question is, yes. Whatever the faults, weaknesses and difficulties of such statements, they nevertheless achieve a number of important things:

- they help to remind patients, service providers, caregivers and the general community that people with mental health problems (including mental illness and mental health disorders) do have special interests and entitlements which ought to be respected and protected;
- they help to inform stakeholders (patients, service providers, caregivers and the community) of what these special entitlements are and thereby provide a basis upon which respect for and protection of these can be demanded;
- they help to delineate the special responsibilities that stakeholders (patients, service providers, caregivers and the community) all have in ensuring the promotion and protection of people's special interests and entitlements in mental health care and in promoting mental health generally;
- they help to remind all stakeholders (patients, service providers, caregivers and the community at large) that their relationships with each other are ethically constrained and are bound by certain correlative duties.

What a consideration of the difficulties outlined above warn, however, is that if a human rights approach to mental health care ethics is to be taken, nurses need to be well informed about the pitfalls of this approach and understand that it may not always be helpful in guiding ethical professional conduct.

Practical ethics in mental health

It is to be expected that in the course of caring for people with mental health problems, nurses will encounter a variety of practical ethical issues. In addition, it is important to understand that these issues will vary both in kind and complexity, depending on:

- who the patient (client) is (for example, whether the 'patient' is an individual, a family, a group or an entire community);
- where the patient is located (for example, whether in a community or institutional setting, a private or public place, whether free or constrained physically, legally or otherwise); and
- what resources are available to assist the patient in whatever form these resources might be required (for example, a patient might be in need of legal aid and accommodation, not merely health care; a patient might also just be in need of 'a friend' — someone who will just sit and listen and reassure them that 'everything will be OK').

These considerations will, in turn, have a bearing on determining the nature of a nurse's given moral responsibilities and the extent to which he or she is obligated to fulfil these.

For instance, it is quite probable that a nurse's responsibilities do not just begin and end with an individual patient. If the whole notion of moral obligation is taken seriously from a professional point of view, then there is considerable room to suggest that the moral responsibilities of nurses extend far beyond their immediate one-to-one professional–client relationships to include other things such as professional and political activism aimed at improving the plight of those who suffer from mental health problems (Johnstone 2002b, 2002c, 2001). Activism of this kind could be aimed at securing such things as: the demystification and destigmatisation of mental health disorders, mental illness and other mental health problems, better mental health care services (to be distinguished here from psychiatric services) for the community, and other general mechanisms which will assist those with mental health problems to be spared the devastating consequences of stigma and discrimination which many continue to suffer.

Given the above, it can be seen that practical ethical issues for mental health nurses can and do involve much more than the commonly discussed moral problems of the right to health care, informed consent and competency to decide, privacy and confidentiality, the political abuse of psychiatry and psychiatric research (see, for example, Beauchamp and Childress 2001; Chodoff et al. 1999; Christensen 1997; Engelhardt 1995; Rave and Larsen 1995; Weinstein 1990; Buchanan and Brock 1989). Other important practical issues concern the moral imperatives of the professional–client relationship (including mutuality, therapeutic alliance, safety, security, trust, compassion and empathy); the moral dimensions and unacceptable consequences of stigma and discrimination; and the moral imperatives of transcultural and indigenous mental health nursing, to name some. Unfortunately, due to the limited scope of this discussion, it is not possible to explore all these issues in a manner that would do justice to them or which would provide nurses working in the mental health care sector with the in-depth understanding they need in order to be able to deal with these issues effectively. Nevertheless, they are identified here to alert nurses to the possible range of ethical issues they need to be informed about and which will, at some stage, have a bearing on their practice.

Advanced directives ('Ulysses contracts') in mental health

Before proceeding there is one practical issue that can be addressed here and which warrants attention, and that is the issue of *psychiatric advanced directives*, or 'Ulysses contracts' as they have been called (Widdershoven and Berghmans 2001; see also Lavin 1986).

People with serious mental illnesses can often experience periods of profound distress during which their capacity to make prudent and rationally competent choices concerning their care and treatment options can be seriously compromised. During such periods, the mentally ill can also be at serious risk of harming themselves and/or others. In either case, timely and effective psychiatric treatment and care is imperative (as the case study given at the end of this chapter demonstrates).

In many instances, people with serious mental illnesses might not comply with and might even refuse outright to accept recommended psychiatric treatment (e.g. oral or intramuscular psychotropic medication, or electroconvulsive therapy). In such instances, because of the psychiatric imperatives to treat their conditions (particularly if extremely distressed and 'out of control'), the mentally ill are vulnerable to having medical treatments imposed on them against their will. Enforced treatments, in such cases, however, may compound their distress and make future treatment difficult, especially if the patient later feels (i.e. during a moment of restored competency to decide) that the fiduciary nature of the professional–client relationship has been violated.

Situations involving the enforced medical treatment of the mentally ill can cause significant distress to caregivers as well who, while wanting to respect the choices of their patients, may nevertheless recognise that without treatment, patients in distress (and their families or supporters) will not be able to be consoled and, worse, may remain unnecessarily in a state of psychiatric crisis. Here very practical questions arise of what, if anything, can be done to strike a balance between respecting the patient's autonomous wishes and constraining their freedom where its exercise could be harmful to themselves and/or to others?

One approach has been to adopt *psychiatric advanced directives*, or 'Ulysses contracts'. Widdershoven and Berghmans (2001, p. 92) contend that:

> By using psychiatric advance directives, it would be possible for mentally ill persons who are competent and with their disease in remission, and who want timely intervention in case of future mental crisis, to give prior authorisation to treatment at a later time when they are incompetent, non-compliant, and refusing treatment

Widdershoven and Berghmans (2001) explain that the general model of psychiatric advance directives is the 'Ulysses contracts'. The name 'Ulysses contracts' derives from Homer's story of the mythological character Ulysses (known as Odysseus in Greek mythology) who escaped being seduced to his death by the 'sweet songs' of the Sirens, the magical women of Cyrene, who cast spells on the sailors of ships so that their vessels would be wrecked and subsequently could be scavenged. Being previously warned of the evil intentions of the Sirens, Ulysses took the precaution of commanding his sailors to bind him to the mast of his ship (effectively restraining him), and to plug their ears with wax so that they could not hear and hence be seduced to their deaths by the Sirens. Ulysses further ordered his sailors not to release him from the mast until they were safely past the Sirens. By taking these steps, Ulysses was able to investigate the power of the Sirens without being seduced to his death by them as well as ensure the safety of his ship and his crew as they sailed past them. This story is used controversially in philosophy to demonstrate the difference between freedom and autonomy: in this case, although Ulysses had his *freedom* constrained (i.e. by having his body tied to the mast of his ship), his *autonomy* (rational preference) was essentially left intact — including during the momentary period of his incompetence while under the bewitching spell of the magical Sirens.

The Ulysses contracts enables respect not only of the patient's wishes, but also their values (i.e. in regard to what is important in life). And while such contracts should not 'replace deliberation about possible future changes in the patients' condition,' they nevertheless have an important role to play in eliciting and guiding communication about such matters (Widdershoven and Berghmans 2001, p. 93; see also Spellecy 2003).

Some worry about the moral authority of psychiatric advance directives (particularly if patients change their minds at some point), and their vulnerability to being abused and misused (Spellecy 2003). These concerns, however, are no more problematic than they are for advanced directives at the end stage of life (discussed in Chapter 12 of this book) and are amenable to a range of processes that can ensure they achieve their intended purpose; namely, ensuring protection of the patient's significant moral interests, welfare and wellbeing. For example, during 'critically reflective periods' or 'cool thinking periods' the opportunity to revoke a previously made psychiatric advanced directive must always be present; treatment options should remain the subject of ongoing critical evaluation, and so on.

In Chapter 6 of this book, under the discussion of competency to decide, the case example was given of an involuntary psychiatric patient who was held down and given an intramuscular injection of psychotropic medication against his will (see pages 152–3). It will be recalled that this incident resulted in the patient being left grossly mistrustful of nursing staff and even less willing to comply with his prescribed oral medication. There is room to speculate that had a Ulysses contract been in force at the time for this patient, clearly setting out his wishes in regard to treatment options, a very different outcome might have resulted.

Future directions in mental health care ethics

This discussion on mental health care ethics would be incomplete without some consideration being given to the future directions in which the field of mental health care ethics should take.

It is of some considerable significance that many of the respondents to the National Inquiry into the Human Rights of People with Mental Illness felt that 'one of the most debilitating aspects of being mentally ill was not the illness itself, but the social stigma it attracts' (Burdekin et al. 1993, p. 443). As one respondent disclosed: 'The horrendous consequences of my illness have been [a result of] public attitudes of ignorance, fear, discrimination and neglect and professional indifference (Gillespie — cited in Burdekin et al. 1993, p. 443). Equally significant is the inquiry's overall finding that what clients of mental health services were largely affected by were not the 'big' ethical issues constructed as being 'paramount' by mainstream bioethics (for example, informed consent, confidentiality, and so forth). Rather, clients were affected by much more 'basic' day-to-day relationship and existential issues which, while perhaps lacking the intrigue of other exotic bioethical issues, nevertheless have a profound moral dimension and warrant just as much attention as do the 'big' ethical issues which have tended to preoccupy contemporary mainstream bioethics discourse. The key issues identified by people with mental health problems were:

- the desperate need for understanding;
- the need to be able to speak openly and to be heard;
- the longing for acceptance by others of the mystery and the unpredictability of their illness, without constantly having to defend and explain to those who have little interest in understanding; and
- the desire to be equal with others and to have basic human rights respected.

(adapted from Burdekin et al. 1993, pp. 439–40)

Similar findings were made by another, although less known, provincial report examining the experiences of women survivors of sexual assault who had been seriously misunderstood and mistreated by mainstream psychiatric services (South East Centre Against Sexual Assault 1994). Although these reports are now over a decade old, their findings remain current (see WHO 2001).

What, then, are some of the lessons to be gained from these findings and what are their implications for the future development of mental health care ethics?

In the introductory comments to this discussion, it was claimed that: If there is to be a genuine promotion and realisation of 'social justice, equity, access and a compassionate society with mental health as a primary goal' (Raphael 1995), what is also required is the development, promotion and practice of a substantive mental health care ethic. Such an ethic must, by its very nature, be one which is responsive to and reflective of the lived experiences of clients with mental health problems, as well as their carers. To achieve this, it is clear that the very first place the development of such an ethic must begin is not the abstract theories and principles of traditional Western moral philosophy. Rather, such an ethic must take as its methodological starting point the lived realities and experiences of those who suffer as a result of their mental health problems as well as the lived realities and experiences of the people who share the primary responsibility of caring for them. Such an approach will also empower those whose lives have been affected by mental health problems to 'speak for themselves' and in so doing to challenge the status quo by virtue of engaging in the positive political act of 'making visible' their experiences and naming their own reality. 'Speaking for themselves' will also enable survivors of mental health problems to provide the foundations needed for achieving the understanding and respect they are so desperately seeking. Finally, such an approach will facilitate the development of our moral thinking generally and will enable a very 'life-rich' contribution to be made to mainstream bioethics discourse which remains largely incomplete because of the many 'moral voices and moral selves' (adapted from Hekman 1995) that have not yet been heard (see also the graphic 'life stories' presented in Glass 1989; Read and Reynolds 1996).

Conclusion

Over the years there has been a scandalous neglect of mental health care ethics in and by the mainstream bioethics movement as well as by the health professions. The reasons for this are varied and complicated and, in many respects, reflect the very stigma and discrimination that has become so characteristic of the field of mental health care in general. Nevertheless, there is increasing evidence that if the field of mental health care ethics has been the most neglected (and it has), it is also the most promising. New and important work is being undertaken which heralds a whole new understanding, acceptance, commitment and approach to mental health care ethics and to the people with mental health problems who stand most in need of the benefits of this work. Whether this work will succeed, however, will depend not on either bioethics or law or government policy. Rather, it will depend on the 'right attitude', and how successful stakeholders in the discourses on mental health care are in demystifying mental health disorders, mental illness and other mental health-related problems, and stripping the stigmatisation from these issues that historically has seen them relegated to the 'too hard basket', not just in mainstream ethics discourse, but in the minds of us all.

CASE SCENARIO AND CRITICAL QUESTIONS

Case scenario[3]

While driving one evening, a woman with an eight year history of paranoid schizophrenia became so disturbed by racing thoughts and altered perceptions of external stimuli that she felt unsafe and abandoned her car in the middle of a busy road. From a nearby telephone booth, she rang a private psychiatric hospital in which she had previously been a patient and sought assistance. She explained to the nurse who received her call that she was 'too frightened to drive' in case she hurt other people, and she was afraid to go home in case her estranged husband (from whom she was being divorced) would have her committed as an involuntary patient at a local psychiatric facility. Unfortunately, the woman no longer had any health insurance and her only source of income was an invalid's pension. Thus she could not be re-admitted to the private hospital where she had been treated previously. Concerned about the woman's safety, the nurse who received the telephone call secured the assistance of a second nurse to keep the woman talking on the phone while arrangements for her safe removal from the telephone booth could be made. One hour later, the woman was finally 'rescued' from the telephone box. When she was found, she was observed to be 'exhausted and sitting on the floor of the telephone booth in tears'. The reason it took so long to assist the woman was because the nurses involved encountered the following difficulties:

- when the local police were contacted for assistance, their initial response was that the woman 'had already requested assistance in person' and that she 'was a "nutter" who wanted a free ride home';
- when the seriousness of the case was explained, the police responded by stating that they had no car available and that one would have to be dispatched via the Police Department's Communication Centre (PDCC);
- minutes later the police called back to advise the nurse that the PDCC had refused to dispatch a car, stating it was the ambulance service's responsibility to transport a psychiatric patient (the traffic hazard posed by the woman's care was ignored);
- when contacted, the ambulance service responded appropriately and took the woman to the emergency department of a local hospital;
- the hospital, however, refused admission to the woman on the grounds that she 'did not live within the hospital's region';
- it was recommended that the woman be subsequently transported to another facility — specifically the one she feared;

- some days later it was revealed that the patient never arrived at the local psychiatric facility on the day in question (she had refused ambulance transport out of fear of the designated hospital and walked home because her car had been hit by moving traffic);
- later the woman was certified because of her 'deteriorating mental state and erratic and dangerous behaviour' and admitted to the very hospital she feared (taken from Johnstone 2001, pp. 205–6).

Critical questions

1. What were the woman's rights in this situation?
2. What corresponding duties were owed to her and by whom?
3. If you were the nurse receiving the woman's telephone call in this case, how would you have dealt with the situation?
4. What are your rights and responsibilities as a professional care giver in regard to caring for people with mental health problems?
5. Is the nursing profession doing enough to advocate and promote the welfare and wellbeing of the mentally ill? If not, what can and should be done to improve the status quo?

---

1 The notions, 'mental disorders', 'mental illness', 'psychiatric disorders' and 'mental health problem' are not synonymous, and thus it would be misleading to use them interchangeably. For instance, a person can have a mental health problem yet not be 'mentally disordered'.

In Australia, 'mental disorder' is a term used to 'describe individuals suffering from some form of psychiatric condition which impairs their functioning' (Tomison 1996, p. 2). Although the terms 'mental disorder' and 'mental illness' are often used synonymously, 'mental illness' is a form of legalese used in legal contexts to refer to persons considered 'patients' under various state and territory Mental Health Acts. In contrast, persons suffering from a 'psychiatric condition' are defined as 'those who have a mental disorder that has had a disabling effect on them' (Tomison 1996, p. 2). Controversially, a mental health problem, in turn, could be distinguished as a 'problem' of a psychogenic sort which causes discomfort — and even a certain degree of distress, but does not interfere with the sufferer's functioning and performance of social responsibilities.

2 See, in particular, the National Mental Health Policy (Australian Health Ministers 1995), the Mental Health Statement of Rights and Responsibilities (Mental Health Consumer Outcomes Task Force 1995), the Evaluation of the National Mental Health Strategy: Final Report (National Mental Health Strategy Evaluation Steering Committee 1997); 'Out of hospital, out of mind!': A Review of Mental Health Services in Australia — 2003 (Groom et al. 2003), The World Health Report 2001. Mental Health: New Understanding, New Hope (WHO 2001), and other reports available via the Mental Health Council of Australia [at *www.mhca.com.au/*] and the Australian Commonwealth Department of Health and Ageing [at *www.mentalhealth.gov.au/*].

3 Taken from Johnstone, M. (2001). 'Stigma, social justice and the rights of the mentally ill: challenging the status quo', *Australian and New Zealand Journal of Mental Health Nursing*, 10, pp. 200–9.

Chapter 8

Ethical issues associated with the reporting of child abuse[1]

LEARNING OBJECTIVES

Upon the completion of this chapter and with further self-directed learning you are expected to be able to:

- Define child abuse.
- Discuss critically the bases upon which child abuse and its prevention stands an important moral issue not just for nurses, but for the community at large.
- Explore common ethical issues associated with the identification and prevention of child abuse.
- Examine critically the moral responsibilities of nurses and the broader nursing profession in regard to the mandatory and voluntary notification of child abuse.

KEYWORDS

- Child abuse
- Child maltreatment
- Child protection
- Confidentiality
- Mandatory reporting
- Voluntary reporting

Introduction

According to the World Health Organization (WHO) globally over 40 million children aged 0–14 years suffer from abuse and neglect each year, and require health and social care (WHO 1999). In countries with reliable mortality reporting, WHO further estimates that as many as one in 5000 and one in 10 000 children under the age of five dies each year as a result of physical violence (WHO 1997). The 'burden of ill health' caused by child abuse-related injuries has been calculated to be 'staggering in terms of cost and socio-economic development' (WHO 1999). For instance, one study from the United States of America alone estimated that 'the costs for 2 million child abuse victims is $US12.4 billion for one year' (WHO 1999).

Child maltreatment (literally the 'wrong handling' of children) and its harmful consequences can and ought to be prevented. Nurses, like others, have a strong professional, legal and moral obligation to take appropriate action to prevent child maltreatment and the burden of suffering that is so demonstrably associated with it. However, the nature and implications of this obligation requires critical examination in order to improve understanding of the conditions under which it might be held to be binding, and to ensure that it is fulfilled in a manner that genuinely maximises the moral interests of vulnerable children.

Historically, the problem of child maltreatment and protection has prompted a variety of responses at a social, political, legal, and professional level (Johnstone 1999b). Notable among these has been the controversial introduction of contemporary mandatory (and permissive) reporting legislation. The introduction of this legislation has had important implications for the broader nursing profession as well as for individual practitioners.

Today, the mandatory and voluntary reporting of child maltreatment constitutes an important ethical issue for members of the nursing profession, and for authorities formally charged with the legal responsibility of regulating nursing standards and practice. Despite this, the issue has received relatively little attention in the nursing (ethics) literature, and has received even less attention in mainstream child abuse, bioethics, jurisprudence, and other related literature. Of particular concern, and the subject of this chapter, is the lack of attention given to examining the nature and implications of the (professional, legal and moral) obligation of *nurses* to report child maltreatment, and the 'special issues' this obligation may raise for individual members of the nursing profession. It is an important aim of this chapter to redress this oversight, and to identify and address key issues warranting attention by individual nurses, nurse registering authorities, professional nursing organisations, and others who are not nurses but whose work may involve liaison and collaboration with members of the nursing profession.

In the discussion to follow, attention will be given to providing a brief overview of the development of the modern child protection movement, to examining why child abuse constitutes a significant moral issue for members of the nursing profession and the community at large, and to addressing some of the key ethical issues raised by mandatory reporting requirements.

The development of the child protection movement in North America: a brief historical overview

In the United States of America, reported cases of child abuse date back to the seventeenth century. In 1655, for example, a master was convicted in a Massachusetts' court and punished for the death of his 12 year old apprentice (Watkins 1990, p. 500). Almost 200 years later, in *Johnson v State* (1840), 'a Tennessee parent was charged with excessive punishment of a child' (Watkins 1990, p. 500). In this case, the court held:

> A parent has the right to chastise a disobedient child, but if he [sic] exceeds the bounds of moderation, and inflicts cruel punishment, he [sic] is a trespasser, and liable to indictment therefor[sic], the excess which constitutes the offence being, not a conclusion of law, but a question of fact for the determination of the jury.
>
> (*Johnson v State* (1840) — cited in Watkins 1990, p. 500)

It is also known that in the early 1820s, public authorities in New York recognised their duty to intervene in cases of child abuse (including parental cruelty and gross neglect). This, however, often resulted in children being indentured (that is, placed into service or an apprenticeship) in conditions as bad or worse than those from which they had originally been removed (Folks 1902 — cited in Watkins 1990, p. 500). The practice of indenture did not fade out until about 1875 following the passage of the 13th Amendment in 1867, which ended not only slavery but 'involuntary servitude within the United States or any place subject to its jurisdiction' (Watkins 1990, p. 500).

Significantly, laws which could be used to protect children from cruelty existed long before the date of the 13th Amendment being passed. As an early commentator on the care of destitute, neglected and delinquent children noted, during the 1800s, 'laws for the prevention of cruelty to children were considered ample, but *it was nobody's business to enforce the laws*' (Folks 1902 — cited in Watkins 1990, p. 501, emphasis added). Although American 'state statutes were adopted after 1825 that established a public duty to intervene in cases of cruelty or neglect of children', these were rarely enforced (Folks 1902; Thomas 1972 — cited in Watkins 1990, p. 501). Further, these statutes stopped short of mandating 'a responsibility to search out children at risk' (Watkins 1990, p. 500). Significantly, it was not until after the landmark (and now legendary) Mary Ellen child abuse case of 1874 (described below) that this situation began to change, largely due to the establishment and development of a formal movement for the protection of children which was initiated as a result of the widespread publicity given to this case. A key feature of this movement was to make it 'somebody's business' to enforce child protection laws.

The Mary Ellen case

The Mary Ellen case involved a small child (of approximately 10 years of age) who had been severely abused by her guardians since the time of her indenture in 1866. A visitor among the poor, Mrs Wheeler, received complaints about the child's maltreatment and, when unable to get assistance from either the police, benevolent societies or charitable gentlemen, approached the president of the society for the Protection of Animals for assistance in gaining protection for the child against further cruelty by her guardians (Lewin 1994, p. 15; Watkins 1990, p. 501). The president of the society ultimately agreed to help and, with his assistance, the case was brought before the New York State Supreme Court. Mary Ellen is reported to have appeared in court 'wrapped in a carriage blanket and wearing ragged garments. Her body was bruised, and she had a gash above her left eye and cheek where she had been struck with scissors' (Lewin 1994, p. 15).

The court case was successful, the outcome of which resulted in Mary Ellen being placed in the protective care of Mrs Wheeler. Mary Ellen's abusive female guardian, meanwhile, was convicted of criminal assault and sentenced to 'one year in the Penitentiary at hard labour' (Watkins 1990, p. 502). Following the publicity given to this case, the New York Society for the Prevention of Cruelty to Children (NYSPCC) was formed in 1874 and 'became the child protection and rescue model for several US states and foreign countries' (Watkins 1990, p. 501; see also Lewin 1994, p. 15; Goddard 1996, p. 96). A century later, in 1976, the first international conference on child abuse was held in Geneva. Among other things, this conference increased the world's understanding that the problem of child maltreatment was not just a local or a national one, but was unequivocally international in its scope (Fogarty and Sargeant 1989, p. 149).

Development of the child protection movement in England and Australia

The North American experience was to be influential in the development of the child protection movement in the United Kingdom, with the first Society for the Prevention of Cruelty to Children in England being established in 1883 and ultimately receiving Queen Victoria's patronage in 1889 (Fogarty and Sargeant 1989, p. 17). Like its North American counterparts, this society aimed, among other things, to achieve specific child protection and rescue law reforms, which up until then had failed to be passed. For example, in the 1870s, attempts to introduce anti-cruelty legislation into the English parliament were 'entirely rebuffed' with the prime minister of the day, Lord Shaftesbury, defending:

> the evils you state are enormous and indisputable, but they are so private, internal and domestic in character as to be beyond the reach of legislation, and the subject would not, I think, be entertained in either House of Parliament.
>
> (cited in Fogarty and Sargeant 1989, p. 17)

Australia, as a colony of England, was very much influenced by British attitudes and political antipathy in dealing formally with the issue of cruelty to children (Renvoize 1993, p. 31; Fogarty and Sargeant 1989, pp. 16–17). Of particular interest to this discussion is the situation in the Australian State of Victoria which was not exempt from the problem of child abuse. For example, in 1863, inquests into the deaths of children under three years of age found that approximately one-quarter had died as a result of causes 'denoting neglect, ignorance or maltreatment' (Gandevia 1978 — cited by Goddard 1996, p. 10). Although child-specific welfare legislation was passed as early as 1864 (the *Neglected and Criminal Children's Act*) and a Society for Prevention of Cruelty to Children (modelled on the British society) established in 1897, as Fogarty and Sargeant comment (1989, p. 16):

Throughout the 19th century the State displayed a deliberate reticence to intervene in family matters. Whereas factory legislation and educational developments increasingly took cognisance of the particular needs of children and there was legislation protecting animals against cruelty, there was a marked antipathy to protect children against maltreatment by their parents or custodians.

A notable example of this antipathy can be found in an argument that was advanced against a proposed Bill introduced into the Victorian parliament in 1891 and which was aimed at 'making incest a criminal offence' (Renvoize 1993, p. 31). In rejecting the passage of the Bill (which was later passed), it was argued 'that it would be better that a few persons should escape than that such a monstrous clause as this should be placed upon the statute book in this colony' (Renvoize 1993, p. 31). Later examples show that this antipathy persisted well into the twentieth century. For example, between 1966 and 1968, concern about child maltreatment and protection in Victoria was again highlighted when two medical researchers, publishing in the *Australian Medical Journal*, recommended the introduction of mandatory reporting laws (Birrell and Birrell 1966, 1968). The government of the day, however, rejected this recommendation on grounds that it would 'run counter to "welfare ideology" and could lead to hysteria and an urge to punish cruel parents' (Hiskey 1980 — cited in Mendes 1996, p. 27). In its stead, a system of voluntary reporting was recommended. A decade later, in 1986, a recommendation for mandatory reporting was again opposed by the government of the day, this time on grounds that 'it was punitive rather than preventive and likely to lead to a large increase in false reports' (Colyer 1986 — cited in Mendes 1996, p. 27).

Today, the issue of child maltreatment and the need for effective child protection services remains problematic and an 'endless challenge' in countries around the world, including Australia (see, for example, the reported commentary by Garbutt 2003). Over the past few years, there has been a sharp increase in reported incidents of child abuse and neglect Australia wide. 'The system' of child protection has not, however, been able to cope with the increase in demands placed upon it. Despite a rise in the reporting of child abuse, significant numbers of children are still maimed and killed each year as a result of abuse received at the hands of their primary carers (Australian Institute of Health and Welfare 1998; Strang 1996). A troubling aspect of this scenario is that in Australia, as has been shown to be the case overseas, very often 'the circumstances leading to the most serious cases of child abuse almost always were known to the authorities, but there was no intervention because *no-one would take responsibility*' (Monash Review 1986, p. 11, emphasis added). In 1996 these failures of the Australian child protection system were described by one critic as a 'national tragedy', and prompted calls by the then Chief Justice of the Family Court, Justice Alastair Nicholson, for the system to be investigated by a royal commission of inquiry (Milburn 1996, p. 3). This call has been largely ignored at both a social and political level (Johnstone, 1999b, 1999c). Arguably, what lies at the basis of this social and political inertia is an even more insidious moral inertia and a culpable lack of moral will to challenge and change the status quo. What will shift this moral inertia remains an open question. What is certain, however, is that this moral malaise will continue until it is recognised and understood that child maltreatment is most profoundly a moral problem and, as such, deserves a sustained and comprehensive moral response.

What makes child abuse a bona fide and significant moral issue?

Child abuse constitutes a significant moral problem and, as such, demands a substantial moral response. Reasons for this are outlined below.

As previously considered in Chapter 3 of this book, it is generally accepted that something involves a (human) moral/ethical problem where it has as its central concern:

- the promotion and protection of people's genuine wellbeing and welfare (including their interests in not suffering unnecessarily);
- responding justly to the genuine needs and significant interests of different people; and
- determining and justifying what constitutes right and wrong conduct in a given situation.

Adjunct to these concerns is an additional consideration, namely, that people have a moral responsibility to not cause unnecessary harm to others and, where able, ought to come to the aid of those who are suffering and in distress. As Amato (1990) notes in his *Victims and values: a history and a theory of suffering* (p. 175):

> There is an elemental moral requirement to respond to innocent suffering. If we were not to respond to it and its claims upon us, we would be without conscience and, in some basic sense, not completely human. And without compassion for others and passion for the causes on behalf of human wellbeing, what is best in our world would be missing.

These considerations all apply in the case of child abuse. As can be readily demonstrated, the problem of child abuse fundamentally concerns:

- promoting and protecting the wellbeing and welfare of children at risk of harm because of the abuse and neglect by more powerful others;
- protecting children from this harm requires a careful calculation and balancing of the needs and interests of 'different people'; for example, the children themselves, their primary caregivers (who are often, although not always, the abusers), others (such as family, friends) who may also have an important relationship with the child, prospective notifiers (who may themselves sometimes experience negative outcomes — including violence and abuse — as a result of their interventions aimed at protecting children at risk), society as a whole and, not least, future generations (who may find themselves unwitting participants in the sequelae of intergenerational abuse); and
- determining and justifying the 'rightness' and 'wrongness' of intervening or not intervening in a case of known or suspected child abuse.

Adjunct to these concerns is an additional consideration involving the moral responsibility people have to not cause unnecessary harm to children and, where able, to come to the aid of children who are suffering and in distress as a result of being maltreated and/or neglected by others.

Underscoring child abuse as a moral problem are a number of other important considerations revolving around the extraordinary vulnerability of children generally. Children are among the most vulnerable members of our community. For the most part, they are unable to protect themselves from the harms imposed on them by people more powerful than themselves. Invariably children have to rely on others for help if their wellbeing and welfare is to be safeguarded. Without intervention and help offered by others, the abuse and neglect of children rarely stops (Child Protection Victoria 1993, p. 9; Goddard 1996). Historically, however, children have not always been able to rely on others (including benevolent citizens, health professionals and public officials) to intervene and help them (Johnstone 1999b). Nor have they been able to rely on legal law and its processes. As has been pointed out elsewhere, children have long been considered 'different' under law and stand as the 'paradigmatic group excluded from traditional liberal rights' otherwise accorded to and protective of autonomous adults (Minow 1990, p. 283). Equally troubling, neither have children been able to rely on ethics/morality to protect them. Historically, as in the case of law, ethics has also treated children as 'different'; specifically, as not deserving the moral respect otherwise accorded to rationally competent adults (usually men) and which, if accorded to children, could have resulted in 'substantial [and unwanted] intrusion' into the lives of parents (especially fathers) and guardians (male benefactors) (adapted from Schrag 1995, p. 357; see also Archard 1993; Radi 1979; Johnstone, 1999b). Because of not being able to rely on others, law or ethics for help, children historically have remained at risk of and have experienced otherwise avoidable harms which, if experienced by adults, would have been (and would be) universally condemned, even by the most rudimentary of moral calculations, as being morally unacceptable.

In light of these and other considerations, it is manifestly evident not only that child abuse is a significant moral problem, but that it warrants a substantial moral response. To be effective this response must include moral initiative and action at an individual, group, community and state/territory level aimed at providing genuine *presence* ('being there') for the children who require the assistance of others in order to get the protection they need from a situation of potential or actual abuse and/or neglect.

The problem of ambivalence toward the moral entitlements of children

In an attempt to redress the historical and legitimated vulnerability of children in the case of child abuse and neglect, governments have responded by enacting either mandatory or voluntary reporting laws obligating certain people (on either legal or moral grounds) to intervene by reporting known or suspected cases of child abuse to child protection services. This response has not been without controversy, however. Pivotal to the controversy have been variant moral beliefs, values and attitudes concerning what constitutes the morally most appropriate response to child abuse given the complex of overlapping relationships, responsibilities and variant moral calculations that are inherent in any potential or actual child abuse situation. So intense has been this controversy that, in some instances, it has resulted in a significant and serious 'backlash' against child protection (see, for example, Myers 1994).

While there is little disagreement among stakeholders in the child abuse debate that it is morally wrong for children to be harmed unnecessarily and that children *should* be protected from the harmful behaviours of others, there is considerable disagreement about the kinds of things that can and should be considered *bona fide* 'harmful' to children, the kinds of acknowledged harms that children ought to be formally protected from, and how best to protect children from the harms deemed both *bona fide* and unacceptable. Thus, while there may appear to be a social consensus about the moral unacceptability of child abuse, quite the reverse may be true. As Lantos (1995, p. 45) points out, an apparent consensus about child abuse may, paradoxically, 'mask profound disagreements' about the nature of child abuse and the apparent responsibilities of various parties (including parents/guardians, health professionals and government authorities) to intervene. An example of this can be found in the tragic Australian child abuse case of Daniel Valerio.

The case of Daniel Valerio

On 8 September 1990, Daniel Valerio, a 2-year-old boy living in the state of Victoria, was bashed to death by his stepfather. During the inquest that followed, it was revealed that 21 professionals (including three general medical practitioners, a paediatrician, nurses, social workers, a psychologist, a community health worker, teachers and police) as well as neighbours and family friends had all observed bruising on Daniel Valerio's body in the months leading up to his death (Farouque 1993a, p. 3; Garner 1993, p. 24; Goddard 1996, pp. 174–5). Despite making these observations, no action was taken and, as a result, the child remained in an abusive situation. In July, before his death, Daniel Valerio was admitted to a local hospital for assessment and treatment of a large haematoma on his forehead and other bruises observed on his body, head and limbs. Despite suspicions about the nature of the boy's injuries, the attending paediatrician, in consultation with a psychologist acting as a social worker at the hospital, 'decided that there were not sufficient grounds to refer to protective services but that Daniel should be monitored' (Goddard 1996, pp. 174–5). Later it was also revealed that a family doctor had suspected the child was being abused a week before he died 'but left it to the boy's mother — a key suspect — to seek specialist medical advice' (Farouque 1993b, p. 3). Upon autopsy, it was found that Daniel Valerio had sustained 104 external injuries, predominantly bruises, on his body (Farouque 1993a, p. 3; Garner 1993).

The Daniel Valerio case received widespread media attention around Australia and sparked public outrage. A burning question on many people's lips was: How could this have happened? One commentator has since suggested that a possible reason for why the case 'happened' is because the professionals concerned were simply 'not convinced of the need to act' (Goddard 1996, p. 180). He has further contended that had a stranger (rather than a primary caregiver) been suspected of beating the child, 'the responses of all the systems would have been entirely different'; quite probably the child would have received 'immediate medical examination and treatment' and the media would have reported the attack 'and provided descriptions of the attacker' (Goddard 1996, pp. 180–1). Instead, Daniel Valerio's case was met initially with silence and disbelief until it was too late.

Is the 'failure of the system' to blame?

It has been suggested that the failure of 'the system' to be convinced of the seriousness of a child's situation and the need to take protective action rests, in complicated ways, on a prevailing social–cultural ambivalence about violence towards children (Goddard 1996). In support of this claim, it is contended that violence towards children is often viewed, controversially, as being merely 'discipline' (and hence socially acceptable) when carried out at the hands of parents/guardians. (Indeed, this point is underscored everyday in supermarkets around the country where children are physically 'disciplined' [read physically abused] into submission by their adult custodians; were adults treated in this abusive way by other adults, it is likely that local security officers or the police or both would be called, and charges of criminal assault possibly laid against an offending adult.) This explanation is, however, incomplete. The 'failure of the system' to intervene appropriately to protect children rests on something far deeper and more complex than an ambivalence about violence per se towards children. There are other underpinning ambivalences at play, including (and perhaps especially) an extraordinary social–cultural ambivalence about the *moral status, moral interests* and *related moral entitlements of children* and the *correlative moral responsibilities* these entitlements impose on others who come into contact with children (Johnstone 1999b). This 'moral ambivalence' has contributed to the 'failure of the system', by undermining the confidence of people in taking what Hoff (1982) calls 'private moral initiative' and 'private benevolence' (read individual moral action) needed to genuinely assist and protect children who are at risk.

If children were genuinely regarded as having moral status and significant moral interests deserving of protection (at least comparable to that otherwise enjoyed by adults), the world's historical response to child maltreatment and protection may well have been very different. For instance, there may have been less of a tendency both privately and publicly to regard the moral interests of children as being subordinate to the interests of adults (in particular, parents). This, in turn, might have resulted in individuals (including professionals), groups, communities and governments responding more effectively to the problem of child maltreatment and protection than has historically been the case. And it might also have resulted in individuals, groups and communities positioning themselves better to break the cycle of intergenerational violence that has become so characteristic of contemporary societies everywhere. Instead, the problem of child abuse has foundered on a bedrock of moral malaise that, arguably, will not shift until there is a concerted effort at both an individual and collective level to challenge and change the status quo.

The ethical implications of child abuse

Whether driven by legal obligation or moral commitment, or both, a health care professional's decision to report child abuse (or not report it, as the case may be) never occurs in a moral vacuum and is never free of moral risk. Even in the face of clinical certainty (insofar as this is possible) and the threat of legal and professional censure for non-compliance with mandatory reporting requirements (insofar as this is probable), there is always room to question: Should I report this particular case of known or suspected child abuse and/or neglect? Underpinning this question are the additional questions of: What are the possible consequences to the child of me reporting or not reporting this case? What are the possible consequences to the child's family/caregivers of me reporting or not reporting this case? and What are the possible consequences to me of reporting or not reporting this case? Possible answers to these questions will depend, in varying degrees, upon an effective harm/benefit analysis of the situation.

The moral demand to report child abuse

Child abuse (often used as 'an "umbrella" term that covers a wide range of activities that harm children in some way' [Goddard 1996, p. 28]), can take a number of forms, including physical, sexual, emotional and spiritual. It can also involve neglect, defined here as 'the failure to provide the child with the basic necessities of life, such as food, clothing, shelter and supervision, to the extent that the child's health and development are placed at risk' (Child Protection Victoria 1993, p. 3). In some instances, all forms of abuse may overlap; for example, a child who is sexually abused is *ipso facto* abused physically, emotionally and spiritually as well (Renvoize 1993, p. 36).

Although there is some disagreement about how child abuse can and should be defined (Johnstone 1999b; Goddard 1996; O'Hagan 1993), this is not sufficient to threaten strong moral arguments against child abuse and its intervention, as some have suggested (see, for example, Lantos 1995, p. 43). Child abuse can be defined in ways that unequivocally distinguishes it from other 'acceptable' behaviours directed at children (for example, play, discipline, 'character building', education) and it is spurious to suggest otherwise. A key feature of child abuse (not carried by other behaviours directed at children) concerns the risk of non-accidental and culpable harm that it poses to a child's genuine welfare and wellbeing. These risks are not merely speculative or imaginary, but substantive and known through the supportive findings of rigorous research, an increasing body of professional literature on the subject, and, not least, by the survivors of child abuse themselves who are increasingly coming forward to share their experiences by making their 'stories' public.

In all its forms, child abuse can cause significant and lasting harm to children and, ultimately, the adults they become. Borrowing from Archard (1993, p. 150): 'A child may be harmed both as a child *and* as a prospective adult. The adult of the future can be harmed by what is now done to the child'. It is this consequence of harm that makes child abuse and neglect morally objectionable. Understanding this, however, requires at least a rudimentary understanding of the notion of 'harm', the way it is linked to human welfare and wellbeing, and why it is morally compelling both *not to cause harm* and *to prevent harm* to others.

The notion of harm and its link with the moral duty to prevent child abuse

As previously considered in Chapter 3 of this text, harm may be taken as involving the invasion, violation, thwarting, or 'setting back' of a person's significant welfare interests to the detriment of that person's wellbeing (Feinberg 1984, p. 34; Beauchamp and Childress 1994, p. 193). Wellbeing, in turn, can include interests in:

> continuance for a foreseeable interval of one's life, and the interests in one's own physical health and vigour, the integrity and normal functioning of one's body, the absence of absorbing pain and suffering or grotesque disfigurement, minimal intellectual acuity, emotional stability, the absence of groundless anxieties and resentments, the capacity to engage normally in social intercourse and to enjoy and maintain friendships, at least minimal income and financial security, a tolerable social and physical environment, and a certain amount of freedom from interference and coercion.
>
> (Feinberg 1984, p. 37)

The test for whether a person's interests and wellbeing have been violated or thwarted rests on 'whether that interest is in a worse condition than it would otherwise have been in had the invasion not occurred at all' (Feinberg 1984, p. 34). For instance, if a person (for example, a child, a young person or an adult survivor of child abuse) is left psychogenically distressed (for example, emotionally unstable, anxious, depressed and/or suicidal) as a result of his/her abusive childhood experiences, our reflective commonsense tells us that this person's interests have been violated and the person him/herself 'harmed'. As the American philosopher Joel Feinberg (1984) explains, the violation of a person's welfare interests renders that person 'very seriously harmed indeed' since 'their ultimate aspirations are defeated too'.

Protecting the interests of children as *children* and as *prospective adults*

It is generally recognised in contemporary bioethical thought that people ought not to cause harm to or to impose risks of harm onto others. It is also accepted that people have a moral obligation to prevent harm to others if this can be done without sacrificing other important moral interests (Beauchamp and Childress 2001; Singer 1993). By this view, acts which violate the interests of others, or fail to prevent the interests of others being violated, are prima facie morally wrong. The abuse of children — and the failure to prevent it — clearly violates the interests of children (both as *children* and as *prospective adults*) and renders them seriously harmed. It is the profound risk of the harmful consequences of child abuse (at all stages of life), and the utter preventability of these consequences, that makes intervention in child abuse at all levels morally compelling. Failure to prevent this harm is morally wrong. Further, the moral unacceptability of child abuse is underscored when it is remembered that the harmful consequences of child abuse do not remain quarantined in a 'lost and forgotten' childhood which a person can leave behind upon entering adulthood. As Briere (1992, p. xvi) points out 'in the absence of appropriate intervention, hurt children often grow to become distressed and symptomatic adolescents and adults' — a morally significant and harmful outcome.

What is not always understood in this debate is that the negative effects of child abuse can be long term and sometimes devastating, affecting, in morally significant ways, not only the individuals who survive their traumatic childhoods, but those with whom they share relationships including family, friends, partners, co-workers, service providers and the community at large (see, for example, Corby 2000; Roy 1998; Mullinar and Hunt 1997; van der Kolk et al. 1996; Phillips and Frederick 1995; Vicki 1995; Loring 1994; Terr 1994; Valent 1993; Elliott 1993; Porterfield 1993; Renvoize 1993; Wilson and Raphael 1993; Briere 1992; Herman 1992; Sanford 1990). This is so, even for those who receive professional help in dealing with their child abuse issues. As one commentator notes:

> Day to day, moment to moment, our feelings and perceptions of the world can change. No matter how long you have been 'working' on your abuse, or how you may feel that at last you can live your life rather than just exist, there are times when you can be overwhelmed quite unexpectedly with painful feelings and memories of your abuse. The 'trigger' can be a smell, a sound, a memory apparently from nowhere. Of this, one survivor says: 'One day, one moment, you can believe that you are all right, that the world and the people in it are all right, and the next be right back down there in the pit of despair'.
>
> (Longdon 1993, p. 59)

This 'reality' is exemplified by one adult survivor of child abuse, who writes:

> The last seven years have been very difficult for me. For nearly two years I was unable to work, simply being traumatised by the memories that kept bombarding me. My ensuing depression put me in a psychiatric hospital for about eight months in total, and during that time I tried to end my life three times by taking overdoses, and continued to self-abuse by slashing myself. It took me eight years to complete a three-year university degree, as I had to keep dropping out when I had breakdowns.
>
> (Mono 1997, p. 40)

These examples (which stand as just two among many [see others included in Mullinar and Hunt 1997]) show that adult survivors of child abuse can be seriously harmed (have their welfare interests and wellbeing violated) by their traumatic childhood experiences. The survivors quoted in these examples are plagued by painful feelings and memories of their past childhood abuse and, as a result, are thwarted in realising their ultimate aspirations, not least to be free of the 'absorbing pain and suffering' and 'emotional instability' that has come to characterise and burden their lives. This outcome is morally wrong and ought to have been prevented.

It might be objected here that many survivors of child abuse do not emerge from their traumatic childhood pasts as 'damaged goods' (Sanford 1990), do go on to live productive and satisfying lives (which indeed they do [see, for example, Higgins 1994]), and therefore are no longer 'harmed' by their childhood abuse. While many survivors of child abuse do go on to live productive and satisfying lives, this is not sufficient to negate or to override the moral obligation to intervene and prevent child maltreatment. There are at least two reasons for this. Firstly, maltreated children are still harmed *as children* by their traumatic experiences irrespective of their survival into adulthood. To deny the suffering of children — or at least to render this suffering as irrelevant — is to discriminate against them in morally unjust ways; it seems to be saying that the suffering of children does not count (or, at least, does not count as much as the suffering of adults) just because it is *children* who are suffering. This 'adultist' view is morally indefensible. Secondly, even though adults who have survived child abuse do go on to live productive and satisfying lives, this is not to say that they do not also suffer in unjustly burdensome ways as a result of their traumatic childhood pasts.

Considerations against the mandatory and voluntary notification of child abuse

Public policy requirements to report child abuse have historically been criticised and even rejected by a range of people including members of the medical profession, community support groups and, not least, members of the judiciary (for example, Family Court judges) (Johnstone 1999b; Goddard 1996; Mendes 1996; Myers 1994; Chandler 1993; Fogarty 1993; Magazanik 1993; MacNair 1992; Fogarty and Sargeant 1989). The grounds for this criticism and rejection have mostly been utilitarian in nature, involving a calculation of harms and benefits to the: (1) professional–client relationship; (2) parents and families of allegedly abused and neglected children; and, lastly (3) allegedly abused and neglected children themselves. Requirements to report child abuse and neglect have also been criticised, controversially, on civil libertarian grounds. Here arguments are advanced to the effect that requirements to report child abuse stands as a fundamental violation of parental rights to be free of state interference and to decide how best to raise their children (Archard 1993). As one commentator observes in relation to the alleged 'dangers' of children's rights discourse, 'taken literally, respect for children's rights may permit substantial intrusion into parents' lives' (Schrag 1995, p. 356). These considerations are not unproblematic, however, and are themselves vulnerable to criticism. Consider the following.

The professional–client relationship

Legitimised requirements to report child abuse and neglect have been viewed as being problematic primarily on grounds that they threaten the sanctity of the professional–client relationship by eroding professional discretion about: (1) duties of confidentiality; and (2) how best to deal with child abuse cases (for example, by discretional and confidential counselling) (Goddard 1996, p. 98; Lantos 1995, p. 44;

Winslade 1995, p. 455; Lewin 1994, p. 15; MacNair 1992, pp. 128–9; Quinn 1992, pp. 86–96). A related concern has been that legitimised reporting requirements can also shift and extend the boundaries of responsibility of the professional–client relationship; namely, to include not just the *adult*–client but the *child*–client as well. This is seen as potentially creating an intolerable tension between the possibly competing and conflicting interests of all stakeholders in question. For example, it could create for an attending health professional the moral dilemma of how best to uphold the interests of an abused child–client without also violating the interests of an abusing adult–client, and vice versa. It may well be that, in the end, it is not possible for the health professional to uphold the interests of both clients equally, prompting the question: What should I do?

Consequential to the shift in boundaries of responsibility, there is also a commensurate change in role for the health professional, namely, from that of clinician-healer/therapist to that of 'statutory protector'. For some, this assumed role of 'statutory protector' could further threaten the therapeutic sanctity of the professional–client relationship, begging the question of the moral acceptability of health care professionals functioning as the 'eyes of the state'; that is, as agents of a 'state surveillance' system.

Parents and families

Legitimised requirements to report child mistreatment have also been criticised and rejected on grounds that these stand to seriously threaten the 'liberal rights' (to privacy and self-determination), welfare interests and wellbeing of parents and families (Archard 1993, pp. 122–32). The risk of this happening is seen to be especially high in the case of false allegations being made, or where health care professionals are either 'overly zealous' or incompetent or impaired in performing their assessments of allegedly abused children and reporting their findings to child protection services. For example, health care professionals may be lacking in the necessary skills or may make the wrong judgments or, because of their own unresolved personal issues, are just not able 'to come to terms fully with any abuse' (Renvoize 1993, p. 152; see also Goddard 1996; Lantos 1995; Tilden et al. 1994; Miller and Weinstock 1987; Giovannoni 1982). Some critics contend that, in the ultimate analysis, the legitimated reporting of child abuse could result in parents and families being left stigmatised, embarrassment and even irreparably damaged — particularly if the family is 'totally dismembered through termination of parental rights' (Giovannoni 1982, p. 108; Lantos 1995, p. 44). Parents and families could, therefore, be harmed as a result of interventions by child protection services. This, in turn, could seriously harm the welfare interests and wellbeing of the children suspected of being mistreated by their parents and families, but who nevertheless remain dependent on them for care. In short, harmed parents/families could *ipso facto* result in harmed children.

Abused and neglected children

Perhaps among the most serious and troubling criticisms of all is the view that legitimated requirements to report child abuse may, paradoxically, cause further harm to abused children themselves (Goddard 1996; Lantos 1995; Lewin 1994; Miller and Weinstock 1987; Giovannoni 1982). The 'harmfulness' of the intervention, in this instance, is thought to derive from and be compounded by a number of processes.

- Through children being separated (sometimes prematurely) from their parents/primary caregivers and surrendered to 'ambiguous substitute family arrangements' (Giovannoni 1982, p. 108; Miller and Weinstock 1987, p. 162).
- Where separation and removal damages the child–parent/guardian relationship, not least through 'interfering with the ability of abusing parents to deal with their problems and reintegrate their families' (Miller and Weinstock 1987, p. 162). Further, if protective processes (for example, court action) are unsuccessful, this could result in an abused child being returned 'unprotected to an unbelieving family which might scapegoat them and blame them for all the disruption' (Renvoize 1993, p. 152).
- Where protective services simply fail mistreated children, for example:
  - where referrals and protective interventions are handled poorly (investigations may be delayed or be ineffective; children may be returned to violent and abusive homes and thus committed to a life of re-abuse, crime and death [see, for example, Fogarty 1993, p. 8; MacNair 1992, p. 129; Pegler 1996, p. 4; Pegler and Farouque 1996, p. 1; Coffey 1996, pp. 1, 4; Daly et al. 1996, p. 1; Hawes and Honeysett 1996, p. 3; Kissane 1993, pp. 24–5, 1995, p. 13; Chandler 1993, p. 28]);
  - where mechanisms for securing child protection may themselves be traumatic and 'abusive' (legal processes [including police involvement and court proceedings] are, for example, characteristically intrusive and 'adversarial' in nature; media coverage is characteristically intrusive and can be harmfully 'exposing' and adversarial in nature) (Lewin 1994); and
  - where protective services are inadequate to meet the needs of mistreated children, resulting in increasing numbers of children being drawn into a child protection system that is 'incapable of caring for them properly' (for example, as can occur in the case of a protective system plagued by budgetary constraints) (Fogarty 1993, p. 7).

Thus, in the final analysis, rather than promoting and protecting the welfare interests and wellbeing of abused and neglected children, mandatory and voluntary reporting requirements might block, thwart, intrude upon, set back, invade and violate these moral entitlements. In short, reporting requirements used as a child protection intervention may ultimately prove to be more harmful than the abuse itself.

Responding to the criticisms

The question remains, however, of whether legitimated demands to report known and suspected cases of child abuse and neglect do stand to 'adversely' affect the nature and boundaries of the professional–client relationship, the 'deserving' interests of parents and families (and, it should be added, other abusing adults) and, not least, the interests of mistreated children. And, if so, what the moral implications of this might be. It is to briefly considering these questions that the remainder of this chapter will now turn.

The problem of maintaining confidentiality

Reporting child abuse, unless consented to by both the abuser and the child (given the child is capable of giving consent), almost always involves a breach of confidentiality and privacy. A key reason health care professionals are reluctant to breach confidentiality concerns a fear that, if abusers cannot rely on or trust professional caregivers to keep secret abuse-related information disclosed in the professional–client relationship, then they (the abusers) may be discouraged from seeking help to remedy their abusive behaviours. In effect, legitimised reporting laws could 'drive people underground' (Goddard 1996, p. 98; Magazanik 1993, p. 18; MacNair 1992, p. 129). It is not clear, however, that this fear is sufficient to justify maintaining confidentiality in favour of an abusing adult. There are a number of reasons for this. The first of these concerns the very nature of the moral demand to maintain confidentiality itself.

Traditionally, as discussed in Chapter 6 of this book, the rule of confidentiality has demanded that information gained in the professional–client relationship ought to be kept secret even when its disclosure might serve a greater public good. Over time, however, real-life examples and moral theorising have repeatedly shown that treating the rule of confidentiality as being *absolute* is morally unjust, indefensible and unreasonable (Bok 1983, 1978). At best, maintaining confidentiality should be treated as only a *prima facie* obligation. What this means is that while, as a general rule, confidentiality ought to be maintained in the professional–client relationship, there may sometimes be stronger moral reasons for overriding this obligation. An example here would be where an abusing adult discloses to an attending health care professional his or her intention to deliberately injure a child. A decision to disclose this information in order to warn and protect the intended child-victim would be justified on grounds that it could help to prevent an otherwise avoidable harm from occurring.

Superficially, the disclosure of privileged information in the above example might appear to be in breach of a disclosing client's 'rights' to confidentiality. However, con-fidentiality was never meant to stretch so far as to compel an attending health care professional to lie or to protect those who have no right to impose their malevolence on innocent victims — in this instance an innocent child (Bok 1978, p. 148). Borrowing from Bok (1978, p. 155), 'only an overwhelming blindness to the suffering of those beyond one's immediate sphere' could justify the maintenance of absolute confidentiality in the case where innocent others are at risk of being harmed. Further, a client's moral entitlements to have certain information about themselves kept secret are forfeited where the maintenance of confidentiality about their case stands to seriously impinge on the moral interests and wellbeing of innocent others. In this instance, morally constrained discretionary breaches of confidentiality are morally justified.

In the case of child abuse, there exists strong moral grounds for justifiably overriding an obligation of confidentiality that might otherwise be due to an abusing adult, and for discretionary disclosures to be made to appropriate people. In regard to the 'possible harm' that discretionary disclosures may cause to abusers (for example, driving abusers 'underground' and discouraging them from seeking help; causing them to feel hurt, embarrassed and stigmatised; dismembering families; and so forth), this is not sufficient to justify the maintenance of *absolute* confidentiality. One reason for this is: it is not clear that discretionary disclosures will necessarily harm the welfare interests of abusers. The aim of protective interventions (of which the legitimated reporting of child abuse is a form) is to 'protect children, not to punish abusers' and to be 'curative and remedial rather than punitive' (Corby 2000; Lewin 1994, p. 16; Fogarty 1993, pp. 86–8; Miller and Weinstock 1987, p. 167; see also Scott and O'Neil 1996). Thus disclosures that are made to appropriate people stand to not only benefit an abused child, but also set in motion a process that could potentially assist the abuser as well. If the abuser is genuinely accepting of responsibility for his or her abusive behaviour toward children and is committed to rehabilitation, then the problem of competing demands to maintain confidentiality can be overcome by the health care provider negotiating the discretionary disclosure of privileged information gained in the professional–client relationship. If, however, an abuser is unwilling to accept responsibility for his or her abusive behaviour and is unwilling to give permission for a discretionary breach of confidentiality to the relevant authorities, the health care professional has an overriding moral obligation to take the action necessary to protect the interests of an at-risk child or children. Discretionary breaches of confidentiality are morally justified in these instances.

The problem of statutory surveillance

Some claim that legitimised reporting requirements could exacerbate the problem of child abuse in another way; namely, by facilitating its 'over-reporting' (including a proliferation of false allegations being made about its incidence) (Goddard 1996, p. 98; Renvoize 1993; Miller and Weinstock 1987). This, it is contended, might result in 'more children and families being drawn into a system which does not have the capacity to provide the necessary services to them' (Fogarty 1993, p. 12). Furthermore, were health care professionals seen to be spearheading this 'over-reporting' through their surveillance role, this could result in a loss of community trust in service providers and, ultimately, 'the system' which, in turn, could work against an effective overall societal response to child abuse and neglect.

It is not clear, however, whether community trust in health care professionals would be eroded by a proliferation in the reporting of child abuse. For one thing, a proliferation in the reporting of child abuse may not necessarily be spurious. An increase in reporting could be directly linked to a genuine increase in the actual incidence of abuse which, in turn, can be further linked to increased professional and community awareness of what constitutes child abuse and its unacceptability (Corby 2000; Goddard 1996; Fogarty 1993). Thus, while being perplexed by an increase in the reporting of child abuse, the community might nevertheless be reassured that 'the system' is working and that children are being protected from unnecessary harm. Contrary to the claims made above, it might be a *failure* by health care professionals to report child abuse that risks undermining community confidence in their services, not the reverse. The Daniel Valerio case (cited earlier in this chapter) is an example of this.

Preserving the integrity of the professional–client relationship

Legitimated requirements to report child abuse do not necessarily threaten the sanctity or integrity of the professional–client relationship. If disclosures are handled in a morally, legally and clinically informed, competent and sensitive manner, this need not involve a collapse of the boundaries between matters of clinical competence and legal and moral prescription/proscription, as some have suggested (Giovannoni 1982, p. 108). To the contrary. Legal and moral prescriptions/proscriptions in the case of child abuse can strengthen the bases and boundaries of clinical competence by reminding health care professionals to always consider carefully the precise impact that their acts and omissions can have on the lives of others (especially children both as children and as prospective adults), and to remain vigilant in regard to their capacity to harm as well as benefit those in their care.

Upholding the interests of parents, families and abused children

It is fully acknowledged that the act of reporting child mistreatment is one which is fraught with difficulties. It is further acknowledged, there are no guarantees that mistakes will not occur. But the risks of *failing* to intervene are equally if not more onerous. By not reporting instances of child mistreatment, there is a risk that abused and neglected children will be 'left forgotten and invisible' (Mullinar and Hunt 1997) and, without help, will go on to be symptomatic adults. There is an additional risk that, without intervention (whatever the risks), the sequelae of child mistreatment could 'continue to wreak havoc generation after generation' (Lord 1997). Appropriate intervention to prevent child abuse (of which reporting may be the first step) can make a significant contribution to breaking the cycle of intergenerational violence.

As suggested earlier, it is not necessarily the case that protective interventions (of which the legitimated reporting of child abuse is a form) will harm the deserving welfare interests of abusing parents and families. It needs to be remembered that a key aim of interventionist strategies is 'to protect children, not to punish the abusers', and, where able, to offer dysfunctional adults and families remediation. Thus appropriate interventions stand to not only benefit an abused child, but also to set in motion a process that could potentially assist and benefit abusers as well.

In the case of children, there is no denying that separation from a primary caregiver can be an extremely traumatic experience for a child — even when the primary caregiver is the abuser. While it might be assumed that an abused child would be 'happy' to get away from an abusive parent, this is not necessarily so. (There are many complex reasons for this which, regrettably, are beyond the scope of this present work to consider [see, for example, van der Kolk 1996, p. 200].) And there is no denying that children can be — and have been — seriously harmed when protective interventions have 'gone wrong'. It is acknowledged that children can be — and are — seriously harmed when the system fails them. What this instructs, however, is not the abandonment of protective services or components of it (for example, reporting requirements). Rather, it highlights the need for protective processes to be improved. In summary, attention ought to be focussed on improving — not removing — the systematic processes that have been put in place to help protect children from the harms of abuse and neglect.

The importance of a supportive socio-cultural environment in child abuse prevention

In her influential text *Trauma and recovery: the aftermath of violence — from domestic abuse to political terror*, the American psychiatrist Judith Herman persuasively argues that (1992, p. 9):

> In the absence of strong political movements for human rights, the active process of bearing witness inevitably gives way to the process of forgetting. Repression, dissociation, and denial are phenomena of social as well as individual consciousness.

Applied in the context of child abuse, there is room to suggest that without a strong political movement for children's right, the process of bearing witness (to child mistreatment) will likewise give way to a communal forgetting. The risk of forgetting is particularly great in an environment which is not supportive of or encourages personal moral initiative and individual acts of benevolence (moral action) aimed at genuinely assisting and protecting children who are at risk.

Herman (1992, p. 8) contends that 'without a supportive environment, the bystander usually succumbs to the temptation to look the other way'. Currently, the social and cultural environment in Australia (as well as overseas) is not generally supportive of child abuse prevention and, to some extent, even supports the position of the 'morally passive bystander' (consider, for example, the positive regard generally given to people who 'mind their own business' and the disparagement made of those who do not). For many health care professionals located in this unsupportive environment, looking the other way may seem a preferable option to 'becoming involved' (Goddard 1996). This 'not becoming involved' might even be seen, controversially, as being a morally preferable option on grounds that it could help to avoid the otherwise unpredictable harmful consequences that can (and do sometimes) flow from intervening or becoming involved in a given child abuse/neglect case. What might not be appreciated, however, is that succumbing to the temptation to look the other way and to avoid involvement is not a morally neutral response. Just because health professionals may have done nothing actively to abuse a child (that is, they may have merely witnessed evidence of possible abuse), this does not mean that they have avoided complicity in the harms to the child caused by his or her initial mistreatment. Borrowing from Joseph Fletcher (1973, p. 675) writing in another context, 'Not doing anything is doing something; it is a decision to act every bit as much as deciding for any other deed'. Thus, a decision to do nothing to intervene in the prevention of child abuse is every bit a decision nevertheless, and still stands as a link in the causal chain of events between an actual instance of abuse and the harm to the child that can and does follow from this abuse.

In their classic report on protective services for children in Victoria, Fogarty and Sargeant conclude that (1989, p. 52):

> basically, the issue [of child abuse] is a public one and one in respect of which each section of the community can and should make a contribution. It would we feel be a fundamental mistake to believe that this community problem can be eliminated by a total concentration upon what the government can do for the community. The issue also is — what can the community and individual members of the community do for the state and the children within it? There is too great a tendency both generally and in relation to this particular matter to sit back and demand that the government do this or that but without appreciation of the wider responsibilities which are involved.

There are not, of course, any 'quick fix' solutions to the problem of child abuse and protection. But there is considerable scope to suggest that a lot more could be done at an individual, familial, group, community and state level to improve the status quo. Health care professionals have a particularly important role to play on account of them being in a prime position to discern and provide evidence of instances of child abuse and neglect, and to legitimately intervene to prevent these instances from continuing. Through their informed and morally judicious interventions, health care professionals could, in turn, make a significant difference to the lives and welfare interests of both abused children and abusing adults. Legitimated reporting requirements should, therefore, not be seen as an intrusion or a violation of the professional–client relationship, but as an opportunity to provide support and care to injured and distressed human beings (both children and adults alike).

A system of child protection is only as good as the people who are charged with the responsibilities of upholding it. All health care professionals have an obligation to become sufficiently informed about the clinical, legal and ethical dimensions of child abuse to enable them to competently participate in child protection processes. And there is small doubt that improving the education of health care professionals about child abuse and protection issues will prepare them to deal better with known or suspected child abuse cases. But, as Judith Herman (cited above) makes plain, commitment and education may not be enough; there also needs to be a supportive social environment and a deeply ingrained cultural commitment to preventing the harms of child abuse and neglect across the board. There are a number of points at which initiatives to improve the socio-cultural environment could begin, two examples of which are given below.

One starting point can be found in the nomenclature commonly used to refer to the child protection intervention of 'reporting'. Rather than speak of 'reporting' child abuse, perhaps it would be less punitive to use the notion of 'making notifications'. The term 'reporting', for example, carries a range of negative connotations, including that of 'making a complaint', 'to lay a charge against a person', 'to present oneself to a person in authority' and variations thereof, something which seems to go against the stated aims of reporting; namely, 'to protect the child, not to punish the abuser' (*The Macquarie Concise Dictionary* 1997). The term 'notification' (meaning 'to tell'), in contrast, does not seem to have the same moralistic loading attached to it. A health care professional could 'notify' a case of child abuse to a relevant authority in much the same way that he or she would notify other 'notifiable' conditions such as an infectious disease or other medical condition.

Another starting point may be the electronic and print media. For instance, television advertisements around Australia remind viewers daily that 'If you drink drive, you are a bloody idiot', 'Every cigarette is doing you harm', and 'Work safety: think it, talk it, work it — some injuries never heal'. The financial costs of running these advertisements are seen to be justified even though the advertisements themselves are only a small (be it so important) part of an overall strategy aimed at changing the health risk behaviours in question. This is because the costs of drink driving accidents, smoking and of work-related injuries have all been deemed unacceptable to our community. It is time that the incalculable costs of child abuse and neglect are similarly deemed unacceptable to our community. Comparable initiatives (to those above) need to be taken to help change community attitudes towards the health-risking behaviours of child abuse generally and towards its own deep responsibility to protect children at risk of abuse. On this note, it is worth speculating what community attitudes might be like today if there had been a concerted advertisement campaign (comparable to the anti-drink driving, anti-smoking and work safety campaigns) along the lines of: 'If you abuse a child, you're a bloody coward' or 'Every act of abuse is doing your child harm' or 'Child protection/safety: think it, talk it, work it — some injuries never heal ...'.

Conclusion

This chapter has attempted to show that the issue of child maltreatment not only raises a number of important ethical issues, but is itself an important ethical issue. It has also attempted to show that health care professionals have a moral obligation to intervene in the prevention of child abuse and neglect and that this obligation rests on considerations of the welfare interests and wellbeing of children. And while it is acknowledged that the act of reporting child abuse and neglect is one which is fraught with difficulties, the risks of not reporting are equally if not more onerous — not just to abused children but to the community as a whole. In the ultimate analysis, and in support of Fogarty and Sargeant (1989) cited above, 'each section of the community [including and perhaps especially health care professionals] can and should make a contribution'.

Children should not have to bear 'silent and unacknowledged witness to their own suffering in many ways throughout their lives' (Valent 1993, p. 4). Everyone has a moral responsibility (irrespective of legal law) to break the culture of silence that surrounds child abuse and which has been so effective in invalidating, marginalising and rendering as invisible its untoward effects. Unless this responsibility is accepted and acted upon at an individual and private level, children will remain at risk of the otherwise avoidable harms caused by child abuse and neglect. To fail in this responsibility is not only to fail the most vulnerable members of our society (children), but to fail ourselves and the community as a whole in which we share membership.

Child abuse does not only affect children, it affects us all. It is, therefore, up to each and every one of us (as co-participating members of a moral community) to do what we can in order to prevent it and the harms that flow insidiously from it. Preventing the harms of child abuse is not merely a charitable cause which people can choose to either support or not support. Rather it is an obligation supported by the deepest of ethical considerations and which is binding on all of us. The ultimate question, then, is not one of *whether we ought to intervene* in the prevention of child abuse, but *how we may better intervene* and achieve the desired moral outcomes of this intervention.

CASE SCENARIO AND CRITICAL QUESTIONS

Case scenario[2]

You are a registered nurse working in a paediatric unit. You have been assigned to care for a 12-year-old girl by the name of Christine who has been admitted for observations and investigation of a recent and severe bout of undifferentiated abdominal pain. Shortly after Christine's admission, while assisting her to have a shower, you notice bruising on her arms and back. After asking her gentle probing questions, Christine confides in you that her mother beats her regularly. She further confides that the bruises on her arms and back are the result of a particularly vicious beating her mother had given her recently using a wooden coat hanger. She also discloses that some weeks earlier she had taken an overdose of aspirin to 'try and maker her mother stop beating her', but that all her mother had done at the time was to laugh at her and tell her 'how stupid she was' and sent her to her room to 'sleep it off'. Christine then begs you not to tell anyone, pleading, 'If my mother finds out that I've told anyone, she will beat me up. It will be much worse for me.'

Concerned for Christine's wellbeing and mindful of your statutory duty to report known or suspected cases of child abuse, you decide to seek advice from Christine's consultant paediatrician. On doing so, the paediatrician tells you: 'Christine is my patient, not yours. You are not to take this matter any further.'

Critical questions
1. What are your moral and legal responsibilities in this case?
2. Are you obliged to uphold Christine's request for confidentiality to be maintained?
3. Are you obliged to honour the paediatrician's directive in this case?
4. What action should you take?

---

1   An earlier version of this chapter was presented under the title *Ethical issues associated with the mandatory and voluntary reporting of child abuse: implications for health professionals in Victoria*, at the Wyeth Health and Nutrition Conference, Hotel Sofitel, Melbourne, 2 August 1997. It has been revised for inclusion in this text.

2   Reprinted with permission from Johnstone, M. and Crock, E. (2001) 'Dealing with ethical issues in nursing practice', in E. Chang and J. Daly (eds), *Transitions in nursing: preparing for professional practice*. MacLennan & Petty, Sydney, p. 141.

BIOETH BIG
BIOE

Chapter 9

Abortion ethics and the nursing profession

LEARNING OBJECTIVES

Upon the completion of this chapter and with further self-directed learning you are expected to be able to:

- Examine critically the definitions of abortion used respectively by pro-abortionists and anti-abortionists.
- Identify two key issues upon which the abortion issue turns.
- Discuss critically the following three positions on abortion:
  - the conservative position
  - the moderate position
  - the liberal position.
- Outline six contemporary developments informing the 'new ethics of abortion' and its possible implications for the abortion debate generally.
- Discuss briefly the common arguments advanced both for and against the view that the fetus is not a person.
- Discuss at least three instances in which the rights of a fetus (once granted) might come into conflict with the rights of others.
- Discuss critically whether the nursing profession should formulate a public position on the abortion issue.

KEYWORDS

- Abortion
- Fetus
- Fetal rights
- Human being
- Maternal rights
- Paternal rights
- Personhood
- Reproductive autonomy
- Reproductive rights

Introduction

It has been estimated that, each year, over 210 million women throughout the world become pregnant and that a significant percentage of these women (22 per cent or 46 million) will have an abortion (World Health Organization 2003). Of the 46 million abortions (representing 35 abortions per 1000 women aged between 15–44) that are performed each year, 20 million are estimated to be unsafe. It has been further estimated that unsafe abortion accounts for at least 13 per cent of global maternal mortality and in some countries (notably developing countries) 'it is the most common cause of maternal mortality and morbidity' (World Health Organization 1998). In response to the issues and challenges raised by this situation, the World Health Organization (2003) has deemed 'preventing unsafe abortion' a strategic priority underpinned by the following two goals:

- In circumstances where abortion is not against the law, to ensure that abortion is safe and accessible.
- In all cases, women should have access to quality services for the management of complications arising from abortion.

Even though the World Health Organization has identified safe abortion as a strategic global priority, abortion as such remains a deeply contentious and divisive issue. Of all the bioethical issues that command public attention today, perhaps none is more controversial than the ethics of abortion. Although abortion has been legal in many countries for several decades now, its moral permissibility continues to be the subject of heated public debate. Significantly, the polarity of values and views underpinning the abortion controversy has threatened to divide nations, has seen abortion clinics firebombed and abortion workers fatally shot by pro-life fanatics, and has even brought down governments (Hadley 1996).

Despite the legislative and moral reforms of the past four decades, women's so-called 'reproductive rights' (including the right to safe abortion) are still constantly being challenged. And despite being 'sensationally and bewilderingly public', abortion for many women remains a deeply private, personal and even taboo subject (Hadley 1996, p. xi). Even in so-called 'liberal' democratic countries where individualism and a person's right to make important life choices (including the right to choose death) is highly respected and even enshrined in law, women are often forced to justify their need of an abortion in a way 'that many find to be degrading and intrusive' (Greenwood 2001, p. ii3). And while there is much rhetoric about women having 'reproductive autonomy', doctors and the courts that legitimate their authority, ultimately have the power to decide if, when, how and under what circumstances a woman's reproductive rights will be exercised (Greenwood 2001; Hadley 1996; see also Gillon 2001; Hewson 2001; Wyatt 2001; Pojman and Beckwith 1994).

In recent years, a 'new ethics of abortion' has emerged (Greenwood 2001; Gillon 2001; Wyatt 2001). This 'new ethic' is rekindling the fires of old controversies surrounding the moral status of the fetus and posing new challenges to modern moral thought about the permissibility and impermissibility of abortion. Processes informing the 'new ethics of abortion' include the following five developments (which Wyatt [2001, pp. ii15–ii18] believes 'have irreversibly altered the ethical debate about abortion in Western societies'):

1. *advances in fetal physiology* (these have made it possible to confirm that fetuses have 'a range of sophisticated abilities with well developed sensory perception in all systems: vision, hearing, touch, taste and smell'; it is now known that even very young fetuses have the capacity to imitate facial expressions, breathe, and initiate hand-face contact, startle, sucking and swallowing movements);

2. *development of fetal medicine as a speciality* (making it possible to discern major abnormalities and to 'provide seamless medical care for the fetus through the intrauterine period and on into the critical first hours and days of birth'; it is now possible to provide such intrauterine treatment as blood transfusions and curative surgery for congenital defects);

3. *development of neonatal intensive care and improved survival of extremely preterm infants* (with developments in specialised neonatal intensive care techniques, it is now commonplace for preterm babies of just 23–24 weeks of gestation to survive; the survival of preterm babies of just 22 weeks weighing less than 500 g at birth has also been described);

4. *changed perspective on the rights of the disabled* (many in the disabled rights movement regard the abortion of fetuses with genetic disorders or other disabling conditions to be discriminatory and as being prejudicial against disabled people);

5. *changes in professional counselling* (research has shown that the way information is given to parents can significantly influence the choices they make; this, in turn, has given rise to a new imperative for so-called 'non-directive counselling').

Another development prompting 'new' debate on the abortion issue is the growth of 'wrongful life' or 'wrongful birth' lawsuits based broadly on the argument that a given infant 'should never have been allowed to be born' (Forrester and Griffiths 2001, p. 205). In such cases, an infant's mother generally seeks compensation on grounds that she was deprived of the opportunity to have an abortion within a relevant time because of a health worker's (e.g. a doctor's or a counsellor's) negligence (e.g. failed abortion; misdiagnosis of fetal abnormality after screening; misdiagnosis of maternal illness which could have resulted in fetal abnormality) (Shapira 1998; Petersen 1997). Just what the outcome of the 'new ethics of abortion' will be, remains an open question. What is clear, however, is that there is 'no Olympian perspective from which these issues can be viewed in benign and omniscient neutrality' (Wyatt 2001, p. ii19).

The abortion issue is not 'new' to the nursing profession. As shown by the examples given in the previous editions of this book, nurses historically have had to face a range of personal, political and professional difficulties (including being discriminated against and losing their jobs) on account of moral disagreements in the workplace concerning the abortion issue. According to recent research, nurses (including those who choose to work in abortion services) also have to face a range of other complexities, tensions and dilemmas inherent in abortion work on account of trying to 'accommodate the requirements of society, the women patients, and their own beliefs' (Huntington 2002, p. 276; see also Ventura 1999). The difficulties experienced by nurses have been compounded by the fact that the 'physical experience, psychological distress and decisions' inherent in abortion work have not been considered from a nursing perspective' (Huntington 2002, p. 276).

Despite the hardships that nurses have had to carry in the past and continue to carry in the present, the nursing profession globally has been relatively silent on the 'abortion question'. Just why this silence has prevailed is a matter for speculation. Nevertheless, one thing is clear: this position cannot be sustained, at least not credibly. Given the World Health Organization's stance on safe abortion as a global health issue, it is becoming increasingly evident that the nursing profession cannot avoid public debate on the matter and must prepare itself to take a stand. This, in turn, demands that attention be given to addressing a number of critical questions including, but not limited to, the following:

1. What is abortion?
2. Is abortion morally right or wrong?
3. If abortion is morally wrong, can members of the nursing profession be decently expected to assist with abortion work and/or care for the women who have had them?
4. If abortion is not morally wrong, can nurses justifiably refuse to assist with abortion work and/or care for the women who have had them?
5. If participating in abortion work, what are the obligations (if any) of nurses toward fathers of a pregnancy who are opposed to their fetus being aborted?
6. In the event of no substantive agreement being reached on whether abortion is morally right or wrong, what, if any, public position should the nursing profession take on the issue?
7. How should the nursing profession decide these things?

It is to addressing these and related questions that this chapter will now turn.

What is abortion?

Before advancing this discussion any further, it is important to first clarify the meaning of the term 'abortion.' Simply put, abortion (from Latin *abortāre*, from *aboriri* to miscarry, from *ab* — wrongly, badly) may be defined as the 'premature termination of a pregnancy by either spontaneous or induced expulsion of a nonviable fetus from a uterus' (*Collins English Dictionary* 1995). Not all participating in the abortion debate subscribe to such a 'simple' definition, however. Instead, most lean toward definitions of abortion that while appearing to be value neutral (objective) are, in essence, ethically loaded and hence at risk of misleading moral debate on the issue. For instance, those who are opposed to abortion typically define abortion in such terms as 'artificially causing the miscarriage of an unborn child', or 'killing an innocent human being' (Fisher and Buckingham 1985). Definitions of abortion using these or similar terms are not just defining the 'act' of abortion, however. They also seem to be conveying the conclusion that *abortion is morally wrong* (at the very least, the terms used — 'unborn child'/'innocent human being' — seem to appeal to our moral intuition that killing another person who is a non-aggressor is a morally terrible action). In contrast, those who support abortion tend to define abortion in such terms as 'terminating pregnancy' or 'ridding the products of unwanted/unviable conception'. Definitions of abortion using these and similar terms seem to imply that abortion is not only *not morally wrong* but may even be *morally neutral* (the terms used 'ridding the products of unwanted conception' seem to invite the 'reasonable' question of: What is so morally terrible about getting rid of something that is 'unwanted' and/or incapable of normal growth and development?).

It is unlikely that a consensus will be reached among contesting parties on a working definition of abortion and that variant ethically loaded definitions will continue to be used. Either way, it is important to remember that the issues at hand need to be decided by careful deliberation, not by definitions; they also need to be examined in a manner that will question rather than reinforce the status quo.

Is abortion morally permissible?

The permissibility of abortion has an interesting history. Anthropological studies suggest that abortion has been widely practised across cultures and throughout human history, and probably dates back even to prehistoric times (Thomas 1986, p. 77). Abortion techniques have been described in early Chinese, Egyptian and Greek texts, and continue to be widely practised in non-industrialised societies and other Third World countries. Muslim traditions permit abortion, so long as it is procured while 'the embryo is unformed in human shape' (Thomas 1986, p. 79). Japan did not introduce anti-abortion laws until the Meiji Restoration (1869–1912).

Contrary to what many Christian fundamentalists believe, opposition to abortion is not justified by appealing to either the Bible (it simply 'does not discuss it' [Badham 1987]), to church traditions or to Christian reasoning. The early religious fathers, including St Augustine, St Jerome and St Thomas Aquinas, did not believe that the embryo was a human being from the moment of conception, and 'all insisted that early abortion could not be classed as homicide' (Badham 1987, p. 11). They also drew a firm distinction between early and late abortions. As far as the personhood of the fetus is concerned, this too 'has virtually no significant support' in the Christian tradition until the teachings of Pope Pius IX (1846–78). And in the Hebrew version of Exodus 21, accidental abortion is seen as an offence (and one punishable by death) 'only if the woman dies' (Thomas 1986, p. 78).

From where then have contemporary views opposing the moral permissibility of abortion arisen? There is much to suggest that it is largely the product of Catholic dogma dating back to the 1854 proclamation of the *Dogma of the Immaculate Conception* and the subsequent series of papal decrees (for example, in 1884, 1889 and 1908), 'which forbade direct termination of a pregnancy even in circumstances where, as in ectopic pregnancies, the result of non-intervention was the certain death of both mother and child' (Badham 1987, p. 12).

Religious dogma aside, the question remains of: Who, if anyone, ought to be permitted to have an abortion? Under what circumstances or conditions might abortion be allowed?

Generally speaking, there are three positions that can be taken on abortion: a conservative position, a moderate position and a liberal position. These three positions (which have changed little since they were first advanced in the early 1970s and 1980s) are considered briefly below.

The conservative position

According to the conservative position (see, for example, Brody 1982; Noonan 1983), abortion is an absolute moral wrong, and thus something which should never be permitted under any circumstances — not even in self-defence, such as cases where a continued pregnancy would almost certainly result in the mother's death. A common concern among conservative anti-abortionists is that, if abortion is permitted, then respect for the sanctity of human life will be diminished, making it easier for human life to be taken in other circumstances. Arguments typically raised against abortion here are almost always based on the sanctity-of-life doctrine. One example of the kind of reasoning which might be employed to argue against abortion is as follows:

> It is wrong to kill innocent human beings; fetuses are innocent human beings; therefore it is wrong to kill fetuses.

> (Warren 1973, p. 53)

Or, to use another example:

> Human beings have a natural right to life; fetuses are human beings; therefore fetuses have a natural right to life and killing them is wrong.

Whether human beings do in fact have a natural right to life, and whether fetuses are in fact human beings, are matters of ongoing philosophical controversy (Pojman and Beckwith 1994).

The moderate position

According to the moderate position (see, for example, Werner 1979; Bolton 1983) abortion is only a prima facie moral wrong, and thus prohibitions against it may be overridden by stronger moral considerations. Werner (1979), for example, argues that abortion is permissible provided that it is procured during pre-sentience (i.e. before the fetus has the capacity to feel). Since a pre-sentient fetus cannot feel, it cannot be meaningfully harmed or benefited. Thus, as with other non-sentient or pre-sentient entities, it makes no sense to say a fetus has rights, much less a right to life. In the case of post-sentience, Werner argues that abortion may still be justified on carefully defined grounds, namely: *self-defence* (for example, where the life or health of the mother would be at risk if the pregnancy was allowed to continue); or *unavoidability* (for example, where abortion cannot be avoided, such as in the case of ectopic pregnancy or accidental injury). Abortions performed on lesser grounds are, according to Werner, unjustified.

Bolton (1983) takes a slightly different line of reasoning. She argues that, since fetuses are not undisputed persons, they do not have the same rights not to be killed as do actual undisputed persons. Thus, in the case of life-threatening pregnancy, at least, a woman's right to life overrides that of the fetus. Bolton also argues, controversially, that if women are not permitted to have abortions, the community might find itself deprived of the beneficial contributions that a woman freed of the burdens of child rearing would otherwise be free to make (1983, p. 335). She concedes, however, that there are also cases 'in which others stand to benefit from the pregnant woman's bearing a child' (Bolton 1983, p. 337), and that this too might contribute to the community's benefit. The bottom line of Bolton's position is that abortion is morally permitted in some situations, and might even be 'morally required' in others, and it is not morally permitted in some other types of situations. Either way, the facts of the matter need to be carefully assessed and analysed before an abortion decision is made.

Another moderate argument raised in defence of abortion is that a woman is under no moral obligation to bring a pregnancy to term, particularly in instances where the pregnancy has been forced upon her (as in the case of rape), or where the pregnancy has not resulted from a voluntary and informed choice (as in cases involving contraceptive failure or ignorance). In her classic and still widely cited article 'A defence of abortion', Judith Jarvis Thomson (1971) contends, for example, that even if it is conceded, for the sake of argument, that a fetus is a person, this still does not place an obligation on a woman to carry it to full term. This is because morality does not generally require individuals to make large sacrifices to keep another alive. Thus, if pregnancy requires a woman to make a large sacrifice — and one which she is not willing to make — it is morally permissible for her to terminate the pregnancy.

It could, of course, be objected that the kinds of sacrifices a woman might ultimately be required to make by giving birth could be avoided by her allowing the unwanted child to be adopted. And, indeed, many view the *adoption option* as a respectable way out of the abortion dilemma — even in cases involving severely disabled fetuses or severely disabled newborns (see, for example, Rothenberg 1987). Thomson, however, rejects the adoption option, arguing that it can be utterly devastating on relinquishing mothers — a claim which finds considerable support in research studies on the subject (see in particular Gillard–Glass and England 2002; Marshall and McDonald 2001; Howe et al. 1992; Else 1991; Lancaster 1983; Harper 1983; Winkler and van Keppel 1983; Shawyer 1979). It can also be utterly devastating on adopted children, who may grow up 'wondering who they are' and spending a lifetime searching for their unknown biological parents (Lifton 1994; Strauss 1994; Health and Community Services 1992). In some countries, babies born out of wedlock (especially 'rape babies') can face a life of shame and rejection (see in particular Doder 1993, p. 8). 'Rape babies' can even be prevented by law from being adopted. After the Bosnia war, for example, it was reported that the government of the day prohibited adoption of the children of rape victims, in the hope that their natural mothers will one day accept them (Williams 1993, p. 8). As these examples show, the adoption option is not as 'simple' as its advocates would have people believe.

The liberal position

The third stance on abortion, the liberal position (see in particular Tooley 1972; Warren 1973; Thomson 1971), holds that abortion is morally permissible on demand. Michael Tooley (1972) argues, for example, that since fetuses are not persons, they cannot meaningfully claim a right to life. He points out that the notion 'person', in this instance, is a purely moral concept, and that the unfortunate tendency by some to use it as if it were synonymous with the notions of 'human being' and 'human life' is grossly misleading. Warren (1973) argues along similar lines. She contends that a fetus is not a *human being* and to claim that it is only begs the question. She points out that it is one thing to use *human* to refer 'exclusively to members of the species *Homo sapiens*', but quite another to use it in the sense of being 'a full-fledged member of the moral community' (p. 53). In other words, it is one thing to be human in the *genetic* sense, but it is quite another to be human in the *moral* sense. These two senses are quite distinct, and care must be taken to distinguish between them. She concludes (p. 53):[1]

> In the absence of any argument showing that whatever is genetically human is also morally human ... nothing more than genetic humanity can be demonstrated by the presence of the genetic human code.

The consequence of this is unavoidable. It has yet to be demonstrated that the genetic humanity of fetuses alone qualifies them to have fully-fledged membership of the moral community.

Judith Jarvis Thomson (1971) also argues that a fetus is not a person. She contends that it is nothing more than a 'newly implanted clump of cells'. In defence of this claim, she argues that a fetus is 'no more a person than an acorn is an oak tree'. The analogy can be extended further to show that, just as stepping on an acorn is significantly different from cutting down an oak tree, so too is aborting a fetus significantly different from killing an actual person.

The conclusion of these and similar views is that, once it is admitted that a fetus is nothing more than a clump of genetically human cells, the abortion issue becomes a non-issue. It would make no more sense to speak of the right of a fetus to life than it would be to speak of some other piece of genetically human tissue's right to life, say, a strand of human hair or a piece of human toenail (both of which are genetically human).

The three positions on abortion discussed so far can be expressed diagrammatically as shown here in Figure 9.1.

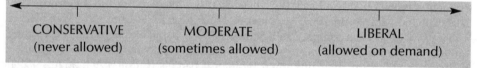

Figure 9.1 Three positions on abortion

Abortion and the moral rights of women, fetuses and fathers

In considering further the above three positions on abortion, it can be seen that the abortion issue rests on two key points: (1) the moral status of the fetus, and (2) the moral rights of pregnant women to control their bodies and their lives (also referred to as 'reproductive autonomy' [Hewson 2001]). To recap, anti-abortionists argue that the human fetus is a human being, and therefore has a right to life at least equal to that of the mother's. Pro-abortionists, however, reject this view, arguing that, while a human fetus is genetically human, this in no way implies that it is morally a *human being* with a full set of rights claims. Neither, they argue, is a fetus a *person*. In defence of this position, pro-abortionists contend that in order for a fetus to be a person it *must* satisfy the moral criteria of *personhood* (which are very different from the criteria of *fetalhood*) — something that a fetus simply does not do. Let us consider this claim further.

In 1973 the reputed North American philosopher, Mary Anne Warren, argued controversially that, for an entity to be a person, it must satisfy a number of criteria, namely (1973, p. 55):

1. consciousness (of objects and events external and/or internal to the being), and in particular the capacity to feel pain;
2. reasoning (the developed capacity to solve new and relatively complex problems);

3. self-motivated activity (activity which is relatively independent of either genetic or direct external control);
4. the capacity to communicate, by whatever means, messages of an indefinite variety of types, that is, not just with an indefinite number of possible contents, but on indefinitely many possible topics;
5. the presence of self-concepts, and self-awareness, either individual or racial, or both.

Warren admitted that there were numerous difficulties involved in formulating and applying precise criteria of personhood. Even so, it could be done. Commenting on the criteria she had formulated, Warren argues that an entity does not need to have all five attributes described, and that it is possible that attributes given in criteria 1 and 2 alone are sufficient for personhood, and might even qualify as necessary criteria for personhood. Given these criteria, all that needs to be claimed to demonstrate that an entity (including a fetus) is not a person is that any entity which fails to satisfy all of the five criteria listed is not a person. She concluded that if opponents of abortion deny the appropriateness of the criteria she has identified, she knows of no other arguments which would convince them. She concludes: 'We would probably have to admit that our conceptual schemes were indeed irreconcilably different, and that our dispute could not be settled objectively' (p. 56).

Michael Tooley (1972), like Warren, also interpreted 'person' in rationalistic terms. He argued that in order for something to be a person it must have a serious moral right to life. And in order to have a serious moral right to life, it must possess 'the concept of self as a continuing subject of experience and other mental states, and believe that it is itself such a continuing entity' (Tooley 1972, p. 44). Since fetuses do not satisfy this basic 'self-consciousness requirement', as Tooley called it, they are not persons — they do not have a serious moral right to life, and therefore to kill them is not wrong.

More recently, in a revised version of her earlier work, Mary Anne Warren (1997) expands on and refines the characteristics which she believes are central to the concept of personhood, namely (p. 84):

1. *sentience* — the capacity to have conscious experiences, usually including the capacity to experience pain and pleasure;
2. *emotionality* — the capacity to feel happy, sad, angry, loving, etc.;
3. *reason* — the capacity to solve new and relatively complex problems;
4. *the capacity to communicate*, by whatever means, messages of an indefinite variety of types; that is, not just with an indefinite number of possible contents, but on indefinitely many possible topics;
5. *self-awareness* — having a concept of oneself, as an individual and/or as a member of a social group; and finally
6. *moral agency* — the capacity to regulate one's own actions through moral principles or ideals.

Although conceding that it is difficult to define these traits precisely, or to specify 'universally valid behavioural indications that these traits are present', Warren (1997, p. 84) nevertheless holds that these criteria of personhood are functional — pointing out that an entity 'need not have all of these attributes to be a person'. She explains (p. 84):

It should not surprise us that many people do not meet all the criteria of personhood. Criteria for the applicability of complex concepts are often like this: none may be logically necessary, but the more criteria that are satisfied, the more confident we are that the concept is applicable. Conversely, the fewer criteria are satisfied, the less plausible it is to hold that the concept applies. And if none of the relevant criteria are met, then we may be confident that it does not [apply].

Warren (1997) suggests that in order to demonstrate that a fetus is not a person, all that is required is to claim that a fetus has *none* of the above six characteristics of personhood.

For some, the personhood argument does little to settle the abortion question. For example, it might be claimed that, even if it is true that a fetus is not a person, it nevertheless has the potential to become one, and therefore it has rights (see also Warren 1977). Thus abortion is still wrong on the grounds of the potentiality of the fetus (Glover 1977, p. 122). Or, to borrow from Warren's analogy cited earlier: even though an acorn is not an oak tree, it nevertheless has the potential to become one; therefore crushing an acorn is tantamount to chopping down an oak tree.

There are a number of obvious difficulties with this view. First, the argument tends to presume that what is potential will in fact become actual. In the case of zygotes, however, this is quite improbable. As Engelhardt points out, only '40–50% of zygotes survive to be persons (i.e. adult, competent human beings)' (1986, p. 111). It might then be better, suggests Engelhardt, to speak of human zygotes as being only '0.4 probable persons'.

Second, the argument strongly suggests that it is not the fetus per se that is valued, but rather *what it will become* (Glover 1977, p. 122). It is difficult to interpret just what kind of moral demand this creates. As Glover points out (p. 122):

> It is hard to see how this potential argument can come to any more than saying that abortion is wrong because a person who would have existed in the future will not exist if an abortion is performed.

If we take the *potentiality argument* to its logical extreme, we are committed to accepting, absurdly, that contraception, the wasteful ejaculation of sperm, menstruation and celibacy are also morally wrong, since these too will result in future persons being prevented from existing (Warren 1977, p. 277).

The main unresolved question, however, is: Can a *potential* person be meaningfully said to have *actual* rights and, if so, can these rights meaningfully override the existing rights of actual persons? Or, to put this another way: Can a fetus (a potential person) have actual rights and, if so, can these meaningfully override the existing rights of its mother (an actual person)? The crux of the dilemma posed here is whether the more immediate and actual rights of the pregnant woman should be recognised before the more remote and potential needs of the fetus, or vice versa.

One answer is that, given our understanding of the nature of moral rights and correlative duties, there is something logically and linguistically odd in ascribing rights to fetuses (non-persons), particularly during the pre-sentient stage. If we were to accept that non-sentient fetuses have moral rights, we would be committed, absurdly, to accepting that all sorts of other non-sentient things have moral rights — including human toenails, strands of hair, or pieces of skin. For argument's sake, however, let us accept that the fetus does have moral rights and, further, that these can meaningfully conflict with the mother's moral rights. The question which arises here is which fetal/maternal rights are likely to conflict?

The most obvious is the fetus' and the mother's common claim to a right to life. This is particularly so in cases where the mother's life would almost certainly be lost if the pregnancy were allowed to continue. In such situations it seems reasonable to claim that the mother's right to life must at least be as strong as the fetus' right to life. And, further, since both stand to die unless the pregnancy is terminated, then surely it is better, morally speaking, that only one life is lost instead of two? It is difficult to see how anyone could reasonably and conscientiously choose an outcome which would see both the mother and the fetus die. Furthermore, as stated elsewhere in this book, morality does not generally require us to make large personal sacrifices on behalf of another, and thus it would be morally incorrect to suggest that the mother has a duty to sacrifice her life in defence of the fetus. In the case of life-threatening pregnancies, then, it seems reasonable to conclude that the pregnant woman's right to life has the weightier claim.

A second set of rights which may conflict is the mother's *right to have control over her body and life's circumstances* versus the fetus' *right to life*. It might be claimed, for example, that a woman's right to choose her lifestyle, career, economic circumstances, standard of health, and similar, override any claims the fetus might have to be 'kept alive'. The mother may then withdraw her 'life support' even if this means the fetus will die in the process (an unfortunate, but nevertheless unavoidable, consequence). Against this, however, it might still be claimed that the inconveniences and other psychological, physical or social ills caused by an unwanted pregnancy are still not enough to justify killing the fetus and violating its right to life (Brody 1982; Noonan 1983). The demand not to kill the fetus becomes even more persuasive when it is considered that there are alternatives available for helping to prevent or alleviate the ills of unwanted pregnancies, such as child welfare and other social security benefits, adoption, counselling, medication, or, as some have suggested controversially, even extracting the fetus and placing it in a surrogate or an artificial uterus (Glover 1977, p. 135). (It should be noted that this latter suggestion is not as far-fetched as it seems. Work has already been carried out overseas on 'maintaining uteri extracted from women outside of a woman's body', and implanting embryos into these wombs [Rowland 1992, pp. 288–9]. Aborted fetuses have been 'kept alive for up to forty-eight hours' in these research projects [Rowland 1992, p. 289].) In cases where alternatives are available, it seems difficult to sustain a claim that the mother's rights ought to be given overriding consideration over those of the fetus.

A third set of rights which might conflict is the mother's *right to health* (and to a quality of life) versus the fetus' *right to life*. In this instance, the mother's health and quality of life are threatened not by her pregnancy but by a progressive debilitating disease, such as Alzheimer's, Parkinson's or diabetes. The mother might, for example, contemplate getting pregnant for the sole purpose of growing tissue which can be harvested and transplanted into her brain or pancreas in an attempt to restore her health. The issue of fetal tissue transplantation has long been the subject of intensive debate (see in particular Engelhardt 1989; Gillam 1989; Griffiths 1988; Mandel 1985). Although governments are striving hard to prevent this type of scenario from occurring, there have already been cases of women getting pregnant and having abortions for the sole purpose of supplying fetal tissue for transplantation — if not for themselves, for others including a fetus' siblings (see for example Morrow 1991; Gibbs 1990).

A fourth set of rights which may cause conflict involves not only the competing claims of a fetus and its mother, but also those of the father (Purdy 1996, pp. 161–7; Teo 1975). During the 1980s there was a number of legal cases (notably in the UK, USA, Canada and Australia) involving fathers undertaking legal action in an attempt to stop their (ex)wives and (ex)girlfriends from having abortions (AFP 1989; Beyer 1989; Lowther 1988; PA 1987; Leo 1983; see also Forrester and Griffiths 2001, p. 203). In 1987, for example, a 23-year-old father was reported to have taken court action in an English court of appeal to try and stop his 21-year-old girlfriend, an Oxford University student, from having an abortion (PA 1987, p. 6). The court was reported to have rejected the father's appeal — significantly, not on the grounds of the woman's right to choose, but on the grounds that the fetus was (PA 1987, p. 8):

> so underdeveloped that, if separated from its mother, it would be unable to breathe either naturally or through a ventilator, was not capable of being 'born alive'.

Upon learning of the court's decision, the 21-year-old Oxford University student is reported to have taken the position that (p. 8):

> It is her decision what she does now, but it is a point of principle that she is now able to control her own body.

The 23-year-old man responsible for her pregnancy is reported to have been 'disappointed and very surprised at the result' (PA 1987, p. 8).

A year later, a similar case occurred in the United States of America. It involved a 24-year-old man who was reported to have 'lost a lower-court appeal for the right to force his estranged [19-year-old] wife to have their baby' (Lowther 1988, p. 8). The court was reported to have ruled against the father, on the grounds that the abortion concerned only the estranged wife (Lowther 1988, p. 8). Rejecting the court's decision, the man decided to 'fight to seek a legal precedent' in favour of fathers — even though his estranged wife had gone ahead and had an abortion after the court's findings. In explaining his decision to take further legal action, the man was reported to have said (Lowther 1988, p. 8):

> I was willing to take full responsibility and raise the baby and take care of it; there's nothing for me to do now but let the wounds heal. Maybe the next guy will have it easier.

Critics of his stance, and advocates of a woman's right to choose, argued, however, that 'it is nothing short of involuntary servitude to order a woman to carry a child she does not want' (Lowther 1988, p. 8). Against this, an Indiana lawyer argued in support of the man's actions that what they were asking the court to do was merely (Lowther 1988, p. 8):

> to find that there should be a balancing of the interests of the father against those of the mother on a case-by-case basis.

In 1989, one year later again, a similar case was reported in Canada. This time it involved a 25-year-old man who took court action to stop his 21-year-old ex-girlfriend from having an abortion (Beyer 1989). The case took a dramatic twist, however, when, with considerable embarrassment, the woman's lawyer announced, before the court case had concluded and all arguments completed, that his client, 'worried that it might be too late for an abortion even if she won the case, had decided not to wait' (Beyer 1989). Commenting on the case, Beyer writes (p. 60):

Defying a lower-court injunction, she had gone ahead with the operation. The court was stunned. But it went on nonetheless to rule unanimously that the injunction barring the abortion was invalid. The court thus seemed to be ending a recent spate of injunctions against abortion sought by angry ex-boyfriends.

Not surprisingly, these cases have been viewed with little sympathy from women who historically have been left alone with the burden and hardships of child-rearing after the fathers of their children have long abandoned them. Some even worry that, if the paternity rights debate is allowed to progress to its logical extreme, it could have paved the way for even rapists to prevent their victims from having abortions, and to press for access rights after the baby has been born. It has also been suggested that recognition of paternal rights may see the courts inviting rapists 'to be present at the birth' (Rogers 1992).

Just what the ultimate outcome of the 'mothers' rights versus fathers' rights' debate will be, remains an open question. To date, the courts in Australia and the UK have not recognised the 'rights' of fathers either to be consulted about a termination of pregnancy or to enforce the rights of an unborn child to be protected against abortion (Forrester and Griffiths 2001, p. 203). In the USA, however, a very different situation exists. As Hadley reports (1996, p. 74):

> the question of spousal consent to abortion has rumbled around for a considerable time, and a number of states have tried to make spousal consent or notification part of their abortion law.

This is an issue which is not going to go away.

Abortion, politics and the broader community

The abortion issue is extraordinarily complex; it is also extremely political, as some spectacular overseas incidents have shown. For example, in 1990, Belgium was thrown into a constitutional crisis after King Baudouin, Belgium's reigning monarch, stepped down from his throne temporarily 'because his conscience would not let him sign a law legalising abortion' (Reuter 1990a, p. 7). As a result, the government had to take over the King's powers and pass the abortion law. It is reported that once the abortion law was passed the King's inability to reign ceased, and he resumed his position on the throne (Reuter 1990a, p. 7).

In the same year, it was reported that disagreement over abortion law threatened to 'derail a treaty on German unity' (Reuter 1990b, p. 7). The disagreement was primarily over whether 'West German women may take advantage of East Germany's liberal abortion laws after unification' (Reuter 1990b, p. 7).

In 1992, Ireland (where abortion is illegal) witnessed political uproar and large public demonstrations after the High Court banned a 14-year-old rape victim from travelling to Britain for an abortion (the girl had been raped repeatedly by a friend's father over a one-year period) (Barrett 1992c, 1992d; Holden 1994). It was reported that many European constitutional lawyers considered the ban a breach of the Treaty of Rome, which had brought the European Community (EC) into being almost four decades earlier, and, among other things, 'permitted the right to free movement within the EC' (Barrett 1992c). The situation reached crisis point when it was evident that the ban threatened the European Community's Maastricht Treaty on European political union, which Irish voters were due to vote on a few months later (*Independent* 1992, p. 6; Barrett 1992a, 1992b, 1992f).

The case is reported to have aroused the concerns of a number of influential groups, including Irish legislators and lawyers and members of human rights and women's groups, and to have raised serious questions about how far the state and its officials should interfere in the fundamental rights of its citizens (*Independent, New York Times* 1992, p. 9). The travelling ban was eventually lifted by the Supreme Court in Dublin, and the girl was able to travel to Britain for an abortion (*Independent* 1992 p. 6). Later in the year, two Dublin counselling clinics appealed successfully to the European Court of Human Rights against the Irish Government's prohibition on women gaining access to information about abortion services overseas (Barrett 1992e, p. 8; Holden 1994). The judges who heard the case are reported to have decided that the Irish Government was 'violating fundamental human rights by preventing women from gaining access to information about having abortions abroad' (Barrett 1992e, p. 8). The counselling clinics were also reported to have been awarded costs and damages of more than $400 000 (Barrett 1992e, p. 8).

Abortion was also a major issue in the American presidential election of 1992, with the then presidential contenders Bill Clinton and Ross Perot both trying 'to lure pro-choice voters to their side' (Barrett, L. I. 1992, p. 54). During the campaign, the Bush camp (whose law reforms saw the loss of civil rights protection for United States abortion clinics [*Baltimore Sun* 1993] and the banning of abortion counselling at federally-funded clinics [Toner 1993]) admitted publicly that anything raising the profile of the abortion issue was 'a problem for us' (Barrett, L. I. 1992, p. 54). Initially, the Clinton camp also wanted to avoid too much attention being paid to the abortion issue. It was reported that basically 'he wanted to avoid the appearance of catering to "special interests", including feminists' (Barrett, L. I. 1992, p. 55).

The abortion debate in the United States took a dramatic and historic turn in 1993, when an anti-abortion protester shot and killed a doctor during a pro-life demonstration outside a lawful abortion clinic (Rohter 1993, p. 7). Abortion rights groups took the shooting of the doctor as a 'symbol of the increasing harassment' of health workers involved in abortion work, which has seen abortion clinics increasingly vandalised and destroyed by arsonists. In one case, a clinic was firebombed and razed (Rohter 1993, p. 7). Since that first shooting in 1993, at least four other abortion workers have been gunned down by anti-abortion fanatics (Hadley 1996, p. xi). Today doctors who perform abortions 'wear bullet-proof vests as they journey to work' (Hadley 1996, p. xi).

Closer to home, Australia has also experienced the politicisation of abortion, with a small number of politicians attempting, unsuccessfully, to introduce legislation aimed at restricting abortion services for women. In 1988, for example, the Reverend Fred Nile, a New South Wales independent MP, attempted unsuccessfully to introduce his *Unborn Child Protection Bill*, which could have seen doctors performing abortions jailed for up to 14 years and fined $100 000 (Ansell 1988, p. 21). The Reverend Nile was reported to have said that the Bill would allow abortion only if the mother's life was in danger, and that 'no exceptions would be made for any threat to the mental health of the mother' (Ansell 1988, p. 21). The medical director of the Family Planning Association of New South Wales is reported at the time to have condemned the Bill on the grounds that it would 'not stop women having abortions — it would just drive them underground' (Ansell 1988, p. 21).

Alistair Webster (a Liberal politician in New South Wales) has also made several attempts over the years to introduce legislation aimed at eliminating Medicare rebates for abortion services. An attempt in 1990 was condemned by the Women's Electoral Lobby, who reminded politicians supporting the move that 'no legislation has ever prevented desperate women from terminating unwanted pregnancies' (Schnookal 1990, p. 2). Further, as one ALP member responded during parliamentary debate on the matter:

> Medicare benefits do not cause abortion. It will not go away if we remove the benefit, just as unemployed people will not disappear if we remove the unemployment benefit ... The best way to reduce abortion numbers is better sex education, family planning and support for pregnant women — from their partners and from the government.
>
> (Dr Ric Charlesworth, cited by Wainer 1990, p. 8)

In 1998, however, the abortion debate reached a new dimension in Australia when Western Australian politicians voted in favour of legislation regarded as creating Australia's 'most liberal abortion laws' (Reardon 1998, p. 7). The legislation (introduced by Labor MLC Cheryl Davenport, and ratified by the upper house of parliament within weeks of passing through the lower house) repealed 'criminal sanctions against women for procuring an abortion' (Le Grand 1998, p. 1; see also Ewing 1998, p. 3; Reardon 1998, p. 7). The legislation was reported as leaving a woman's *informed consent* as the 'minimum requirement for doctors to perform lawful abortion' — literally, *abortion on demand* (Le Grand 1998, p. 11). It was speculated at the time that the abortion law reforms in Western Australia would 'trigger a review of abortion laws' in other Australian states (Ewing 1998, p. 3). Four years later, the Australian Capital Territory (ACT) removed abortion from the Criminal Code.

At a broader international level perhaps one of the most controversial examples of an attack on abortion comes from the Pope. In February 1993, the Pope is reported to have told Bosnian women pregnant as a result of wartime rape that 'they should not seek abortions, but give birth to the children' (*Bioethics News* 1993, p. 3). It is estimated that between 20 000 and 70 000 women had been raped — the majority of violated women being Muslims (Corlett 1993, p. 4). It is reported that the Pope addressed the women in a letter as follows: 'Do not abort. Your children are not responsible for the ignoble violence you have undergone'. He asked the women to 'accept the enemy' into them, and make him the 'flesh of their own flesh' (*Bioethics News* 1993, p. 3).

The Pope's comments subsequently became the subject of much criticism by Muslims and Catholic theologians alike. One outspoken German Catholic theologian (a woman) is reported to have said that the Pope 'had no right to get involved in matters of which he can have no understanding' and that 'no bachelor ... could decide on matters such as these. A decision can be made only by those who have been raped' (*Bioethics News* 1993, p. 3).

There remains much more to be said on the politics of and the moral controversies surrounding abortion than there is space here to do. For example, we have yet to address the problems of:

- restrictive abortion laws and the real suffering these have caused — and continue to cause — girls and women who find themselves trapped by an unwanted and/or intolerable pregnancy (see, for example, the *Bobigny case* [Henderson 1975], the *Roe v Wade* case [McCorvey 1994], the *Irish 'X'* case [Holden 1994], and Messer and May's [1988] *Back rooms: voices from the illegal abortion era*);

- sex-selected abortions, practised widely in countries where a patriarchal and misogynist preference for sons results in the 'sex-selected' abortions of female fetuses (a form of gendercide) in those countries (see, in particular, Mary Anne Warren's [1985] *Gendercide: the implications of sex selections*);
- homophobic-selected abortions — otherwise referred to as 'gay gene abortions' — proposed in the event of a 'sexuality gene' being discovered (it has been seriously suggested by a leading geneticist and Noble laureate that if a gay gene is discovered, and a fetus is found to be 'gay-gene identified', a mother ought to have the option of aborting a fetus if 'she doesn't want a homosexual child' [Loudon and Wilson 1997; Joyce 1997);
- rape-abortions, and the dilemmas associated with terminating pregnancies resulting from rape and sexual abuse (see also Holden 1994);
- eugenic-abortions, and the dilemmas associated with aborting fetuses with disabilities ranging from the very minor to the extremely severe (for instance, there is both formal and anecdotal evidence that fetuses have been aborted for relatively minor 'cosmetic' deformities, for example, having one leg shorter than the other, or having a cleft lip [Hager 2002]);
- the role of 'fetal police' (comprised of registered medical practitioners, 'risk managers', legislators, lawyers and judges) who take steps to coerce, detain and even incarcerate women who engage in health-injurious behaviours (such as cigarette smoking, illicit drug taking, alcohol consumption, and the like) during pregnancy (see, in particular, Ruth Macklin's [1993] discussion on 'The fetal police: enemies of pregnant women' included as Chapter 4 of her text *Enemies of patients*; Gallagher 1995; Hadley 1996; Pojman and Beckwith 1994);
- the nature and implications of the 'hard choices' women have to make when choosing abortion (Cannold 1998; Hadley 1996); and, not least,
- the traumatic consequences to women of having abortions, including the terrible complications that abortion procedures themselves can have such as 'sepsis, haemorrhage, uterine perforation, kidney failure and even coma' (Cannold 1998, p. 16; Fisher and Buckingham 1985).

Other problems yet to be examined include the following:

- determining the point at which a fetus actually becomes a person — for example, is it at conception/syngamy, upon achieving viability, or at birth? (see also Gillon 2001; Kissling 2001; Buckle and Dawson 1988; Warren 1988; Glover 1977, pp. 123–6);
- 'slippery slope' arguments which reason that, if abortion is permitted, our moral characters and expectations will seriously decline; that is, if we allow abortion today, we will allow infanticide tomorrow and the next day we will allow euthanasia of other 'useless' persons.

Consideration of these and similar problems must be left for another time.

Conclusion

As has been shown by the discussion advanced in this chapter, abortion is a highly complex and controversial issue, and one which is unlikely to be resolved to the satisfaction of all the parties involved. This means that nurses will invariably encounter moral disagreements in abortion contexts — many of which may not be able to be reconciled. The discussion here also warns the nursing profession that it cannot afford to be complacent or indecisive about developing a formal (policy) position on abortion practices and procedures, or the questions of social justice these raise. Equally important, the discussion here demonstrates the need for the abortion issue to be opened up for formal and informed discussion within the ranks of the nursing profession. It can never be assumed that nurses have had a trouble-free path to conscience-free participation in abortion work. If we do not know what experiences nurses have had in this area, we will never be in a position to advance a nursing perspective on the moral permissibility of abortion, much less on the extent to which nurses can be reasonably expected — against their moral conscience, and also against their emotional health — to assist with abortion work. In formulating policies on the abortion issue, however, the nursing profession must be careful not to lose sight of its moral commitment to respecting women's personal choices (no matter how disagreeable these might appear to be). Individual nurse clinicians, meanwhile, must take care not to fall into the moralising trap of imposing their personal values on others — in this instance, women who have decided, for whatever moral reason, to abort a pregnancy which, if carried to full term, promises intolerable consequences. The point remains, however, that so long as the nursing profession remains indecisive about reaching a just position on the subject, women contemplating abortion will not be able to rest assured that they will receive safe and quality nursing care before, during and after an abortion procedure. Nurses choosing to work in abortion services, meanwhile, will continue to carry the emotional burdens of their distressing work silently, personally, and without the level of professional support that their peers receive in other ('more acceptable') distressing areas.

CASE SCENARIOS AND CRITICAL QUESTIONS

Case scenario 1

A registered nurse and midwife was allegedly refused employment at a large New South Wales rural hospital because she was conscientiously opposed to participating in abortion and sterilisation work (Broekhuijse 1988). The nurse had apparently been offered a position at the hospital concerned, and had written back accepting the offer. In her letter of acceptance, however, she pointed out that she was conscientiously opposed to abortion and sterilisation procedures, and that if she was asked to participate in such procedures she would exercise her right to refuse. To this, the director of nursing is reported to have replied: 'It would be quite impractical for you to be excluded from any involvement in the care of these patients' (Broekhuijse 1988, p. 13). After several more letters had passed between the nurse and the director of nursing, and after the nurse had declined the offer of an alternative position, the original offer of employment was withdrawn.

Case scenario 2

Nursing and midwifery staff involved in an abortion procedure carried out at a private hospital were astonished to discover that the expelled fetus, which was of 21–22 week gestation, 'cried and moved and had an obvious heartbeat' upon delivery (Schulz 1999, p.2). A nurse subsequently contacted the doctor on call advising him that the abortion procedure had resulted in a 'live birth'. Because the fetus was regarded as being of a 'non-viable age', however, the doctor allegedly advised that nothing further needed to be done. Since the fetus was not expected to live, it was covered in a stainless steel dish without medical attention. It was claimed that the fetus lived for 80 minutes after being aborted (Schulz 1999, p.2). The staff involved were distressed about the situation and reported it to hospital management. The case later became the subject of a coronial inquiry to determine 'why no care was given to a baby who obviously was alive' (Schulz 1999, p.2). The coroner was reported to have clarified that 'the inquest was not concerned with the rights and wrongs of abortion. It was about the child's rights during the 80 minutes it lived' (Schulz 1999, p.2).

Critical questions

1. Is it reasonable for nurses who are opposed to abortion work to seek employment in organisations that provide abortion services?
2. In instances in which abortion procedures result in the delivery of a 'live birth' (an outcome that is not uncommon with late trimester abortions), what actions would you take and why?
3. In what circumstances might a nurse validly claim a 'right' to refuse to assist with abortion procedure and, conversely, a 'duty' to refuse?
4. What, if any position, should the nursing profession take on the abortion issue?

Chapter 10

Euthanasia, assisted suicide and the nursing profession

LEARNING OBJECTIVES

Upon the completion of this chapter and with further self-directed learning you are expected to be able to:

- Define and differentiate between the terms 'euthanasia', 'assisted suicide' and 'mercy killing'.
- Explain why dictionary definitions of euthanasia can be misleading when considering the ethics of euthanasia and assisted suicide.
- Outline five conditions which must be satisfied in order for an act to count as an instance of euthanasia.
- Differentiate between six types of euthanasia commonly discussed in the bioethics literature.
- Discuss critically at least:
  - five arguments commonly raised in support of euthanasia and assisted suicide; and
  - seven arguments commonly raised against euthanasia and assisted suicide.
- Examine critically the *killing/letting die* distinction.
- Discuss critically the issue of terminal sedation associated with the withholding of artificial hydration and nutrition at the end stage of life.
- Construct critical arguments for and against the proposition that the nursing profession should support the legalisation of euthanasia and assisted suicide.

KEYWORDS

- Assisted suicide
- Doctrine of double effect
- Euthanasia
- Involuntary euthanasia
- Killing/letting die distinction
- Mercy killing
- Passive euthanasia
- Non-voluntary euthanasia

- Sanctity of life
- Slippery slope
- Voluntary euthanasia

Introduction

In 1990, in the United States of America, Janet Adkins, a victim of Alzheimer's disease, died after pushing a red button on a suicide machine — or 'mercitron', as it has been called — designed by a retired pathologist, Dr Jack Kevorkian, whom she had approached for assistance to die (Gibbs 1993, 1990). Adkins, who is reported to have 'feared an excruciating future', soon came to be viewed as a 'symbol of all those patients who confront a horrible disease and vow to maintain some dignity in death' (Gibbs 1990, p. 70). Dr Kevorkian, meanwhile, found himself in the forefront of the pro-euthanasia debate and, as *Time Magazine* put it:

> a standard-bearer for all those who fail to see a moral difference between unplugging a respirator and plugging in a poison machine.
>
> (Gibbs 1990, p. 70)

Despite being dubbed 'Dr Death', Dr Kevorkian continued his crusade for the legalisation of euthanasia/assisted suicide, or, as he called it, 'medicide' in the United States of America (Gibbs 1993, p. 52; see also Brovins and Oehmke 1993; Kevorkian 1991). As part of this crusade, in December 1998 Dr Kevorkian was successful in getting authorities in the state of Michigan (USA) to charge him with first-degree murder after he admitted, for the first time, having *directly administered* a fatal injection to one of his patients (Riley 1998a, 1998b, 1998c; see also Magnusson 2002, pp. 28-32). In all other cases (130 in total), Dr Kevorkian admitted only to *presiding over* the suicides of his patient, that is, 'instructed the patients and supervised them while they activated an injection from his so-called "suicide machine" ' (Riley 1998c, p. ii; see also Riley 1999a and 1999b).

Dr Kevorkian's case went to trial in March 1999, representing the fifth time he had been tried over the deaths of his patients. On 26 March, 1999, the jury returned a verdict of second degree murder and he was sentenced to serve 10–25 years in the Michigan State Prison (Magnusson 2002, pp. 28–32). In passing her sentence, the Judge presiding over the case stressed that the trial was not about 'the political or moral correctness of euthanasia', but about lawlessness and murder (AFD, DPA 1999). Referring to a national television broadcast several months earlier in which Dr Kevorkian dared legal authorities to arrest him for his actions, the Judge responded:

> You had the audacity to go on national television, show the world what you did and dare the legal system to stop you. Well, sir, consider yourself stopped.
>
> (Judge Jessica Cooper, reported comments cited by AFP, DPA 1999)

In the Netherlands, during the same period, a very different scenario was at play. In contrast to the United States of America, euthanasia and assisted suicide was, at the time of Janet Adkins' medically-assisted death, legally tolerated (although still a criminal offence) in the Netherlands. By the time Dr Jack Kevorkian had facilitated his first 'assisted suicide' in 1990, Dutch doctors had already participated in thousands of medically-assisted deaths. In 1986, for example, the Royal Dutch Medical Association reported that there were between 5000 and 6000 cases of voluntary euthanasia each year in the Netherlands (British Medical Association 1986). In 1990, the overall incidence of euthanasia was estimated by formal sources to be between

4000 and 6000 deaths annually (de Wachter 1992, p. 24). In 2001 it was reported that approximately 2500 cases of euthanasia were notified to authorities in the previous year, with another 1000 cases going unreported 'because of "grey" areas in the law' (Mann 2001, p. 17). Some contend that the overall incidence of euthanasia is, in reality, unknown and, if informal sources are to be relied upon, could range from between 2000 and 20 000 cases a year (de Wachter 1992; Keown 1992; ten Have and Welie 1992).

Currently, in the Netherlands, under certain clearly defined conditions that have undergone 'subtle elaborations over the past three decades', euthanasia and assisted suicide — although still illegal under Dutch criminal law — are not viewed by the courts as a punishable offence (Magnusson 2002, pp. 64–5; see also Jochemsen 1994; Keown 1992; Browne 1990; Vervoorn 1987). In 1993, legislation was passed clarifying and affirming the strict conditions under which euthanasia and assisted suicide were permitted. The passage of this new law was reported at the time as giving the Netherlands the world's most lenient policy on 'mercy killing' (Hirschler 1993, p. 7). Seven years later, the leniency of the Dutch 'mercy killing' laws was expanded even further when statutory support was given for the first time to the defence of 'necessity' (passed by the Lower House of the Dutch Parliament in November 2000, and the Upper House in April 2001) (Magnusson 2002, p. 65). The defence of 'necessity' permits a doctor to avoid legal liability for assisted deaths on the grounds of professional duty; that is, 'to reduce suffering and respect the autonomy of the patient' and provided that he or she (the euthanasing doctor) can demonstrate that 'due care' was exercised in determining that the patient's request 'was voluntary and well-considered, that the patient's suffering was unbearable, and that there is no prospect of improvement' and no 'reasonable' alternative (Magnusson 2002, p 65). Significantly, under the 'due care' requirements:

> it is not necessary for the patient to be suffering physical pain: unbearable mental anguish is sufficient. Similarly, there is no requirement for the patient to be in a terminal phase of an illness, or indeed to be suffering from any (physical) condition at all. A physical disability, or a condition of 'untreatable misery' … will suffice.
>
> (Magnusson 2002, p. 65)

The above legislative reforms have not only given the Netherlands the world's most lenient policy on euthanasia and assisted suicide, but has also given the world a 'laboratory' for 'testing' and 'observing' these practices— and one which has attracted many onlookers from both ends of the moral spectrum in regard to the moral permissibility of euthanasia. Certainly, the Netherlands is currently the only country in the world which is able to offer retrospective studies of substance concerning the practice of euthanasia and any emerging patterns or trends associated with it. Consider the following.

In 1995, in a nationwide study of euthanatic practices in the Netherlands, and which involved a survey of physicians who had attended over 6000 certified deaths, the following statistics were revealed: of the certified deaths evaluated, approximately 43 per cent occurred in persons over the age of 65 years; of these, around 29 per cent were as a direct result of euthanasia, around 31 per cent as a result of physician–assisted suicide, and around 40 per cent as a result of a decision to forego treatment (van der Maas et al. 1996; van der Wal et al. 1996). In contradiction to an earlier 1990 study, van der Maas et al. (1996, p. 1703) found that euthanasia was more common among female patients than males, that decisions to forego treatment tended to be made more often in the case of older females, and that the decisions to forgo treatment were made 'relatively often by nursing home physicians'. Meanwhile, a 1996 study of homosexual men with AIDS found that in the population under study, patients with AIDS experienced death by euthanasia or physician–assisted suicide at a rate 12 times higher than the frequency among all deaths (Bindels et al. 1996). While researchers continue to find no evidence of an increase in euthanasia since laws proscribing it have been relaxed (see, for example, Bindels et al. 1996, p. 503), it is estimated that 59 per cent of euthanatic deaths still go unreported, with cases of physician–assisted death without the patient's explicit request being the most under-reported of all (van der Wal et al. 1996). Hendin (1998) warns that, despite the legal safeguards, active euthanasia has been and continues to be widely abused in the Netherlands. Two years later, Jochemsen and Keown (1999, p. 16) likewise contended that although there had been improved compliance with procedural requirements in the Netherlands, 'the practice of voluntary euthanasia remains beyond effective control' (see also Keown and Jochemsen 1999). While there is considerable scope for caution in translating the meaning of these figures and associated warnings for cultural contexts outside of the Netherlands, they nevertheless offer some 'cautionary tales' — not least, that even the best of legal safeguards may still be inadequate.

In 1996, Australia became the subject of international attention when it became the first country in the world to fully legalise active voluntary euthanasia. This followed the passage, in May 1995, of the Northern Territory's controversial *Rights of the Terminally Ill Act* 1995, which came into effect on 1 July 1996. Almost one year later, however, the Act was overturned by the Australian Federal Government — although not before five people had sought assistance to die under the Act. Of these people, four were successful in achieving legally assisted deaths; the only person not successful in achieving his wish was eligible for assistance to die under the Act but was 'unable to find a specialist who was prepared to be one of the three doctors required under the Act' to certify eligibility for an assisted death (Senate Legal and Constitutional Legislation Committee 1997, p. 11). To date, despite the success of the Australian Federal Government in overturning the Northern Territory's euthanasia legislation, proponents of euthanasia speculate that it will only be a matter of time before euthanasia and assisted suicide will be legal in not just one, but possibly all jurisdictions in Australia.

In 2002, in what has been described as an unprecedented and 'landmark legal case', a British High Court Judge ruled that a competent 43 year old woman with quadri-plegia and unable to breath unaided, had the 'right to die' and to have the 'machine keeping her alive' switched off (*Herald-Sun* 2002, p. 7). This ruling stands just less than a decade after a House of Lords Select Committee report released in 1994 opposed legalising euthanasia in England (Magnusson 2002, p. 66). A year later in Australia, in what has also been described as a 'landmark decision', a similar ruling was made. In what has become known as the 'tube woman case', a Victorian Supreme Court judge ruled that a 68-year-old woman (known only as BMW) suffering from a rare and fatal brain disease, and who had been kept alive for three years by artificial tube feeding, be allowed to die (Davies 2003, p. 5). The judge is reported to have said that her ruling would now make it possible for the woman's advocate 'to decide, on behalf of BMW, whether it is now time to allow her to die with dignity' (Davies 2003, p. 5). It was noted, however, that once the tube feeds were stopped, it could take between one and four weeks for the woman to die. Margaret Tighe of Right to Life Australia is reported to have criticised the court decision, arguing that it was 'not an act of love to kill somebody by dehydration and starvation' (Davies 2003, p. 5).

Euthanasia and assisted suicide continues to receive widespread attention both locally and globally, and remains the subject of much controversy. Central to the controversy is the fundamental question of whether a doctor should intentionally and actively assist a patient to die, and, if so, by what means. These same questions can (and should), of course, also be asked of nurses — particularly given the fundamental role nurses play in caring for and promoting the dignity of patients who are incurably ill, suffering intolerably and dying (Daverschot and Van Der Wal 2001; Crock 1998; Asch 1996).

In this chapter, attention is given to examining the nature and moral implications of the euthanasia/assisted suicide question for nurses. Attention is also given to clarifying what euthanasia is, how it differs from assisted suicide and 'mercy killing', and the kinds of moral arguments that can be raised both for and against the legitimation of euthanatic practices. It is hoped that by examining these and related issues, members of the nursing profession will move a step closer toward answering the following kinds of questions.

- How significant or important is the euthanasia/assisted suicide issue for the nursing profession?
- Should the nursing profession take a formal position either way on the euthanasia/assisted suicide question (for example, should nursing organisations adopt formal position statements advocating a particular view on the moral permissibility or impermissibility of euthanatic practices, or is this a matter that should be left to individual nurses to decide conscientiously)?
- To what extent, if at all, should the broader nursing profession participate in public debate on the euthanasia/assisted suicide question (for example, should nursing organisations actively lobby for the legalisation of euthanasia/assisted suicide)?
- In the event of euthanasia/assisted suicide being decriminalised, what (if any) should be the role of nurses in regard to assisting with or actually performing euthanasia and/or assisted suicide?
- How best can the nursing profession proceed to answer these and related questions (see also Johnstone 1996a)?

Euthanasia and its significance for nurses

Next to abortion, euthanasia is probably one of the most controversial bioethical issues to have captured the world's attention. And, like the abortion issue, it is unlikely to be resolved to the satisfaction of all concerned.

Euthanasia and the so-called 'right to die' are not new issues for nurses. In Australia, one of the first articles addressing the subject was published as early as 1912 in the *Australasian Nurses Journal*. Reprinted from the *British Medical Journal*, the article contains concerns and viewpoints which remain current — including the agonising question of whether euthanasia should be legalised. Citing an 1873 essay on the subject, the article contends that 'a modified *harikari* should be made lawful in England' (and, one presumes, her colonies, including Australia), and, quoting the essay's author, that: 'on the whole it cannot be doubted that the benefits resulting from a change in the law would be simply enormous' (Lionel Tollemache, cited in the *Australasian Nurses Journal*, 16 September 1912, p. 304).

While euthanasia may not be a new issue for nurses, it has nevertheless become a more complex, intense and significant one. Evidence of this can be found in the increased attention being given to the experiences of nurses in regard to euthanasia in both the professional and lay press over the past 20 years. In 1987, for example, the English nursing periodical *Nursing Times* carried a provocative report on the fate of four Dutch nurses who had been arrested in Amsterdam after it was alleged they had practised euthanasia on three hopelessly ill patients. The report concluded that, if the nurses were found guilty of killing the patients, they could face prison sentences of up to 20 years (*Nursing Times*, 25 March 1987, p. 8).

Almost a decade later, in another (although unrelated) case in 1995 in the Netherlands, a 38-year-old Dutch registered nurse was given a two-month suspended prison sentence for performing active voluntary euthanasia on a patient suffering end-stage AIDS (Staal 1995, p. 7; van de Pasch 1995; van der Arend 1995; see also Daverschot and Van Der Wal 2001). What was particularly significant about this case was that the sentence was passed despite the fact that:

- the patient (who was a friend and colleague of the nurse) had specifically requested that the nurse perform the act of assisted death; and
- the procedure fully complied with legal regulations governing euthanatic practices in the Netherlands (for example, the patient had competently requested assistance to die, he was suffering from an end-stage illness, a second medical opinion had been obtained, and the procedure was fully attended to and supervised by a qualified medical practitioner [who, significantly, escaped sentence] (van de Pasch 1995, p. 108).

As I have discussed elsewhere (Johnstone 1996c, pp. 21–2), this case helped to demonstrate the tenuous position of nurses in relation to euthanatic practices — even in countries where euthanasia and assisted suicide are 'legally tolerated'. In this case, the court's decision seemed to hinge on the view that euthanasia and assisted suicide were *medical procedures* of a nature that could not (and should not) be delegated to nurses. More specifically, the court clarified that the deed of 'ultimate care' (the procedure that is the act of euthanasia itself) could only be performed by a doctor and could not be delegated to anyone else (Daverschot and Van Der Wal 2001; Staal 1995, p. 7).

Nurses in the United Kingdom have also experienced significant problems in relation to the euthanasia issue. For example, in 1991, a UK registered nurse experienced threats of violence and obscene phone calls, was vilified by some sections of the media, and was made a scapegoat in the eyes of the public after reporting to the appropriate authorities that a terminally ill patient had died possibly as a result of being administered 10mmol of potassium chloride by a consultant physician, Dr Nigel Cox (Hart and Snell 1992, p. 19). The incident was discovered after nurses noted the blatant documentation of the drug administration in the patient's case history which 'had been left in the nurses' station for all to see' (Hart and Snell 1992, p. 19). The registered nurse's attempts to contact Dr Cox about the matter were unsuccessful. Not wishing to implicate other staff in the matter and recognising her professional duties as prescribed in the United Kingdom Central Council for Nursing, Midwifery and Health Visiting (UKCC) (1992) *Code of Professional Conduct*, the registered nurse decided that she 'had no choice but to report the incident'. Accordingly she notified the director of nursing services and the unit general manager. One month later, Dr Cox was convicted of attempted murder at Winchester Crown Court, after the Justice hearing the case rejected the argument that 'Cox's intention in injecting lethal quantities of a drug which lacked analgesic properties was to relieve pain, rather than to kill' (Magnusson 2002, p.26). He subsequently received a one-year suspended prison sentence (Hart and Snell 1992, p. 19). He was not deregistered by the General Medical Council (UK), however, and continued to practise medicine. The registered nurse meanwhile carried a disproportionate burden of suffering for her actions.

Besides sometimes finding themselves unwitting witnesses to the illegal euthanatic practices of others, there is anecdotal evidence, some published research and a number of court cases suggesting that a small percentage of nurses (e.g. in the United States of American, Hungary, Australia, England, and the Netherlands) have also taken active steps to bring about the death of a patient themselves (Rozsos 2003; Magnusson 2002; Crock 1998; Kitchener 1998; Asch 1996; Walsh and Pirrie 1996; Staal 1995; Stevens and Hassan 1994; Kuhse and Singer 1992, 1993; Turton 1992). One commentator has even alleged controversially that British nurses are 'often' involved in performing euthanasia on patients:

> British nurses are often involved in euthanasia; but that due to the illegality of euthanasia practices, it is difficult to assess the exact extent of the problem — particularly in a culture which prescribes that nurses should not 'tell on colleagues'.
>
> (Turton 1992, pp. 92–3)

Euthanasia and assisted suicide is, however, a controversial issue for nurses in the United Kingdom (Johnstone 1996c). Significantly, the prestigious Royal College of Nursing (RCN), a leading professional nursing organisation in the United Kingdom, has historically and unequivocally rejected the role of nurses in participating in euthanasia. This position has been made explicit in an issues paper on living wills. In this paper, the RCN takes the following position (RCN 1994):

> The RCN believes that this [euthanasia] is contrary to the public interest and to the medical and nursing ethical principles as well as to natural and civil rights.

It further asserts:

> The RCN is opposed to the introduction of any legislation which would place on doctors or nurses a responsibility to respond to a demand for termination of life from any patient or from their relatives.

In 2003, the RCN's opposition to euthanasia was reaffirmed by its General Secretary, Dr Beverly Malone, who stated in a RCN media release:

> The RCN is against euthanasia and assisted suicide. Euthanasia is illegal and the RCN does not condone it. The RCN believes that the practice of euthanasia is contrary to the public interest, to nursing and medical ethical principles as well as patients' civil rights. The RCN is opposed to the introduction of any legislation which would place the responsibility on nurses and other medical staff to respond to demand for termination of life from any patient suffering from intractable, incurable or terminal illness.

The euthanasia/assisted suicide question has also proved to be a significant professional issue for Australian nurses. For example, in January 1995, recognising the seriousness of the euthanasia issue for members of the nursing profession, the Royal College of Nursing, Australia (RCNA) took the unprecedented step of releasing for comment a discussion paper entitled Euthanasia: an issue for nurses (Hamilton 1995). As I have discussed elsewhere (Johnstone 1996b), the RCNA received over 70 responses to this discussion paper from concerned and interested nursing organisations, groups and individuals from around Australia. The responses received represented nurses working in a variety of clinical areas and fields of nursing (including education) and reflected a great diversity of knowledge, opinion, values and beliefs about euthanasia and assisted suicide. In some cases, the responses also demonstrated an overwhelming need for information and guidance on how best to respond to the uncertainty, controversy, complexity and perplexity that has become so characteristic of the right to die movement generally. Perhaps most confronting of all, however, was the emerging difficult question of whether the nursing profession should formally and publicly support the legalisation of active voluntary euthanasia. Related to this was the equally confronting question of whether representative nursing organisations should adopt a formal position statement either supporting or rejecting the role of nurses in active voluntary euthanasia and assisted suicide. Not surprisingly, while the responses demonstrated the need to raise and address these troubling questions, they fell far short of offering a definitive answer to them. Recognising the complexity and perplexity of the issue, the RCNA subsequently commissioned, as part of its professional development series, a monograph entitled: *The politics of euthanasia: a nursing response* (Johnstone 1996a). The purpose of this monograph was not to provide nurses with definitive answers to the difficult questions posed by the euthanasia debate. Rather, it was to advance a discussion that would enable nurses 'to formulate their own thinking and viewpoints on the subject and to be able to contribute to broader professional discussion on the whole issue of the right to die' (Johnstone 1996b, p. 22). In July 1996, the RCNA also issued its first position statement on voluntary euthanasia and assisted suicide — subsequently revised and reaffirmed in 1999 (Royal College of Nursing, Australia 1996, 1999). This position statement primarily focuses on clarifying the illegal status of euthanasia/ assisted suicide in Australia, acknowledging that there exists a diversity of moral viewpoints on the euthanasia issue, reminding nurses of their professional responsibility to be reliably informed about the ethical, legal, cultural and clinical implications of euthanasia and assisted suicide, and recognising and supporting the appropriateness of nurses taking a 'conscientious' position on the matter.

The RCNA's initiatives (just outlined above) were to prove extremely timely, coinciding as they did with the enactment of the Northern Territory of Australia's controversial *Rights of the Terminally Ill Act* 1995 which came into effect on 1 July 1996. As already stated in the opening paragraphs of this chapter, the passage of this legislation earned Australia the controversial distinction of being the first country in the world to legalise active voluntary euthanasia. Of significance to nurses (and to this discussion) is that the legislation anticipated and provided for nurse participation in active voluntary euthanasia and assisted suicide (either by way of preparing, or being delegated the task of actually administering, a substance to terminate life [see section 16(1)]; see also Trollope 1995 p. 21). What, arguably, was troubling about the legislation's provisions in regard to nurse participation was that they had been enacted even before the broader nursing profession itself had:

- clarified its position on the euthanasia/assisted suicide question (at the time, the issue had not been widely discussed in the Australian nursing literature, and policy statements on the subject were either non-existent, inadequate or only at draft stage); and
- taken the necessary steps to ensure that its membership had been fully informed about and adequately prepared to deal with the complex range of political, social, cultural, moral, legal and clinical issues raised by public policy innovation and legal ratification of active voluntary euthanasia and assisted suicide (Johnstone 1996b).

Significantly, in May 1996, less than two months before the *Rights of the Terminally Ill Act* 1995 (NT) came into effect, the Nurses' Board of the Northern Territory took the unprecedented step of formulating and ratifying a formal position statement on euthanasia (see *Nurses' Board of the Northern Territory Position Statement on the Nurse's Role in Euthanasia*, included in full as Appendix 5 in Johnstone 1996a). This position statement was keyed to the *Rights of the Terminally Ill Act 1995* (NT) and sought to clarify the role and function of nurses in relation to the Act's provisions. Specifically, the position statement supported:

- the role of nurses assisting in the voluntary euthanasia of competent patients; and
- the rights of nurses to conscientiously refuse to participate in the euthanasia of patients (Johnstone 1996c, p. 36).

The position statement also outlined the obligations of nurses in regard to the ethical and legal aspects of euthanasia, employment policies, professional competence and education (Johnstone 1996c, pp. 36–7).

As stated earlier, the decriminalisation of euthanasia and assisted suicide in the Northern Territory of Australia was short lived. Almost one year after its enactment, intense political pressure resulted in the *Rights of the Terminally Ill Act* 1995 (NT) being overturned by the Australian Federal Government. Currently, euthanasia and assisted suicide is illegal in Australia, and anyone who wilfully assists a person to die would be viewed by the courts as having committed the criminal offence of homicide (Wallace 1991, p. 265, ss. 14–65; Magnusson 2002). As Dix et al. warn (1996, p. 339, s. 1223):

> It should be made very clear from the outset that the law does not allow mercy killing. Where a person takes steps to end, or hasten the end of another person's life with the intention or the knowledge that this is likely to be the consequence of his or her actions, such a person may be liable for murder or, should death not eventuate, attempted murder. The sentence for murder is imprisonment for life, although in some jurisdictions (NSW, Vic, ACT) there is a discretion in the trial judge to order a sentence of less duration ...

Despite the current legal prohibition against euthanasia and assisted suicide in Australia, Magnusson (2002, p. 272) asserts that it is a 'virtual certainty' that many medical practitioners are 'heavily involved in assisted death'. Magnusson (2002, pp. 24, 32) points out, however, that 'doctors are rarely punished for their involvement in assisted death' — even when making 'front page news' with admissions of having performed euthanasia. This is the situation not only in Australia, but also in Britain and the United States. For example, in the United States, between 1950 and 1991, only eleven doctors were prosecuted for euthanasia (Cox 1993, p. 234). Thus, while euthanasia as such is illegal, it nevertheless seems to be tolerated where it can be shown that the intention was 'therapeutic' (i.e. to alleviate suffering) rather than homicidal (i.e. to kill).

In Australia, proponents of euthanasia/assisted suicide speculate that it will only be a matter of time before euthanasia and assisted suicide will be legal in all jurisdictions in Australia. Given this prediction, there is ample room to speculate that it will only be a matter of time before Australian nurses will once again have to grapple with the complex and perplexing questions raised by the legalisation of euthanasia/assisted suicide, and, in particular, the possible and actual implications of this for nurses at a personal, professional, and political level (Johnstone 1996a).

Public opinion on the euthanasia/assisted suicide issue

In reaching a position on the euthanasia/assisted suicide issue, it might be tempting to appeal to and/or be persuaded by public opinion on the matter. Consider the following.

Over the past two decades, public opinion in Australia, Europe and the United States suggests majority support (around 75 per cent) for the legalisation of euthanasia and physician-assisted suicide (VES 2003; Somerville 1996; Kuhse 1991; *Australian Dr Weekly*, 10 August 1990, p. 9; Kuhse and Singer 1988; Humphries 1983; Radic 1982). In Australia, for example, opinion polls conducted by Morgan and Newspoll respectively during 1995 and 1996 showed 75–78 per cent public support for physician-assisted suicide. A Newspoll conducted in July 1996 also found that 39 per cent strongly favoured and 24 per cent (making a sub-total of 63 per cent in favour) partly favoured changes to the law allowing doctors to perform active euthanasia via the administration of a lethal injection (Senate Legal and Constitutional Legislation Committee 1997, pp. 81–3). In 2002, a UK public opinion poll indicated that 81 per cent of those surveyed supported the legalisation of euthanasia for people suffering unbearably from a terminal illness (VES 2003). Similar support has also been indicated by public opinion polls conducted in France (88 per cent), Belgium (72 per cent), Germany (75 per cent), Italy (75 per cent), the Netherlands (85 per cent), Spain (70 per cent), and the United States (75 per cent) (VES 2003). Just what is to be made of this public opinion, however, is open to question. As discussed earlier in Chapter 2 of this book, public opinion is not a reliable guide to moral conduct; all that it tells us is that a certain group of people *hold a particular opinion*, not that the opinion held is 'morally right' all things considered. In short, it tells us nothing about the moral acceptability or the moral authority of the opinion held. We must therefore look elsewhere (that is, beyond public opinion) to guide our deliberations on whether euthanasia and assisted suicide are morally right or wrong. It is to looking 'elsewhere' that the remainder of this chapter will now turn. This exploration will begin firstly by clarifying what euthanasia is, and how, if at all, it differs from other end of life practices such as assisted suicide and 'mercy killing'. This, in turn, will be followed by a critical examination of views popularly raised for and against the legitimation of euthanasia and assisted suicide.

Definitions of euthanasia, assisted suicide and 'mercy killing'

Euthanasia

The term euthanasia comes via New Latin from Greek *eu* (meaning 'easy', 'happy' or 'good') and *thanatos* (meaning 'death'); it is translated literally as 'good death' or 'happy death'. Contrary to popular opinion, the Greeks did not use the term euthanasia (or equivalents) to imply either 'a means or method of causing or hastening death' (Carrick 1985, p. 127). Rather, it was used in a broader and somewhat metaphorical sense 'to describe the *spiritual state* of the dying person at the impending approach of death' (Carrick 1985, p. 127). Historical evidence also suggests that euthanasia, as we understand it today, was in fact prohibited in ancient medical circles (Carrick 1985, p. 81). Plato, for one, even went so far as to suggest that physicians who attempt to poison another 'must be punished by death', whereas the lay person who attempted such a thing should only be fined — indicating that physicians were regarded as having the greater burden of responsibility to refrain from causing death (Carrick 1985, p. 83). Carrick comments that 'if someone's life was terminated without his (sic) consent, normally this was prima facie a case of homicide' (p. 128).

Contemporary English definitions of euthanasia vary. *The Oxford English Dictionary*, for example, defines it as 'the action of inducing a quiet and easy death', and the *Collins English Dictionary* as 'the act of killing someone painlessly, especially to relieve suffering from an incurable illness'. *Webster's Dictionary*, similarly, defines euthanasia as 'an act or practice of painlessly putting to death people suffering from incurable conditions or disease'.

Whether euthanasia *is* any of these things, however, is a matter of some controversy. For example, we can imagine a case of 'inducing a quiet and easy death' which is a case not of euthanasia but of cold-blooded murder. I could, for example, slip a calming and sleep-inducing sedative into my fit grandmother's nightcap, and the moment she starts blissfully sleeping in her armchair administer to her a lethal dose of intravenous morphine. My sole intention might be nothing more than to secure her premature death so that I may receive the large inheritance I know she has left me in her will. There is something about this example which, to borrow from Beauchamp and Davidson (1979, p. 295) 'omits all the subtle aspects of our notion of euthanasia'. Likewise, we can imagine cases involving patients with incurable diseases or conditions who would nevertheless not be candidates for euthanasia. Diabetes, for example, is an incurable disease, and colour blindness an incurable condition. Yet, we would not, I think, regard either of these incurable states as grounds for euthanasia.

The notion of 'painlessly' inducing death is also unhelpful. We can, for example, imagine a *painless means* of causing death (for example, injecting a lethal substance through the side arm of an intravenous line, or removing someone from a life-support system or withholding food and fluids) but where the *death itself* is nevertheless painful and/or distressing (for example, where a patient is acutely aware of the sensations of suffocation after being taken off a respirator or after being given a large dose of narcotics, or is aware of both hunger and thirst sensations when food and fluids have been withheld). Just because the *means* of death was 'pain-free', it does not always follow that the *death itself* was a 'good death'.

All three dictionary definitions are also inadequate in that they say nothing about the kinds of reasons which should be considered for killing another person, leaving it wide open for motivations of self-interest to be admitted (Beauchamp and Davidson 1979, p. 295). The questions remain: How should euthanasia be defined? How can we be sure that a given act is an act of euthanasia rather than some other kind of act, such as murder or unassisted suicide?

In a classic article on defining euthanasia, Beauchamp and Davidson (1979) argue that for an act to be an instance of euthanasia, it must satisfy at least five conditions.

1. *Intentionality*. Death must be intended and not be merely accidental, and further must be intended by at least one other human being.
2. *Suffering and evidence of suffering*. Here suffering may be in the form of conscious pain, mental anguish, and/or serious self-burdensomeness (as may occur in cases of high quadriplegia, or

tetraplegia, or the like). This interpretation of suffering fully upholds the view that ending a person's pain is not always tantamount to ending that person's suffering (see also Cassell 1982, 1991; Kuhse 1982; Hill 1992; Starck and McGovern 1992). In assessing a person's level of suffering, every effort must be made to gain 'sufficient current evidence' (Beauchamp and Davidson 1979, p. 301); in this instance, it is simply not enough to rely on mere guesswork or on supposition based on ignorance.

3. *Reasons for death and the means of death.* Beauchamp and Davidson contend that death-causing acts must be motivated by beneficence or other humanitarian considerations (such as the demand to end suffering). Killing acts which are not motivated by these things are not acts of euthanasia, but murder. Further to this, any means of death chosen must also be of a nature that does not cause more suffering than is already being experienced (Beauchamp and Davidson 1979, p. 302).

4. *Painlessness.* This condition is related to the previous one and demands, quite simply, that any death act performed must be as painless and as merciful as possible. Beauchamp and Davidson (1979, p. 303) explain that if the means of bringing about death causes more suffering than if that particular means was not used, then the individual will be effectively deprived of a 'good death'.

5. *Non-fetal humanity.* Beauchamp and Davidson (1979, p. 303) contend that if this simple qualification is not included then we would not be able to distinguish acts of abortion from acts of euthanasia.

Beauchamp and Davidson maintain that the five conditions they have formulated supply a 'non-prescriptive definition' of euthanasia, and thus one which avoids dictating a particular moral conclusion. Whether they have succeeded, however, is another matter. The definition still seems ethically loaded, and therefore carries prescriptive meanings. Nevertheless, the five conditions given supply an important step towards the formulation of an operational definition of euthanasia, and one which can be meaningfully applied in the euthanasia debate.

Having defined euthanasia, there now remains the task of distinguishing between the different types of euthanasia that can be practised. The bioethics literature typically distinguishes between six different types of euthanasia: (1) voluntary active euthanasia, (2) voluntary passive euthanasia, (3) involuntary active euthanasia, (4) involuntary passive euthanasia, (5) non-voluntary active euthanasia, and (6) non-voluntary passive euthanasia. In the case of *voluntary euthanasia*, a fully competent patient makes an informed and voluntary choice to have a medically assisted death, asks for assistance to die, and gives an informed consent for the actual procedure of euthanasia to be performed. In short, the patient explicitly requests a doctor or a nurse to administer a lethal injection to hasten his/her (the patient's) death. This is also sometimes referred to as 'consensual euthanasia'. The Dutch case cited earlier, involving a registered nurse who was prosecuted for performing euthanasia on a patient, is an example of this. *Involuntary euthanasia* (or non-consensual euthanasia), in contrast, involves the exact opposite, namely, killing a patient without the patient's informed consent and/or contrary to that patient's expressed wishes (where these are known or could be known) (Lewins 1996, p. 114). The involuntary killing of patients as part of the Nazi medicalised killing programs during the second world war is an example of this. *Non-voluntary euthanasia* (also a form of non-consensual euthanasia) stands in contrast again and involves the act of killing a patient whose wishes cannot be known either because of immaturity, incompetency or both. As McGuire (1987) explains, whereas the term 'involuntary' implies an action which is carried out against the wishes of the patient, 'non-voluntary' simply implies that there is no voluntariness — in the sense that the patient is not capable of either denying or giving consent (as in the case of the permanently comatose or brain-injured patient). In the case of the permanently comatose, McGuire contends, euthanasia would be 'neither voluntary nor involuntary, but is simply non-voluntary' (p. 12). The killing of severely disabled newborns (albeit with parental consent) would be an example of this.

Active euthanasia, meanwhile, typically involves a deliberate act (or commission) which results in the patient's death. The deliberate act of administering a lethal injection or a lethal dose of pills is an example of active euthanasia. This type of euthanasia is sometimes referred to as positive euthanasia. *Passive euthanasia*, on the other hand, involves a deliberate omission or the withholding of certain life-supporting cares and treatments. Withholding antibiotics, nutrition and fluids, mechanical life supports, or other life-supporting measures from terminally or chronically ill patients are examples of *passive euthanasia*. This type of euthanasia is sometimes referred to as negative euthanasia (Glaser 1975).

The six types of euthanasia just outlined can be expressed diagrammatically, as shown in Figure 10.1.

	Passive	Active
VOLUNTARY [Consensual]	Voluntary passive euthanasia	Voluntary active euthanasia
INVOLUNTARY [Non-consensual]	Involuntary passive euthanasia	Involuntary active euthanasia
NON-VOLUNTARY [Non-consensual]	Non-voluntary passive euthanasia	Non-voluntary active euthanasia

Figure 10.1 Six categories of euthanasia

Assisted suicide

The term 'euthanasia' (and, more specifically, voluntary active euthanasia) is sometimes used interchangeably with the term 'assisted suicide'. As I have explained elsewhere (Johnstone 1996c), this interchanging usage is not, however, strictly correct. While it is acknowledged that there may be no morally significant difference between voluntary active euthanasia and assisted suicide (see Brock 1993, p. 204; Parker 1994, pp. 34–42), there is nevertheless a qualitative (experiential) difference between them. With assisted suicide, a qualified medical practitioner supplies the patient/client with the means (for example, a prescription for a lethal dose of drugs) of taking his or her own life but, unlike in the case of voluntary active euthanasia, it is the *patient/client* (not the doctor) 'who acts last' (Brock 1993, p. 204; Campbell 1992, p. 276). To put this another way, in the case of active euthanasia it is the *qualified medical practitioner who kills the patient/client*; whereas in the case of assisted suicide, *the patient/client kills him or herself.* Interestingly, while there may indeed be no morally significant difference between voluntary active euthanasia and assisted suicide (in both instances the ultimate choice rests with the patient/client, both involve assistance from a qualified medical practitioner [or his or her proxy, for example, a nurse] and both result in the foreseeable and intended death of the patient/client suffering from an irreversible medical condition), the law, public policy and public opinion have all distinguished between them (Brock 1993; Glick 1992). A notable US example here can be found in the 1994 *Oregon Death with Dignity Act* (known as 'Measure 16') which legalised physician–assisted suicide (in the form of prescribing a lethal dose of medication), but not active voluntary euthanasia (Magnusson 2002, p. 64; Kuhse 1995). It has also been argued controversially that physician–assisted suicide is more defensible and hence preferable to active euthanasia since with the former 'the willingness [by the patient] to commit suicide gives compelling evidence of the patient's desire to die' (Dixon 1998, p. 29).

'Mercy killing'

A third terminology which has found usage in discussions on euthanasia is that of 'mercy killing'. Although this term is also sometimes used interchangeably with the term 'euthanasia' it can nevertheless be distinguished from euthanasia on a contextual basis. Specifically, as Glick explains (1992, pp. 81–2):

> Mercy killing is not the same as voluntary active euthanasia since many killings are committed without patient request or consent — typically an elderly husband shoots his terminally ill and unconscious or Alzheimer's disease-stricken wife. But the cases almost always exhibit wrenching long-term personal suffering and sacrifice and financial ruin ... They evoke sympathy for both killer and victim and perpetuate interest in the legalisation [sic] of voluntary active euthanasia, which some believe might eliminate the compelling need that desperate people feel for killing their hopelessly ill spouses.

A classic example of a 'mercy killing' scenario can be found in the highly publicised Australian case of Raymond Riordan, a 71-year-old man, who admitted trying to kill his 71-year-old wife who was suffering from advanced Alzheimer's disease (Haslem 1998, p. 3). Although pleading guilty and convicted of attempted murder (which could have carried a jail sentence of up to 25 years), Riordon was freed after being placed on a three year good behaviour bond. Justice Cummins of the Victorian Supreme Court is reported to have said that while Riordan had acted illegally, he had 'sought to relieve (his) wife of her terrible suffering and indignity' (Haslem 1998, p. 3). Describing Riordan as a 'person of compassion and selflessness, totally devoted to his wife', Justice Cummins stated that Mrs Riordan's 'deteriorating health had had a "catastrophic" effect on her husband, who sought treatment for depression' (Haslem 1998, p. 3). Mr Riordon's son, meanwhile, is reported to have told the court that he had 'never seen two people more devoted to each other than his parents'. He is reported to have described how (Haslem 1998, p. 3):

> Every morning they would rise at six o'clock and have brekkie [breakfast] and go for walks ...They would probably cover 30km [sic] and there probably was not more than 100m they weren't hand-in-hand.

Outside the court, Mr Riordan's son was further reported as stating (Haslem 1998, p. 3):

> It's dad's wish that not one other person ... has to go through what he's been through. He would like to see the law-makers of this country ... do something about laws covering euthanasia.

Views for and against euthanasia/assisted suicide

Like other controversial bioethical issues, euthanasia and assisted suicide have proponents and opponents. Attitudes towards them range from liberal and moderate acceptance to absolutist conservative prohibition. It is to examining some of the various viewpoints for and against euthanasia and assisted suicide that this discussion will now turn.

Views in support of euthanasia

Those who support euthanasia typically take the view that it is morally wrong to allow people to suffer unnecessarily. As one author writes:

> the most horrible thing in the world for us, living and sentient beings, is inexorable suffering pain, without any possible compensation when it has reached this degree of intensity; and one must be barbarous, or stupid, or both at once, not to use the sure and easy means now at our disposal to bring it to an end.
>
> (Reiser 1975, p. 28)

Popular views advanced in support of euthanasia (and, in particular, in support of legalising it) fall roughly under four main augmentative categories:

1. arguments from individual autonomy and the right to choose;
2. arguments from the loss of dignity and the right to the maintenance of dignity;
3. arguments from the reduction of suffering;
4. arguments from justice and the demand to be treated fairly.

(adapted from Beauchamp and Perlin 1978, p. 217)

A fifth and controversial category of argument raised in support of euthanasia is that, in some instances, patients have a 'duty to die' (Hardwig 1997; Beloff 1992, pp. 52–6) and furthermore that it might even be a violation of a person's 'freedom of conscience' not to respect this duty (Lewis 2001, pp. 60–2).

ARGUMENTS FROM INDIVIDUAL AUTONOMY AND THE RIGHT TO CHOOSE

We generally accept that people have a right to choose. And, as we have already seen in Chapter 3, the moral principle of autonomy demands that we respect other people's choices, even if we consider them to be mistaken or foolish. The only grounds upon which a person's autonomous choices can be justly interfered with is if they stand to impinge seriously on the significant moral interests of others. Proponents of voluntary euthanasia argue that the right to choose includes the right to choose death (abbreviated as 'the right to die'). Given the right to die, this means that others (including the state) should not interfere with a person's decision to die, and in some instances may even entail a positive duty to assist a person to die — as in cases where a person desires death but is physically unable to end his or her own life. Voluntary euthanasia is thought to be justified here on grounds of autonomy and the demand to respect a person's autonomous wishes.

An important example of this can be found in the comments of Baume (1996, p. 17) who writes that voluntary euthanasia is justified because 'it is a self-regarding victimless action from an individual decision in a matter which affects individuals alone'.

ARGUMENTS FROM THE LOSS OF DIGNITY AND THE RIGHT TO THE MAINTENANCE OF DIGNITY

Related to the demand to respect a person's autonomous choices is the further demand to respect and maintain a person's dignity. Advances in medical technology have increased medicine's capacity to prolong a person's life. Its methods, however, are not always humane, and can seriously erode a person's self-concept, character, sense of self-worth and self-esteem, and the like. As Beauchamp and Perlin (1978) point out, some patients 'are not only subjected to intense and abiding pain, they are often aware of their own deterioration, as well as of the burden they have become to others' (p. 217). They conclude that under these conditions 'it seems uncivilised and uncompassionate' not to allow patients to choose their own death. Euthanasia in some pain states as well as in some chronic disease states may well be the most dignified option.

ARGUMENTS FROM REDUCTION OF SUFFERING

Suffering is generally regarded as morally unacceptable and, as discussed in Chapter 3 of this work, morality demands that, where possible, people (including the very young as well as others across the life span) should be spared or prevented from suffering unnecessarily. In cases where patients' suffering is intense, protracted, unendurable and intractable, it seems cruel to deny them the choice of death as a means of release from their suffering. Euthanasia in these kinds of cases is said to be justified on grounds of 'prevention of cruelty' or 'mercy' (Beauchamp and Perlin 1978, p. 217). It is also thought to be justified on the grounds that people have the indisputable right to judge their suffering as unbearable, and the concomitant right to request euthanasia to end their unbearable suffering (see, for example, Admiraal 1991, p. 11). This, in turn, is grounded in the fact that, despite the achievements of modern medicine, doctors still cannot relieve all suffering (Magnusson 2002; Pool 2000; Admiraal 1991; Cassell 1991).

ARGUMENTS FROM JUSTICE AND THE DEMAND TO BE TREATED FAIRLY

It is argued that everybody is entitled to be treated fairly and to share equally the benefits and burdens of life. To deny patients the option of being spared intolerable and intractable suffering is to treat them unfairly, and to make them carry a burden which others do not have to carry. Furthermore, to deny patients the right to die (that is, in a manner and time of their choosing) is to impose unfairly on them the values of others. Only patients, or those intimately involved with them (for example, family and friends), can judge what is in their own best interests. For others to deny patients the right to choose death is therefore to violate unfairly these patients' autonomy, dignity and entitlement to be spared the harms that will flow from suffering intolerable and intractable pain. Where euthanasia is the only thing that can end patients' intolerable and intractable pain and/or suffering, it stands as a morally just alternative.

ARGUMENTS FROM ALTRUISM AND THE 'DUTY TO DIE'

It is argued that in certain circumstances (such as in the case of old age, chronic illness, or when medical treatment is futile) it may be a person's duty to volunteer for euthanasia (Hardwig 1997; Kilner 1990; Beloff 1992; Schwartz 1993) and that it might also be a violation of a person's right to freedom of conscience to interfere with the exercise of this duty (Lewis 2001, pp. 60–2). Beloff (1992, p. 53), for example, apparently finds it quite plausible that:

the mere thought of becoming a burden to others, not to mention a drain upon society, would suffice to make [some] choose voluntary euthanasia as the only honourable course of action still open to them.

In situations where a person's primary caregivers are burdened to the point where they cannot live their lives fully and are themselves beginning to suffer as a result of their burden of care, euthanasia, argues Beloff, is not only permissible, but required. Beloff (1992, p. 54) explains that this is because:

If there *is* a duty to die it is one that arises from our basic human predicament, the fact that we are dependent on others, and it is a duty we owe to those we cherish.

Hardwig (1997, p. 57) holds a similar position, contending that sometimes ending one's own life is 'simply the only loving thing to do'. He writes (pp. 56–7):

I may well one day have a duty to die, a duty most likely to arise out of my connections with my family and loved ones. Sometimes preserving my life can only devastate the lives of those who care for me. I do not believe I am idiosyncratic, morbid or morally perverse in believing this. I am trying to take steps to prepare myself mentally and spiritually to make sure that I will be able to take my life if I should one day have such a duty... Tragically, sometimes the best thing you can do for your loved ones is to remove yourself from their lives. And the only way you can do that may be to remove yourself from existence.

In regard to the assumed *right to freedom of conscience*, it might be argued that 'the decision whether or not to commit [assisted] suicide is essentially a matter of conscience' – the terms of which can be formulated on either religious or secular terms – which must be respected (Lewis 2001, p. 61).

Counter-arguments to views supporting euthanasia

Not surprisingly, those who are against euthanasia are not moved by these kinds of arguments. The anti-euthanasia response typically entails three main approaches: (1) to assert a number of counter-claims and counter-arguments against the views put forward in support of euthanasia; (2) to assert a number of distinctive arguments against euthanasia; and (3) to reject altogether the notion of passive euthanasia (killing by omission) on the grounds that there is a morally significant difference between directly killing a person and merely letting a person die 'naturally' (referred to in the bioethics literature as the 'killing/letting die distinction').

AUTONOMY AND THE RIGHT TO CHOOSE DEATH

While the moral principle of autonomy is well established in Western moral thinking, it nevertheless has limits. Whether 'autonomy' was ever meant to stretch so far as to impose a moral duty on a doctor or a nurse to comply with a patient's request for euthanasia — to intentionally and actively assist that patient to die — is an open question. If complying with a patient's request for euthanasia has the foreseeable consequence of harming or affecting prejudicially the significant moral interests of others (for example, the doctor[s] or nurse[s] receiving the request, or the patient's family and friends), there is considerable scope for arguing that the doctor(s) and nurse(s) in question have no duty to perform euthanasia, no matter how autonomous the patient's request for it. Further, given the complex nature of the morality of euthanasia, it is rather simplistic to hold that euthanasia can be justified on the grounds of patient autonomy *alone* without consideration being given to other important moral considerations which might also have a significant bearing on a patient's choosing active or passive euthanasia, and on a doctor's, a nurse's, a family member's or a friend's providing it.

Appeals to autonomy to justify euthanasia and assisted suicide are, however, problematic on another account. Paradoxically, acts of euthanasia/assisted suicide carried out in response to a patient's autonomous request, destroy the very basis of their justification. According to Safranek (1998), while autonomy is necessary for the existence of a moral act, it is not *sufficient* to justify an act. As he explains (p. 34):

> The justification of the act will hinge on the end to which autonomy is employed: if for a noble end, then it is upheld; if depraved, then it is proscribed. It is not autonomy per se that vindicates an autonomy claim but the good that autonomy is instrumental in achieving. Therefore an individual cannot invoke autonomy to justify an ethical or legal claim to acts such as assisted suicide; rather he [or she] must vindicate the underlying value that the autonomous act endeavours to attain.

Since autonomous requests for euthanasia and assisted suicide are socially threatening (they threaten human survival), it is appropriate that the autonomy of individuals requesting such threatening acts (euthanasia/assisted suicide) be circumscribed — at least until such time it is clarified and agreed just what kinds of 'goods' autonomy should be invoked to achieve (Safranek 1998, p. 34).

(It is important to note here that autonomy discourse is extremely powerful, making challenges to it difficult. So successful has been the promotion of autonomy, and the assumed sovereign rights of individuals to exercise self-determining choices, that the imperatives of these things — especially in the case of euthanasia/assisted suicide — have come to seem 'so self-evident to all "right thinking people" that to question them seems almost perverse' (Moody 1992, p. 50). Those who do question them risk being publicly ridiculed and dismissed by opponents as ill-informed and 'illogical', or worse as being 'insulting' to vulnerable and oppressed groups [see, for example, the reported comments in the Senate Legal and Constitutional Legislation Committee 1997 at pp. 71, 176].)

DIGNITY AND THE RIGHT TO DIE WITH DIGNITY

Dignity and dying with dignity does not necessarily entail choosing death over the artificial prolongation of life. The demand to respect and maintain a person's dignity might equally entail respect for a person's autonomous wish that 'everything possible be done' to prolong or sustain her or his life — and to sustain a sense of hope that is fundamental to living that life meaningfully, even though (and when) dying. Here, it is important to understand that the ethical controversies surrounding the care of dying patients are not just about management at a technological, medical or institutional level. As Campbell (1992, p. 255) points out, they should also be seen 'as a sign of a deeper crisis of meaning in our culture', and as an indication of how impoverished our society has become in 'assessing the significance of suffering, dying and death as part of a whole human life'. Given this, as Campbell goes on to explain (p. 255):

> The emergence of the individual asserting inviolable rights to self-determination becomes intelligible in this void as a way to create meaning through a freely-chosen style of life and an authentic manner of death.

One way to respond to this crisis of meaning is to 'provide compassionate presence to the sufferer', not to 'end the suffering by killing the sufferer' (Campbell 1992, pp. 269, 276). Another is to deny altogether the philosophical bases for a 'right to die' (see, for example, Kass 1993).

SUFFERING AND THE DEMAND TO END IT

Suffering is not just a medical problem; it is also an existential problem involving profound questions concerning the meaning and purpose of human life and destiny (Neimeyer 2001; Spelman 1997; Attig 1996; Campbell 1992; Starck and McGovern 1992; Amato 1990; Klemke 1981). To 'end suffering by killing the sufferer' is, to borrow from Campbell (1992, p. 276), to misunderstand 'both suffering and ourselves in a way that threatens [infinitely] our moral integrity'.

JUSTICE AND THE DEMAND TO BE TREATED FAIRLY

To deny patients the right to *choose treatment* — including the artificial prolongation of 'hopeless life' — is as unjust as to deny patients the right to choose death. Denying patients' requests for 'everything possible to be done', where this conforms with their notions of dignity, meaning, value and quality of life, is to impose unfairly on them the values of others. As in the case for euthanasia, only patients (or those close to them) can judge what is in their best interests, and they must be permitted to make these judgments.

ALTRUISM AND THE 'DUTY TO DIE'

In some circumstances, people may have a conscientious 'duty to live' in order to spare the pain of their grieving loved ones, who desire their ill loved one to live 'as long as possible'. Being dependent on others is not necessarily being a burden on them (see, for example, Kanitsaki 1994, 1993). Even if dependency does become burdensome — either for the dependent person or her or his carers — it is not clear how, if at all, this gives rise to a so-called 'duty to die'. At best, it may only substantiate 'our basic human predicament' that:

> the very experience of illness, and more fundamentally the process of aging that inevitably culminates in death, not only reveals our shared vulnerability and dependency, but also that we are all subject to some kind of ultimate powers beyond our control. Through our knowledge and technology we may aspire to a mastery of nature and the immortality of the gods, but we continually receive reminders of our dependency and finitude. From this it follows that any control we assert over our dying is already limited, and that dependency and dignity are not mutually exclusive.
>
> (Campbell 1992, p. 270)

At worst, to embrace a 'duty to die' may be to embrace an all-pervasive sense of pessimism and hopelessness which would blind people to understanding that 'the lives of even the terminally ill are precious and matter, right up to the last second of breath' (Mirin, reported by Gibbs 1993, p. 53). And it may risk blinding people to the fundamental insight which has been articulated so well by the late French philosopher and feminist, Simone de Beauvoir (1987, p. 92), that, while all people must die, death is still an accident, and that, even if people know this, and consent to it, death remains 'an unjustifiable violation' (de Beauvoir 1987, p. 92). By this view, therefore, to embrace a duty to die emerges as an embracement of the unjustifiable violation of human life and all that it stands for. It also risks the perversion of morality — and of its ultimate aim, notably, how best to live the 'good life'. Finally, if currency is given to the notion of people having a 'duty to die', this might have the undesirable effect of adding 'to the distress and guilt [conscience] of those who wondered whether they were too great a burden on others' (Muirden 1993, p. 14).

Specific arguments against euthanasia

Specific arguments commonly raised against euthanasia (and the need to legalise it) include:

1. arguments from the sanctity-of-life doctrine;
2. arguments from clinical uncertainty, misdiagnosis and possible recovery;
3. arguments from the risk of abuse;
4. arguments from non-necessity;
5. arguments from discrimination;
6. arguments from irrational or mistaken or imprudent choice;
7. the 'slippery slope' argument.

ARGUMENTS FROM THE SANCTITY-OF-LIFE DOCTRINE

A popular argument raised against euthanasia draws heavily on the sanctity-of-life doctrine and contends that, since life is sacred and inviolable, *nothing* (not even intolerable and intractable suffering) can justify taking it. Sanctity-of-life arguments against euthanasia run something like this:

1. human life is sacred, and taking it is wrong;
2. euthanasia is an instance of taking human life; therefore
3. euthanasia is wrong.

Whether human life is sacred, and whether taking it is always wrong is, however, a matter of philosophical controversy (Singer 1993; Kuhse 1987).

ARGUMENTS FROM CLINICAL UNCERTAINTY, MISDIAGNOSIS AND POSSIBLE RECOVERY

An argument often used against euthanasia is that which speaks to the risk of clinical uncertainty (ambiguity), misdiagnosis and the possibility of recovery. Doctors diagnosing life-threatening medical conditions are not infallible and can (and do) make mistakes (Craig 1994; Wilkes 1994). Furthermore, patients can sometimes recover spontaneously and unexpectedly from devastating and/or terminal illnesses — for reasons not always understood or accepted by medical scientists (for an insightful exploration of people's capacity to heal and to recover unexpectedly from life-threatening conditions, see Gawler 2001; Dossey 1993, 1991; Chopra 1989). A poignant example of this can be found in the case of the noted best selling author of the *Women's Room*, Marilyn French. In 1992, French was diagnosed belatedly with metastasised oesophageal cancer. Her treating doctor at the time was extremely pessimistic about her prognosis, advising French that she had 'terminal cancer, that there was no hope for cure or remission, and that [she] was not to think of that' (French 1998, p. 34). Of this moment, French writes (p. 34):

> What was he saying? Hope, but not too much? Hope, but don't expect a cure? What was I to hope for, then? He emphasized that mental attitude was crucial to anything they did. I spoke up, assuring him that I had strong powers of concentration and that I wanted to hope ... But he wasn't listening; he was talking over me. There was no hope for a cure, he said ...

French, however, rejected the pessimism of her physician and simply 'decided' to survive. Accordingly she 'twisted' what medical information she had on oesophageal cancer to her purpose. For example, she seized on an article that stated 'one in five people treated with extreme measures survive non-metastasised esophageal cancer for five years' and decided those figures applied to her (despite her metastases). In French's words, 'I decided I had one chance out of five. I simply made it up' (French 1998, p. 35). By the end of that day, she had obliterated the word 'terminal' from her memory; and within a couple of days, she had increased her odds of survival to be one in four and had 'repressed any sense that [she] was deluding herself' (French 1998, pp. 35–6). After going through what French describes as a 'season in hell' involving years of pain, dread and severe illness, she reached 'a plateau of serenity' (French 1998, p. 237). At the time of writing an autobiographical account of her experience of survival (published in 1998), French stated that, although suffering from a number of symptoms related to the damage caused to her bodily systems by the intense radiotherapy and chemotherapy treatment she received, she was feeling 'relatively well' and secure in the knowledge that the aches and pains she felt were not an indication of cancer (which had been cured).

There is also the possibility that new cures might be found for certain life-threatening conditions. For example, scientists have shown that the 'human spinal cord may have the capacity to reconnect and regenerate, and that treatment for spinal injuries may be tested on humans within a couple of years' (Ewing 1994, p. 1). If a cure for serious spinal injuries were found, quadriplegics, for example, might not request assistance to die as they are now doing.

Finally, an important example of how a misdiagnosis can misinform the choice of euthanasia as a 'treatment option' can be found in the much publicised Australian case of Nancy Crick. Mrs Crick, a 69-year-old grandmother, died in a blaze of media publicity after having 'one last smoke, a sip of Baileys Irish Cream liqueur and a drug overdose' (Davies 2002; Griffith 2002, p. 4; Hudson 2002, p. 1). Her death (witnessed by 21 relatives who were at her bedside) followed a campaign by pro-euthanasia supporters 'to allow Mrs Crick, who had suffered bowel cancer, the right to die at a time of her own choosing' (Franklin et al. 2002, p. 1; see also Hudson 2002). The case took an unexpected turn when a forensic pathology report following autopsy revealed no evidence of bowel cancer (Franklin et al. 2002). Dr Nitschke, a euthanasia campaigner who supported Mrs Crick in her quest for assistance to die, was reported as 'not being surprised' by the report stating 'The only definite way cancer could have been established was through surgery and she flatly refused to have it' (Franklin et al. 2002, p. 2). He later admitted being present when Mrs Crick's doctors had informed her two months before her assisted suicide that she probably did not have cancer (Jackson 2002). Nitschke is reported to have further admitted that 'Now I think we should have perhaps stressed it [the uncertain diagnosis] more … *it was a mistake in emphasis*' [emphasis added] (Jackson 2002, p. 2). Mrs Crick's son, meanwhile, was reported to have said that he would be 'massively shocked if the tests showed there was no cancer' (Franklin et al. 2002, p. 2). Other commentators were quick to point out that whether Mrs Crick had cancer was irrelevant, since there were no arguments as to why she should not have had the assistance she wanted, that is 'to end her life with others present' (Syme 2002; Komersaroff 2002).

What is of concern about the euthanasia option (and what the above cases highlight) is that once euthanasia is performed it cannot be reversed. Once done, it is done. The risk of error is unacceptable, and overrides any other considerations which might favour euthanasia in a particular case.

ARGUMENTS FROM THE RISK OF ABUSE

The possibility of euthanasia being abused is an argument frequently raised against euthanasia. For example, Dr Nell Muirden, of the Peter MacCallum Cancer Institute in Melbourne, has emphasised the danger of euthanasia being abused by unscrupulous relatives (Muirden 1993; Athersmith 1986). Others, however, are more concerned about legislation giving one group (notably doctors) the power to terminate life. Such power could be particularly problematic in contexts heavily influenced by coercive (negative) social and political processes. In the United States, for example, Margaret Pabst Battin, one of the foremost experts on end of life issues, warns (1991, p. 399):

> This [the United States] is a country where 1) sustained contact with a personal physician is decreasing, 2) the risk of malpractice action is increasing, 3) much medical care is not insured, 4) many medical decisions are financial as well, 5) racism is on the rise, and 6) the public is naïve about direct contact with Nazism or similar totalitarian movements. Thus, the United States is in many respects an untrustworthy candidate for practicing active euthanasia.

For the anti-euthanasiasts, the risk of abuse is unacceptable and underscores the need to reject the moral permissibility (as well as the legalisation) of euthanasia.

ARGUMENTS FROM NON-NECESSITY

Some contend that it is simply 'not necessary' to legislate or to support euthanasia. The reason commonly offered (particularly by those working in palliative care) is that the medical, nursing and allied health professions have been successful over the years in allowing patients to 'die with dignity' (Mendelson 1997; Ashby and Stoffell 1991). Since patients are 'dying well' or are having 'good deaths' anyway, why take the matter any further?

ARGUMENTS FROM DISCRIMINATION

It is sometimes suggested that euthanasia entails blatant discrimination, notably by treating some lives as less worthy than others. Margaret Tighe, president of the Victorian Right to Life, for example, repeatedly argues that euthanasia is detrimental to terminally ill, sick and incompetent people. She has long maintained that euthanasia 'reinforces the concept that there are some lives not worthy to be lived' (Harari 1987; Maslen 1986). Others worry that were euthanasia and its counterpart assisted suicide to be legitimated, 'people with disabilities will be subtly coerced to accept death prematurely' (Mayo and Gunderson 2002, p. 14).

By this view, just as any other act of discrimination is morally offensive, so too is euthanasia.

ARGUMENTS FROM IRRATIONAL, MISTAKEN OR IMPRUDENT CHOICE

It is sometimes argued that any person requesting euthanasia is not really exercising a rational or prudent choice, and that, for this reason, among others, an individual's request for euthanasia should not be taken seriously. One of the staunchest supporters of this view is the Vatican. In its 1980 *Declaration on euthanasia*, it states (1980, p. 7):

> The pleas of gravely ill people who sometimes ask for death are not to be understood as implying a true desire for euthanasia; in fact it is almost always a case of an anguished plea for help and love.

There is also the risk that a person's lawful representative might 'get it wrong'. Just as someone who is in unbearable and untreatable misery might make irrational or imprudent choices, so too might their advocates — who, even though well intended, might nevertheless be misguided in their beliefs and actions. For example, Professor Peter Singer, one of the world's most controversial philosophers and foremost advocates of euthanasia, has long argued that it is morally justifiable and even morally desirable (on utilitarian grounds) to kill severely disabled newborns and other 'non-persons' (e.g. children, adults and older people who, because of being brain injured or suffering from a severe organic brain disease, such as end stage Alzheimer's, are incapable of making rational and autonomous life choices) (Singer 1993; Kuhse and Singer 1985). In 1999, however, it was reported that Professor Singer's beliefs about euthanasia and the grounds upon which euthanasia might be justified and/or morally required in certain cases, were seriously challenged by a personal tragedy, notably, that of his mother becoming a 'non-person' (by his own definition) on account of developing advanced Alzheimer's disease (Churcher 1999). When asked whether his personal situation would cause him to abandon his beliefs, he is reported to have replied (p. 19):

> I think this has made me see how the issues of someone with these kinds of problems are really very difficult. Perhaps it is more difficult than I thought before, because it is different when it's your mother.

The question of whether a death request is necessarily the product of irrational or imprudent or mistaken choice, however, is likely to remain a matter of controversy.

'SLIPPERY SLOPE' ARGUMENT

Also popular in the anti-euthanasia debate, as it is in the anti–abortion debate, is the 'slippery slope' contention. It will be recalled that the slippery slope argument holds that we risk a decline in our moral standards once we permit the taking of human life. For example, if we permit abortion today, we will permit infanticide the next day, and euthanasia the next. In the case of euthanasia, a slippery slope argument might run as follows: once we allow euthanasia for consenting persons, we will permit euthanasia for unconsenting and non-consenting persons, such as infants, the intellectually impaired and the severely brain-injured. Once we compromise the standards for protecting human life, we compromise all other standards pertaining to human life and wellbeing. Euthanasia, then, should never be justified.

An instructive example of the risk of 'slippery slope' action in the context of euthanasia being practised can be found in the 1991 Dutch case involving a psychiatrist who medically assisted the suicide of a female patient who was suffering emotionally but who was otherwise physically healthy; that is, she had no somatic illness (Klotzko 1995; Ogilvie and Potts 1994). Although deemed by her psychiatrist not to be suffering from a psychiatric illness, the patient was nevertheless regarded as being clinically depressed. The social history of this woman is as follows and worth quoting at length:

> She was a 50-year-old social worker. She was also a painter in her spare time. She was divorced. She had been physically abused by her former husband for many years. She had two sons. One son, Peter, died by suicide in 1986, at the age of 20. She then underwent psychiatric treatment for a marriage crisis following his suicide. At the time, she strongly wished to commit suicide, but decided that her second son, Robbie, age 15, needed her as a mother.

> Her son, Robbie, died of cancer in 1991, at the age of 20. Before his death, she decided that she did not want to continue living after he died. She attempted suicide, but did not

succeed. On July 13, 1991, she wrote to a social worker at the academic hospital where her second son died of cancer; she asked for a contact and for pills, so that she could kill herself. She had bought a cemetery plot for her sons, her former husband, and herself; her only wish was to die and lie between the two graves of her sons.

(Klotzko 1995, pp. 240–1)

Subsequently, the patient wrote to Dr Boudewijn Chabot, a psychiatrist, requesting assistance to die. On 28 September 1991, Dr Boudewijn Chabot, after assessing the patient, provided her with a lethal dose of medication and remained with her while she swallowed the medication and died (Klotzko 1995, p. 239). He subsequently reported the death to the relevant authorities following which he was prosecuted by the Supreme Court of the Netherlands. On June 21, 1994, in what has been described as a 'historic ruling', the Supreme Court of the Netherlands found Dr Chabot guilty, but declined to punish him. Significantly, in reaching its verdict, the court rejected the contention that 'help in assistance with suicide to a patient where there is no physical suffering and who is not dying can never be justified' (Ogilvie and Potts 1994, p. 492). To the contrary. As Ogilvie and Potts report (p. 492), the court:

> explicitly accepted that euthanasia and assisted suicide might be justified for a patient with severe psychic suffering due to a depressive illness and in the absence of a physical disorder or terminal condition.

Significantly, the court found that Chabot's guilt lay not in his providing a medically-assisted death to his patient, but in his failure to obtain a second psychiatric opinion on the woman, and his failure to secure independent expert evidence that an 'emergency situation existed' — regarded as providing 'the normal mitigating defence in such cases' (Ogilvie and Potts 1994, p. 492).

Responses to the Chabot case have been mixed. Some have cited the case to underpin their sympathy for the view that (Ogilvie and Potts 1994, p. 493):

> in severe and persistent depressive illness, when all appropriate physical treatments, including polypharmacy, electroconvulsive therapy, and psychosurgery, have apparently been exhausted, voluntary euthanasia may sometimes seem to be as justifiable an option as it does in intractable physical illness.

Others, however, take the Chabot case as underscoring the fears of those advancing the slippery slope argument. As Ogilvie and Potts (1994, p. 493) point out, the Chabot case of 'psychiatric euthanasia' has demonstrated that the 'slippery slope' exists. They conclude:

> However well any legislation is hedged about with guidelines and protections against abuse, the slippery slope predicts an inevitable extension of those practices to other, more vulnerable, groups, such as those who are demented, mentally ill, chronically disabled, frail, dependent, and elderly — and perhaps even simply unhappy.

A further example of the slippery slope leading to an 'inevitable extension' of euthanatic practices can be found in the Dutch legislative reforms, referred to in the opening paragraphs of this chapter. The new legislation 'now permits persons aged between sixteen years or older to make an advance directive requesting euthanasia if they later become incompetent' (Magnusson 2002, p. 65). Children aged 16 to 17 years are also authorised to request assistance to die, provided their parents are 'involved in the decision process' [emphasis added]; in the case of children 12 to 15 years, however, parental approval is required before a request for euthanasia can be honoured (Magnusson 2002, p. 66).

The arguments for and against euthanasia considered here are not the only arguments raised in bioethics literature, but they are nevertheless common, and nurses need to become familiar with them. It should be pointed out that none of these arguments is uncontroversial, and that much more remains to be said about them than there is space here to do. Nevertheless, the discussion so far provides a starting point from which nurses can begin to address questions relating to the moral permissibility of euthanasia and assisted suicide.

The killing/letting die distinction

Another response to the euthanasia debate is to argue that there is a morally significant difference between 'killing' and merely 'letting die'. Opponents of euthanasia claim that so-called *passive euthanasia* is merely 'letting die'; it is not euthanasia at all, and is therefore morally permissible. Let us explore this view further.

It is sometimes suggested that where medical treatment is relatively 'expensive, unusual, difficult, painful or dangerous' (sometimes referred to as 'extraordinary' treatment), no moral obligation exists to use it in order to prolong a person's life (Beauchamp 1997; Gert et al 1997; Singer 1993; Vatican 1980, pp. 10–11; Glover 1977, pp. 195–6). Furthermore, where a given life-prolonging treatment is unduly 'burdensome' to the patient, or even costly, it may, in conscience, be withdrawn (Vatican 1980, pp. 10–11). Even though the withdrawal of life-restoring or life-prolonging therapy may causally result in a patient's death, this need not be regarded as an intentional termination of a life, and therefore an act of passive euthanasia, but rather as merely 'letting nature take its course'. To put this another way, it is merely 'letting die', not direct and intentional killing. Withholding or withdrawing burdensome life-saving or life-prolonging treatment is therefore not, strictly speaking, euthanasia.

Bonnie Steinbock (1983) has argued classically that withdrawing or withholding burdensome life-prolonging treatment should not be viewed as the intentional termination of life, but as 'the avoidance of painful and pointless treatment' (p. 293) — a position also upheld in law (Forrester and Griffiths 2001). Where decisions are made to withdraw treatments, these are really decisions about 'the most appropriate treatment for a given patient', not about killing that patient. She further contends that if a case of ceasing treatment is to hold as a case of euthanasia, it must first be shown that a particular treatment has been withdrawn with the *intention of causing death*. Where this cannot be shown, a claim of killing simply does not hold.

There are cases in which a doctor is simply 'not at liberty', argues Steinbock (1983), to continue treatment — such as where a competent patient has explicitly refused a recommended life-saving therapy. In such cases it seems odd to hold the doctor culpable for failing to provide treatment or for causing the patient's death. Similarly, in cases involving hopelessly ill patients, where 'nothing more can be done', it seems implausible to hold that the discontinuation of a given treatment directly *caused* a patient's ultimate death (Steinbock 1983, p. 294). Here it is *disease* which has provided the causal link to a patient's death, not some act or omission on the part of a doctor or a nurse (see also Forrester and Griffiths 2001).

The ultimate conclusion of Steinbock's argument is that the discontinuation of life-prolonging treatment cannot be considered the intentional killing of another — that is, an act of euthanasia. At best, it is merely 'allowing nature to take its course' or allowing the 'natural flow of events to continue'.

The case for 'letting die' fails to consider, however, that deliberately *not acting* in life-threatening situations is itself a kind of act (see also Weinryb 1980). In this respect, a conscious decision to withdraw or withhold life-saving therapy still amounts to a 'deliberate inducement of death' (Trammell 1978). As Fletcher points out (1973, p. 675):

> It is naive and superficial to suppose that because we don't 'do anything positively' to hasten a patient's death we have thereby avoided complicity in his [sic] death. Not doing anything is doing something; it is a decision to act every bit as much as deciding for any other deed.

By this view, it can be seen that withdrawing or withholding life-saving treatment still involves deliberate choice, just as positively administering treatment does, and as such still has 'a place among events' (Green 1980, p. 204). In this respect discontinuing or withholding burdensome life-saving treatment may hold as at least one way of intentional killing.

The view that withholding or withdrawing life-saving treatment is tantamount to intentional killing becomes even more compelling when considering the very nature of medical/health care contexts, which generally have the facilities to restore and/or prolong life. As Gruzalski (1981) points out, failing to treat in a medical setting is one way of killing *precisely because* in such settings there are the means to prolong life; where these means are not used, then a *failure to treat* can be differentiated from *disease* as a causal factor in a patient's death. A good example of this is the highly publicised United States case of Clarence Herbert (cited in Veatch and Fry 1987, p. 175). Mr Herbert, a 55-year-old security guard, suffered a respiratory arrest following an uneventful closure of an ileostomy. He was subsequently intubated and transferred to intensive care for treatment. There was, however, some controversy about whether Mr Herbert should be maintained on a ventilator. Nevertheless, the decision was made to discontinue his respiratory support. Although unconscious, Mr Herbert continued to breathe spontaneously and his vital signs stabilised. Despite this stabilisation, a second decision was made to withdraw all intravenous and nasogastric fluids, and to transfer Mr Herbert from the intensive care unit to a room in the hospital's surgical unit. Six days after his respiratory arrest, Mr Herbert died. An autopsy listed 'anoxia and dehydration as two of the causes of death' (Veatch and Fry 1987, p. 175). Here then is one case in which a failure to treat (namely the withdrawal of respiratory support and hydration) contributed causally to a patient's death; in this case a *failure to treat* was clearly distinguishable from mere *disease*.

The killing/letting die distinction is vulnerable to criticism on other grounds as well. Tooley (1980), for example, argues that there is no morally significant difference between *intentionally* killing and *intentionally* letting die, and that it is therefore just as wrong to 'intentionally refrain from interfering with a causal process as it is to initiate it' (p. 58). One of the consequences of this view is that, if there is no significant distinction between intentionally killing and intentionally letting die, it is probably the case that there is also no real distinction between active and passive euthanasia, since, like killing and letting die, these share the same intention — that of bringing about or hastening a patient's death. This, suggests Tooley, forces us to conclude that either euthanasia is somehow justified and therefore not morally wrong, or that we are morally confused or insincere in our thinking about it being wrong.

Arguing along similar lines, James Rachels (1975) contends that not only is there no distinction between killing and letting die, but that letting die 'has no defence' (p. 496), particularly where the period of letting die entails a period of prolonged and intolerable suffering (see also Beauchamp 1997; Singer 1993). Cases involving the withdrawal or withholding of nutrition and hydration from severely disabled newborns and severe stroke patients who are not at the end stage of life are examples of this. Rachels further argues (p. 495) that where letting die is allowed for so-called 'humane reasons', it amounts to much the same thing as killing; that is, the *cessation of treatment* amounts to *intentionally terminating another's life*. Consider, for example, the practice of withholding nourishing fluids from severely disabled newborns. As a result of this practice, the severely disabled newborn almost always dies (mostly as a result of dehydration and starvation). The decision to withhold fluids from a severely disabled infant is usually considered a 'humane' course of action, since if the infant were to live it could only look forward to a 'burdensome' life. In these kinds of cases, withholding fluids from a severely disabled newborn amounts to exactly the same thing as administering lethal injections to it, since both acts have the same intention (and outcome) — that is, of hastening the newborn's death and thereby preventing it from living or having to live a 'burdensome' life.

If we accept these views, against the proponents of the killing/letting die distinction, we are also committed to accepting that there is no morally significant difference between withholding nourishment and fluids and administering a lethal injection. This is particularly so in cases where both have as their intention the hastening of a patient's death, the ending of a patient's suffering, and where both ultimately stand as a causal link to the patient's death when it actually occurs. If we accept this, we are further committed to accepting that in the ultimate analysis there is no intrinsic difference between active and passive euthanasia.

Intentional killing versus alleviating pain

At this point some comment needs to be made on the issue of narcotic administration to chronically and terminally ill patients. Is this, in some cases, tantamount to killing patients? I have spoken to many nurses who feel that their actions in administering prescribed narcotic analgesia to some patients have been tantamount to 'murder'. The question which arises here is: Is the administration of narcotics in some cases the same as intentional killing? If so, is this always morally wrong?

It must be remembered, first, that many cases of medically prescribed narcotic administration are *not* cases of intentional killing, and in fact may prolong life. Second, it is also likely that some cases fall somewhere between prolonging life and intentional killing. Third, it is probably true that some cases of medically prescribed narcotic administration are cases of intentional killing (see earlier discussion in this chapter on nurse involvement in euthanasia). Let us refer to these three kinds of cases respectively as analgesia without death; analgesia with unintended death; and analgesia with intended death.

ANALGESIA WITHOUT DEATH

There are some pain states which can only be relieved by the administration of narcotic agents. An effective narcotic regime — even when entailing enormous doses — can, however, control pain without necessarily 'doping' or debilitating the patient. Indeed, many patients receiving large doses of narcotics remain alert, pain-free and as active as their disease will allow. Muirden (1993), for example, cites the case of a 55-year-old man who had cancer and who, at one stage of his illness, was receiving up to 3600 milligrams of morphine by injection (the usual dose is about 10 milligrams every four hours, a total of just 60 milligrams a day). She writes: 'He did not die of an overdose, and did not remain in a drowsy or drugged state' (Muirden 1993, p. 18). In such cases the administration of narcotics is clearly nowhere near tantamount to intentional killing. In fact, it may be quite the reverse. As pain specialists have long pointed out, the correct prescription of narcotic agents (for example, morphine) as well as the use of sedatives is more likely to prolong patients' lives than shorten them, because patients are 'able to rest, sleep, eat more and take a renewed interest in life' (Twycross and Lack 1984, p. 183; see also Sykes and Thorns 2003; Mendelson 1997; Muirden 1993). In regard to this matter — particularly in the context of palliative care — Ashby and Stoffell (1991, p. 1323) conclude that there is 'no evidence that the skilled and appropriate delivery of palliative measures (in particular the use of opioid analgesics and anxiolytic drugs) shorten life' and that by operating within a 'therapeutic ratio' treating physicians are able to balance 'symptom relief against a risk of death' (see also Sykes and Thorns 2003).

ANALGESIA WITH UNINTENDED DEATH

There are other pain states which can only be relieved by the administration of narcotic analgesia. However, unlike the previous type of case, these pain states require the administration of narcotics at a level which *may* compromise patients' alertness and physical ability (including the ability to eat and drink), and may even render them semi-comatose. In these types of cases, death may be hastened, even if not directly intended. Although the precise incidence of this type of case occurring is not known (McStay 2003), they do occur frequently enough to be of concern to some nurse clinicians — particularly when associated with the withdrawal or withholding of life-sustaining nutrition and hydration (to be discussed later in the chapter under the subheading 'Medical directives to withhold or withdraw nutrition and hydration').

ANALGESIA WITH INTENDED DEATH

In another type of case, ill or debilitated patients do not have an organic pain state, or have only trivial pain states, but are nevertheless prescribed potentially lethal narcotic regimes. Pat Turton (1992, 1987), for example, cites the case of an elderly stroke patient who was prescribed what one nurse considered an 'unnecessary and dangerous' dose of morphine. The nurse's views were shared by the hospital pharmacy. When the nurse questioned the drug order, however, she was asked by the prescribing doctor 'Is this your first ward?', the implication being that the nurse was naive. Turton comments that the drug was given by another nurse and the woman died within hours. Similar cases occur every day in residential care homes and in some general hospital wards. In other cases, analgesia is given to seriously ill patients who have neuropathogenic pain states which conventional medicine is unable to alleviate. The drug regime given is clearly intended to hasten death, although this intention may be 'disguised' in some way — for example, by stating a rationale to 'alleviate pain', even though it is known that the pain cannot be alleviated. It is difficult to avoid the impression that in all these cases the administration of a given narcotic regime is tantamount to intentional killing or the intentional shortening of life.

Given these three situations, the question remains: Is the administration of potentially lethal doses of narcotics always morally wrong?

The case of *analgesia without death* is morally uncontroversial. Here narcotic regimes enhance not only patients' wellbeing but also patients' lives. Since no moral standards are compromised, the administration of enormous doses of narcotics in this instance is morally permissible.

The case of *analgesia with unintended death*, however, is not so morally clear-cut. Although a patient may well be spared intolerable suffering by the administration of large and potentially lethal doses of narcotics, this cannot be achieved without compromising the patient's sanctity of life. For some nurses, the conflict between the demand to alleviate a patient's pain and the demand to respect and preserve a patient's life is the most troublesome of all. When caught in such a conflict, these nurses generally find the preservation-of-life principle too compelling to override and, rightly or wrongly, opt for withholding the analgesia.

Like analgesia with unintended death, *analgesia with intended death* is morally controversial. It also needs to be remembered that administering analgesics for the intended purpose of bringing about death is illegal and would be viewed by the courts as tantamount to homicide. This is an issue which requires open and honest intellectual debate, as indeed the entire debate on euthanasia and assisted suicide makes plain (Magnusson 2002; Crock 1998).

THE DOCTRINE OF DOUBLE EFFECT

Catholic theologians have long recognised the dilemma posed by intolerable pain and the use of potentially lethal doses of narcotics as a means of suppressing pain. Interestingly, although the Vatican prohibits euthanasia, it nevertheless permits the use of narcotics as a means of alleviating pain — and, furthermore, permits dosages which might suppress a patient's level of consciousness and even shorten a patient's life (Vatican 1980, p. 9). There are, however, clearly defined conditions which must be met. First, there must be no other means of alleviating the patient's pain; in other words, potentially lethal doses of narcotics must never be prescribed except as a last resort. Second, the intention of using narcotics must be to only *alleviate pain*, not to cause death.

The first condition, that of last resort, is consistent with the general principles governing effective and safe pain management and, as it stands, is relatively uncontroversial. The second condition, however, that of intentionality, takes its force from the controversial 'doctrine of double effect', and thus is vulnerable to the same criticisms as is the doctrine itself.

The doctrine of double effect was developed by Catholic theologians. It states, roughly, that it is always wrong to do a bad act for the sake of good consequences, but that it is sometimes permissible to do a good act even knowing it might have some bad consequences. To illustrate this doctrine, consider the case of a patient suffering intolerable and intractable pain. In this case, ending the patient's life would also result in ending the patient's intolerable and intractable pain. While ending the patient's *pain* would be a 'good thing', ending the patient's *life* would not. Indeed, given the sanctity-of-life doctrine, deliberately ending an innocent patient's life would be a morally evil thing to do. Thus, we could say here, it would always be wrong to end an innocent patient's life (a bad act) in order to alleviate that patient's pain (a good consequence).

Given the 'good' of alleviating pain, however, we are morally permitted to give the patient analgesia — even though this might have the foreseeable and unfortunate consequence of shortening the patient's life. This is permitted since, even though the act of narcotic administration is associated with the foreseen possibility of hastening death, ending the patient's life is not the conscious intention behind the act. In short, the decision and action of giving the narcotics was not done with 'murder in your heart'. To express the doctrine of double effect another way, we could say: it is always wrong to end patients' lives for the sake of alleviating their pain, but it is sometimes permissible to give potentially lethal doses of narcotics to alleviate pain, even though this might result in the patient's death — as long as the patient's death is not the intended outcome.

Significantly, although primarily originating from Roman Catholic religious tradition, the doctrine of double effect has influenced secular legal reasoning in regard to end of life decision-making (McStay 2003, pp. 53–6; Mendelson 1997, p. 112). One US legal commentator has even suggested that:

> the double effect principle represents sound public policy to the extent that it allows physicians to provide adequate palliative care without engaging in clearly illegal conduct.
>
> (McStay 2003, p. 54).

The doctrine of double effect has been the subject of much philosophical criticism, however, most notably on account of its over-reliance on what is called the foreseeability/intentionality distinction. This distinction holds roughly that foreseeing that a bad consequence will occur as a result of a given act is not the same thing as intending that bad consequence. For example, foreseeing that a patient will die as a result of being given large doses of narcotics is not the same thing as intending to end that patient's life; therefore the person who administers the narcotic is not morally culpable.

Critics reject this, however, and argue that the distinction drawn here is misleading. They contend that foreseeing a bad consequence of an action is exactly the same as intending it, since the agent knows that a bad consequence is pending but deliberately refrains from preventing it. To some extent, this position is also upheld in legal law. As Kuhse (1984) points out, the law presumes: 'everyone must be taken to intend that which is the natural consequence of his [sic] actions' (p. 26).

Given these criticisms, then, it seems that we cannot rely on the distinction between merely alleviating a patient's pain and intentionally ending a patient's life. Although it might perhaps be psychologically more tolerable to admit this distinction, it is not morally tolerable to do so. Where does this leave us?

The position is clear — nurses must all pursue a path of rigorous moral analysis of their actions. Acts involving narcotic prescription and administration must satisfy the ultimate standards not only of medicine, nursing and law, but also of ethics.

First and foremost, narcotic administration must accord with patients' considered preferences. This means that every effort must be made to establish what patients' preferences are, and to what extent patients are prepared to tolerate or not tolerate pain. Nurses must be open to the possibility, for example, of some patients preferring to suffer a certain degree of pain rather than compromise their mental alertness and physical ability. While a nurse might not agree with this kind of decision, it is nevertheless the patient's prerogative to make it.

Second, pain management must be guided by moral as well as clinical and legal considerations (for a helpful outline of the agreed principles/standards of lawful narcotic administration see Mendelson 1997, p. 112).

Lastly, those involved in the administration of narcotics must be free conscientiously to refuse to administer drug regimes which they judge to be morally controversial or unacceptable.

Implications for nurses of narcotic administration

Narcotic administration (particularly in the case of terminal sedation) will always remain a controversial issue for some nurses, as it does for other clinicians (McStay 2003). Nevertheless it is not insurmountable. In the case of legally prescribed narcotic pain management regimes, a sound knowledge of the principles of pain management, proper pain assessment, and correct drug administration will help to reduce the likelihood of moral dilemmas occurring. In other cases, a clear articulation of relevant moral standards and values will help to reduce or at least adjudicate many of the moral problems associated with effective pain management and drug administration. Either way, the position nurses are morally obliged to take is clear: the patients are always the nurses' primary concern. If nurses have good reason to believe that a patient's safety, dignity, autonomy and wellbeing will be compromised by a given drug order or regime, then they must question it. This is not only a moral requirement, but also a legal requirement. It is far better to question a narcotic order and be wrong than not to question a narcotic order and be wrong — with the former, what is at stake may be only a little self-pride; with the latter, at stake may be a patient's life.

'Nursing care only' directives

A common, although not widely acknowledged, euthanatic practice — and one that has significant implications for nurses — is that of doctors prescribing 'nursing care only' for patients deemed 'medically hopeless'. In many instances (although, of course, not all), this medical prescription has become a euphemism for non-voluntary and involuntary passive euthanasia since what is in fact being ordered is not *nursing care*, but rather the *withdrawal* of both *competent nursing care* and *life-sustaining (medical and nursing) care*. To illustrate this point, consider the widely discussed Dr Leonard Arthur case (Kuhse 1984), and the Danville case (Robertson 1981). Although these two cases are now somewhat dated, the issues they raise remain current in contemporary nursing care contexts — particularly in regard to the common practice of prescribing terminal sedation in association with the withdrawal or withholding of nutrition and hydration (for a comprehensive account of the 'terminal sedation' issue, see McStay 2003).

THE DR LEONARD ARTHUR CASE

On 1 July 1980, in a small English city, a Down's syndrome infant named John Pearson died in the arms of a nurse. The case would have escaped public attention had it not been for a member of staff reporting the circumstances of the case to Life, an anti-abortion organisation. On the basis of the information obtained by Life, John Pearson's attending physician, Dr Leonard Arthur, was charged with murder. The charge was based on the prosecution's claims that:

1. Dr Arthur had ordered the administration of the drug DFl18 with the intention of bringing about the baby's death;
2. the fact that Dr Arthur had ordered 'nursing care only' showed that he had intended the infant to die.

(Kuhse 1984, p. 22)

Dr Arthur's 'nursing care only' order in this instance directed the feeding of *water only* to the infant, and the administration of the drug DFl18 '*at the discretion of the nurse in charge* but not more than every four hours' (Kuhse and Singer 1985, p. 2, emphasis added). Since John Pearson had no organic pain syndrome as such, it would seem that the DF118 was prescribed for the purposes of sedating him and suppressing his hunger sensations.

However we look at this case, it is clear that what Dr Arthur ordered was *not* nursing care, or, if it was, it was highly negligent nursing care. For example, feeding only water to an infant who is demonstrably able to take and tolerate a full and nourishing fluid regime falls far short of reasonable and acceptable standards of nursing care, as does the administration of a narcotic to an infant who does not have a pathological pain state. It also falls far short of accepted medical standards of care and is highly questionable legally (McStay 2003; Craig 1996, 1994; Ashby and Stoffell 1995, 1991; Wilkes 1994). Let us explore this claim further.

Nurses are formally educated to assess individuals' fundamental health needs, to diagnose needs deficits (i.e. health problems) and to plan nursing interventions aimed at helping people to meet their own health needs. Nurses are also formally educated to evaluate the outcomes of their nursing interventions and to modify their plans of care if an individual's health needs and health goals have, for some reason, not been met. Among the ten or so basic health needs which nurses are taught to assess are nutrition (including hydration), comfort (including being pain-free) and safety (including being kept free of the harms that might be caused by the over-prescription or inappropriate prescription of certain drugs). The formal education given to nurses in this area provides the minimal legal standard of reasonable and acceptable nursing care. Any nurse who fails to assess and diagnose correctly a person's health problems and plan nursing interventions to help meet the health needs of a patient is practising below a reasonable and acceptable standard of nursing care, and is thus practising negligently.

Even if hunger is conceded as a genuine 'pain state', this still does not justify the administration of large doses of narcotics or sedatives, nor does it rescue nurses administering these from culpability (McStay 2003). There are at least two reasons for this. First, it is not normal practice to administer large doses of narcotics or sedatives to alleviate hunger pain. If it were, patients hungry from, say, pre- and post-operative fasting would be routinely administered narcotics or sedatives as part of their care. As we know, this is not done. Nurses should be rightly suspicious of medical prescriptions directing the administration of potentially lethal doses of narcotics or sedatives to infants who are not dying from the natural progression of a life-threatening disease, who do not have a genuine pathological pain state, and who are suffering hunger only from not being fed adequately.

A second reason why narcotic or sedative administration is not justified in the case of hungry severely disabled newborns is that there is no clinical basis for preferring a narcotic agent or a sedative agent over a bottle of milk for alleviating these infants' so-called 'pain states' and associated distress. As a general rule, narcotics are prescribed only for extreme pathological pain states or where other non-narcotic agents are known to be ineffective in alleviating a given type of pain. In less extreme pain states, the tendency is to prescribe non-narcotic agents (such as aspirin or paracetamol), or even to avoid prescribing analgesia altogether, with preference being given to other methods of pain management such as exercise, change of bodily position, massage, physiotherapy, transneuronal stimulation, the administration of antacids, and, in the case of babies and infants, simply nursing them on one's lap and spending time with them. Since hunger is not generally regarded as an extreme pain state (in fact hunger is not even listed as a pain state in general analgesic guidelines and manuals), it is again highly suspect that narcotics should be chosen as a preferred 'treatment' option over the simple administration of a bottle of milk or other means of artificial nutrition and hydration which could be provided safely — even at the end stage of life (see, for example, Steiner 1998). Similarly, sedatives are usually prescribed for children only as a last resort. Where children's distress can be easily resolved by feeding them and/or nursing them on one's lap, there seems little to justify the administration of potentially lethal doses of a given sedative or narcotic analgesic.

It is, I think, fairly obvious that 'nursing care only' orders, as given by doctors in the case of severely disabled newborns (as well as other cases), are prescriptions for deliberately 'hastening death'. It is also clear that, by so ordering 'nursing care only', doctors are placing nurses in a position of legal negligence and possibly of even committing homicide. Obvious as these points are, however, they have been conveniently ignored by some courts. In the case of Dr Leonard Arthur, the suggestion that John Pearson had been killed by the *nursing care only* order was dismissed. Significantly, the defence council's success was largely based on showing that ordering 'nursing care only' was *proper medical practice* (Kuhse and Singer 1985, p. 9). In this case, the judge ignored any thought that the attending nurses had acted negligently by giving 'water only' to a hungry infant otherwise capable of feeding, and had effectively committed homicide by giving potentially lethal doses of narcotics to an infant who did not have a genuine organic pain syndrome (see also Gunn and Smith 1985). Following his trial at Leicester in November 1981, Dr Arthur was acquitted of the criminal charges brought against him. His acquittal is reported to have sparked 'rejoicing' (Kuhse and Singer 1985, p. 10).

THE DANVILLE CASE

On 6 May 1981, Siamese twins were born at a hospital in Danville, Illinois. The babies were joined at the waist with three legs. Upon seeing the deformity, the attending anaesthetist passed the order: 'Don't resuscitate, let's just cover the babies' (Robertson 1981, p. 5; Horan 1982). The father of the twins, also a doctor, gestured support for the anaesthetist's decision. It was later revealed that the decision to let the infants die had been made on little more than a visual impression of the infants' condition. Robertson (1981) writes that in fact no assessment was made to check whether there was any brain damage, whether the twins could be separated, or what their prognosis was. No effort was made to explore either adoption or institutional alternatives for the babies. The decision was made in ignorance, and furthermore was made at the most stressful point in time — at delivery. Nevertheless, an order was written in the medical notes not to feed the babies, and they were taken to the newborn unit to die.

Nurses involved in caring for the twins, not surprisingly, became increasingly uncomfortable with the decision to withhold feeds from the babies. And it is claimed that at least one of the nurses 'fed the babies several times' (Robertson 1981, p. 5). The case received public attention after an anonymous caller reported it to the Illinois Department of Children and Family Services. Upon receiving the call the department immediately investigated the caller's claim, and the babies were transferred to another hospital for assessment and care. Later, in an unprecedented step, criminal charges were filed against both the parents and the doctors for 'conspiracy to commit murder and endangering the life and health of children' (Robertson 1981, p. 5). In the legal case that followed, nurses described how the twins 'cried in pain because they were hungry; how the cries dwindled down to whimpers as they were starved to death, how the skin started to wrinkle ...' (Robertson 1981, p. 6; see also Horan 1982).

As in the Dr Arthur case, nurses were once again placed in a legally and morally intolerable position on account of a 'routine' medical order to withhold nourishment. What made the medical directives in both cases seriously problematic was that they both required nurses to administer terminal sedation to, and to withhold feeds from, babies who were otherwise able to tolerate 'normal' feeding; who were not in a terminal phase of an illness; and who, with appropriate care and treatment, had a good prospect of recovery and living. Even if the babies were in a terminal phase of illness, the medical directives were still morally and legally wrong. Consider the following.

MEDICAL DIRECTIVES TO WITHHOLD OR WITHDRAW NUTRITION AND HYDRATION

People in the terminal phase of their illness, because of being in pain or severe distress and/or being sedated, may invariably reach a point where they cannot take food and fluids 'naturally' — that is, voluntarily by mouth, with or without assistance, in order to satisfy their hunger and thirst (Ashby and Mendelson 2003, p. 262). Here the question arises of: *How should clinicians (doctors and nurses alike) respond to this situation?*

The issue of withholding or withdrawing nutrition and hydration from patients at the end stage of life has been one of the most contentious issues in palliative care (see, in particular, the vitriolic debate between Craig 1994, 1996 and Ashby and Stoffell 1991, 1995). Basically there are two points of view:

1. hydration and nutrition should be administered (artificially, if necessary) to patients regardless of the terminal phase of their illness (Craig 1996, 1994);
2. there should be a gradual reduction and eventual cessation or non-initiation of treatment as the patient's condition deteriorates (Ashby and Stoffell 1995, 1991).

Those who argue that hydration and nutrition should continue to be provided — even at the end stage of life — contend that if fluids are withheld or withdrawn from patients they will inevitably enter into a state of dehydration which, in turn, will result in 'circulatory collapse, renal failure, anuria and death' (Craig 1994, p. 140). In short, without hydration and nutrition, patients who are heavily sedated will die — *whatever the underlying pathology* (Craig 1994, p. 140). Furthermore, dehydration can lead to severe complications that may unacceptably alter the patient's quality of life while they are dying; such complications can include: 'increased asthenia, nausea, postural hypotension, fever with no underlying infectious process, increased risk of bed sores, and constipation' as well as the 'accumulation of opioid metabolites, grand-mal seizures, and hyperalgesia' (Steiner 1998, pp. 8, 12).

Another complication of dehydration is that of patients suffering from intolerable thirst and hunger during the terminal phase of their illness (see McCann et al. 1994). On this, Craig argues (p. 142):

> It is widely assumed that a terminally ill patient is not troubled by hunger or thirst but this is difficult to substantiate as few people return from the grave to complain.

Finally, some worry that doctors might 'get it wrong' (i.e. make diagnostic errors) and accordingly patients might not only die 'poorly', but needlessly. On this point Craig contends (1994, p. 140):

Diagnostic errors can also occur. A reversible psychosis or confusional state can be mistaken for terminal delirium, aspiration pneumonia for tracheal obstruction, obstruction [of the bowel] due to faecal impaction for something more sinister, and so on. The only way to ensure that life will not be shortened is to maintain hydration during sedation in all cases whereby inability to eat and drink is a direct consequence of sedation, unless the relatives request no further intervention, or the patient has made his/her wishes known to this effect.

Not all, however, share these views and argue that a gradual reduction and eventual cessation or non-initiation of treatment as the patient's condition deteriorates is not only clinically indicated, but also ethically mandated (Ashby and Stoffell 1995, 1991; see also Ashby and Mendelson 2003; McStay 2003). Proponents of this view argue that if and when a patient is in the terminal phase of illness:

> no form of artificial hydration or alimentation is undertaken, all measures not required for comfort are withdrawn, and no treatment-related toxicity is acceptable unless the effects of this are less than the benefits achieved by the treatment. For example, artificial hydration may be required in the terminal phase to satisfy thirst or other symptoms attributable to lack of fluid intake.
>
> (Ashby and Stoffell 1995, p. 136)

The view that hydration and nutrition should not be continued to be provided during the terminal phase of an illness rests on concerns that such treatment is more likely to *add* to the distress of the dying person, rather than provide relief. For example, research has shown that artificial hydration provided intravenously can lead to a range of associated medical conditions and complications including: vital organ failure from fluid overload (this can lead to such conditions as pulmonary and cerebral oedema and their associated complications); infection and bacteremia from catheter and cannulation sites; arterial perforation, thrombosis, cardiac arrhythmias, cardio-pulmonary arrest and pneumothorax during/following insertion of central venous lines; and pulmonary emboli (Steiner 1998, pp. 8–9). Fluids administered long term (i.e. for periods longer than 2–3 weeks) via either nasogastric tubes of gastrostomy (e.g. percutaneous endoscopic gastrostomies or 'PEG' tubes) have also been associated with serious complications such as: diarrhoea due to osmotic load; aspiration pneumonia (due to tube displacement/the regurgitation and aspiration of gastric contents); metabolic abnormalities; mechanical difficulties (e.g. blocking of the tube, nasal irritation or erosion, tube displacement) (Steiner 1998, pp. 11–12). Research in this area remains limited, however, and it is conceded by all parties that until a sound body of 'gold standard' research (including randomised controlled trials as well as rich qualitative studies) is available, and key questions answered about both the physiology and lived experiences of the administration of fluids to terminally ill (and sedated) patients, it is unlikely that the strongly polarised views on the matter will be resolved, or, at least, satisfactorily adjudicated. As Steiner (1998) notes, however, conducting such research may be difficult because of the ethical issues involved.

Disputes aside, there does appear to be a consensus in the field that a gradual reduction and eventual cessation of artificial hydration and alimentation (AHA) is appropriate during *the terminal phase of care* (Ashby and Mendelson 2003; McStay 2003; Steiner 2003; Parkash and Burge 1997; Ashby and Stoffell 1995, 1991; Craig 1994; Ahronheim and Gasner 1990; Belcher 1990; Sykes 1990; Lynn 1989). The critical issue here, however, is identifying and deciding correctly *the point at which a patient is, on the balance of probabilities, in the 'terminal mode phase in which death seems inevitable and imminent'* (Ashby and Stoffell 1991, p. 1323) — bearing in mind that 'identifying the time of actual dying' is easier in retrospect than prospect (Gillon 1994, p. 131).

Concurring with Ramsey (1976), Dyck (1984) and Grisez and Boyle (1979), Ashby and Stoffell (1995) contend that it is possible to distinguish between 'those persons who are dying and those who are not'. Objective clinical standards enabling determinations to be made that 'death is imminent' include: demonstrated disease progression, vital organ failure, and the subjective (psychological, emotional and intuitive) responses of the patient and/or those close to them indicating that the 'end is near' (Ashby and Stoffell 1995, 1991). During this stage, the intake of food and fluid decreases 'naturally', although 'both are always available (that is — they are never withdrawn)' if the patient wants it. Ashby and Stoffell suggest that reassurance may also need to be provided to the family/support carers during this phase 'that dying people usually want only enough food and drink to keep them comfortable — and frequent mouth care' (Ashby and Stoffell 1991, p. 1323; for a helpful qualitative study on family perspectives on the issue of hydration in terminal care, see Parkash and Burge 1997).

Essential hydration (i.e. hydration necessary to control the symptoms of thirst) as well as analgesia can be provided safely and simply during the terminal phase by subcutaneous fluid infusion (or hypodermoclysis). This 'rediscovered' technique (first used in the 1940s and 1950s, but which was largely superseded by intravenous therapy technology that was developed at the time) is generally well tolerated, has a low incidence of adverse events, and last *in situ* longer (Steiner 1998, pp. 9–11). Accordingly, it has gained considerable acceptance in palliative care in recent years and is used widely (Steiner 1998, pp. 9–11; Ashby and Stoffell 1995, p. 136; Bruera et al 1990). To some extent, the use of hypodermoclysis has resolved some of the practical dilemmas and disputes about the provisions of food and fluids during the terminal phase of an illness; moral questions remain, however. Whether starting, stopping or not starting artificial hydration and alimentation, the criteria for deciding what to do ultimately rests on whether the dying person's moral interests are being served by the decisions that are made. Here the critical question arises of: *How best to decide what those moral interests are?* (an issue that will be considered further in the following chapter on 'End of life decision-making and the nursing profession').

Position statements on euthanasia/assisted suicide and the nursing profession

A pressing question currently facing the nursing profession concerns what, if any, formal position nurses ought to take on the euthanasia/assisted suicide issue? For many, this question remains an open one. For some, the failure by some nursing organisations to formulate a firm position, either way, on the euthanasia/assisted suicide question is untenable and paradoxical — paradoxical since even a 'non-position' is a position (Johnstone 1996a).

Significantly, there is no universally agreed nursing position on the ethics of euthanasia/assisted suicide; different nursing organisations in different countries hold quite distinct and sometimes opposing views on the matter, and on whether it is appropriate for nurses to assist with euthanatic procedures (Johnstone 1996b, pp. 32–43). For example, whereas some nursing organisations (such as the Royal College of Nursing in the United Kingdom, and the American Nurses' Association in the United States of America) have stated positions firmly rejecting the role of the nurse in participating in or assisting with active voluntary euthanasia and/or assisted suicide, others (such as the National Nurses' Association in the Netherlands) have stated positions supporting the role of the nurse in assisting with euthanasia/assisted suicide (Johnstone 1996b, pp. 32–43). While there does seem to be some agreement among nursing organisations on the matter of patients rights to self-determination, and to die with dignity and peace (Johnstone 1996b, p. 38), this support has stopped short of being translated into a frank pro-euthanasia/assisted suicide position with the matter tending to be left to individual nurses to decide on the basis of conscience (see for example, International Council of Nurses 2000; Royal College of Nursing, Australia 1999).

In several respects it is not surprising that there exists moral uncertainty and disagreement among members of the nursing profession about the 'rightness' and 'wrongness' of euthanasia/assisted suicide; about the kind of position the nursing profession should take, if at all; and, in the event of euthanasia/assisted suicide being decriminalised, about what kind of role nurses should play in the medically assisted deaths of patients. Many people hold differing views on these and related issues, and there is no reason why nurses should be any exception in this regard. Furthermore, it is important that this moral uncertainty and disagreement exists — a point that is not always understood. Nurses like other members of the community should not fear moral uncertainty. Appropriately placed it fosters what I shall call here 'moral vigilance' — a moral 'watchfulness' that can and does provide an important check against moral complacency. Neither should nurses fear moral disagreement or the diversity of opinion underpinning it (provided, of course, this does not spill over into violence, as has happened with the abortion debate where, it will be recalled, pro-life supporters have murdered pro-choice supporters in the name of upholding their 'pro-life' beliefs). As has long been recognised in philosophy, disagreement is the beginning of our thinking, not its end. Philosophical disagreement can help to stimulate our moral imagination, and to sharpen and refine our moral thinking. In this respect, moral disagreement can, paradoxically, be creative and protective, not destructive; it can enable us to discover new solutions which might otherwise have alluded us — to see not just new things, but to engage in a new way of thinking about the things we have discovered. Moral uncertainty and disagreement, therefore, can both provide important beginning points for developing our moral thinking and finding sustainable and satisfying moral stances from which to view the world and guide our moral conduct. Consider the following case scenario.

A few years ago I was participating in a panel discussion on euthanasia and assisted suicide which had been scheduled during a one day seminar on the topic. During the panel discussion (in which a number of distinguished guests participated) I noticed a young woman (a nurse) crying silently in the audience. Concerned about this young woman's obvious distress, I approached her during the morning tea break to ask if she wished to discuss with me what was troubling her. This she agreed to do. Upon hearing her story, I asked whether she would be willing to share her situation with the rest of the seminar participants once the proceedings recommenced after the morning tea break. This she also agreed to do. When the proceedings of the seminar recommenced, I had the opportunity to call on the young woman to share her feelings about the topic under discussion. She bravely faced her audience and related the following:

> I am sitting here listening to you all. And I am so envious because you all seem to be so sure about where you stand on the [euthanasia] issue. You are either *for* or *against* it. But I do not have the benefit of such certainty. I simply do not know where I stand and this makes me feel very upset. You see, it is like this: I am a 'good Catholic girl', with a good Catholic education. My church tells me 'euthanasia is wrong' and that I must not support

it. But then, I am also a nurse. I believe I am a good nurse and I believe in nursing. And my profession tells me I must support patients' rights — I must be an advocate for my patients' rights. And then there are my patients. Sometimes my patients want to die and ask for assistance to die. And I want to do what is right by them. And then there is me, the human being, torn between what my church tells me I should do, what my profession tells me I should do, and what my patients want me to do. I just feel so torn, because I really feel so uncertain about what *is* the right thing to do. I just don't know. I just don't know which side of the fence I should be on. And I feel that somehow maybe I am stupid or deficient because of this — especially when I listen to all of you here being so sure about the positions you are holding.

With this brave and frank admission came other admissions from other people in the audience: significantly, and contrary to superficial appearances, most of the people attending the seminar felt the way this nurse did, but had been unable to say so publicly. We then spent some time exploring the permissibility of feeling 'uncertain' about new and previously unexplored ethical issues, of taking the time necessary to consider other points of view and to explore possible answers to the difficult questions raised, and to ultimately reach a position on the issues identified that the person in question could 'live with'.

Some time later the nurse in question contacted me. She had reasoned the issue through and had reached a position about which she felt confident at both a personal and professional level. What had helped her most in reaching this position was peer support, and the 'permission' her peers had given her to take the time she needed to 'think through' the issues at hand. She also particularly valued the opportunity the seminar had provided in regard to exposing her not just to the issues raised but to the many different points of view expressed in response to them. But most important of all, she valued being able to share her story, and in this sharing to 'make visible' a problem that she was soon able to discover was not hers alone.

Coming to terms with the complex questions raised by the euthanasia/assisted suicide issue requires a systematic response by both individual nurses and the broader nursing profession. Specifically, it requires of nurses to gain knowledge and understanding of the profound ethical, legal, cultural, clinical and political dimensions of euthanasia/assisted suicide, and the influence these dimensions have on the profession and practice of nursing (Johnstone 1996a). Equally important, it requires peer support and understanding among nurses and a recognition that the euthanasia/assisted suicide question is not — and never has been — simple and clear-cut.

In concluding this section, it is my considered view that in order for a position statement on euthanasia/assisted suicide to be meaningful to members of the nursing profession, it must minimally reflect that euthanasia and assisted suicide are controversial moral issues, that there exists a diversity of opinion on whether euthanasia and assisted suicide are morally justified, and that nurses are likely to encounter this diversity of opinion during the course of their work. Further, such a position statement must also reflect that there exists a diversity of opinion on whether nurses have a legitimate role to play in providing medically assisted deaths to patients and that all nurses have a responsibility to ensure that they are reliably informed about the ethical, legal, cultural, political and clinical dimensions and implications of euthanasia and assisted suicide as a 'health care' option.

Conclusion

Euthanasia and assisted suicide are issues that have obvious significance for members of the nursing profession. While nurses can choose to accept or reject the findings of public debate on the euthanasia/assisted suicide issue, they cannot ignore them since, to do so, would be to risk not just their own moral interests, but importantly the interests of patients for whose care they share responsibility.

The issues of euthanasia and assisted suicide have not been widely discussed in the nursing literature, and the need to do so is long overdue. If this neglect is not redressed, it will be to the peril of the nursing profession, as the experiences of nurses in the Northern Territory of Australia and the Netherlands (discussed in this chapter) reminds us. It will be recalled, for instance, that in 1996, Northern Territory nurses had to confront the reality of being enabled by law to participate in euthanasia and assisted suicide *before* the broader nursing profession had reached a position on the matter and had determined what it regarded as 'acceptable standards of nursing practice' in relation to the actual practice of euthanasia/assisted suicide. In the Netherlands, meanwhile, nurses had to confront the reality that they could be successfully prosecuted for performing euthanasia even when such an action was in accordance with legally prescribed criteria. Nurses are — and have always been — in a tenuous position in regard to their role in participating in end of life practices. It is timely that this tenuous position is addressed in the interests of reducing not just the vulnerability of nurses, but of the patients otherwise reliant on nurses for quality care at the end stages of their lives.

CASE SCENARIO AND CRITICAL QUESTIONS

Case scenario

In 1996, in what is believed to be the first case of its kind in Australia, a nurse was charged with murder after he turned off the life support machine sustaining the life a 37-year-old woman (and mother of three) who was suffering from a rare and crippling brain disease. Although there was some suggestion that the woman was 'brain dead', she had not been 'formally declared dead' (Donovan 1996, p.2). It was also alleged in media reports that 'the appropriate documents required to remove treatment from a comatose patient had not been signed at the time of the woman's death' (Walsh and Pirrie 1996, p. 1). Media reports also claimed that the nurse took the action he did on the grounds that he 'believed that he was acting in the patient's best interests' (Walsh and Pirrie 1996, p. 2) and that he believed he had the permission of the woman's husband (Das 1996, p. 7).

The case was reported to have focussed 'national attention on the care and treatment of incompetent and severely brain damaged patients' and to have revived 'the whole euthanasia question'; the case was also reported to have focused attention 'on hospital guidelines and regulations on the care of brain-damaged patients' (Walsh and Pirrie 1996, p. 2). Later media reports further suggested that the case had shown 'that there was a "demarcation dispute" about who had the right to disconnect life support machines.' (Das 1996, p. 7).

Critical questions

1. Were the nurse's actions in this case tantamount to an act of euthanasia, assisted suicide, 'mercy killing', or homicide?
2. Accepting for arguments sake that the nurse's actions were not homicidal (the nurse was in fact acquitted of the charges against him), were they morally justified? If so, on what grounds? If not, why not?
3. If euthanasia and assisted suicide were legalised, should provisions be included to legitimate the role of nurses to assist in patient deaths? If so, what role specifically should nurses have?
4. Should the nursing profession formally support the legalisation of euthanasia and assisted suicide and engage in political activism to achieve law reform in this area? Upon what basis do you rest your arguments in support of your views?

Chapter 11

Ethical issues in suicide and parasuicide

LEARNING OBJECTIVES

Upon the completion of this chapter and with further self-directed learning you are expected to be able to:

- Discuss the distinction between suicide and parasuicide and why making this distinction is important.
- Provide an overview of key religious and cultural processes that have historically influenced the development of punitive and stigmatising attitudes toward people who have suicided or attempted suicide.
- Examine critically at least five criteria that must be met in order for an act to count as *suicide* rather than some other form of death (e.g. euthanasia).
- Consider arguments both for and against the proposition that people have a 'right to suicide'.
- Examine critically the conditions under which a person's decision to suicide ought to be respected.
- Discuss critically the ethics of suicide prevention, intervention and postvention.

KEYWORDS

- Parasuicide
- Self annihilation
- Self harm
- Suicide
- Suicide intervention
- Suicide postvention
- Suicide prevention

Introduction

Suicide is recognised internationally as being a major public health issue. Defined by the World Health Organization (WHO) as 'the result of an act deliberately initiated and performed by a person in the full knowledge or expectation of its fatal outcome', suicide accounts for an average of 15.1 per 100 000 deaths across 53 countries for which complete data are available (WHO 2001, p. 37). Significantly, the suicide rate for males (24 per 100 000) is universally higher than for females (6.8 per 100 000) (WHO 2001, p. 37). Although suicide occurs in all ages across the lifespan (including the very young and the very old) and in people from all walks of life, it stands universally as a leading cause of death among young adults. Although the probable 'causes' of suicide vary across cultures and countries, depression and substance abuse have both been implicated as critical factors leading to suicide (Rudnick 2002, p. 151; WHO 2001, p. 39).

The figures given above do not include attempted suicide rates. While reliable data on the incidence of attempted suicide are difficult to obtain, according to Australian estimates, for every male suicide there are approximately 30–50 attempts; and for every female suicide there are approximately 150–300 attempts (Suicide Prevention Victorian Task Force 1997, p. 21). It has been further estimated that of those who engage in suicidal behaviour (attempt suicide), 15 per cent will ultimately succeed in ending their own lives (Suicide Prevention Victorian Task Force 1997, p. 21).

In Western countries, suicide is ranked amongst the top ten causes of death (Suicide Prevention Victorian Task Force 1997, p. 9). In the Australian State of Victoria, suicide deaths were once reported to have even outnumbered the state's road fatalities (Ryle 1993). The probability that some road fatalities are also 'autocides' (i.e. deaths as the result of premeditated [suicidal] automobile accidents [Donnelly 1990, p. 8]) increases the significance of these statistics.

According to the National Advisory Council on Youth Suicide Prevention (2000, p. 1) more than 2500 Australians die from suicide each year — many of them young people. Today, Australia has one of the highest rates of suicide among young people aged 15–24 years, with rates in this age group having tripled over the past 40 years (National Advisory Council on Youth Suicide Prevention 2000, p. 6). Suicide data also show that youth suicide (particularly among males) is over-represented in remote and rural areas; youth suicide is also over-represented among gay and lesbian youth (especially those living in remote and rural areas), possibly accounting for up to 30 per cent of completed youth suicides each year) (Suicide Prevention Victorian Task Force 1997, pp. 19, 40). Explaining this statistical over-representation, one commentator has written that 'homosexual orientation, cultural homophobia and geographical/social isolation are clearly a lethal mixture' (Christian 1997, p. 9). Other high risk groups include: men over 80 years of age, Aboriginal and Torres Straight Islander people (rates have been estimated to be approximately 40 per cent higher than the general population), the homeless, people with HIV/AIDS, and people in custody (National Advisory Council on Youth Suicide Prevention 2000, p. 7; Suicide Prevention Victorian Task Force 1997, pp. 38–40).

Suicide figures in the United States of America are comparable with those in Australia. According to official estimates, there are approximately 30,000 certified suicides in the United States each year, with many other probable suicides classified as 'accidental deaths' (Beauchamp and Childress 2001, p. 188). Youth suicide rates in the

United States are also alarmingly high with suicide standing as the third leading killer of young people and accounting for '14 per cent of all deaths in the teenage-range' (Remafedi 1994b, p. 7; Davis 1992, p. 92; Donnelly 1990, p. 9). There is also consistent evidence showing 'unusually high rates of attempted suicide among gay [and lesbian] youth, in the range of 20–30 per cent, regardless of geographic and ethnic variability' (Remafedi 1994b, p. 7). As in Australia, gay and lesbian youth may comprise 'up to 30 per cent of completed youth suicides annually' in the United States of America (Gibson 1994, p. 15). These rates are thought to be causally linked to these youths' traumatic experiences of coming to terms with their sexuality in contexts (such as families, communities, society as a whole) that are for the most part unsupportive, alienating and aggressively homophobic (see in particular Remafedi 1994a).

The magnitude of the suicide problem in the United States was highlighted in 1993 with the reported suicide of a six-year-old girl, believed to be the youngest recorded suicide in the State of Florida (Power 1993, p. 9). The child was killed after she deliberately placed herself in front of an oncoming train. Her death was witnessed by three other children aged six, seven, and eight years old respectively — all of whom 'tried to move her as the train approached' (p. 9). The engineer was unable to stop the train 'until nearly a kilometre after impact' (p. 9). It is believed that the little girl wanted to die so that she could 'become an angel and be with her mother', who was dying of cancer (p. 9).

(As a point of interest, contrary to popular thought, child suicide is not an isolated or new phenomenon. During the late Middle Ages and early modern period, for instance, children under the age of 15 years were regarded as being at increased risk of suicide owing to the violent and abusive ways in which they tended to be treated during this period [Williams 1997, p. 153]. Today, while suicide rates are relatively low in children under 15 years of age, there has been some suggestion these may be increasing. In 1995, for example, in the Australia state of Victoria, four deaths by suicide were of children aged between 10 and 14 years [Suicide Prevention Victorian Task Force 1997, p. 16].)

Suicide, by its very nature, is an extremely difficult and complex issue to address. At a personal level, the suicide of a loved one, a friend or an associate can be a devastating experience. Those 'left behind' may find themselves struggling 'to make sense of the suicidal act and the causes of suicidal behaviour' (Davis 1992, p. 90). They may also find themselves overwhelmed by feelings of grief, shame, remorse, anger, despair, and possibly even guilt at the thought that 'perhaps they could have done more' or that 'if only they had been there ... it might never have happened'. It has been estimated that for every suicide, between six and ten people (including family, friends and co-workers) are directly and strongly affected by the event (Suicide Prevention Victorian Task Force 1997, p. 25; Williams 1997, p. 224). Significantly, people bereaved by suicide are themselves ten times more likely than the general population to die from self-inflicted deaths (Suicide Prevention Victorian Task Force 1997, p. 25).

Suicide is also difficult to address at a professional/therapeutic level. Even the very best of psychotherapies may still fail to prevent a person suiciding; and even the very best of medical and nursing care may still fail to restore someone who has attempted suicide to a life that is 'worthwhile' and worth living. Equally if not more problematic are the difficulties of addressing the suicide issue at a moral level. Included among these difficulties is the challenge suicide and attempted suicide pose to fundamental moral notions about the value, sanctity and meaning of life. An important question here is not 'how to achieve a better more fruitful [good] life' — a central question in Western moral philosophy — but, as Heyd and Bloch (1981, p. 185) point out, 'whether to live at all'. More seriously, suicide challenges morality itself, and not least the values, standards and principles comprising it which might otherwise be appealed to for guiding deliberation on such issues as the entitlements and responsibilities of people contemplating suicide; the moral permissibility and impermissibility of suicide prevention; the entitlements and responsibilities of others toward those contemplating or attempting suicide; and other similar issues. Compounding the moral complexity of these issues is the additional consideration that, unlike other causes of death, suicide (or, more specifically, death from suicide) is relatively preventable (Baume 1988, p. 43).

Nurses who have either cared for a person who has attempted suicide, or who have been involved in the care of family members and friends of someone who has attempted suicide or succeeded in suiciding, will be only too familiar with the deep emotional agony that inevitably comes with this kind of situation. They will also be very aware of the complex moral problems that are commonly associated with implementing interventions aimed at preventing suicide, with caring for those who have attempted unsuccessfully to suicide, and with the difficulties of addressing these problems in a satisfying and helpful way.

It is not the purpose of this discussion to examine or present a treatise on the clinical aspects of suicide (its underlying causes, and means of prevention), or, indeed, on the philosophy or sociology or anthropology of suicide. Such a task would require major works in their own right — as has already been undertaken (see, for example, Battin 1982, 1996; Battin and Mayo 1980; Clemons 1990; Colt 1991; Durkheim 1952; Farberow 1975a; Firestone 1997; Hendin 1998; Kaplan and Schwartz 1993; Miller 1992; Stengel 1970). Rather, the task here is to assist nurses to gain an understanding of the moral aspects of suicide and suicide prevention, and the nature of nurses' moral obligations when caring for people who are contemplating or who have attempted suicide. In undertaking this task, attention will be given to examining briefly:

- the history of suicide in different cultures and societies;
- definitions of suicide, and possible criteria that must be met in order for an act to count as suicide; and
- some important moral concerns that are raised by the suicide question, and which have significant implications for the profession and practice of nursing.

Socio-cultural attitudes to suicide: a brief historical overview

Concepts of and attitudes toward suicide have varied enormously across different cultures and throughout time (see in particular Farberow's [1975a] *Suicide in different cultures*). Just what was regarded as an act of suicide and whether suicide was approved or disapproved depended on a range of factors, including cultural norms and mores, religion, law, politics, and personal and social morality (Alvarez 1980; Amundsen 1989; Battin 1982, 1996; Beauchamp 1989; Beauchamp and Childress 2001; Beauchamp and Perlin 1978; Brody 1989b; Cooper 1989; Farberow 1975b; Ferngren 1989; Hendin 1998; Miller 1992; Stengel 1970). These factors have seen Western attitudes toward suicide shift dramatically from those of socio-cultural approval through to religious prohibition, criminalisation, and ultimately the medicalisation of suicide (see Figure 11.1).

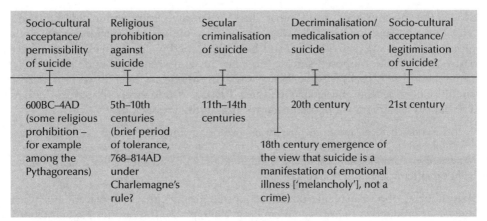

Figure 11.1 The transformation of attitudes to suicide

Socio-cultural acceptance of suicide, 600 BC – 4 AD

In the introduction to *Suicide: the philosophical issues*, Battin and Mayo (1980, p. 1) note that 'suicide has not always been assumed to be tragic or a phenomenon that is always to be prevented'. They go on to point out that, in both the early Greek and the Hebrew cultures, 'suicide was apparently recognised as a reasonable choice in certain kinds of situations', and that for some early North African Christians, 'suicide — like martyrdom — was a mark of religious devotion practised as a way of insuring attainment of immediate salvation' (Battin and Mayo 1980, p. 1).

In Ancient Greece and Rome, suicide was viewed as permissible (at least for the upper classes[1]) if it was chosen for 'the best possible reason' (Alvarez 1980, p. 18). The 'best possible reasons' included to preserve honour; to avoid dishonour or ignominy; as an expression of grief or bereavement; and for high patriotic principle or for a patriotic cause (Farberow 1975b, p. 5; Alvarez 1980, p. 18). There are many famous examples of suicide deaths in the history and mythology of ancient Greece and Rome. Notable among these are the Greek mythological character Jocasta (the mother of Oedipus, King of Thebes), who hanged herself to avoid the grief and shame she felt upon learning of her unwitting complicity in the sins imposed on her by fate (Sophocles 1911, vv. 1213–86); Socrates, the famed ancient Greek philosopher, who killed himself patriotically by drinking hemlock after he was sentenced to death for corrupting the minds of the youth of Athens with his philosophical ideas (see Plato's *Euthyphron, Apology, Crito,* and *Phaedo* in Church's [1903] translation *The trial and death of Socrates,* and in Tredennick's [1969] translation *The last days of Socrates*); and the Roman matron Portia, who, upon learning of the death of Brutus at Philippi, killed herself by swallowing red-hot coals in what French (1985, p. 142) suggests was a kind of *suttee*. Zeno, the founder of Stoic philosophy (who apparently supported Seneca's view that suicide was permissible, but only as a last resort in the case of intractable suffering), also suicided. He apparently hanged himself in disgust at the age of 98 after falling and dislocating a toe! (Farberow 1975b, p. 5). The Roman view of suicide was perhaps among the most liberal during this period. Alvarez comments (1980, p. 23):

> the Romans looked on suicide with neither fear nor revulsion, but as a carefully considered and chosen validation of the way they had lived and the principles they had lived by ... To live nobly also meant to die nobly and at the right moment. Everything depended on the dominant will and a rational choice.

Not all the ancient Greeks and Romans had a permissive attitude to suicide, however. The Pythagoreans, for example, were vehemently opposed to suicide on religious grounds (Wennberg 1989, p. 41). And both the famed ancient Greek philosophers Plato and Aristotle opposed suicide, on religious and secular grounds respectively (Wennberg 1989, p. 42). While Plato was sympathetic to suicide 'when external circumstances became intolerable' (Alvarez 1980, p. 20), Aristotle (Aristotle 1976, p. 130 [1116a 12–15]) was opposed even to this, on the grounds that:

> to kill oneself to escape from poverty or love or anything else that is distressing is not courageous but rather the act of a coward, because it shows weakness of character to run away from hardships, and the suicide endures death not because it is a fine thing to do but in order to escape from suffering.

Aristotle also opposed suicide on the economic grounds that it deprived 'society of one of its productive members' (Wennberg 1989, p. 42). Interestingly, extant taboos against suicide in the city of Athens saw the corpse of the suicide victim 'buried outside the city, its hand cut off and buried separately' (Alvarez 1980, p. 17). Alvarez points out, however, that suicide taboos and the treatment of corpses in these instances were linked not so much as might be thought to religious prohibition or to Aristotelian notions of one's duty to contribute productively to the state. Rather, they were linked 'with the more profound Greek horror of killing one's own kin. By inference, suicide was an extreme case of this, and the language barely distinguishes between self-murder and murder of kindred' (Alvarez 1980, p. 18).

In Rome, on the other hand, while permissive attitudes towards suicide were enshrined in law (Alvarez 1980, p. 22), there were exceptions based on practical and economic grounds. For example, it was a criminal offence for a slave to suicide, since it deprived the master of his capital investment (if this offence was committed within the first six months of a slave being purchased, he could be returned dead or alive to the original master and a refund obtained) (Alvarez 1980, p. 23). Soldiers who suicided were also deemed to have committed a serious offence — 'desertion'. This was because a soldier was 'considered to be the property of the state [a chattel] and his suicide was tantamount to desertion' (Alvarez 1980, p. 23). Finally, it was considered an offence for a criminal to suicide 'in order to avoid trial for a crime for which the punishment would be forfeiture of his estate' (Alvarez 1980, p. 23). Relatives were, however, entitled to defend the accused in his absence. If successful, they would retain property rights to the deceased's estate; if unsuccessful, they would forfeit all property rights, and the deceased's estate would go to the state. Thus, as Alvarez concludes (p. 23):

> suicide was an offence against neither morality nor religion, only against the capital investments of the slave-owning class or the treasury of the state.

There are many other examples of old and ancient cultures in which suicide was tolerated, permitted and even esteemed: the Druids, for example, viewed suicide as a passport to paradise, and as a means of accompanying their departed friends (Alvarez 1980, p. 13); in Japan, suicide was ritualised in the form of *seppuku* or *hara kiri* (more commonly known in the variant spelling *harikari*) (Farberow 1975b, p. 3; Smith and Perlin 1978, p. 1622); and in India and China, the ceremonial sacrifice of widows (of which the Hindu custom of *suttee* is an example) was also common (Wennberg 1989, p. 39). (Whether this 'ceremonial sacrifice' should be viewed as *suicide* rather than *homicide* is, however, a contentious point — see, for example, Daly 1978, pp. 114–33.)

Perhaps some of the most poignant examples of the tolerance, if not the permissibility, of suicide can be found in the early Jewish and Christian traditions. Suicide in the orthodox Jewish tradition has been and continues to be viewed as an abhorrent and heinous sin, and is expressly forbidden (Smith and Perlin 1978, p. 1622; Kaplan and Schwartz 1993). Historically, suicides in Jewish communities have resulted in the people who have suicided being denied full burial honours and other associated rituals, for example, mourning (Farberow 1975b, p. 4; Wennberg 1989, p. 48). There have, however, been some interesting and heart-rending exceptions to this attitude of prohibition. Possibly one of the most famous of these was the mass suicide in 73 AD of 960 Zealots (men, women and children) at Masada, on the western shore of the Dead Sea. In this instance, the Zealots preferred to die at their own hands rather than submit to the Roman legions surrounding their sanctuary (Wennberg 1989, pp. 49–50; Battin 1982, p. 166; Alvarez 1980, p. 17; Farberow 1975b, p. 4). Significantly, the Masada victims are honoured, not condemned in the Jewish tradition (Wennberg 1989, p. 50). In more recent history, in what has been referred to as 'the incident of the ninety-three maidens' (Wennberg 1989, p. 50), 93 Jewish female students and teachers (including the head teacher) chose to suicide rather than to submit themselves to the infamous Gestapo for 'immoral purposes'. Describing the incident, Battin writes (1982, p. 166):

> During the Second World War, the directress of an orthodox Jewish girls' school in a Nazi-occupied city came to understand that her girls, ranging in age from twelve to eighteen, had been kept from extermination in order to provide sexual services for the Gestapo. When the Gestapo announced its intention to avail themselves of these services — ordering the directress to see that the girls were washed and prepared for defloration by 'pure Aryan youth' — she called an assembly and distributed poisons to each of the students, teachers and herself. The ninety-three maidens, as they came to be called, swallowed the poison, recited a final prayer, and died undefiled.

Commenting on this mass suicide, Wennberg (1989, p. 50) explains that, like the suicide of the 400 children facing defilement in the Talmud, rather than this act being viewed as a sin it would be viewed as 'an act of faithfulness to God'; that is, of the victims submitting themselves to God's purpose, rather than to the immoral purposes of the men who would violate them.

The Christian religion, and more specifically its sacred writings, the Bible, also offers some interesting examples of tolerant if not permissible attitudes toward suicide (Farberow 1975b, p. 4; Rauscher 1981, pp. 105–7; Smith and Perlin 1978, p. 1622; Wennberg 1989, p. 47). The first and perhaps most poignant example of all is what Wennberg (1989, p. 45) describes as the Bible's 'curious silence' on the subject of suicide. Indeed, as Smith and Perlin (1978, p. 1622) also observe, 'the Bible contains neither an explicit word for suicide nor an explicit prohibition of the act'.

Despite the apparent omission of an explicit condemnation of suicide, there are a number of significant and famous incidents of suicide mentioned in the Bible:

- Samson, who pleaded 'Let me die with the Philistines' as he toppled the temple filled with God's enemies and was crushed to death (Judges 16: 30);
- Saul, who 'took a sword and fell on it' (1 Samuel 31: 4);
- Saul's armour-bearer, who 'also fell on his sword' (1 Samuel 31: 5);
- Ahithophel, who 'hanged himself, and died' (2 Samuel 17: 3);

- Zimri, who 'burned the King's house down upon himself with fire, and died' (1. Kings 16: 18);
- Judas, who 'went and hanged himself' (Matthew 27: 5).

Another (although less certain) Biblical example of suicide (contrary to popular thought, it may in fact be more an example of euthanasia) is the case of Abimelech (Judges 9: 52), who, in the course of attempting to set fire to a tower in which men and women had locked themselves for protection, was seriously injured after a woman in the tower 'dropped an upper millstone on Abimelech's head and crushed his skull' (Judges 9: 53). Fearing that his manner of death would tarnish his posthumous reputation, he begged his young armour-bearer:

'Draw your sword and kill me, lest men say of me, "A woman killed him". ' So his young man thrust him through, and he died.

(Judges 9: 54)

Some even suggest that the death of Jesus Christ is an example of suicide (Alvarez 1980, p. 12; Rauscher 1981, p. 107). Whether Jesus' death can be regarded as suicide, however, depends entirely on how suicide is defined.

The Bible's apparent failure to prohibit or condemn suicide explicitly, while significant, should not be taken as implying Christian approbation of the act. As Wennberg (1989, p. 46) points out, acts of suicide are — and have long been — incompatible with Christian theology (see also Amundsen 1989, pp. 77–153; Beauchamp 1989, pp. 183–219; Boyle 1989, pp. 221–50; Ferngren 1989, pp. 155–81; Kaplan and Schwartz 1993). The only apparent exception to this prohibition, at least until the teaching of St Augustine, was if suicide was the only option available in order to 'protect one's virginity or to avoid forced apostasy' (Battin 1982, pp. 3, 70–1).

Attitudes of religious prohibition against suicide

Until about 250 AD, attitudes towards suicide were largely permissive, and suicide was common even among the early Christians (Farberow 1975b, p. 6; Alvarez 1980, p. 12; Battin 1982, p. 71). In fact, the rise of Christianity as a persecuted religion brought with it an 'almost epidemic rate of self-destruction', justified as martyrdom (Heyd and Bloch 1981, p. 191). The reasons for this martyrdom are said to have included (Farberow 1975b, p. 6):

pessimism, longing for a better life, a struggle for redemption, and a desire to come before God and live there forever.

The religious fathers of the day were, however, appalled by the 'squandering of human life', and sought to halt it immediately by making it the subject of explicit and absolute religious prohibition (Wennberg 1989, p. 54). Thus, writes Farberow (1975b, p. 6):

As the 4th century began, changes appeared, with the Church adopting a hostile attitude that progressed from tentative disapproval to severe denunciation and punishment. Antagonism toward suicide developed. Suicide became proof that the individual had despaired of God's grace, or that he [sic] lacked faith and was rejecting God by rejecting life, God's gift to man [sic].

The church's emphatic and official prohibition saw a marked decline in the incidence of suicide, with one writer commenting that, by the twelfth century, 'while the Catholic Church held sway in Europe, suicide became practically unknown' (Farberow 1975b, p. 6).

Two highly influential figures in the fight against suicide/martyrdom were the Christian theologians St Augustine (354–430 AD) and St Thomas Aquinas (1225–74). St Augustine's principal theological argument against suicide rested on his interpreting the sixth commandment ('thou shalt not kill') as applying not only to *homicide* (the killing of another), but to *suicide* (the killing of the self) (Heyd and Bloch 1981, p. 191). Rejecting the popular view at the time that suicide was a way of avoiding sin and gaining a passport to eternal paradise, St Augustine countered that 'suicide is itself the gravest sin' (Heyd and Bloch 1981, p. 191). Thus St Augustine denounced suicide 'as a crime under all circumstances' — a view that was quickly ratified as the official view of the Church (Stengel 1970, p. 68). In 452 AD, for example, the Council of Arles declared the act of suicide to be 'an act inspired by diabolical possession'; one century later, the Church set another disincentive to suicide, this time by ordaining that 'the body of the suicide be refused a Christian burial' (Stengel 1970, p. 69).

St Thomas Aquinas' views against suicide were as absolute and as uncompromising as were St Augustine's (Wennberg 1989, p. 65). His arguments were, however, more systematic (Heyd and Bloch 1981, p. 191) and less vulnerable to criticism (Wennberg 1989, p. 66). Central to Aquinas' position were the arguments that suicide constituted an offence to and a violation of one's duty to oneself, the community, and God; he also regarded suicide as 'contrary to the natural law and to charity', and hence wrong (St Thomas Aquinas 1978, pp. 103–4). Whether suicide is, in fact, any of these things has been and remains the subject of much controversy, which will not be settled here (see, for example, Barrington 1983; Battin 1982, 1996; Battin and Mayo 1980; Beauchamp 1978a, 1978b; Brandt 1978, 1980; Brody 1989a; Donnelly 1990; Hume 1983; Kant 1983; Margolis 1975; Szasz 1988; Wennberg 1989).

As Christian religious prohibition against suicide spread across Europe, so too did 'the acts of violence and indignity perpetrated against the dead body' — partially, at least, because of 'fears of evil spirits released by the suicide' (Stengel 1970, p. 69). In some countries, for example, 'a stake was driven through the body and it was buried at the crossroads' (Stengel 1970, p. 69; Farberow 1975b, p. 7); an alternative to skewering the body with a stake was to place a stone on the face of the corpse, which would have the same effect as a stake — namely, it would prevent the victim from 'rising as a ghost to haunt the living' (Alvarez 1980, p. 8). The last degradation of the corpse of a person who had suicided occurred as recently as 1823 in England, when a Mr Griffiths was buried at the crossroads of Grosvenor Place and King's Road, Chelsea (Stengel 1970, p. 69; Alvarez 1980, p. 8). For 50 years after this, however, the bodies of suicide victims were still not treated with full respect, and, if unclaimed, were donated legitimately to schools of anatomy for dissection (Alvarez 1980, p. 8).

In France, as in England, it was also common practice to treat the corpse of a suicide victim in a violent and undignified way. Alvarez writes (1980, p. 9), for example, that:

> varying with local ground rules, the corpse was hanged by the feet, dragged through the streets on a hurdle, burned, thrown on the public garbage.

As well as this, as in other European countries, the property of suicide victims was legally confiscated, and their memories legitimately defamed (Alvarez 1980, p. 9; Stengel 1970, p. 69). Perhaps worst of all, especially for followers of the Christian faith, was the punishment of being denied a proper Christian burial within the consecrated grounds of the church — a punishment which existed around the world right up until the 1960s and 1970s, and which may still exist in some countries even today. In 1968, for example, a United States study of Roman Catholic and Greek Orthodox priests in Los Angeles found that suicide victims were still sometimes — albeit rarely — denied Christian burial (Demopolous 1968, cited in Farberow 1975b, p. 12). Apparently the many sympathetic priests who were burying suicide victims essentially overcame canonical prohibitions against providing Christian burials to suicide victims by accepting that the deaths in question were either 'accidental', 'natural', or the 'irresponsible act of an unsound mind', and hence not a culpable sin (Farberow 1975b, pp. 12–13; Donnelly 1990, p. 9). In the mid-1970s, a similar situation existed in Catholic Italy. In an article examining the psycho–cultural variables in Italian suicide, Farber noted (1975, p. 179):

> Suicide is more severely disapproved and regarded with more horror than in many other countries. A suicide cannot be buried in sacred ground; the family is grievously shamed. On a practical level, for example, an applicant will be rejected by the police force if there has been a suicide in the family. It is understandable, therefore, that a sympathetic doctor, priest, or police official will collaborate in having a suicide reported as a death from some other cause. Such behaviour is widely accepted in the Italian culture, in which family loyalty outweighs the value of civic responsibility.

Significantly, this collaboration has resulted in what Farber describes as a 'severe distortion of official statistics on suicide and the reasons for suicide', with 'mental illness' being cited as the main reason (p. 179). This is because (p. 180):

> in the eyes of the Church, only suicide by a sane person, who is responsible for his [sic] decision, is a sin. The label of mental illness allows for normal, religious burial and provides a shield for the family.

The criminalisation of suicide

Prohibitions against and punishments for suicide were not only enshrined in and made a part of canon law. Under the influence of religious views, sanctions against suicide were also enshrined in (secular) common law (Stengel 1970, p. 70). Opinion varies on when suicide was first deemed a crime in England; some suggest that it could have been as early as the tenth century, while others contend that it was not until as late as 1485 (Stengel 1970, p. 70). By around 1554, however, suicide was definitely 'equated with murder as a criminal offence (*felo de se*) and attempted suicide a misdemeanour' (Stengel 1970, p. 71). Legislation in other European countries also viewed suicide as a crime equivalent to murder, and worse. In 1670, for instance, pressure from the Church saw secular legislation enacted making suicide 'not merely murder but high treason and heresy' (Farberow 1975b, p. 9).

Anti-suicide legislation, like its counterpart in canon law, brought with it inordinate prejudice and penalties against suicide. This resulted in bizarre treatment of those unfortunate enough to be caught surviving a suicide attempt. An example of the gross inhumanity that anti-suicide legislation could both prescribe and enforce can be found in what was probably a public execution held some time during the 1860s in London and reported in the contemporary press. (Note: executions in England were public until 1868 [Carr 1961, p. 336].) Nicholas Ogarev, a Russian exile staying in London at the time, described the incident in a letter to his beloved, Mary Sutherland:

> A man was hanged who had cut his throat, but who had been brought back to life. They hanged him for suicide. The doctor had warned them that it was impossible to hang him

as the throat would burst open and he would breathe through the aperture. They did not listen to his advice and hanged their man. The wound in the neck immediately opened and the man came to life again although he was hanged. It took time to convoke the aldermen to decide the question what was to be done. At length the aldermen assembled and bound up the neck below the wound until he died. Oh my Mary, what a crazy society and what a stupid civilisation.

(quoted in Carr 1961, p. 336)

This example of gross inhumanity and absurdity — and the 'weird vindictiveness [of] condemning a man to death for the crime of having condemned himself to death' (Alvarez 1980, p. 8) — was sanctioned by both the church and the state. Further, this 'weird vindictiveness', as Alvarez (1980, p. 8) describes it, did not end until almost 100 years after this incident occurred. Stengel (1970, p. 71) comments, for example, that even as late as 1946–55 in England and Wales, 5794 people were brought to trial for attempting suicide. Of these, 5447 were found guilty; and of these, 5138 were fined or put on probation, and 308 were sentenced to prison without the option of a fine or probation (Stengel 1970, p. 71). The capricious way in which the law was implemented is exemplified by a 1955 English case in which a 'sentence of two years' imprisonment was imposed on a man for trying to commit suicide in prison' (Stengel 1970, p. 71).

As religious and social opponents of suicide began to lose their influence, the old, cruel, prejudicial, religiously based superstitious attitudes against suicide and attempted suicide gradually changed. Medical dogma replaced religious dogma, and suicide came to be viewed as the act of a 'diseased mind', rather than a diseased ('diabolically possessed') soul. Laws prescribing the desecration of corpses and the confiscation of property were abolished (Farberow 1975b, p. 12). In 1961, England decriminalised suicide (Stengel 1970, p. 71; Glover 1977, p. 170; Browne 1990, p. 10). In Canada, suicide was decriminalised in 1972; and in the United States, while attempted suicide continues to be illegal in some states, suicide itself 'is not illegal in any state' (Browne 1990, p. 10).

Just over 200 years ago, in 1790, France emerged as the first country to repeal its anti-suicide legislation (Stengel 1970, p. 71). Two centuries later, 'both suicide and attempted suicide are not criminal events in any civilised society' (Browne 1990, p. 10).

The medicalisation of suicide

The pressure to reform anti-suicide legislation came mainly from doctors, followed by sympathetic magistrates, and lastly members of the clergy (Stengel 1970, p. 71). However, the medical profession's political lobbying in this instance achieved considerably more than mere legislative reform; it also achieved legitimation of the medicalisation of suicide. In England, for example, soon after the 1961 *Suicide Act* was passed, the Ministry of Health in London advised all doctors and relevant health authorities that:

> attempted suicide was to be regarded as a medical and social problem and that every such case ought to be seen by a psychiatrist.

(Stengel 1970, p. 72)

Whether this 'reform' has been, as Stengel (1970, p. 72) claims, a less 'moralistic and punitive reaction' than that expressed in former legislation remains to be seen. Those who attempt suicide are still frequently the subject of 'negative attitudes', even on the part of attending health care professionals (Bailey 1998; Baume 1988; Donnelly 1990;

Dunleavey 1992; Knight 1992; Lindars 1991; Morse 2001); further, they can still find themselves incapacitated involuntarily by the law. As Beauchamp and Childress (2001, p. 190) point out:

> Although suicide has been decriminalised, a suicide attempt, irrespective of motive, almost universally provides a legal basis for public officers to intervene as well as grounds for involuntary hospitalisation.

As well, social and religious taboos still necessitate a degree of secrecy about the circumstances of a person's 'unexpected illness' or 'accidental death'. Donnelly (1990, p. 9) claims that the legacy of past taboos concerning suicide still sees doctors and coroners pressured into using euphemisms when officially certifying or describing the cause of death of a suicide victim. In one notable example, a British report described as 'accidental' the death of a man 'who just happened to shoot himself while cleaning the muzzle of his gun with his tongue!' (Donnelly 1990, p. 9).

The 'medical gaze' of 'the clinic' (Foucault 1973) may well prove ultimately to be a more humane alternative than the punitive gaze of criminal law — thought to be justified as a system of 'moral accounting' (Foucault 1977, p. 250). When I think of the many people — young and old, vulnerable and desperate — who have been admitted to hospital following a failed suicide attempt, and in whose care I have been involved (mostly in accident and emergency departments or intensive care units), I am inclined to think that the anti-suicide law reforms we inherited in the twentieth century have not really changed the status quo. These law reforms have resulted not so much in the *decriminalisation of suicide* as in the *medicalisation of the law*: where once suicide victims and their families were made to account to the law, now they must account to medicine (psychiatry); where once suicide victims were made to prove their innocence before the law, now they must prove their competence; and where once those who attempted suicide were imprisoned for the crime of stealing the gift of life from God, now they are hospitalised involuntarily for violating the gift of civil liberty from society. As Alvarez observes (1980, p. 31):

> modern suicide has been removed from the vulnerable, volatile world of human beings and hidden safely away in the isolation wards of science. I doubt if Ogarev [the Russian exile] and his ... mistress would have found much in the change to be grateful for.

Over the past few decades there has been a renewed interest in the moral aspects of suicide, prompted largely by the euthanasia/euthanatic suicide (assisted suicide) debate (discussed in Chapter 10 of this book), and increasing public demand for the 'right to die' to be enshrined in law. This renewed interest has, arguably, marked the beginning of a trend back (rightly or wrongly) to permissive attitudes toward suicide and, more specifically, the socio-cultural normalisation of suicide — particularly in cases of intolerable and intractable suffering (see Figure 11.1). It is no small irony, however, that whereas in the ancient world economic considerations provided the grounds for the legal prohibition of suicide (particularly among the poor and working classes) and for the just punishment of those who attempted suicide, in the modern world economic considerations will probably provide many of the grounds for legalising suicide (and more particularly, euthanasia/assisted suicide). This is especially likely in the contexts where the financial and other material costs associated with caring for people with end-stage illnesses becomes burdensome and go beyond what can be 'reasonable sustained' (examples of which were given in Chapter 6 of this book; see also Battin 1982, 1996).

Defining suicide

Before examining some of the moral issues raised by the suicide question, it is necessary first to establish at least a working definition of *suicide* — a term which, incidentally, entered the English language only in 1651 (Wennberg 1989 p. 17; Battin 1982, pp. 22–58).

The word *suicide* comes from the Latinate *sui*, 'of oneself' and *cidium*, 'a slaying' (from *caedere*, 'to kill'). Like many other terms used in moral discourse, *suicide* is not easy to define; indeed, there is no universally agreed definition of what suicide is, or of what criteria should be met in order for an act to count as an instance of suicide. As Margolis (1978, reprinted in Beauchamp and Perlin 1978, pp. 92–3) explains, the 'culturally variable character of suicide' has given rise to many competing views on what it is, with the unhelpful consequence that some acts have been included as suicide and others firmly excluded. This, in turn, has had some important practical consequences, including the difficulty of ascertaining accurate and comparable statistics on the incidence and causes of suicide (Beauchamp 1980, pp. 68–9).

For Wennberg (1989, p. 17), wrestling with the problem of defining *suicide* is to be taught a lesson in 'linguistic humility'. Nevertheless, our commonsense notions of what suicide is, our ability to recognise instances of suicide and to distinguish these from other kinds of death (for example, homicide, patricide, matricide, fratricide, sororicide, infanticide, regicide and euthanasia or euthanatic suicide [Battin 1982, p. 20]), and the very existence of terms in our language which make it possible to speak of suicide as a distinctive kind of death, all provide grounds for optimism about our ability to achieve at least a working — if not a universal — definition of suicide.

According to Stengel (1970, p. 77), a commonsense notion of suicide can be expressed in the following terms:

> A person, having decided to end his [or her] life, or acting on a sudden impulse to do so, kills himself [or herself], having chosen the most effective methods available and having made sure that nobody interferes. When he [or she] survives he [or she] is said to have failed and the act is called an unsuccessful suicide attempt. Death is the only purpose of this act and therefore the only criterion of success. Failure may be due to any of the following causes: the sense of purpose may not have been strong enough, or the act may have been undertaken half-heartedly because it was not quite genuine; the subject was ignorant of the limitations of the method; or he [or she] was lacking in judgment and determination through mental illness.

This definition is not, of course, without controversy. For example: What constitutes a 'genuine' suicide attempt? When is a suicide attempt to be regarded as 'half-hearted' as opposed to 'whole-hearted'? (see also Knight 1992). Further, as Stengel himself points out, the definition may not do justice to what has become 'a very common and varied behaviour pattern' (1970, p. 77). Nevertheless, it provides an important insight into the kinds of criteria that should be met in order for an act to count as suicide. One such criterion is that of *intention* — specifically, the *intention to end one's life* (Margolis 1975, reprinted in Beauchamp and Perlin 1978, p. 95). As Beauchamp points out (1980, p. 70), central to what is called the 'prevailing definition' of suicide is the following premise: 'Suicide occurs if and only if there is an intentional termination of one's own life'.

Beauchamp (1980, pp. 73–9) suggests that other criteria should be met in order for an act to count as suicide, including the following:

1. death is chosen voluntarily (that is, is free of coercive or manipulative influences);
2. an active means of death is chosen;
3. death is caused by the person desiring death (one dies by 'one's own hand');
4. death is *self-regarding* (rather than altruistic or *other-regarding*); and
5. the person seeking death does not have a fatal or terminal illness.

Windt suggests similar criteria of suicide (all of which have been mentioned in the suicide literature). These are:

1. death [must be] caused by the actions or behaviour of the deceased;
2. the deceased wanted, desired, or wished death;
3. the deceased intended, chose, decided or willed to die;
4. the deceased knew that death would result from his [or her] behaviour; and that
5. the deceased was responsible for his [or her] own death.

(Windt 1980, p. 41, tabulations added)

At first glance, these and similar criteria of suicide appear helpful. On closer analysis, however, a number of problems quickly become apparent — not least the problem of so-called 'exceptional cases', and whether the criteria listed are relevant to or can be applied appropriately and meaningfully to these cases. Consider, for example, the cases of people engaging in dangerous and potentially life-threatening ('suicidal') sports (for instance, bungee jumping, mountain climbing, racing car driving, hang gliding); dangerous work activities (being a member of a bomb disposal squad or a combat soldier are paradigm examples here); or other life-threatening activities such as cigarette smoking, eating and drinking excessively, illicit drug taking, and so on. In all these cases, it is probably true that the people concerned chose the activities in question; were aware of the potential threats the activities posed to their lives and wellbeing; voluntarily engaged in the activities chosen; and, were they to die as a result of engaging in these activities, were 'responsible for their own deaths', insofar as they were witting accomplices to the activities and their associated risks. Further, while the people concerned might not have intended their own (accidental) deaths, they nevertheless foresaw their deaths as a possibility associated with the risky activities they had engaged in, and thereby, ipso facto, can be said to have intended their own demise. Given the criteria for suicide outlined above, it seems we are committed to accepting that people who die as a result of their deliberately engaging in dangerous sporting activities, work activities or lifestyles have, in essence, suicided. Yet, this does not seem to accord with our intuitions on the matter — nor does it sit comfortably with what we would perhaps ordinarily regard as suicide. Let us examine another example to see if this will clarify the matter.

In 1982, Barney Clark, aged 62, became the first human being to receive an artificial (mechanical) heart (Beauchamp and Childress 2001, p. 188; Rachels 1983). Recognising that this medical experiment had the potential to make Barney Clark's life burdensome, his doctor, Willem Kolff, gave him a key that could be used to turn off the compressor sustaining the artificial heart's action. Defending his decision to supply this key, Dr Kolff argued that if Barney Clark:

suffers and feels it isn't worth it any more, he has a key that he can apply ... I think it is entirely legitimate that this man whose life has been extended should have the right to cut it off if he doesn't want it, if life ceases to be enjoyable.

(cited in Beauchamp and Childress 2001, p. 188)

The conceptual dilemma which arises here is this: if Barney Clark had chosen to use the key he had been given, and had turned off the compressor driving his artificial heart, which of the following statements would have been the most accurate description of his action and the cause of his death:

1. forgoing extraordinary means of life-sustaining treatment;
2. withdrawing from an experiment;
3. letting nature take its course;
4. natural death;
5. euthanasia;
6. suicide?

To complicate the issue, as Beauchamp and Childress point out (2001, p. 188):

If [Clark] had refused to accept the artificial heart in the first place, few would have labeled his act a suicide. His overall condition was extremely poor, the artificial heart was experimental, and no suicidal intention was evident. If, on the other hand, Clark had intentionally shot himself with a gun while on the artificial heart, the act would have been characterised as suicide.

And, to complicate the issue still further, what if Barney Clark had consented to receiving the heart in the belief that the risks associated with the experiment were so great that a hastened death would be assured? Could this be classified as a kind of suicide?

Part of the difficulty in sorting out the conceptual confusion surrounding the development of an adequate definition of and criteria for suicide can be linked to the lingering legacy of varying socio-cultural historical and religious taboos against suicide. Beauchamp and Childress (1989, p. 223) suggest, for example, that we often shield acts of which we approve (or at least acts of which we do not disapprove) from the stigmatising label of 'suicide' — preferring instead to use terms that are more socially acceptable, such as 'euthanasia' or 'withdrawing extraordinary life-saving treatment', and similar notions. If this is correct, it is ironic, considering that the term 'suicide' was first adopted in the seventeenth century as a more 'acceptable' alternative to the then contemporary usages 'self-murder' and 'self-slaughter', which were regarded by more liberal-minded people of the day as having unacceptably negative connotations (Battin 1982, pp. 22, 58).

In the light of these considerations, perhaps an important first step in developing a workable definition of and criteria for suicide is to demystify suicide, and to strip it of the taboos and stigmatisations which still seem to linger around it — and which may encourage people to be less than intellectually honest when speaking of its incidence and cause. A second and related step is to modify the negatively connoted language that tends to be used in referring to and discussing suicide. In this instance, the problem of language is highly significant, and should not be underestimated. As Wennberg explains (1989, p. 17):

'suicide' is not a neutrally descriptive term like 'cat', 'car', or 'flower'. Rather, it carries with it a strong negative connotation, especially when it is part of the phrase 'commit suicide'.

For one typically does not *commit* X where X is either something approved or something of neutral standing (cf. 'commit murder', 'commit a felony', 'commit a crime', 'commit adultery', 'commit a sin', 'commit treason', 'commit a *faux pas*', etc.).

The lesson here is important and obvious: the use of the phrase 'committed suicide' (as opposed to using the term *suicided*) is misleading and unhelpful — not least because it seems to imply the commission of a crime, or even a sin, when clearly there has been none.

A third and final step toward developing a working definition of and criteria for suicide is to reinstate the authority of our own ordinary commonsense experience of the world, and our collective experience-based knowledge of what is and is not an act of suicide or attempted suicide. One reason for this is that, in the ultimate analysis, the distinction between suicide and other types of death (for example, euthanasia) may rest not on sophisticated philosophical criteria, but on our fine intuitions informed by life-experience. I suspect, however, that in the main, conceptual clarity in regard to what is and is not an act of suicide will rest on something far more substantial than abstract criteria or even well informed intuition. Rather, the matter will be decided by appealing to:

1. the known intentions and motivations of the person who has died (for instance, whether the death was pursued as 'an alleged solution for the ills of dying' [euthanasia], or pursued as an 'alleged' cure for the ills of living [suicide] [Donnelly 1990, p. 9]);
2. the context in which the person died;
3. whether the person who died genuinely believed there was no other alternative besides death in order to alleviate his or her suffering, or to transcend the life circumstances which for him or her had become unbearable.

The problem remains, however, that ascertaining these things may be just as difficult as establishing reliable criteria for suicide. Nevertheless, it is important that suicide be defined. One reason for this is that without an adequate definition of suicide it will remain extremely difficult to assess accurately the incidence, cause and appropriate means of preventing suicide. It will also be difficult to eradicate the spurious distinction which is sometimes drawn between 'genuine' and 'non-genuine' suicide attempts, with the tragic consequence that some who are suffering and needing help will be dismissed as malingerers, and worse, as not suffering or needing help at all.

(To advance understanding on the raw suffering and despair that suicidal people experience, see in particular: Williams [1997] *Cry of pain: understanding suicide and self-harm*; Heckler [1994] *Waking up alive: the descent to suicide and return to life*; and Knight's [1992] discussion on the suffering of suicide.)

Finally, without an adequate definition of suicide it will make it difficult to engage in substantive moral debate on the ethical aspects of suicide, and to respond effectively and appropriately to the many moral problems raised by the suicide question, some of which are considered below.

Before continuing, however, a brief clarification is required on the working definitions of the terms 'suicide' and 'parasuicide' to be used in the remainder of this chapter, and on the distinction which might otherwise be drawn between 'suicide' (as presently being considered in this chapter) and 'euthanasia' (as considered in the previous chapter).

Although there is no universally agreed definition of suicide, and, as shown, the term itself is difficult to define (see also Soubrier 1993), suicide is generally recognised as being one of the five medical–legal classifications of modes of death, which are taken to include (in addition to suicidal death): accidental, natural, homicidal, and undetermined death (Colt 1991, pp. 263–4). Furthermore, while acknowledging the many difficulties associated with formulating a precise and universally agreed definition of suicide, there is a strong sense in which suicide (at least in the Western world) can be meaningfully understood as:

> a conscious act of self-induced annihilation, best understood as a multidimensional malaise in a needful individual who defines an issue for which the suicide is perceived as the best solution.
>
> (Shneidman 1985, p. 203)

A more elaborate explication of this view is as follows (advanced by Edwin Shneidman [1993, p. 3], popularly regarded as the 'father' of contemporary suicidology [Leenaars 1993, p. xi]):

> My principal assertion about suicide has two branches. The first is that suicide is a multifaceted event and that biological, cultural, sociological, interpersonal, intrapsychic, logical, conscious and unconscious, and philosophical elements are present, in various degrees, in each suicide event.
>
> The second branch of my assertion is that, in the distillation of each suicide event, its essential element is a *psychological* one; that is to say, each suicidal drama occurs in the mind of a unique individual. Suicide is purposive. Its purpose is to respond to or redress certain psychological needs. There are many pointless deaths but there are no needless suicides. Suicide is a concatenated, complicated, multidimensional, conscious and unconscious 'choice' of the best possible practical solution to a perceived problem, dilemma, impasse, crisis, or desperation.

Parasuicide (a term which came into usage in the late 1960s in an attempt to overcome the confusion associated with using the term 'attempted suicide' [see Kreitman 1969; Williams 1997, p. 68]) can, in turn, be defined as:

> An act with non-fatal outcome, in which an individual deliberately initiates a non-habitual behaviour that, without intervention from others, will cause self-harm, or deliberately ingests a substance in excess of the prescribed or generally recognised therapeutic dosage, and which is aimed at realising changes which the subject desired via the actual or expected physical consequences.
>
> (Williams 1997, p. 69)

For the purposes of this discussion, both suicide and parasuicide are taken here as being the 'unequivocal expression of raw suffering' (and it might be added 'psychache' [Shneidman 1993]) of individuals — a suffering from which, for a variety of reasons (not always known or understood by others), these individuals have not been able to secure relief (Heckler 1994, p. xxiv). Suicide ideation (suicidal thoughts) and suicidal behaviour are also taken here as being 'the result of extreme and unusual human predicaments' which require our deepest and most empathic understanding (Heckler 1994, p. xxv), not our derision as has so frequently been the case (see Bailey 1994, 1998).

Suicide, as being considered in this chapter, is taken here as referring to a different kind of death that might otherwise be brought about by voluntary active euthanasia or physician–assisted suicide. While euthanasia, physician–assisted suicide and 'unassisted' suicide (the topic of this chapter) share many features in common, as we will go on to see, there are also some significant differences between them. One such difference was captured recently by the following insightful comments made in class by an on-site overseas student undertaking a Bachelor of Nursing (post-registration) degree at RMIT University in Melbourne, Australia:

> As I see it, in the case of euthanasia/assisted suicide, the person wants to live, but *cannot* (and it is too hard to die); whereas in the case of 'suicide proper', the person can live, yet *does not* want to (it is too hard to live).
>
> (Su Chia Hsian, personal communication)

Other differences will become more apparent as the discussion in this chapter is advanced. One key difference, however, warrants mention here: whereas euthanasia and physician–assisted suicide tends to be conducted in the context of a breakdown in physical health and wellbeing, suicide (as being considered here) tends to occur in the context of a breakdown in mental health and wellbeing; that is, it is linked in important ways to a lethal combination of the psychogenic distress states of depression, hopelessness, despair, and apathy (Colt 1991; Firestone 1997; Heckler 1994; Hendin 1998; Leenaars 1993; Lester and Tallmer 1994; Remafedi 1994a; Shneidman 1993; Williams 1997).

Suicide: some moral considerations

As discussed earlier under the subheading 'Socio-cultural attitudes to suicide: a brief historical overview', the Judaeo-Christian traditions have, for the most part, regarded suicide as the gravest sin imaginable, and as constituting the most serious violation of one's duties to oneself, to others and to God. These views have been extremely influential and, not surprisingly, the subject of much philosophical debate. Today, however, as Knight (1992, p. 262) correctly points out, 'religiously speaking, the notion of suicide as an unforgivable sin has few, if any, defenders in contemporary moral philosophy'. Further, unlike the days when religious prohibition saw suicide condemned as a grossly immoral act, it is difficult today to find tenable moral arguments against the suicide of people who are able to choose autonomously to end their own lives (Knight 1992, p. 262). Nevertheless, a number of troubling questions remain about the ethics or morality of suicide, such as: Is there a right to suicide? If so, what conditions must be satisfied before this right can be claimed? What are the obligations of others in regard to those contemplating or attempting suicide? Is there a duty to prevent suicide? If so, under what conditions should a suicide be prevented? It is to briefly answering these questions that the remainder of this discussion now turns.

Autonomy and the right to suicide

Fundamental to Western moral thinking is the principle of autonomy. As discussed in Chapter 3 of this book, the moral principle of autonomy prescribes that a person's considered choices should be respected — even if others disagree with them or regard them as foolish — provided they do not interfere with or harm the significant moral interests of others. If we accept this principle, we must also accept that people who choose autonomously to suicide are entitled to have their choices respected, and further, that it would be morally indefensible to prevent these people from exercising their choices. By this view, as Beauchamp explains (1980, p. 100):

If people are autonomous, then they have the right to be left alone and to do with their lives as they wish, so long as they are sufficiently free of responsibilities to others. From this perspective, the intervention in the life of a suicide is simply an unjust deprivation of liberty.

Jonathan Glover argues along similar lines (1977, p. 171), explaining that once it is admitted that suicide need not always be regarded as an 'irrational symptom of mental disturbance' (see also Wennberg 1989, p. 39), then:

[it] is a matter for each person's free choice: other people should have nothing to say about it, and the question for someone contemplating it is simply one of whether his [or her] future life will be worth living.

It is far from certain, however, that people contemplating or attempting suicide are, in fact, entitled to be 'left alone and to do with their lives as they wish' (Beauchamp 1980, p. 100), or that 'other people should have nothing to say about it' (Glover 1977, p. 171). There are a number of reasons for this. First, an act of suicide is never without moral consequences: not only does it have an impact on the significant moral interests of the person suiciding, but it can significantly affect the important moral interests of others (as stated earlier, between six and ten people can be directly and significantly affected by the suicide of another). As experience tells us, suicide can shatter, injure and destroy the lives of other people; it can also cause substantial loss to society (see also Battin 1982, 1996). Where suicides do affect the significant moral interests of others, there are at least prima facie grounds for justifying paternalistic intervention to prevent those suicides occurring. As well as this, where other people's significant moral interests are at stake, there may even be an obligation on the part of people contemplating suicide not to proceed with planned actions aimed at ending their own lives (Brandt 1978, p. 128) — although it is an open question just how realistic this demand is in the case of people suffering severe psychological distress.

In the light of these circumstances, it is evident that claims to autonomy *alone* are not sufficient to justify an unequivocal acceptance of a person's decision to suicide, or to justify non-intervention or 'non-postvention' (counselling and therapy after a suicide attempt [Battin 1982, p. 16]) in the case of contemplated or attempted suicide. Of course, there is always the possibility that the concerns or interests of others may not be strong enough to override a person's autonomous choice to suicide. This, however, is something which must be determined by careful evaluation and a 'balancing of considerations' of all the moral interests involved (Beauchamp and Perlin 1978, p. 91), not just by an uncritical deontological acceptance of the moral principle of autonomy. Such a calculation might even show that a contemplated suicide, once carried out, should indeed be permitted in the interests of others. For example, the suicide of a long-term abusing spouse might be shown to be more permissible morally than the homicide of his abused wife and children. Whether this would really be a morally desirable outcome, however, is a contentious point and unfortunately one which is beyond the scope of this work to address.

A second reason why it is not clear that people contemplating or attempting suicide should not have their choices interfered with is that the *quality* of the autonomy behind the choice may not be optimal. As discussed in Chapter 3 of this book, as a *concept* (to be distinguished here from a *principle*), autonomy refers to a person's independent and self-contained ability to decide. At issue in the case of suicide is the question of whether a person contemplating suicide is really capable of making the evaluative, deliberative and reflective choices that are fundamental to a 'rational' and autonomous decision to suicide. While it is true that even so-called 'incompetent' people are still capable of making self-interested choices (see, for example, the discussion on competency in Chapter 6 of this book), the extent to which the choices of these people should be respected is not something that can be decided solely on the basis of the demands prescribed by the moral principle of autonomy; there are other moral considerations that need to be taken into account — including the moral demand to prevent otherwise avoidable harm to people, which a suicide-death could cause.

The issue of the quality of a suicidal person's autonomous choice to kill himself or herself is an important one and, even when considered from a clinical as opposed to a philosophical perspective, has an important bearing on deciding the ethical acceptability of paternalistic interventions aimed at preventing people from suiciding (see also Rudnick 2002).

It has been suggested that depression 'is a substantial part of the picture of at least 50 per cent of suicides' (Knight 1992, pp. 249–50). Research in the United Kingdom, however, has shown that *70 per cent* of suicides involve people suffering from major depression (Williams 1997, p. 51). While depression alone may not result in suicide, when it is coupled with abiding and intolerable feelings of hopelessness about the future, despair and apathy, the risk of suicide is extremely high (Firestone 1997; Heckler 1994; Hendin 1998; Knight 1992; Williams 1997). Of importance to the discussion at this point is the consideration that feelings of depression, hopelessness, apathy and despair can have a significant and far-reaching impact on a person's ability to make 'truly' autonomous choices. As has long been recognised in the bioethics literature, these feelings can:

- restrict people's abilities to evaluate and calculate correctly the range of possibilities and probabilities available when planning and making judgments about their lives and future prospects (Brandt 1978, p. 131; Beauchamp 1980, p. 101);
- skew calculations of the probable harms and benefits that may flow from suicide (as Beauchamp [1980, p. 101] points out, 'without depression, persons might make quite different calculations even when their situation is dire');
- result in suicidal people overestimating the magnitude and insolubility of their problems (Knight 1992, p. 266);
- result in impulsive and imprudent choices which might otherwise not have been made (Heyd and Bloch 1981, p. 187).

In short, feelings of depression, hopelessness, apathy and despair can undermine in very significant ways a person's ability to make sound autonomous choices. The question remains, however, of whether these feelings and a possible associated diminution in the ability to make sound autonomous choices are of a nature that justifies paternalistic intervention to prevent a person suiciding — including using invasive procedures to resuscitate someone who has attempted suicide. Or would such intervention — no matter how benevolent — still constitute an unacceptable violation of the moral principle of autonomy?

The short answer to these questions is that intervention may not only be justified, but may even be required, in the interests of both promoting a person's autonomy and saving a worthwhile life. On this point, Jonathan Glover explains (1977, pp. 176–7):

> Where we think someone bent on suicide has a life worth living, it is always legitimate to reason with him [or her] and to try and persuade him [or her] to stand back and think again. There is no case against reasoning, as it in no way encroaches on the person's

autonomy. There is a strong case in its favour, as where it succeeds it will prevent the loss of a worthwhile life. (If the person's life turns out not be worthwhile, he [or she] can always change his [or her] mind again.) And if persuasion fails, the outcome is no worse than it would otherwise have been.

Glover goes on to contend that where suicidal tendencies are the product of temporary depressive mood-swings — for instance, where the person 'alternates between very much wanting to go on living and moods of suicidal depression' — then intervention aimed at overriding a decision to suicide 'is less disrespectful of autonomy than overriding a preference that plays a stable role in a person's outlook' (p. 178). If, for example, a person repeatedly and persistently attempts suicide, and the underlying preference (that is, to die) informing these attempts remains constant, then the onus is on would-be 'rescuers' or interveners to reconsider their own judgments about whether the life of the person attempting suicide is, in fact, worthwhile and worth living, or whether they have been mistaken in their views. Unpleasant as it may be, the demand in the latter instance may be an overriding one in favour of *not* intervening to save the person's life (Glover 1977, p. 178). Before this position is accepted, however, there are at least prima facie grounds for asserting that the following five conditions must be met:

1. that the decision to suicide is based on a realistic assessment of the life-circumstances or situation at hand (Motto 1983, pp. 443–6; Knight 1992, p. 254);
2. that the person contemplating suicide has made an 'exhaustive examination' of all available options and has taken into account the 'various possible "errors" and [made] appropriate rectifications of his [or her] initial evaluation' (Brandt 1978, p. 132);
3. that the thought processes used in reaching the decision to suicide have not been impaired by severe emotional distress, feelings of hopelessness and despair, mental illness or the adverse side-effects of drugs (Knight 1992, p. 254);
4. that the degree of ambivalence between wanting to live and wanting to die is minimal (Motto 1983, pp. 443–6; Glover 1977, p. 178; Donnelly 1990, p. 8); and
5. that the desire and motivation to suicide is of a nature that 'uninvolved observers from their community or social group [would find] understandable' (Knight 1992, p. 254).

While the satisfaction of these criteria may not always result in the prevention of morally undesirable consequences in situations involving people wanting to suicide, it may nevertheless result in more appropriate assessments of when it is right and when it is not right to paternalistically override a person's autonomous decision to suicide.

One problem which emerges here, however, is that, even if these criteria are not satisfied, does that necessarily justify paternalistic intervention to prevent a person suiciding? What if the suicidal person in question is in a state of intolerable suffering as in the *Chabot case* discussed in the previous chapter? Here the additional question arises: Can those who are suffering intolerably and intractably (whether on account of physical or mental illness or some other state of physical or psychogenic distress) be expected decently to go on living? Or should people in these situations be released from the 'obligation to live' — if, indeed, it is an obligation — irrespective of their ability to decide autonomously what is in their own best interests? Are others entitled morally to force a person to go on living a life characterised by excruciating feelings of depression, hopelessness, apathy, despair and a sense that life has lost all meaning and purpose?

It is not unreasonable to hold that a person in this state would prefer death to life. As Glover points out (1977, p. 174):

> Most of us prefer to be anaesthetised for a painful operation. If most of my life were to be on that level, I might opt for a permanent anaesthesia, or death.

Margolis (1978, p. 96) argues, however, that while prolonged anaesthesia may indeed be 'prudentially preferable to enduring pain', the desire to reduce pain in itself 'cannot justify suicide to end pain as a decision of a prudential sort'. One reason for this is that enduring even intolerable pain may, in the ultimate analysis, still be preferable to no life at all (Margolis 1978, p. 96; see also Glover 1977, p. 174). Another reason is that to allow suicide as a means of alleviating suffering is to compound the hopelessness underpinning the suffering of suicide; it is also to abandon as hopeless those who have abandoned themselves as hopeless, and thereby to violate a fundamental professional ethic of care and responsibility to aid the distressed (see also Murphy 1983, p. 442).

If suicide is viewed as a 'violent statement about human connections, broken and maintained' (Lifton 1979, p. 239), and not simply as a matter of exercising an autonomous choice (as Hauerwas [1986, p. 107] reminds us, 'life has a purpose beyond simply being autonomous'), perhaps our moral obligations toward those contemplating or attempting suicide will become clearer. In particular, as Knight's (1992) discussion on the suffering of suicide clarifies, there needs to be a much greater understanding of the excruciating sense of hopelessness and despair that underlies and motivates many a decision to suicide. Drawing on the remarkable work by Heckler (1994), there also needs to be a much greater appreciation by others that behind every suicide and parasuicide is a life story of 'overwhelming circumstances'. As Stubbs (1994, p. xii) reminds us, in the foreword to Heckler's insightful study *Waking up alive: the descent to suicide and return to life*:

> Suicide is caused by feelings not by facts — a similar event may be borne by one person and may lead another to suicide or attempted suicide. Events, feelings and experiences add strands to a net that can drag you under. The final straw can be the weight of gossamer but the combined effect can be devastating. Or the final straw can weigh like an iron girder ... Unless we have stood on the edge of the precipice of our own life, we can only begin to grasp how it feels.

Once these and related considerations are understood, it may become clearer that the way to remedy the suffering underlying a decision to suicide is not to do away with the sufferer, but to do away with the sense of hopelessness and despair fuelling the suffering. This, however, requires great compassion, empathy and commitment on the part of those intervening and preventing people suiciding. As Knight puts it (1992, p. 266):

> Intervention in suicide involves walking down that 'dark road' and immersing oneself into that world in which the suicidal person is living. One soon discovers that most suicidal persons have a predisposition to overestimate the magnitude and insolubility of their problems. Coupled with this, as has been emphasised by those 'who have been there', is an exaggerated negative view of the outside world, of themselves, and of the future. An

awareness of what and how a suicidal person is thinking and feeling may lead those intervening to see quickly that the suicidal person's plight has a way out, and soon hope begins to dawn.

Suicide prevention: some further considerations

It is probably true that most health care professionals feel obliged to:

- try and persuade people contemplating suicide to change their minds;
- counsel those who have lost their sense of hope, purpose and meaning in life, in order to modify their perceptions and regain a more optimistic outlook on the future;
- resuscitate people who have attempted suicide and who are on the brink of death; and
- treat the injuries of people whose suicide attempts have failed.

Whether health care professionals do, in fact, have these obligations may, in the end, be a matter to be decided not by moral theory, or even by law, but by empathy, compassion, kindness and wisdom, informed by a profound understanding of human vulnerability and suffering, together with a commitment to take each case on its own unique and individual merit. Either way, it is important not to forget that our obligation to render aid to a person contemplating or attempting suicide is as strong as it would be to aid any person in distress (Brandt 1980, pp. 129–31), and that this may require more than merely protecting a person's autonomy; it may require the more substantive task of protecting a person's genuine human welfare, and restoring in them a sense of hope that, often due to circumstances quite beyond their control, has abandoned them.

Conclusion

Some may find it amenable to view suicide as the manifestation of a mental illness, and hence something that is 'irrational' and 'irresponsible' and ipso facto quite beyond the realms of moral inquiry (see, for example, Beauchamp and Childress 2001; Heyd and Bloch 1981; Margolis 1978; Stengel 1970; Wennberg 1989). This discussion has shown, however, that even if suicide is the product of mental illness or extreme emotional distress, depression, or other psychogenic pain states, it still has a profound moral dimension, and still requires those involved in suicide prevention and intervention to justify their views and actions, and not to merely assume that these are in themselves morally correct just because they have as their end the preservation of life or the maximisation of autonomy.

Suicide and parasuicide is an issue of importance and concern to *all* nurses, not just to those working in the area of mental health. How well nurses and others respond to the moral issues raised depends, however, on a variety of factors — including the success with which suicide is stripped of the taboos which still surround it, and the degree to which suicide is demystified as a desperate act aimed at transcending a situation which a distressed person has come to perceive as hopeless.

Some years ago I was involved in the care of a woman who had attempted suicide by pouring a can of petrol over herself and setting fire to it. She arrived in casualty with 100 per cent burns to her body. Incredibly, despite the horrendous injuries her body had sustained, her eyes were unharmed. The extent of her burns made it impossible to insert an intravenous line in the usual way, and a cut-down (which involves a surgical incision to expose a deeply situated vein) had to be performed. I remember the doctor looking at me while he was performing the cut-down, and gasping in horror as the woman's burnt flesh parted in his hands. Nevertheless, this compassionate man succeeded in inserting the intravenous line, and consoled the woman as he did so. As we all worked diligently to retrieve this injured life, the woman looked on smiling, and reassuring us all with the words, 'Don't worry dears, I will be all right'. I remember looking up at this woman and, on observing her terrible injuries, thinking how desperate she must have been to have engaged in such an act. She, however, looked back at me with eyes that were clear and shining, and, bizarre as this whole scene was, I could see that she had found incredible peace within herself. The image of her burnt and tortured body did not sit well with the peace expressed in her eyes, but I knew that she had achieved her goal, and that it would be only a matter of time before she would be released from the suffering that had motivated her to undertake such a desperate act. Her death a day or two later was no surprise. Yet I still cannot help thinking that this woman paid a terrible price for the peace she eventually found in death, and could not find in life.

During the same year, I was involved in the care of a man who had also attempted suicide, in this instance by placing the muzzle of a gun in his mouth and shooting himself. He failed in his attempt to kill himself, however, and succeeded only in destroying one side of his face. After receiving plastic surgery to repair the serious gunshot wound sustained, he was admitted to intensive care. Unlike the woman who had set fire to herself, however, he was not at peace within himself. As he lay corpse-like on his bed, I remember noting that his eyes were like the eyes of a dead man — fully dilated, dull, and unresponsive to light. It was as though his soul had died, and nothing mattered any more. Once, when his plastic surgeon visited to check his wounds, the man handed the doctor a note. Written on the note were the words: 'Dear Dr X — did you do this [the surgical repair] for your sake or mine?'. Understandably, the surgeon, who was a compassionate and gentle man, was devastated. Shortly after being transferred out of the intensive care unit to a general ward, the man climbed out through a toilet window and plunged to his death several storeys below. Many of the staff were left feeling that they had failed this man. The circumstances motivating his initial suicidal attempt had not seemed insurmountable to them, and they sincerely believed he was 'better'. But he was not better, and eventually he too achieved his goal of death. As I recall the case of this desperate and hopeless man, I cannot forget the costly suffering and distress of those he left behind — especially his wife and young children. How different things would have been if he, like the people caring for and about him, could have perceived that his problems were not as overwhelming as he thought, and that it was not necessary to take the desperate action that he ultimately took. To this day, I am reminded by this case of the importance of never underestimating the capacity of human beings to feel deeply and to suffer profoundly on account of things which seem (though they may not necessarily be) insurmountable, and of how feelings of desperation and hopelessness associated with problems perceived as insurmountable can so easily override the desire to go on living.[2]

In June of 1993, a Victorian coroner's court was reported to have found that the suicide of five severely depressed patients at Larundel Hospital was, among other things, a regrettable consequence of a well-intended but nevertheless misguided priority being given to upholding patients' rights to confidentiality (i.e. the 'right' not to be observed too closely) at the expense of patient care. Further, there had been a less than optimal level of commitment to 'patient–centred *continuity of care* rather than changes in treating medical personnel due to patient progress' (Pegler 1993, p. 26, emphasis added). The coroner is reported to have also found that 'the most important issue arising from the inquests was family and carer involvement in treatment', and that 'a policy needed to be developed on the conflict between patient rights and patient care' (Pegler 1993, p. 26).

Whether matters such as these can — or, indeed, should — be the subject of institutional policy is a debatable point. As experience tells us, even the very best of policies may still fail to prevent this kind of situation from occurring. Nevertheless, it is clear that there is room for improvement in the care and treatment of those contemplating or attempting suicide, and, more importantly, in understanding the moral issues involved in caring for those who, for whatever reason, are unable to care about themselves. It is also clear that, in securing these improvements, nurses must ensure that, in attempting to uphold the moral rights of their emotionally distressed, severely depressed and mentally unwell patients, they do not lose sight of the importance of also protecting and promoting their patients' *welfare and wellbeing* — something which may not always be secured by paying homage to abstract moral rights and principles. By doing this, nurses, and others involved in caring for people who are contemplating suicide or who have already attempted suicide, may well succeed in helping to prevent and remedy the terrible sufferings and tragedies that have become so characteristic of the whole phenomenon of suicide in our community and in the world.

CASE SCENARIO AND CRITICAL QUESTIONS

Case scenario

'Gabby', a woman in her early forties and married with children, was admitted to a general medical ward of a metropolitan hospital after taking an overdose of anti-depressant medication. Gabby had suffered from depression since she was 15 years old. Her suicide attempt in this instance occurred during a period of what she described as 'acute depression' (Morse 2001, p. 235). While in hospital, Gabby was extremely sensitive to the prejudicial way she was being perceived and treated by nursing staff on account of her being an 'OD' (overdose). Reflecting on the experience she stated:

> I got the feeling that, was, *you bloody idiot, you shouldn't have, you know, you need to be in a nut ward, not up [here]. We've got really genuinely sick people here* … and I felt that they [the nurses], that's what they thought, that I wasn't genuinely ill. [emphasis added]
>
> (quoted in Morse 2001, p. 238)

When recounting her experience she was able to recall only one instance where she felt she was shown any sort of care:

> ... and, you know, when you cry, I mean 'cause you're so depressed, you cry ... only one male nurse came up to me and said, he put his arm around me and he said, 'Look, it can only get better, sweetheart'.
>
> (quoted in Morse 2001, p. 240)

Critical questions

1. What are your responsibilities as a professional caregiver in regard to caring for people who have attempted unsuccessfully to suicide?
2. How might you have maximised Gabby's moral interests, welfare and wellbeing in this situation?
3. What action, if any, would you take if you encountered a caregiver treating patients hospitalised for care and treatment following a failed suicide attempt in a contemptuous and dismissive manner as experienced in this case?

---

1   Initially, suicide was prohibited on religious grounds. As religious forces weakened, however, attitudes to suicide changed. Farberow (1975b, p. 4) explains: 'while the attitudes of horror and condemnation for suicide were preserved in the lower classes, the upper classes seemed to develop a different religion and different morals, expressing tolerance and acceptance [of suicide]'.

2   Names and details of times and places have been suppressed, but these are true stories that reflect the experience of all nurses everywhere.

Chapter 12

End of life decision-making and the nursing profession

LEARNING OBJECTIVES

Upon the completion of this chapter and with further self-directed learning you are expected to be able to:

- Discuss critically 'Not For Treatment' (NFT) and 'Do Not Resuscitate' (DNR) directives.
- Discuss critically the moral criteria that might be used to justify an NFT or DNR directive.
- Examine critically the ethical dimensions of NFT and DNR directives.
- Discuss critically ways in which DNR policies and procedures could be improved.
- Discuss the notion 'medical futility' and its implications for the profession and practice of nursing.
- Explain why medical futility has been abandoned as a decisional criteria in end of life decision-making.
- Examine critically the criterion 'quality of life' and its relevance to end of life decision-making.
- Discuss critically three senses in which the notion quality of life might be used.
- Explore the possible risks to patients of making faulty quality of life judgments.
- Define 'advance directives'.
- Discuss critically how advance directives work.
- Examine critically the risks and benefits of advance directives.
- Explore how nurses can make a significant contribution to care and treatment decisions at the end stage of life.

KEYWORDS

- Advance directives
- Do Not Resuscitate (DNR) directives
- End of life decision-making
- Enduring Power of Attorney (Medical Treatment)
- Living wills
- Medical futility

- Not For Treatment (NFT) directives
- Quality of life
- Withdrawal of treatment

Introduction

At the end stages of life there invariably comes a point at which decisions have to be made about whether to start, stop or withdraw life-sustaining treatment. The life-sustaining treatment in this instance can include the use of 'aggressive' (invasive) treatments (such as mechanical ventilation/life support machines, surgery, emergency cardiopulmonary resuscitation, haemodialysis, and chemotherapy), or the use of 'less aggressive' (less invasive) treatments (such as the administration of antibiotics, cardiac arrhythmic drugs, blood transfusions, and intravenous and/or nasogastric hydration). Whether involving 'aggressive' or 'non-aggressive' treatments, decisions have to be made either way (i.e. to treat or not to treat) *even* when it is 'obvious' (or at least highly probable) that their administration will not result in improved clinical outcomes for the patient — for example, the patient will continue to experience 'grievous bodily deterioration' (Cantor 1995, p. 1364) and/or will ultimately die, regardless of the treatment given (Cantor 1995; Morreim 1995; Walter 1995). The question remains, however, of who should decide these things and on what basis?

The question of who ultimately should decide whether to provide, withhold or withdraw life-sustaining treatments at the end stage of life, as well as when, where and how best to decide, are all matters of moral controversy. In clinical contexts, controversies surrounding these issues can also give rise to serious conflict and moral quandary among those involved. Conflict, in this instance, can take the form of health care providers being asked to 'do everything' when they believe that a withdrawal of treatment is more appropriate, or, their being asked to 'do nothing' (or, at least, to withdraw treatment) when they believe that it should be continued. When 'unable to agree to either request', this situation can pose a significant and distressing moral dilemma for decision-makers — and one that is not easily resolved (Fine and Mayo 2003, p. 744; see also Council on Ethical and Judicial Affairs, American Medical Association 1999; Hammes and Rooney 1998). The dilemmas and distress among decision-makers in these instances can be compounded when there is also disagreement among clinicians about: the nature and stage of a patient's illness; how responsive a patient's illness might be to treatment; and whether proposed therapeutic measures are 'worth it' if 'the gain in weeks or months that might reasonably be expected' by a given therapeutic intervention are significantly outweighed by the loss of quality of life due to the toxic side effects of the treatment (Ashby and Stoffell 1991, p. 1322).

At the forefront of the moral controversies and dilemmas about end of life decision-making are the issues of Not For Treatment (NFT) directives, withholding/withdrawing food and fluids (already discussed in the previous chapter) and Do Not Resuscitate (DNR)/Not For Resuscitation (NFR) directives, and the criteria or bases used for justifying these directives such as 'medical futility', quality of life considerations, and advanced directives. The practical and moral significance of these issues for attending health care providers (particularly those working in hospitals) is underscored when it is considered that most deaths occur in hospitals and that a significant majority of these deaths occur after a decision has been made — often by someone else — to forgo life-sustaining therapy (e.g. cardiopulmonary resuscitation)

(Hammes and Rooney 1998; Asch et al. 1995; Lynn and Teno 1995; Loewy and Carlson 1993; Ayres 1991). Since these issues have important moral implications for the profession and practice of nursing, some discussion of them here is warranted.

Not For Treatment (NFT) directives

Sometimes, during the course of end of life care, an explicit medical directive might be given to the effect that a patient is Not For Treatment (NFT). Sometimes the patient or his or her proxy will agree with (and may even have requested) the NFT decision that has been made, sometimes they will not. It is when there is disagreement about a treatment choice — that is, where a decision is 'contested' — that the matter becomes problematic. Here an important question arises, namely: When is it acceptable, if ever, to provide, withdraw or withhold life-sustaining medical treatment at the end stage of life?

The problem of treatment in 'medically hopeless' cases

In the past, decisions about what treatments to provide — when, where and by whom — were made autonomously (some would say paternalistically) by attending doctors. This sometimes lead to a situation in which people were being 'aggressively' treated even when their cases were deemed 'medically hopeless'. In other words, people were treated 'aggressively' even where it was evident to experienced bystanders that such treatment would not make a significant difference to their health or life expectancy. Sometimes treatment of this nature was imposed without the patient's knowledge or consent (for example, those in a so-called 'persistent vegetative state'), and gave rise to varying degrees of suffering by both patients and their families/friends.

This situation began to change, however, as the public started to become weary of and started to question the wisdom of people being 'hopelessly resuscitated'. This public questioning saw a number of key cases reaching the public's attention. Rosemary Tong (1995, p. 166) explains:

> As a result of various factors, the withholding and withdrawing cases that captured the imagination of the public in the 1960s and 1970s were ones in which patients or their surrogates resisted the imposition of unwanted medical treatment. The media portrayed dying patients as routinely falling prey to physicians who, out of fear of subsequent litigation ... or out of obedience to some sort of 'technological imperative' ..., insisted on keeping them 'alive' irrespective of the quality of their existence.

Tong (1995) suggests that during the 1960s and 1970s, economic resources permitted everything possible to be done. During the 1980s and 1990s, however, it became increasingly evident that neither individuals nor society as a whole could sustain the 'technological imperative' to treat regardless of the outcomes. Thus communities in the Western world entered into a new era that was characteristically 'burdened with new obligations of social justice' in health care (Tong 1995, p. 167). Whereas end of life issues in the 1960s and 1970s were more concerned with *patient autonomy versus medical paternalism*, in the 1980s and 1990s they had become chiefly concerned with *patient autonomy versus distributive justice* (Tong 1995, pp. 166–7). Since the 1990s, however, a key question that has come to dominate bioethical thought is: Are people at the end stages of their lives (or their proxies) morally entitled to request 'medically inappropriate' 'non-beneficial' and 'expensive' (futile) medical treatment? Is it right to refuse such requests? At stake in answering these questions is not just the entitlements of dying individuals but, as Tong concludes (p. 167):

the future wellbeing of the health care professional–patient–society relationship — a relationship best understood not in terms of competing rights (though that is an aspect of it), but in terms of intersecting responsibilities.

Disputes about futile or useful treatments at the end stages of life invariably represent 'disputes about professional, patient and surrogate autonomy, as well as concerns about good communication, informed consent, resource allocation, under-treatment, over-treatment, and paternalism' (Kopleman 1995, p. 109). They also represent dispute about 'how to understand or rank such important values as sustaining a life, providing appropriate treatments, relieving suffering, or being compassionate' and the bearing these values may have on deciding questions of resource allocation (Kopleman 1995, p. 111).

Who decides?

The question of who and how to decide end of life treatment options is a difficult one to answer. Choices include:

- the medical practitioner (unilateral approach);
- the health care team (consensus approach);
- the patient or his/her surrogate (unilateral approach);
- society (consensus approach).

While all plausible, neither of the above approaches are without difficulties (even in the case of a consensus being reached, this alone is not enough to confer moral authority on the decisions made). For example, while all may entail respect for the autonomy of individuals, they nevertheless risk decisions being made that are arbitrary, biased, capricious, self-interested and based on personal preferences. This is unacceptable (especially in contested cases) since, as Kopleman points out (1995, pp. 117–18,119):

> If one ought to do the morally defensible action in the contested case, then the final appeal cannot be solely preferences of someone or some group. Preference or agreements may be unworthy because they result from prejudice, self-interest or ignorance. In contrast, moral justification requires giving and defending reasons for preferences, and by doing so relying on methodological ideals of clarity, impartiality, consistency and consideration of all relevant information. Other important, albeit fallible, considerations in making moral decisions include legal, social, and religious traditions, stable views about how to understand and rank important values, and a willingness to be sensitive to the feelings, preferences, perceptions and rights of others. The evolution of contested cases often illustrates the pitfalls of failing to take the time and clarify people's concerns, problems, feelings, beliefs or deeply felt needs or even to consider if people are treating others as they would wish to be treated ... Over-treatments may be burdensome to patient and costly to society, yet under-treatments can compromise the rights or dignity of the people seeking help.

In the case of requests being made for 'everything possible to be done' some have suggested that there is no obligation to comply with such requests in so-called medically hopeless cases. Jecker and Schneiderman (1995, p. 160) clarify, however, that 'saying "no" to futile treatment should not mean saying "no" to caring for the patient'. They conclude (p. 160):

> [saying 'no'] should be an occasion for transferring aggressive efforts away from life prolongation toward life enhancement. Ideally, 'doing everything' means optimising the potential for a good life, and providing that most important coda to a good life — a 'good death'.

Decisions about whether or not to initiate or to withhold and/or remove medical treatment on patients deemed 'medically hopeless' will rarely be without controversy (sometimes referred to in the bioethics literature as the 'not starting versus stopping' debate [see, for example, Gert et al. 1997, pp. 282–3]). Nurses are not immune from the controversies surrounding these decisions, and may even find themselves unwitting participants in them. It is essential therefore that nurses are well appraised of the relevant views for and against decisions aimed at limiting or withdrawing the medical treatment of patients deemed (rightly or wrongly) to be 'medically hopeless'.

Do Not Resuscitate (DNR) directives[1]

At some stage during their clinical practice, nurses will be confronted with the difficult moral choice of whether to follow a Do Not Resuscitate (DNR) directive (also called Not For Resuscitation (NFR), No Code, or No CPR directives). This type of directive is usually given by a doctor in an attempt to 'avoid over-treatment and CPR (cardiopulmonary resuscitation) abuses' — particularly in cases involving hopelessly ill patients 'who would be otherwise hopelessly revived' (Humphry and Wickett 1986, p. 209). DNR is thus a form of NFT, and probably is the most common NFT directive given in health care contexts. Typically, a DNR directive directs that: 'in the event of a cardiac arrest, neither basic nor advanced life support measures will be instituted by physicians, nurses, or other hospital staff' (Cushing 1981, p. 22; Honan et al. 1991, p. 54).

A decision not to resuscitate a person is popularly thought to flow from a medical judgment concerning the irreversible nature of that person's disease and their probable poor or hopeless prognosis (see, for example, Haines et al. 1990, p. 228). The validity of this view has, however, been increasingly challenged as critics have shown that the DNR decision is neither a *medical* decision nor a legal decision per se, but rather a *moral* decision since it is based primarily on *moral values* such as those concerning 'the meaning, sanctity, and quality of life' (Yarling and McElmurry 1986, p. 125).

Despite its significant moral and legal implications for nurses, the issue of DNR directives has, on the whole, been poorly addressed by the nursing profession. Just why this state of affairs has occurred is a matter for speculation. It may be that nurses have come to view the DNR directive as constituting a lawful and reasonable medical directive, and thus not something warranting any special or particular concern. Or it may be that nurses *are* troubled by current practices in this area and do wish to speak out, but genuinely do not know how to go about articulating their concerns.

Up until the late 1990s, few health care organisations had operational DNR policies and guidelines — and those that did had poor compliance rates — a situation that placed both patients and staff at risk (Johnstone 1999a, pp. 379–96; Kerridge et al. 1994). Today, a very different situation exists with most health care institutions having policies and guidelines on DNR. Little is known, however, about the quality of these policies or the degree to which hospital staff comply with them. There is some anecdotal evidence to suggest that while DNR policies exist, they nevertheless vary significantly across and even within different organisations. There is also some suggestion that staff do not always comply with the guidelines that are in operation (see, for example, MinterEllison 2001; *Northridge v Central Sydney Area Health Service* 2000; Collier 1999). Thus, while the policy situation has improved, there are still risks (moral, legal and clinical) associated with current DNR practices.

Raising the issues

There is an obvious need to have carefully formulated and clearly documented guidelines and policies governing DNR practices. Without such guidelines:

- patients' rights and interests will be at risk of being unjustly violated (for example, patients could be resuscitated when they do not wish to be, or not resuscitated when they do wish to be);
- nurses and other allied health workers will be at risk of having to carry a disproportionate burden of responsibility and possible harm in regard to actually carrying out DNR/CPR directives (although a DNR directive might be given in 'good faith' medically speaking, it may nevertheless be vulnerable to criticism and censure — not just on moral grounds but on legal grounds as well, especially if it contravenes a patient's expressed wishes) (see, for example, *Northridge v Central Sydney Area Health Service* [2000]).

The following two cases, those of Mr H and Mr X, illustrate the kinds of problems that can be encountered when DNR policies are inadequate or attending staff fail to uphold best practice standards in relation to DNR/CPR practices. These cases both occurred in the cultural context of Australia.

CASE STUDIES

Case 1: Mr H

Mr H[2], 60 years old, was admitted to the intensive care unit of a major city hospital with a provisional diagnosis of septicaemia. At the time of admission he was pale, markedly short of breath, and had an axillary temperature of 40°C. Mr H's past medical history included severe coronary artery disease and a malignant condition. The malignant condition had, however, been successfully treated with chemotherapy, and Mr H was presently in a state of remission. In the light of his provisional diagnosis, a regime of intravenous antibiotics was commenced.

A few hours after Mr H's admission, the on-coming nursing staff for the afternoon shift gathered for 'hand-over'. During hand-over, the charge nurse informed the nursing staff present that she had just received a telephone call from Mr H's physician confirming that the patient was Not For Resuscitation (NFR). As she proceeded to give the afternoon report, a second consulting physician — also involved in Mr H's medical care — approached the assembled nursing staff and reaffirmed her colleague's initial NFR directive. The physician then wrote up her clinical assessment of Mr H and made other important documentations on his medical history chart. She did not, however, make any attempt to document the NFR directive which she had just given to the nursing staff. This 'oversight' was later dealt with by the nursing staff writing the initials 'NFR', in pencil, on the top left-hand corner of Mr H's nursing care plan, which was held in his medical history chart.

A short time later, a nurse who had been sent to help in the unit became involved in a deep conversation with Mr H. During the conversation, Mr H spontaneously and emphatically exclaimed: 'Oh, I wish they would operate on me!' (referring to coronary artery bypass surgery, the opportunity for which he had recently been denied). In response to this the nurse gently asked Mr H whether he had discussed the possibility of bypass surgery with his doctor.

To this Mr H replied quite openly: 'Sure I have, many times, but they won't do it because they say there's only a 50–50 chance of success ...'. He went on to say: 'What can you do? You can't hit them over the head with a bottle and make them do it, can you?'. The nurse enquired further: 'So even though you'd only have a 50–50 chance — you'd still want this coronary bypass surgery?'.

Mr H replied, sombrely:

> Oh, yes. I'd do anything to buy some time. You see, my wife's very ill at home. She has cancer which can't be operated on. She's always been totally dependent on me — even more so since she's been sick. She doesn't have very long to live, and all I want is to live long enough for her, because she's so afraid of being left alone. We can't do much, and we each stay in separate rooms at home. But at least we're reasonably independent and together. I can bring her a cup of tea when she wants it and things like that. I don't care about me, but I want to live long enough for her ... she's so afraid of being left alone ...

Smiling, Mr H concluded: 'It's such a comfort knowing that you and the doctors are doing all that you can for me here ...'.

Realising that Mr H clearly had no knowledge of the NFR directive against him, the nurse went immediately to discuss the matter with the other nurses, who were still in the nurses' bay, having not yet moved to care for their respective patients. There, she discreetly asked whether Mr H or his relatives had been involved in making the NFR decision. To this question one nurse replied: 'Oh! Surely that's silly to include the patient or the relatives ...' and, almost simultaneously, another nurse replied: 'No. We don't do that in this hospital. It's the doctors' decision, and we're obliged to obey their orders ...'.

The nurse caring for Mr H then attempted to point out that her patient had indicated that he very definitely wished to risk the odds of active resuscitation. She then asked further whether the doctors were aware of Mr H's desires. To this, the nurse in charge replied sternly: 'Of course the doctors know! It's their decision, and it's the policy of this hospital to follow such orders'.

As the afternoon shift progressed, Mr H experienced a number of bradycardiac episodes, with the cardiac monitor showing his heart rate dropping to as low as 34 in some instances. The arrhythmia could have been treated relatively easily by the attending nurse administering a prescribed bolus dose of intravenous atropine. When the nurse caring for Mr H went to have the drug checked with the nurse in charge (as was required by unit policy), she was told: 'You don't need to worry about that, he's NFR ...'. Despite the attending nurse's protests, the nurse in charge still refused to check the atropine. Fortunately, during the time of intense debate between the attending nurse and the nurse in charge, Mr H's cardiac rhythm reverted spontaneously to a rate of between 80 and 90 beats per minute. Mr H had several more bradycardiac episodes throughout the shift, but each time spontaneously reverted to a safe rate of 80–90 beats per minute.

A few days later, Mr H's temperature dropped significantly to within normal limits. He stated that he felt better and was looking forward to going home. His blood cultures came back negative (negating his provisional diagnosis of septicaemia), his heart rate was more stable, and his breathing continued to improve. Despite this, however, the NFR directive was not rescinded. Mr H's condition dramatically improved even further one afternoon when he was given a stat dose of intravenous lasix (a diuretic). Following this, it was decided that the presenting medical condition had not, in fact, been septicaemia but pulmonary congestion (secondary to his heart disease) and pneumonia.

Just six days after his initial admission into the intensive care unit, Mr H was judged sufficiently well recovered to be discharged home. He left, happy, thanking the nursing staff for all that they had done and expressing his eagerness to leave and be reunited with his dying wife.

Rightly troubled by the incident, the nurse made an appointment to discuss the matter with the then director of nursing. During the conversation, the nurse indicated that in future she would override any nurse in charge and would contact the prescribing doctor to clarify an existing NFR directive. To this the director of nursing replied:

> Well, of course, if you had contacted the doctors involved in this case, you would probably have found that they wouldn't be very forthcoming anyway. In fact, they would probably have told you it was not your concern. You will find here that it is really the doctor's decision in cases like these, since it is *they* who have the contract with the patient, not the nurses ...

Case 2: Mr X

The second case to be considered here is taken from the Victorian State Government Social Development Committee's *Inquiry into options for dying with dignity: second and final report* (1987). It involves the case of Mr X, who was also cared for in a major city hospital.

Mr X, 78-years-old, was admitted to hospital with a provisional diagnosis of 'Transitional Cell Carcinoma, with metastatic spread to the lungs, liver and spinal cord and brain' (Social Development Committee 1987, p. 111). On admission, Mr X was observed to be lethargic, disorientated and suffering a greater degree of pain than on previous admissions. He had lost weight and admitted to having lost his appetite. The nurse relating the case stated that (p. 112):

> it was apparent to me that Mr X's disease process had insidiously created a decline in his overall wellbeing, to a point where it had now affected his quality of life.

On Friday morning, upon consultation with the ward's resident medical officer, it was stated that Mr X 'had now reached the terminal stage of his illness' and that, apart from keeping him comfortable, nothing more could be done for him, medically speaking. On Friday evening, Mr X's deteriorating condition was discussed with his relatives. It was reported that (p. 112):

> His relatives were distressed over the deterioration they had observed over the past few weeks in Mr X's condition and wellbeing. At this time they emphatically expressed their wish that should Mr X arrest while in hospital, they in no way wanted an emergency procedure of resuscitation performed on him, and wished for him to be allowed to die peacefully with a degree of dignity assured.

Later that same evening, Mr X himself requested (via the hospital chaplain) that 'should he die that evening he had no wish to be actively resuscitated and would prefer to die peacefully' (p. 113).

Mr X's condition continued to deteriorate. On Saturday morning, the nurse in charge called the covering resident medical officer to examine Mr X medically so that it could be formally established that Mr X 'would not be for resuscitation' in the event of his suffering a cardiac arrest. The Social Development Committee (1987, p. 113) further reports:

> The doctor examined Mr X, and agreed that he should not be for cardiopulmonary resuscitation. However, he also stated that he could not instigate that decision until Monday morning, until he had consulted the Registrar and Consultants of the unit, thereby allowing his decision to be reached as a team decision. On this note, Mr X was still for resuscitation should he arrest, in spite of his and his relatives' wish to allow him to die with peace and dignity.

Over the next 24-hours, Mr X's condition declined even further, and at 5 pm on Sunday, in the presence of his relatives, he suffered a cardiac arrest. As the covering resident medical officer had requested that Mr X should still be resuscitated — at least until the matter could be discussed with the unit team — an immediate resuscitation code was called. Full resuscitation procedures were instigated and continued for approximately 20 minutes. No positive outcome was achieved, however, and Mr X was declared clinically dead. Understandably, Mr X's relatives were very distraught about the incident and 'even more so', as the report goes on to quote, 'about the fact that Mr X had been resuscitated both against his and their wishes' (p. 113).

The issues raised by these and other case scenarios can be broadly categorised under three general headings:

1. problems concerning DNR decision-making criteria, guidelines and procedures;
2. problems concerning the documentation and communication of DNR directives; and
3. problems concerning the implementation of DNR directives.

Problems concerning DNR decision-making criteria, guidelines and procedures

CRITERIA AND GUIDELINES USED

Despite the existence of DNR policies and guidelines, different doctors and nurses may nevertheless appeal to different *criteria* (to be distinguished here from *procedures*) for making DNR/CPR decisions (see also Stewart and Rai 1989; Thom 1988). For example, some doctors and nurses might appeal to *quality of life* criteria (to be discussed later in this chapter), while others might appeal to *sanctity of life* criteria when making DNR/CPR decisions. Although DNR/CPR decisions based on either of these criteria might well be in accordance with a patient's preferences, they might equally be in contravention of them. For example, in one case in which quality of life criteria were applied, a previously fit 90-year-old man who required admission to hospital for multiple medical problems was not resuscitated following a cardiac arrest. The decision not to resuscitate him was made by attending medical staff even though both the patient and his wife had clearly indicated that they wished 'everything possible' to be done to try and preserve his life — including cardiopulmonary resuscitation in the event of a cardiac arrest (Hastings Center 1982, pp. 27–8). In contradistinction to this case, in another case this time involving an appeal to sanctity of life criteria, a 70-year-old woman 'was resuscitated over 70 times within a few days' (Annas, in Bandman and Bandman 1985, p. 236). In another similar case, a patient was resuscitated 52 times before 'family members literally threw themselves across the crash cart to prevent the team from reaching the patient' for the 53rd time (Dolan 1988, p. 47).

In still other cases, doctors and nurses might appeal to little more than a personal sense or 'gut feeling' of right and wrong when making DNR/CPR decisions. What is troubling about this is that, while attending doctors or nurses might 'feel' that a particular DNR or CPR decision is right (or wrong, as the case may be), it does not follow that the decision in question is morally sound.

Another troubling practice is that of hospital staff deeming patients to be DNR on the basis of a DNR decision made during a previous hospital admission. For example, if a patient is made DNR during an admission to hospital in March, is discharged, but comes back into hospital in April, the patient is made DNR again on the basis of the March hospital admission decision. The rationale behind this is not entirely clear. What is clear, however, is that such a practice is in contravention of acceptable standards of safe and quality care and should be abandoned.

Equally disturbing is the over-reliance on age as a decisional criterion when making DNR/CPR decisions. Many residential care homes for the aged, for example, have a universal policy of not resuscitating their residents in the event of either a cardiac or respiratory arrest. Persons entering these homes are asked whether they wish to be cremated and where they wish to be buried, but are not always asked whether they wish to be resuscitated if and when they should cardiac arrest. This practice is disturbing for two main reasons: first, it stands to violate the residents' autonomy; second, it relies on what research has shown to be an unreliable and invalid decisional criterion — notably *age* (see in particular Sage et al. 1987).

As a point of interest, one American study investigating the implementation of a Do-Not-Resuscitate (DNR) policy in a nursing home found that, of the 48 residents (who were of a mean age of 81.7 years) who were deemed capable of deciding whether they wanted CPR/DNR, 30 (62.5 per cent) 'chose to be resuscitated in the event of a cardiopulmonary arrest', compared with only 18 (37.5 per cent) who 'decided in favour of DNR' (Fader et al. 1989, p. 545).

In a later British study involving 100 inpatients (mean age 81.5 years) in an acute hospital elderly care unit, 73 per cent of those patients questioned indicated that they would want CPR in the event of a cardiac arrest; this compared with 18 per cent of those questioned indicating that they would not want CPR in the event of a cardiac arrest, and nine per cent who indicating that they were unsure (Mead and Turnbull 1995). However, in another North American study (involving 287 elderly people with a mean age of 77 years), a team of researchers found that, in contradiction to most other studies suggesting that a majority of elderly patients would want to undergo CPR in the event of a cardiac arrest, once respondents were informed about the probabilities of survival following CPR, their preference for CPR declined significantly (that is, almost halved) (Murphy et al. 1994). These two studies were nevertheless unanimous in their conclusions: elderly people are capable of being — and should be — consulted about their CPR status in health care contexts. This conclusion has been validated by the findings of other more recent research (see, for example, Cherniack 2002; Phillips and Woodward 1999).

THE EXCLUSION OF PATIENTS FROM DECISION-MAKING

Despite the widespread acceptance of the principle of patient autonomy and informed consent, some doctors and nurses continue to genuinely believe that patients or their relatives should not be included in the process of making DNR/CPR decisions (Cherniack 2002; Phillips and Woodward 1999; Loewy 1991; Schade and Muslin 1989; Perry et al. 1986). Responding to the case of the 90-year-old man (mentioned above), Carson (1982, p. 28) argued that the admitting hospital in that case had an official policy which effectively took the position 'that entering patients should not be bothered with the details of resuscitation policy but should assume that they will be well cared for and coded if necessary'. Commenting on the same case,

Siegler (1982, p. 29) went even further arguing that where a physician knows ('within limits of uncertainty that characterise all medical knowledge') that CPR would be of no possible benefit to the patient, it should not be initiated — *regardless* of a patient's preferences to the contrary.

Excluding patients or their proxies from participating in DNR/CPR decisions can, however, result in unnecessary suffering for the patient (if he/she survives) and their loved ones. For example, when informed that no attempt had been made to resuscitate her husband, the wife of the 90-year-old man (referred to above) reportedly stated that the decision was 'against her wishes' and that:

> Doing everything [...] is the difference between life and death. The doctor was playing God when he decided he should not try to save my husband. You're not playing God when you've tried everything and exhausted all methods. All I wanted was for them to try. My husband knew how to love and be loved. That was his quality of life. That suited him and it suited me.

(Hastings Center 1982, p. 28)

Many health care professionals believe that patients should not be 'burdened' with having to decide whether they should be resuscitated in the event of a cardiac arrest — particularly if the patient's condition is 'medically hopeless' and any further treatment — including CPR — would be 'futile' (Cherniack 2002; Lo 1991; Loewy 1991; Scofield 1991; Haines et al. 1990; Tomlinson and Brody 1990). This has resulted in patients (or their proxies) sometimes not being consulted about a DNR directive even though institutional policy has required that their consent be obtained and even though research has consistently shown that a majority of patients and their proxies want to be involved in decision-making concerning DNR/CPR directives (Cherniack 2002; Mead and Turnbull 1995; Honan et al. 1991).

MISINTERPRETATION OF DIRECTIVES AND QUESTIONABLE OUTCOMES

Another difficulty associated with current DNR policies and guidelines is that they are vulnerable to being misinterpreted which, in turn, can result in the under-treatment and substandard care of patients (Johns 1996). For example, in the case of Mr H, described at the beginning of this discussion, the DNR directive was interpreted, controversially, as also including the non-treatment of a potentially fatal but relatively easily treatable cardiac arrhythmia. This interpretation is even more troubling when it is considered that the patient was, after all, being cared for in an *intensive care unit*, where the imperative is normally to treat not to withhold treatment from patients presenting with treatable life threatening conditions.

Another disturbing example of the way in which a DNR directive can be misinterpreted can be found in the case of a dying patient who had pulmonary congestion and pneumonia, and, associated with these two conditions, copious mucus production. In this case, the nurses (mis)interpreted the DNR directive to include withholding oropharyngeal/nasopharyngeal suctioning. As a result, the patient was left, quite literally, to drown in his own secretions — until another nurse detected the error and took immediate action to correct the other nurses' misinterpretation of the directive. The lesson to be learned from this case — and others like it — is that 'No Code' does not mean 'no care' (Saunders and Valente 1986; see also Lo 1991).

Problems concerning the documentation and communication of DNR directives

A second issue of concern in the DNR debate involves the means by which DNR directives are documented and communicated to members of the health care team.

In the past, DNR directives were communicated using the following questionable processes:

- DNR directives being given verbally only (i.e. they were not formally documented in the patient's medical or nursing notes). This practice came about largely because doctors were 'loathe to indicate in written notes in patient records that a patient [was] not for resuscitation' (Social Development Committee 1987, p. 108).
- DNR directives being 'confirmed' by sticking coloured dots (usually black ones) or scribbling an asterisk either on the patient's medical history chart and/or by the patient's name on the ward's bed allocation board. As a point of interest, in 1988 the Association of Medical Directors of Victorian Hospitals recommended to the Victorian Hospital Association that 'a round white sticker with "sky" blue border and an oblique "sky" blue stripe be adopted by hospitals to denote Not For Resuscitation'. They advised that the sticker should be 'placed on the front of the patient record, on the bed card and on the patient's wristband' (*Victorian Hospital Association Report* 1988, p. 3).
- DNR directives being 'confirmed' by pencilling the initials 'DNR' or 'NFR' or some other equivalent in an inconspicuous place on the patient's medical history or nursing care plan, or both.
- DNR directives being written euphemistically as 'routine nursing care only', or 'cares for comfort only' (Cushing 1981, p. 24).

While once commonly accepted throughout institutional health care settings, these modes of communicating DNR directives were (and are) highly questionable. For instance, as with *any* verbal directives, verbal DNR directives are vulnerable to being misinterpreted. More seriously, a person who originally gave a verbal DNR directive could later deny that any such directive was given at all. An instructive example of how very serious errors can be made on account of verbal DNR directives being given and, equally instructive, how easily an attending doctor can deny ever having given a verbal DNR directive is provided below.

The case in question involved a patient, identified as Mrs M, who suffered a cardiac arrest while being cared for in an intensive care unit. A medical student covering the unit was called. After initiating CPR he is alleged to have stopped, saying: 'What am I doing? She's a no-code,' and then stopped performing cardiac massage (Adams 1984, p. 54). The case was eventually brought before a grand jury after a nurse anonymously informed Mrs M's daughter that 'her mother had died "unnecessarily" because "a no-code was sent out" ' (Adams 1984, p. 55). As a point of interest, the medical student testified that he never made the comment. When the medical student was later asked in an informal situation why he treated Mrs M as a 'no-code', he replied that the directive to do so had been given to him verbally by a cardiologist (Adams 1984, p. 55).

It is sometimes mistakenly assumed that a verbal DNR directive will 'convey the directive without attaching any legal liability' (Cushing 1981, p. 27). Cushing warns, however, that (1981, p. 27):

while many hospitals allow no code orders to be "unofficial", it is difficult to justify a continuation of this practice. Once the medical decision has been made, the order should be written as any other medical directive.

In addition to verbal directives, there have been other questionable methods used for communicating DNR directives, such as the use of coloured dots, asterisks and pencilled initials and abbreviations. Like verbal directives, however, coloured dots, asterisks and pencilled initials and abbreviations are 'high risk' practices that could result in serious errors being made. It seems quite inconceivable that important and competent medical decisions concerning the life and death of a human being were once reduced to something so careless as a simple black dot, an asterisk, or a set of pencilled abbreviations. It is also inconceivable that competent health professionals once relied so readily on these crude symbols for determining whether or not the interventions needed to aid a seriously ill or dying patient should, in fact, be initiated. The additional dangers of dots were (and are), of course, that they could be bought and placed on charts by almost anybody; they could also become dislodged, stick to the wrong chart, or be placed by the wrong person's name on the bed allocation board, and so on (Adams 1984; Macklin 1993, pp. 34–6).

The use of abbreviations such as 'DNR', 'NFR' and variations thereof, is also problematic. In one case, for example, a nurse informed me that a doctor had once ordered her to write the initials 'NFR' on a patient's chart. When she queried this directive, she was politely told: 'Don't worry. If there are any problems, we'll just say it means "Not for Referral" ...'. In another case, the initials 'NFR' were written on a patient's nursing care plan, which was left hanging on the end of his bed. During visiting hours, a family member visiting the patient took the liberty of examining the nursing care plan and noticed the initials 'NFR' on it. She asked a passing nurse what the letters meant. To this question the nurse replied: 'Oh, don't worry about that. It just means 'Nice Fellow Really ...'.

In yet another case, a dietician writing in a patient's integrated case notes (that is, where all members of the health care team — doctors, nurses, and other allied carers — write up their notes) wrote the initials 'NFR' meaning 'not for referral'. Understandably, the dietician was very distressed when the significance of what she had written was pointed out to her.

A last concern to be considered here is the practice of ordering 'nursing care only' or 'cares for comfort only' when it is considered that nothing more can be done medically for the patient. The professional — not to mention the moral — acceptability of using 'nursing care only' as a euphemism for withdrawing life-saving medical treatment warrants questioning, however. For one thing, in situations where all means have not, in fact, been exhausted, there is always room to question whether CPR (or any other life-supporting measure, for that matter) should, in fact, be rightfully withheld from a patient. On this point it is worthwhile to consider Veatch's helpful comments. In his book *Death, dying and the biological revolution*, Veatch writes (1977, p. 8):

> The question should never be, 'When should we stop treating this patient?' as if the patient were an object to be repaired or discarded. Rather the moral question must be, 'When, if ever, should it be morally and/or legally possible for the patient to decide to refuse medical treatment even if that may mean that dying will no longer be prolonged?'

Problems concerning the implementation of DNR directives

Even when all proper processes have been followed, a nurse might still be left in a quandary about whether to uphold a given DNR directive and may, in practice, experience difficulties implementing a directive even though 'medically indicated' and lawfully prescribed.

Most nurses probably have no difficulty carrying out DNR directives — indeed, in some instances, they may even be largely responsible for encouraging doctors to prescribe them. Some nurses, however, may suffer significant hardships on account of various institutional demands to follow established DNR policies and guidelines.

For instance, there have been a small number of cases in which nurses have been dismissed from their places of employment because of deciding not to initiate resuscitation on a patient even though no DNR directive was in place. In one noted English case, for example, a registered nurse 'who chose to let an elderly man die rather than call in a resuscitation team' was dismissed for gross misconduct (*Nursing Times* 1983, p. 20; see also Johnstone 1994b, pp. 258–9). The fact that the man had lung cancer, was 78 years old and essentially died of 'natural causes' was not deemed relevant to the case (Buchanan 1983; Regan 1983). In another case, this time in Australia, a registered nurse was likewise dismissed from her job and also faced disciplinary action for allegedly 'disobeying a written directive to continue medical treatment' on a seriously ill elderly woman and, on her own volition, deciding that the patient should be 'classified as not for resuscitation' (Collier 1999). Although the patient's physician is reported to have later agreed that a 'not for resuscitation order' would have been given, hospital authorities apparently took the position that the dismissal was justified on the grounds that the nurse had contravened hospital policies (Collier 1999).

The issue of implementing DNR directives is of particular concern to nurses since, quite simply, they are the ones often left with the ultimate decision of whether or not to initiate CPR in an arrest situation. They are thus also invariably left with the burden of having to accept the responsibility for the consequences of both their actions and their omissions in arrest situations.

Improving DNR practices

It is acknowledged here that DNR practices have improved significantly over the past two decades. Nevertheless there are still areas that stand in need of improvement. To this end the following recommendations are made:

1. There needs to be a recognition that DNR decisions have a profound moral dimension, and are not just medical, nursing or legal in nature, and because of this must be made by appealing to sound moral criteria and standards as well as to relevant clinical information.
2. Any DNR decision made ought to reflect the *patient's informed choice* (given informed choice in its most stringent sense here).
3. DNR decisions/directives should be *clearly written* on patients' medical and nursing charts, and should include all the relevant information upon which the decisions have been based (including descriptions of the patients' statements relevant to their request that given life-saving measures be withheld). Alternatively, a 'DNR authorisation' or a

LIMITATION OF MEDICAL TREATMENT (Northern Health)	AFFIX PATIENT IDENTIFICATION LABEL HERE U.R. NUMBER: _____ SURNAME: _____ GIVEN NAME: _____
DATE: ____/____/____ WARD: _____	DATE OF BIRTH: ____/____/____ SEX: ____

The Limitation of Medical Treatment form must be completed in conjunction with the Consultant. The form is to be used to clarify the following:

• Limitation of treatment during present admission

• Withdrawal of current treatment

An alert that a Limitation of Medical Treatment form has been initiated must be documented on the alert sheet, which is located at the front of the patient's medical record. Upon discharge, this document ceases and must therefore be cancelled on the alert sheet.

REASON FOR INITIATION OF THIS FORM

DIAGNOSIS:

PROGNOSIS:

RESULT OF DISCUSSION WITH PATIENT (IF APPROPRIATE), AGENT AND/OR RELATIVES

SPECIFIC DEFINITIVE THERAPY/THERAPIES TO BE WITHHELD

AUTHORISATION OF LIMITATION OF MEDICAL TREATMENT

MEDICAL REGISTRAR	NURSE IN CHARGE	CONSULTANT
Name: _____	Name: _____	Name: _____
Signature: _____	Signature: _____	Signature: _____
Date: ____/____/____	Date: ____/____/____	Date: ____/____/____

REVIEW OF LIMITATION OF MEDICAL TREATMENT WITHIN ADMISSION

The Unit during the episode of care must review the Limitation of Medical Treatment order:

This patient was reviewed by me on ____/____/____ and the previous limitation of medical treatment orders *still apply / do not apply.

Name: _____ Signature: _____ Date: ____/____/____

* Please delete as appropriate

FORM 11150 JULY '03D

LIMITATION OF MEDICAL TREATMENT

MR 6a

THIS ORDER CEASES ON DISCHARGE ☞

HOSPITAL   NORTHERN   THE

Figure 12.1 An example of a form authorising a 'Do Not Resuscitate' directive

(reproduced with permission from Northern Health, 201 Bell St, Preston, Vic)

(**Figure 12.1** continued)

GUIDELINES

FOR WHICH PATIENTS SHOULD THIS BE CONSIDERED
1. The competent patient who has requested a limitation of medical therapy which would otherwise have been considered. These patients should have completed a certificate under the "Medical Treatment Act" (Victoria).
2. The patient who has an illness for which advanced life-support therapies will neither significantly prolong life expectancy, nor improve the quality of life.
3. A patient for whom such therapy carries a far greater risk of complications than possible benefit.

WHICH THERAPY/THERAPIES MAY BE CONSIDERED
1. Emergency cardiopulmonary resuscitation.
2. Ventilatory support for respiratory failure.
3. Inotropic (or invasive) support for cardiovascular failure.
4. Haemodialysis for renal failure.
5. Transfusion of blood or blood products.
6. Operative surgery.
7. Admission of ICU or HDU wards.
8. Antibiotics.

WHICH 'THERAPIES' SHOULD NEVER BE WITHHELD
1. Respect for the dignity of every patient, irrespective of physical or mental condition.
2. Relief from pain, suffering and discomfort.
3. Reasonable provision of fluid therapy and nutrition.

WHO SHOULD BE INVOLVED IN THE DISCUSSION PROCESS
1. Patient (if appropriate).
2. Family, next of kin, significant other.
3. Agent holding Enduring Power of Attorney - Medical Treatment.
4. Designated care givers, e.g. nursing, medical, pastoral, community care givers.
5. Guardianship Board where appropriate.
N.B. Adequate time must be allowed for the patient and family to consider and discuss these issues.

DOCUMENTATION
Decisions to limit medical treatment should be documented on the Pro-forma on the reverse.

CAVEAT
1. No appropriate therapy will be withheld from any patient.
2. Each person must be treated individually - universal or prescriptive statements cannot be made.
3. No decision should be made without adequate consultation with, and agreement between, all parties.
4. Decisions should not be made without consultation with the Unit Specialist.
5. "Quality of life" is a subjective and potentially dangerous criterion for the withdrawal of therapy, when used by health care professionals.
6. This hospital does not advocate nor condone either euthanasia or assisted suicide, and this document is not be used for patients desiring such.
7. These guidelines should be used as such, to assist medical decision making.

'Limitation of Medical Treatment' form could be signed; an example of the latter is shown in Figure 12.1.

4. Mechanisms must be established to ensure the *correct interpretation* of non-treatment directives.

5. Once a DNR decision has been made, it should be *reviewed and reaffirmed* in writing at intervals which are appropriate to the patient's changing condition.

6. A DNR directive should be *able to be revoked* at 'any time at the request of the competent patient, or in the case of the incompetent patient, by the cited next-of-kin or legal representative', or as is morally appropriate (Clinical Ethics Committee 1984).

7. A DNR decision should be carried out only by those who have freely, and possessing the necessary information, agreed to carry out such directives. Where nurses or doctors have genuine conscientious objection to following a DNR directive, morally they ought to be *permitted to abstain* from being actively involved in caring for the patient in question.

By incorporating these and other similar considerations in DNR policies and guidelines, nurses and doctors can rest assured that they truly have done all that is possible to ensure that patients' rights and interests have been properly respected in life-threatening situations, and that they have not overstepped their authority as health care providers. Members of the community at large can also rest assured that their assumptions about being well cared for upon coming into hospital or other related health care agencies are not misplaced, and that they can indeed trust and rely on those people who will most probably care for them during those delicate, life-threatening moments which are all too often characterised by intense personal need and human vulnerability.

Medical futility

One of criterion that is commonly used to justify non-treatment (e.g. NFT/DNR) decisions is that of 'medical futility'. The concept of 'medical futility' (from the Latin *futtilis*, meaning pouring out easily, worthless) is generally used to refer to medical treatment that 'fails to achieve the goals of medicine' in that it offers no discernible benefit to the patient (i.e. it fails to overcome the patient's medical problem, or results in the patient surviving, but only to lead a 'useless life') (Nelson 2003; Jecker 1993).

The notion of medical futility first began being debated in the mid–1980s and was advanced largely in an attempt to convince the public of the need to establish a public policy that would enable treating doctors to 'use their clinical judgment or epidemiological skills to determine whether a particular treatment would be futile in a particular clinical situation' (Helft et al. 2000, p. 293; see also Taylor and Lantos 1995). Underpinning this movement was the idea that:

> once such a determination had been made [that a particular treatment was futile], the physician should be allowed to withhold or withdraw the treatment, even over the objections of a competent patient.
>
> (Helft et al. 2000, p. 293)

The notion of medical futility proved to be extremely controversial, however, and sparked a debate of unprecedented vehemence in the medical literature (Nelson 2003; Helft et al. 2000). Interestingly, this debate peaked in 1995 and then waned, largely because a consensus on the matter could not be achieved: for every thoughtful definition of 'medical futility' that was put forward, critics successfully raised counter-objections, pointing out exceptions that made broad acceptance of the notion and its operationalisation impossible (Nelson 2003; Helft et al. 2000).

Linchpin to the objections raised against the notion of medical futility — including both its objective biophysiological (quantitative) and subjective quality of life (qualitative) elements — were arguments that convincingly showed judgments about medical futility primarily involved 'moral judgments about right and good care', rather than clinical judgments about what was 'medically indicated' and therefore 'medically warranted'. Even when medical (clinical) judgments were based on rigorous clinical and epidemiological data, it was acknowledged by proponents of the medical futility movement that such data 'could not be used [reliably] to determine the level of probability that would justify calling a treatment futile' since such data tended to represent groups not individuals (Helft et al. 2000, p. 294). These data and related systems of prognostication that were devised during this period could not be used for another reason, namely, they failed to take into account the 'existential' goals that various treatments might be capable of achieving, such as enabling a patient to remain alive 'to see a loved one again' (Helft et al. 2000, p. 294). Finally, it was recognised that while doctors 'may be more qualified than patients to make technical judgments about medical treatment, they have no particular expertise in making decisions about such subjective matters as futility' or the subjective values, views, and goals of patients on which judgments of futility were heavily reliant (Helft et al. 2000, p. 294).

Since the mid-1990s, with the notable exception of the texts by Zucker and Zucker (1997) and Rubin (1998), there has been relatively little published on the subject of medical futility. For example, a search of the CINHAL data base in 1995 located 134 articles on medical futility (Helft et al. 2000); in contrast, in October 2003, a ProQuest search of multiple data bases for the preceding 12 month period located only 21 articles on the topic and, of these, only five carried the term 'futility' in the title. Despite this apparent decline in interest in the topic, the problem of how best to decide treatment options that are of limited benefit to patients at the end stage of life remains problematic. Furthermore, even though debate on the notion of *medical futility* has waned, there is much to suggest that local definitions of medical futility are nevertheless very much in use and indeed are operationalised in hospitals everyday to inform (non)treatment decisions (as has been shown by the discussion above, this is especially evident in the case of Not For Treatment (NFT) and Do Not Resuscitate (DNR) directives). A notable example of this can be found in the controversial case of the St Francis Medical Center, in Honolulu, which has recently developed and operationalised a specific and targeted 'medical futility policy' — reprinted in full in Tan et al. (2003). This initiative has, however, been viewed with some concern by observers external to the organisation (see in particular Hamel and Panicola 2003) and might yet see a rekindling of the medical futility debate.

Quality of life

A key decisional criterion commonly appealed to when making decisions about care and treatment for patients at the end stages of life is that of *quality of life*. Quality of life considerations are deemed to be particularly important in situations where a patient's life 'might be saved only to be lived out in severely impaired conditions' (Walter 1995, p. 1352). In such situations, quality of life considerations might be used, albeit controversially, to justify withholding or withdrawing life-sustaining medical treatment from a particular patient.

Despite being frequently appealed to when making treatment decisions, the quality of life criterion is not without controversy. One reason for this is that quality of life is difficult to define and can be used to refer to different though equally valid (subjective) realities. In short, as Welch-McCaffrey (1985, p. 151) points out: 'Quality of life is not a term that has unequivocal meaning nor is it unambiguously determinable in any given case'.

Defining quality of life

Defining quality of life can be a lesson in linguistic humility. One reason for this is that what is at issue here is not just defining '*quality* of life', but '*life*' itself. In the case of the term 'life' (from Old Norse, *lif* meaning body), this can be used to refer to two different realities, namely the:

> (1) vital or metabolic processes that could be called "human biological life"; or (2) "human personal life" that includes biological life but goes beyond it to include other distinctively human capacities, for example, the capacity to choose and to think.

> (Walter et al. 1995, p. 1353)

Likewise with the term 'quality' (from Latin *quālitās*, meaning state, nature), which can refer to several different realities, including: a formal state of excellence; the attributes or properties of either a personal or biological life; the minimum attributes necessary for a personal life (e.g. the capacity or potential capacity to have human relationships/ to pursue human purposes/to live life independently); the value (worth) of life itself (Walter et al. 1995; Kuhse 1987). Each of these realities, in turn, can be variously interpreted, and their interpretations variously interpreted, and so on *ad infinitum*, further demonstrating the complexities involved in trying to devise an agreed operational definition of the criterion.

To date, no consensus has been reached on how 'quality of life' should be defined or interpreted. There is, however broad agreement that the criterion essentially defies precise definition, or at least a definition which could be regarded as being universally acceptable. Nevertheless, as Downie and Calman (1987, p. 190) argue:

> Most ... would agree that quality of life relates to the individual person, that it is best perceived by that person, that conceptions of it change with time, and that it must be related to all aspects of life.

Different conceptions of quality of life

When appealing to quality of life considerations in health care contexts it is important for health care professionals (including nurses) to recognise that 'quality of life' can mean very different things to different people. For example, a class of students undertaking a post-registration Bachelor of Nursing course at RMIT University were once asked for their views on what they regarded as constituting a 'quality of life'. In response to this question, they identified the following (differing) characteristics:

- enjoyment and being happy, further defined as:
  - feeling contented;
  - having no worries;
  - being stress free;
  - feeling fulfilled;
- being healthy (and not having to suffer in any way);
- being valued and respected;
- having freedom and independence (being self-determining);
- being able to function effectively;
- actual achievement and/or being able to achieve important goals;
- having the love of family and friends.

The fact that these students held differing views about what constitutes quality of life is not, in itself, problematic. However, were these students to impose their personal views on their patients and/or to use their personal views to influence care and treatment decisions involving patients with life-threatening illnesses, this would be a different matter. Of particular concern would be the risks that such an imposition of views could pose to patients, especially if they were to influence treatment decisions that could be shown later not to have accorded with the patient's quality of life views. To illustrate the kind of risks involved, consider the following.

In a study on quality of life following spinal cord injury (SCI), a team of researchers found that emergency health care providers' (including nurses') attitudes about quality of life following SCI were substantially more negative than the attitudes expressed by those who had actually sustained such an injury. For instance, whereas only 18 per cent of emergency health care workers 'imagined they would be glad to be alive with a severe SCI', a substantial 92 per cent of those who had a true SCI were glad to be alive (Gerhart et al. 1994). And whereas only 17 per cent of emergency health care workers 'anticipated an average or better quality of life' following an imagined SCI, 86 per cent of those who had a true SCI had an average or better quality of life (Gerhart et al. 1994). Other studies have yielded similar results (Gerhart et al. 1994).

Health care providers (nurses among them) sometimes assume that people who suffer devastating injuries (or illnesses) have — or will have — a poor quality of life. Further, this belief is sometimes translated into the judgment that 'those who cannot lead normal lives would be better off dead' (Gerhart et al. 1994, citing Dunnum 1990). Not infrequently, these kinds of judgments influence decisions about whether or not to treat patients deemed 'medically hopeless' and who, if treated, could at best live only an 'impaired life'. As the above research shows, however, those who provide health care and those who receive it may not always share the same view about the conditions under which a quality of life is possible.

Quality of life judgments can have a significant bearing on *quality* (and *quantity*) of *care/treatment* decisions. The views and attitudes of health care providers may not only significantly affect the care they provide, but may also 'influence patients and families struggling with critical treatment decisions' (Gerhart et al. 1994, p. 807). It is therefore vital that health care providers exercise great care when making quality of life judgments, and act in a morally responsible way when using these judgments to inform clinical decisions. Anything less could result in morally undesirable consequences. For example, a prejudicial judgment about a spinal cord injury patient's quality of life could result in needed care and treatment being withheld or withdrawn prematurely, and the patient dying prematurely as a consequence.

Using quality of life considerations to inform treatment choices

As the discussion thus far has shown, quality of life as a decisional criterion can only be interpreted subjectively and, at the end of the day, can mean quite different things to different people. This finding is important since, among other things, it warns that using quality of life as a decisional criterion when making end of life treatment choices is not without risks (e.g. what might be an appropriate non-treatment decision for one person, might be quite inappropriate and even wrong for another). It also warns that members of the health care team involved in making end of life treatment decisions need to take great care to ensure that what *they* consider to be 'quality of life' is congruent with what their *patients* consider to be 'quality of life' and, further, that such considerations are in fact relevant to deciding the care and treatment options in the situation at hand.

Although quality of life defies precise definition, there are nevertheless three different senses in which it can be used when deciding care and treatment options: *descriptively, evaluatively,* and/or *prescriptively* (that is, morally) (Walter et al. 1995; Morreim 1995; Reich 1978).

Reich (1978, p. 830) explains that where the term quality of life is used as a descriptive statement, an observation is being made merely about the properties or characteristics of a human individual. In other words, quality of life in this sense simply refers to an *observable* and *'objective' description* about certain features or traits a person might have, and thus is morally neutral. An example of a descriptive quality of life statement would be: 'this person has pain', or 'this person has lost her or his functional ability', or 'this person is totally dependent on others for care'. By this view, to say someone has lost quality of life would be to say nothing more than that she or he has lost a particular property or characteristic (or set of characteristics) of life, not the value of life itself.

Quality of life in the evaluative sense, however, is quite different. Here a quality of life statement would express that 'some value or worth is attached to the characteristic of a given individual or to a kind of human life' (Reich 1978, p. 831; see also Walter et al. 1995). For example, an evaluative quality of life statement might assert that 'the pain suffered by this person is bad' and 'the absence of pain in this person is good', or that 'the loss of functional ability experienced by that person is bad' and 'the regaining of function by this person is good', or that 'this person's dependency on others for care is bad' and the 'regaining of independence by this person is good', and so on. To say a person has lost quality of life in this sense would be to assert merely that some property or aspect of her or his life has lost value, not that life itself has lost value — although the attachment of value to certain qualities or characteristics, in this instance, often becomes the very basis upon which an individual human life might be judged worth living or not worth living, and clinical decisions made accordingly (Walters et al. 1995, p. 1353).

Quality of life in the morally normative or prescriptive sense, on the other hand, is quite different again. Here, a quality of life statement would entail a *moral judgment* on a given (already evaluated) quality or set of qualities of an individual human life. Quality of life expressed as a moral judgment in this instance would seek to prescribe what would be a good or bad, right or wrong way of regarding a given individual human life or, more specifically, on the basis of its qualities, what ought and ought not to be done 'to support and protect' it. An example of a morally prescriptive quality of life statement would be:

- a life marked by intense pain is a life which it is not in an individual's best interests to go on living; ending such a life would thus be a morally just thing to do; or
- a life free of pain is a minimally decent life, and thus one worth living; to take such a life would be morally objectionable; or
- a life which cannot be lived independently is a life not worth living; therefore, ending such a life would be a morally decent thing to do; or
- a life which can be lived independently of others is a minimally decent life and therefore a life worth living; taking such a life would be morally objectionable.

In this instance, a statement concerning the loss of quality of life could be interpreted as indicating that the life in question no longer has worth and thus is dispensable. Alternatively, a statement concerning an increase in quality of life could be interpreted as indicating that the life in question has improved worth and thus warrants preservation and protection.

In the light of these three different senses of quality of life, it can be seen that there is enormous potential for making mistakes when deciding end of life treatment options based on quality of life considerations. This observation raises a number of important points for nurses. First, it wisely instructs the need for nurses to distinguish carefully the senses in which they might be using, or rather misusing, quality of life statements. This is particularly important in situations where decisions need to be made about which interventions should be implemented in order to enhance or promote the objective qualities of a person's life, and, further, about which quality or qualities ought to be enhanced or restored over others. For example, once it is identified that a person is in a state of pain which can be observed and described 'objectively' and that the pain in question is evaluated negatively by that person, an attending nurse will be in a relatively strong position to assert that interventions aimed at alleviating pain ought to take priority in that situation. If, however, it is determined that the person in question does not regard the pain as a disvalue, or at least regards its relief as being less valuable than, say, maintaining mental alertness, an attending nurse might be in quite a different position. Chosen interventions aimed at alleviating pain might assume quite a different priority, and indeed might take on quite a different form.

A second important point is that, by distinguishing the different senses in which the term quality of life can be used, the nurse may become more aware of the logical leap between making a *descriptive* judgment on the quality or qualities of a person's life and then making a *prescriptive* judgment (on the basis of that descriptive judgment) concerning what ought or ought not to be done in relation to that person's life. For example, if we distinguish between the different senses of 'quality of life', it soon becomes apparent that it is one thing to say a given person has lost one or two objective (descriptive) *qualities* or *properties* of their life, but it is quite another to say that, on the basis of those lost properties or qualities, the *life* itself of the person in question has less moral value or ought to be treated in one particular way rather than another.

Lastly, when we examine the fragile connection between the descriptive, evaluative and morally prescriptive senses of quality of life, the fundamental questions emerge of *who should decide* which values ought to be given to certain qualities or properties of life, and, further, on the basis of these ascribed values, of whether an individual human life in a particular context ought to be regarded as having one type or degree of moral value rather than another.

In relation to this last point, there is little doubt, at least from a moral point of view, that only the people whose lives are in question can authentically decide what values to ascribe to their qualities (properties) of life and what moral value to ascribe to their lives generally. For example, only the sufferers of their own pain can know what pain or dependency levels they can tolerate, and accordingly only they can identify the boundaries within which their pain or dependency states will be ascribed either positive or negative value. Only the sufferers of their own pain can know the point beyond which pain or dependency on others would render their life intolerable, and the point at which they would judge their life as being either morally less or morally more worthwhile. Bear in mind here that, while some might view pain as diminishing life's worth, others might hold quite a different view. Likewise, some might consider dependency on others as diminishing their life's worth, while others might consider it quite irrelevant to either the meaning or value of their life. What is important to understand is that, no matter how well-intentioned a nurse might be, or how knowledgeable or experienced, this probably will not be enough to enable that nurse to judge correctly either the evaluative or the morally prescriptive aspects of another person's (that is, that patient's) 'quality of life'. Even the descriptive aspect, for that matter, is difficult to judge, given the highly subjective nature of some so-called 'objectively observable' qualities, such as pain or loss of function. Since describing qualities is also very much a matter of interpreting them, there is always room for making judgment errors. It is for this reason that the people whose quality of life is at issue must be respected as the ones who ultimately are the best judges of what is to count as being in their 'best interests', and, further, as the ones who are best able to judge correctly what is to count as being their quality of life. In instances where people are unable (for reasons of incompetency or incapacity) to judge their own quality of life or best interests, this task should rightly fall to those (for example, close family members and/or friends) who intimately know the person in question and who know thoroughly their world views (values, beliefs and wishes).

It can be seen that in using the notion of quality of life, nurses must be very careful to distinguish the exact sense in which they are using it. They must also be aware of how easy it is to leap from a *descriptive statement* concerning a person's qualities of life to a *prescriptive statement* on what should be done for that life — morally, medically, or otherwise. Furthermore, they must take steps to guard against making this leap in judgment, particularly in instances where doing so might result in another not only losing a minimally decent *level* of life, but losing *life* itself.

Advanced directives

Under common law, every person has an overriding right to refuse any treatment, including life-sustaining/saving treatment (Ashby and Mendelson 2003, p. 261; see also Lewis 2001). Underpinning this common law right is the presumption that every adult has the mental capacity to consent or refuse to consent to any medical intervention 'unless and until that presumption is rebutted' (Ashby and Mendelson 2003, p. 261 supra note 11). Sometimes, however, people who are suffering from serious illnesses and/or who are dying will not be able to exercise their right to decide on account of having lost their capacity to make prudent and responsible life choices (i.e. they have become incompetent). In such situations, treatment decisions invariably fall to someone else — for example, the patient's proxy (family/friends) or the health care team. Proxies and health care professionals who find themselves in this surrogate decision-making role may not, however, know what to decide. This is especially so in cases where the patient's wishes are not known or, if known, are open to a variety of interpretations and hence dispute. Problems can also arise where proxies 'express certainty' regarding the preferences of the patient when, in fact, there is no clear basis for their opinions and/or where preferences collide with the values and beliefs of care givers (Johns 1996). A critical question to arise here is: How best to deal with this situation and the dilemmas it poses?

There is an emerging consensus in the medical literature that 'advanced planning' has a constructive role to play in — and can be an effective guide to — end of life decision making, and that the most appropriate instrument for communicating such planning is the *advanced directive* (Martin et al. 2000; Council on Ethical and Judicial Affairs, American Medical Association 1999; Hammes and Rooney 1998). Furthermore, not only can an advanced directive provide guidance on '*how* decisions are to be made, but also *who* is to make them' (Buchanan and Brock 1989, p.95).

What is an advance directive?

The *advanced directive* (also called a 'living will') is a relatively modern phenomena dating back to the late 1960s in the cultural context of the United States of America. Based on the principles underpinning the doctrine of informed consent and its related respect for the sovereignty of the individual to decide what is to count as being in his or her own best interests (see discussion on informed consent in Chapter 6 of this book), advanced directives take as their starting point the right of the individual to be self-determining in the matter of medical treatment when incapacitated — especially at the end of life.

In common law countries there is an increasing acceptance of the view that:

> the most direct way in which a competent person can seek to control what treatment he or she is to receive when incompetence supervenes is to give instructions on the subject before becoming incompetent.
>
> (Lanham 1993, p. 54)

To this end, most common law countries now have 'living wills' legislation of some kind upholding the entitlement of individuals to make known in advance their wishes about, and to provide instructions regarding, what medical care and treatment they would or would not want should they become incompetent (Forrester and Griffiths 2001; Lanham 1993).

How do advance directives work?

An advance directive works by 'directing' one or all of the following things:

- designate another person to make decisions (a proxy directive);
- provide instructions about a person's values and goals or treatment preferences (an instructional directive);
- both of the above (a combined directive) (Lynn and Teno 1995, p. 573 [bullet points added]; see also Sass 1998).

In either case, the directives can be expressed formally or informally. Whereas formal advanced directives take the form of a *signed and legally authorised written document* (such as a living will, an enduring power of attorney), informal advanced directives take the form of *unwritten oral communications* between the patient and his or her family, friends and/or attending health care professionals (Lynn and Teno 1995; Sass 1998). Although both can be used to inform treatment choices at the end stage of life, the formal (written) advanced directive is thought to be preferable since it can:

- provide documentary evidence of the patient's preferences;
- reduce opportunities for fraud and duress;
- reduce ambiguity about what has been authorised;
- authorise the termination of treatment that 'commits all future decision-makers to a course of action and offers legal enforcement for the patient's preferences' (Buchanan and Brock 1989, p. 118; Lynn and Teno 1995, p. 573).

Risks and benefits of advance directives

Although morally warranted, advanced directives (both formal and informal) are not free of difficulties. As Buchanan and Brock (1989) persuasively argue, advanced directives are vulnerable to a number of 'weighty objections' on account of the following considerations:

- a person's previously expressed preferences (no matter how well informed) can change as therapeutic options and hence prognosis change;
- people may not always be the best judges of their interests (interests anticipated to be at stake when an advanced directive was made initially might change radically under future unforeseen conditions);
- 'important safeguards that tend to restrain imprudent or unreasonable contemporaneous choices are not likely to be present, or, if present, to be effective' in contexts involving advance directives (e.g. if a competent patient refuses life-sustaining treatment his or her caregivers can urge the patient to reconsider this choice — which, in some cases, can 'prevent a precipitous and disastrous decision'; in the case of advanced directives being activated, however, the same protective response is less likely);
- the expected condition of a patient when a treatment decision is required may be substantially different to that envisaged when an advanced directive was originally made; in instances where the patient's actual condition is substantially different to what was expected, the authority of the advanced directive is called into question (adapted from Buchanan and Brock 1989, pp. 152–3; see also Sass 1998; Dresser and Robertson 1989).

Advance directives can also be problematic on account of imprecise language being used (leaving them vulnerable to a variety of contentious interpretations) and/or designated proxies disagreeing among themselves about what was in fact meant by statements contained in a directive. Underscoring this difficulty is the additional problem that advance directives of similar content can be the subjects of quite disparate degrees of discretion in regard to whether they are binding upon surrogates. Taking into account all of the above, it can be seen that rather than promoting 'good' end of life decision-making, an advance directive could inadvertently lead to disastrous (non-)treatment choices being made.

Despite these and other difficulties (see in particular Buchanan and Brock 1989), advanced directives are nevertheless regarded as having significant moral importance and authority in clinical contexts, not least on account of serving the following important values:

- preserving patient wellbeing by protecting patients from intrusive and futile medical treatments;
- promoting patient autonomy and self-determination; and
- serving altruism by 'authorising the termination of treatment that would impose financial or emotional costs on others' (Buchanan and Brock 1989, p. 152).

Other values that can be served include:

- enabling patients to plan for death and dying
- strengthening relationships by facilitating communication among loved ones and the settling of 'unfinished business' (Martin et al. 2000; Singer et al. 1998).

The moral authority of advance directives is thought to be particularly strong in cases where it can be shown that:

> The patient clearly understood the clinical situation that was likely to occur, the directive itself is readily understood, the treatment possibilities have not changed substantially since the patient's directive was written (e.g., by an advance in medical therapy possibilities), the discretion allowed to contemporaneous decision makers is clear, and the choices articulated are congruent with what is otherwise known about the patient.
>
> (Lynn and Teno 1995, p. 573)

Significantly, despite the demonstrable moral benefits of advanced directives, both research and practical experience suggests that, for the most part, they are under-utilised in clinical contexts and, to date, appear not to play a major role in guiding treatment decisions to withhold or withdraw life-sustaining treatment (Ashby and Mendelson 2003; Dembner 2003; Cook et al. 2001; Martin et al. 2000; Johns 1996; Lynn and Teno 1995). Reasons for this have included: (1) patients not having made an advance directive; and (2) caregivers not respecting an advance directive that has been made. (As a point of interest, when I have asked students — ranging in number from 10 to 300 — whether they have given Enduring Power of Attorney (Medical Treatment) to someone under the Victorian *Medical Treatment Act 1988*, less than 10 per cent indicate that they have done so.) There is, however, some emerging evidence that this situation is changing. In a study by Hammes and Rooney (1998), for example, the prevalence of advance directives among 540 decedents was found to be 85 per cent. Of these, 95 per cent of the advance directive documents were located in the patients' medical records. The median time between an advance directive being documented and patient death was 1.2 years. In almost all of the advance directives, a request had been made that treatment be forgone as death neared. The treatment preferences expressed seemed to have been consistently followed while making end of life decisions, with treatment being forgone in 98 per cent of the patient deaths. Drawing on the findings of their study, Hammes and Rooney (1998, p. 383) conclude that 'advance planning can be prevalent and can effectively guide end of life decisions'.

Whatever the risks and benefits of advance directives, it is likely that they will gain increasing authority in health care domains to guide end of life decision-making. To ensure that they achieve their intended purpose, it is vital that those making advance directives ensure that they are carefully written and clearly understood by those who may be left to implement them. It needs to be acknowledged, however, there will still be cases in which patients 'may not want or benefit from articulating preference in an instruction directive' and that, ultimately, the most anyone can do is to simply 'identify their preferred surrogate decision-maker' and ensure that this person is fully attuned to their interests, welfare and wellbeing (Lynn and Teno 1995, p. 574).

Conclusion

There is an emerging consensus on the practical and moral importance of communication at the end stages of life and the use of a 'fair process' for dealing with end of life decision-making (Martin et al. 2000; Johns 1996). Fundamental to the 'fair process' being advocated are the following six steps:

1. prior deliberation on the values of the physician, patient, and family;
2. joint decision-making at the bed-side with reference to outcome data and the intention or goals of treatment;
3. facilitated discussion and conflict resolution within the accepted limits of all parties;
4. the use of institutional ethics committees in the event of unresolved disputes;
5. transfer to another treating institution in the event that patients' wishes cannot be upheld;
6. court intervention in the case that another treating institution cannot be found and the patient's or the proxy's request is offensive to the agreed and accepted ethical standards of a majority of health care professionals.

> (adaptation with tabulations, Council on Ethical and Judicial Affairs, American Medical Association 1999)

It is acknowledged that nurses are 'not the final decision-makers in relation to overall medical care planning' (Byrne 2002, p. 15) and that they do not have legitimated authority to make life and death decisions in clinical contexts (Johnstone 1994). Nevertheless, on account of the time they spend communicating with patients and their families/friends, nurses have an important role to play in initiating discussion about future treatment options, particularly in regard to end of life treatment; they also have an important role to play in ensuring that planned end of life care and treatment accords with the patient's values, beliefs and preferences — where these are known and are not in contravention of the law. While not always preventing the dilemmas commonly associated with end of life decision-making, the involvement of nurses — and the communication processes that they can facilitate — may nevertheless provide an important safety and quality check that could help to prevent disastrous care and treatment choices from being made.

CASE SCENARIO AND CRITICAL QUESTIONS

Case scenario

At a seminar on ethical issues in clinical nursing practice, an experienced intensive care nurse asked for advice on 'what more she could have done' in the situation which she then related as follows.

She had been involved in the care of a middle-aged woman who, after suffering a massive myocardial infarction, had been admitted (deeply unconscious) into the local intensive care unit. The woman had been intubated before admission to the unit, and was placed immediately on a respirator. A few days later the medical hopelessness of the patient's condition was confirmed, and a medical decision was made to remove the artificial life-support system that was sustaining her life.

The woman's husband, who had been present most of the time since his wife's admission, objected strongly to this decision, however, and became very aggressive towards the medical and nursing staff. He also threatened to sue the hospital. Recognising the husband's reaction as a manifestation of extreme grief, the intensive care nurse approached the woman's adult children, who were also present, and, in a private setting, discussed with them what *they* thought should or could be done to help their father deal with the situation better. The children were unanimous that what was required was 'extra time' — specifically, that the removal of the life-support system be delayed so that they could console their father and help him to see that the situation really was 'hopeless'; that, tragic as it was, nothing further could be done.

Upon learning of the family's wishes, the nurse offered to act as a mediator between them and the medical staff, to herself remove the life-support from their mother at the appropriate time, and to seek support for their wishes from the attending medical staff. This the family accepted. Over the next hour, the nurse was able to fulfil her role as 'mediator', and succeeded in obtaining full support from the medical staff involved in the case. This support included the medical staff agreeing to the nurse deciding when and how to remove the life-support system from the patient. As a result of this mediation, extra time was 'bought', and the woman's husband and children were able to come to terms with the tragic decision that had been made. The family were all able to sit with the woman as the nurse progressively turned off the artificial life-support system. Later, the husband returned to the intensive care unit and thanked the nurse for her intervention.

Critical questions

1. What are your responsibilities as a professional caregiver in regard to caring for people at the end stages of life?
2. How would you have handled this situation?
3. What advice would you have given the intensive care nurse in response to her request for advice on 'what more she could have done'?

1   An earlier version of the discussion on 'Not For Resuscitation' (NFR) directives was originally presented under the title: 'The nature and moral implications of "Not For Resuscitation [NFR]" directives' at the *Nursing law and ethics, First Victorian State Conference. Theme: 'Matters of life and death'*, Monash University, Melbourne, 30 September 1988 (organised by the School of Nursing, Phillip Institute of Technology). The paper has been revised for publication in this text.

2   Details of this case have been altered to disguise the identity of the patient, the staff and the hospital concerned. Any resemblance the case of Mr H might have to an actual case is therefore purely coincidental.

Chapter 13

Taking a stand: conscientious objection, clinical ethics committees and whistleblowing

LEARNING OBJECTIVES

Upon the completion of this chapter and with further self-directed learning you are expected to be able to:

- Discuss critically the nature of conscience and its role in guiding ethical nursing conduct.
- Outline five conditions that must be met in order for a claim of conscientious objection to be genuine.
- Examine critically arguments both for and against the view that nurses ought to be permitted to conscientiously refuse to participate in certain procedures in nursing and health care contexts.
- Examine critically the role and function of clinical ethics committees.
- Discuss critically what decision-making authority clinical ethics committees should have.
- Discuss critically the implications of clinical ethics committees for the nursing profession.
- Define whistleblowing.
- Discuss the possible adverse consequences to nurses of blowing the whistle.
- Examine critically the conditions under which whistleblowing might be justified.

KEYWORDS

- Clinical ethics committees
- Conscience
- Conscientious objection
- Discrimination
- Hospital ethics committees
- Nursing ethics committees
- Patient care ethics committees
- Whistleblowing
- Whistleblowers

Introduction

At some time during the course of their professional practice there will come a time when nurses must take a stand on what they consider, after careful thought and critical reflection, to be morally important. Taking a stand can involve either individual or collective action. Individual action may involve a nurse refusing conscientiously to participate in a controversial medical procedure; reporting a troubling incident to a superior or some other authority (including an external statutory authority); seeking representation on or advice from a clinical ethics committee or some other decision-making committee; or speaking out in either a conference or some other public forum. On rare occasions, a nurse might decide to approach the media to have his or her concerns aired. Collective action, on the other hand, may involve groups of nurses embarking on an organised lobbying campaign aimed at particular target groups. Or, as has become increasingly common around the world, it may involve strike action — particularly in situations involving substandard working conditions that are placing patient safety at risk (see, for example, Johnstone 2002a, 1999a; Salladay 2002).

Whatever action is taken, it is never free of moral risk. There are many examples in the nursing, legal and bioethics literature (too numerous to list here) of nurses having suffered both personally and professionally because they took a stand on what they deemed to be an important professional or moral issue. For example, nurses conscientiously refusing to participate in certain morally controversial medical procedures have sometimes lost their jobs or have been made to resign 'voluntarily' (some examples of which will be given shortly).

Despite the associated hazards and risks, nurses have a moral obligation to take a stand on important ethical issues. Nevertheless, there are some misconceptions about the nature of this obligation, the options open to nurses for taking a stand, and even about whether it is right to take a stand at all. Some nurses even fear that some of the options open to them (such as conscientious objection, appealing to a clinical ethics committee, lobbying, strike action or whistleblowing) are incompatible with their broader professional obligations as nurses and are therefore 'unprofessional'. For some nurses this has caused enormous personal conflict, and has served more to compound the moral problems they face in the workplace than to help resolve them.

This chapter attempts to clarify some of the confusion surrounding various options open to nurses for taking a stand on a moral issue, and to show that these options might not only be compatible with professional nursing obligations, but may even be prima facie professional nursing obligations in themselves. It is to discussing the particular options of conscientious objection, clinical ethics committees, and whistleblowing that this chapter now turns.

Conscientious objection[1]

Nurses have been 'conscientiously objecting' to workplace practices and related processes for years (for example, by sidestepping a particular patient assignment, changing shifts, declining to work in a particular ward or area, or taking a 'sick day' off work). Their objections, however, have rarely gained public attention. Indeed, it has only been in extreme situations, such as when a nurse has been dismissed or denied employment, or has been threatened in some way, have issues involving conscientious objection come to the attention of others outside of the unit or organisation where they have arisen. Those who have had the courage to formally voice their conscientious refusal to participate in certain medical procedures or organisational processes, or to carry out certain directives given by an employer or superior, have sometimes done so at great personal and professional cost. One of the most famous examples of this can be found in the much cited United States case of Corrine Warthen.

Corrine Warthen, a registered nurse of many years experience, was dismissed from her employing hospital of 11 years for refusing to dialyse a terminally ill bilateral amputee patient. Warthen's refusal in this instance was based on what she cited as ' "moral, medical and philosophical objections" to performing this procedure on the patient because the patient was terminally ill and ... the procedure was causing the patient additional complications' (*Warthen v Toms River Community Memorial Hospital* (1985, p. 205).

Warthen had apparently dialysed the patient on two previous occasions. In both instances, however, the dialysis procedure had to be stopped because the patient suffered severe internal bleeding and cardiac arrest (*Warthen's case* 1985, p. 230). It was the complications of severe internal bleeding and cardiac arrest that she was referring to in her refusal. Her dismissal came when she refused to dialyse the patient for a third time.

Believing she had been wrongfully and unfairly dismissed, Warthen took her case to the Supreme Court, where she argued in her defence that the Code for Nurses of the American Nurses' Association (ANA) justified her refusal, since it essentially permitted nurses to refuse to participate in procedures to which they were personally opposed (*Warthen's case* 1985, p. 229).

The court did not find in her favour, however, and she lost her case. In making its final decision, the court made clear its position on a number of key points (*Warthen's case* 1985):

1. An employee should not have the right to prevent his or her employer from pursuing its business because the employee perceives that a particular business decision violates the employee's personal morals, as distinguished from the recognised code of ethics of the employee's profession ... (p. 233).
2. [In support of the hospital's defence] it would be a virtual impossibility to administer a hospital if each nurse or member of the administration staff refused to carry out his or her duties based upon a personal private belief concerning the right to live ... (p. 234).
3. The position asserted by the plaintiff serves only the individual and the nurses' profession while leaving the public to wonder when and whether they will receive nursing care ... (p. 234).

Another famous example of the personal and professional cost a nurse can play for taking a stance on an issue can be found in the case of Frances Free (also from the United States). Free, an experienced registered nurse, was dismissed by her employer after she had refused to evict a seriously ill bedridden patient. Free's refusal (*Free v Holy Cross Hospital* (1987), p. 1190), in this instance, was based on grounds that to evict the patient would have been:

> in violation of her ethical duty as a registered nurse not to engage in dishonourable, unethical, or unprofessional conduct of a character likely to harm the public as mandated by the Illinios Nursing Act.

The patient in question had been arrested for possession of a hand gun. Meanwhile, an order had been given for her to be transferred to another hospital. The police officer guarding the patient pointed out, however, that because of certain outstanding matters, the other hospital would probably not accept the patient and it was likely that she would be returned to Holy Cross Hospital. Free communicated this information to the hospital's chief of security who responded by telling her that the patient was to be removed from the hospital 'even if removal required forcibly putting the patient in a wheelchair and leaving her in the park' which was across the road from the hospital (*Free's case*, p. 1189). Although Free disagreed with removing the patient, she gave the necessary instructions for the patient's transfer to the other hospital.

As part of the process of dealing with this situation, Free contacted the vice-president of her employing hospital to discuss the matter with him. It is reported that the vice-president 'became agitated, shouted and used profanity in telling Free that it was he who had given the order to remove the patient' (*Free's case*, p. 1189). After this incident, Free contacted the patient's physician who stated that 'he opposed the transfer' and instructed Free 'not to touch the patient but to document his order that the patient should remain at the hospital' (*Free's case*, p. 1189). After checking the patient and 'calming her down', Free received a telephone call 'ordering her to report to the office of the vice-president'. When she arrived at the vice-president's office Free was advised 'that her conduct was insubordinate and that her employment was immediately terminated' (*Free's case*, p. 1189). Free subsequently took court action arguing that her dismissal was 'unfair'. Free lost her case, however. Significantly, during the court proceedings, Free's actions were characterised 'as being of a *personal* as opposed to a *professional* nature and therefore as falling outside the scope of the *Illinios Nursing Act*' (Johnstone 1994, p. 256).

These and similar cases (see also the case of the New South Wales registered nurse who was allegedly denied employment as a midwife because of her conscientious objection to abortion and sterilisation, presented as a case study in Chapter 9 of this book) demonstrate that the issue of conscientious objection by nurses is by no means trivial and deserves sustained attention by all concerned. In particular, attention needs to be given to clarifying the nature and authority of conscience, distinguishing between genuine and bogus claims of conscientious objection, and determining the kinds of policy there should be towards those who conscientiously refuse to perform or to participate in morally controversial medical and/or nursing procedures. As well as this, attention needs to be given to the question of: When, if ever, can a superior decently direct nurses to perform tasks which they are conscientiously opposed to performing? An additional question is: Can nurses decently refuse to assist with tasks which others do not regard as morally problematic? These and other key concerns raised by the conscientious objection debate are addressed in the following sections.

The nature of conscience explained

The *Oxford English dictionary* (2003) defines 'conscience' as:

> the internal acknowledgment or recognition of the moral quality of one's motives and actions; the sense of right and wrong as regards things for which one is responsible; the faculty or principle which pronounces upon the moral quality of one's actions or motives, approving the right and condemning the wrong.

The *Collins English dictionary* (2003) defines 'conscience' as a 'sense of right and wrong that governs a person's thoughts and actions'. These definitions, however, are inadequate to answer questions concerning the legitimacy and power of conscience as a bona fide moral authority. In short, while they help to describe what conscience is, these definitions say nothing about whether individuals should always obey their conscientious senses of right and wrong, or whether others can reasonably be expected to respect another's conscientious claims. In order to find answers to these and related questions, a philosophical analysis is required, such as will now be advanced.

Philosophical accounts of conscience fall roughly into three categories: as *moral reasoning*, as *moral feelings*, and as a *combination of moral reasoning and moral feelings* (see also Beauchamp and Childress 2001, pp.37–9; Rawls 1971, pp. 205–11, 368–9; Mill 1962, pp. 281–4; Kant 1930, pp. 129–35; Hume 1888, p. 458).

CONSCIENCE AS MORAL REASONING

A reasonable or rationalistic account of conscience regards rational moral principles and reason as the source of one's moral convictions. Conscientious judgments, by this view, are really critically reflective moral judgments concerning right and wrong (Garnett 1965; Broad 1940). Rational insight can be either religious or non-religious in nature, depending on what a person's world views are. Either way, a rational conscience typically manifests itself as 'a little voice inside one's head saying what one should and should not do'. Or, to put this in moral terms, it tells us what our moral obligations and duties are. Statements of conscientious objection then are, by this view, merely statements of moral duty which individuals recognise and commit themselves to fulfil. Whether the duties or obligations identified impose overriding or absolute demands, or only prima facie demands on the individual is, however, another matter entirely, and one that is considered shortly.

CONSCIENCE AS MORAL FEELINGS

There are two possible versions of a 'moral feelings' account of conscience — emotivist and intuitionist. Both consist of a tendency to spontaneously experience either emotions or intuitions 'of a unique sort of approval of the doing of what is believed to be right and a similarly unique sort of disapproval of the doing of what is believed to be wrong' (Garnett 1965, p. 81).

It is generally recognised that these feelings are quite different from the sorts of feelings we might have when, for example, looking at a beautiful painting (aesthetic approval) or an awful painting (aesthetic disapproval), or eating a favourite food (the feelings of mere liking) or smelling an awful smell (feelings of mere disliking), or witnessing an act of remarkable human achievement (feelings of admiration) or an act of extraordinary human failure (feelings of disdain). By contrast, in the case of wicked acts or the violation of duty, conscience may manifest itself in strong and distinguishable feelings of moral loathing, shame, remorse, or even guilt, or, as Beauchamp and Childress (1989) suggest, the unpleasant feelings of 'a loss of integrity, wholeness, peace, and harmony' (p. 387). To borrow from Fletcher (1966), conscience can manifest itself as 'a sharp stone in the breast under the sternum, which turns and hurts when we have done wrong' (p. 54). In the case of virtuous acts, conscience may manifest itself as strong feelings of reassurance or moral goodness (Fletcher 1966, p. 54; Kant 1930, p. 130), or, as Beauchamp and Childress (1989) suggest, as feelings of integrity, wholeness, peace and harmony (p. 387). Either way, moral feelings instruct individuals on what they ought and/or ought not to do. As with the rationalistic account, statements of conscience emerge as statements of obligation and duty.

CONSCIENCE AS MORAL REASON AND MORAL FEELINGS

The concept of conscience as a combination of reason and feelings basically involves an integrated response to 'moral catalysts' in the world. It does not rely on 'blind emotive obedience', as Kordig (1976) calls it, nor on an exclusive and blind devotion to reason. Rather, it relies on the mutually guiding and instructive forces of both *moral sensibilities* and *moral reasoning*. This account of conscience is, in my view, the most plausible of the three given, and is thus the one that underpins this discussion.

How conscience works

Now that we have briefly examined the essential nature of conscience, the next question is: How does conscience function as a moral authority?

It is generally recognised that conscience functions as a *personal* (internal) *sanction* and as a *personal moral authority* (Beauchamp and Childress 2001; Childress 1979). Claims of conscience typically identify individual people with their self-chosen or autonomously chosen standards and principles of conduct (Nowell-Smith 1954, p. 268). Further, they *commit* individual people to act in accordance with those principles. In other words, claims of conscience commit the individual person to act morally (Timms 1983, p. 41). Thus, when conscience is said to be 'personal' or 'one's own', all that is being claimed is that a particular set of autonomously chosen moral standards has authority over a particular person — not, as is sometimes mistakenly thought, that the person has a unique and different set of moral standards from everybody else, and thus is a kind of 'moral freak'.

Conscience can be appealed to both as a kind of 'reviewer' or 'judge' of past acts, and as an 'authority on' or as a 'guide to' future acts. Whether conscience is appealed to as judge or guide, however, it is important to understand that conscience is not *morality itself*, nor is it the *ultimate standard* (or even *a* standard) of morality. Rather, as Gonsalves explains (1985, p. 55), it is:

> ... only the intellect itself exercising a special function, the function of judging the rightness or wrongness, the moral value, of our own individual acts according to the set of moral values and principles the person holds with conviction.

Or, as Childress explains (1979, p. 319), it is merely 'the mode of consciousness resulting from the application of standards'.

Gonsalves' and Childress' views make it plain that statements of conscience are not statements of a unique moral faculty or of unique moral standards. Rather, they are statements of a *particular application of adopted moral standards*. Conscientious objection, by this view, essentially translates into a case of *moral disagreement* in regard to which moral statements apply and what one's moral duty is in a particular situation. If this is so, the case for respecting a conscientious objector's claims becomes compelling — particularly in instances where there are no clear-cut moral grounds for settling a specific disagreement (as sometimes occurs in the cases of abortion, organ transplantation, assisting with the involuntary administration of ECT or psychotropic medication, administering blood to Jehovah's Witness patients, and similar cases) (see also Wicclair 2000).

It should be noted here that, once it is accepted that claims of conscience translate into claims of duty, it is conceptually incorrect to speak of conscientious objection as a *right* (as some nursing position statements on the subject do). To assert this would be to assert that an individual has a 'right to have a duty', which is conceptually incorrect. It is more correct to speak of others being bound to respect another's claim of conscience, just as they are bound to respect another's claim of moral duty.

The problem remains, however, that consciences are fallible and can make mistakes (Seeskin 1978). As Nowell–Smith (1954, p. 247) points out, some of the worst crimes in human history have been committed by people acting on the firm convictions of conscience. Hitler, for example, believed he was fulfilling a supreme moral duty by purging the German race of its 'Jewish disease' (Kordig 1976). Others also point out that, in some instances, what appears to be a claim of conscience may be nothing more than a claim of prudence or self-interest or convenience. This invariably raises the question: Should I always obey my conscience? Further to this, claims of conscience can be insincere or counterfeit, raising the additional questions of: How can I distinguish between genuine and bogus claims of conscientious objection? Should I always respect another's conscientious claims? It is to answering these questions that this discussion now turns.

Bogus and genuine claims of conscientious objection

For a conscientious objection to be genuine, it must satisfy at least five conditions.

1. It must have as its basis a *distinctively moral motivation*, as opposed to the motivations of mere self-interest, prudence, convenience or prejudice. By this is meant:
    a. that the action has as its aim the maintenance of sound moral standards, and the achievement of a moral end (Garnett 1965);
    b. that the person performing the act sincerely believes in the moral characteristics of the action in question, and sincerely desires to do what is right (Broad 1940, p. 75; Childress 1979, p. 334); and
    c. that the desire to do what is right is sufficient to override considerations of fear, cowardice, self-interest, and prejudice.
2. It must be performed on the basis of *autonomous, informed, and critically reflective choice*. By this is meant:
    a. that the action must be the agent's 'own', so to speak — that is, it is not the product of coercion or manipulation; and
    b. that that action has been carefully considered — that is, that the person has taken into account all the relevant factual as well as ethical information pertaining to the situation at hand, possible alternatives to the action being contemplated, and predicted moral outcomes of the action once it is taken (Broad 1940, p. 75).
3. Conscience should be appealed to only *as a last resort* — that is, in defence of one's moral beliefs. A claim of conscientious objection is a last resort when all other means of achieving a tolerable solution to a given moral problem have failed. Here conscientious objection is justified on grounds analogous to those justifying self-defence, which permit people to use reasonable force in order to preserve their integrity (in this case, their moral integrity) (Machan 1983, pp. 503–5).
4. The conscientious objector must admit that *others might have an equal and opposing claim of objection*. For example, a nurse refusing on

conscientious grounds to assist with an abortion procedure must be prepared to accept that the aborting surgeon may feel obliged as a matter of conscience to go ahead with the abortion. To quote from Broad: 'What is sauce for the conscientious goose is sauce for the conscientious ganders who are his [sic] neighbours or his [sic] governors' (Broad 1940, p. 78).

5. *The situation in which it is being claimed must itself be of a nature which is morally uncertain*; that is, there are no clear-cut moral grounds upon which the matter at hand can be readily and satisfactorily resolved, and competing views can be shown to be equally valid.

If we accept these criteria, the task of distinguishing bogus from genuine claims of conscientious objection becomes considerably easier. To illustrate this, consider four types of situations in which nurses commonly claim conscientious objection: the lawful but morally controversial directives of a superior; a conflict of personal values between a nurse and a patient; personal fear of contagion; and unsafe working conditions.

CONSCIENTIOUS OBJECTION TO THE LAWFUL BUT MORALLY CONTROVERSIAL DIRECTIVES OF A SUPERIOR

Nurses as employees are compelled by the principle of employment law to obey the lawful and reasonable directives of an employer or superior. The problem is, however, that nurses might not always agree morally with the lawful directives they have been given, and thus may sometimes find themselves in the uncomfortable position of having to perform acts which violate their reasoned moral judgments (Johnstone 1998, 1994).

There are many examples of nurses having been caught in both personal and professional dilemmas on account of legal demands to obey the lawful though morally controversial directives of doctors and nurse superiors. Examples have typically involved situations in which nurses have been directed, against their will, to assist with morally controversial procedures such as abortion, euthanasia, electroconvulsive therapy (ECT) and organ transplantation. The difficulties nurses have encountered in such situations have been compounded by the fact that they have had little, if any, avenue for officially expressing their conscientious refusal without fear of losing their jobs or facing other threats.

Situations involving nurses' conscientious refusal to follow lawful but morally questionable directives invariably pose the age-old question of whether an individual can, all things considered, be decently expected to follow morally controversial or morally bad, although legally valid, laws — or, in this case, lawful directives.

As I have stated elsewhere (Johnstone 1988), the problem of legal–moral conflict is not new to philosophy. Questions of, for example, what is the proper relationship of morality to law, what is to count as a *good* legal system, or whether individuals ought to be compelled to obey immoral laws, have long been matters of philosophical controversy. Hart, an Oxford scholar and professor of jurisprudence, for example, argued almost half a century ago that existing law must not supplant morality 'as a final test of conduct and so escape criticism' (Hart 1957). He also argued that the demands of law must be submitted to the scrutiny and guidance of sound morality before they can be justly enforced (Hart 1961). Not surprisingly, these kinds of views have sparked intense debates in both philosophy and law. It is beyond the scope of this text to discuss Hart's views and address the interesting questions concerning the philosophy of law that they raise. Nevertheless, it is assumed for argument's sake here that any law which fails the test of sound moral scrutiny should be either adjusted or rejected; it is also assumed that to punish autonomous moral agents for refusing to obey lawful but morally questionable directives is *morally unjust*.

A number of other important considerations are worthy of attention here. First, there is the persuasive view that forcing nurses to act against their reasoned or conscientious judgments is to not only ignore or diminish their moral autonomy, but also to violate the principles of morality itself — not least those of autonomy and reflectivity (Muyskens 1982, p. 61). Perhaps even more troubling is the possibility that violating nurses' consciences would also unjustly violate their integrity as moral agents (see also Wicclair 2000; Childress 1979).

Second, it is generally recognised that if people are forced constantly to violate their conscience then their conscience will gradually weaken and lose its authority (Kant 1930). This in turn makes it easier for individuals to avoid fulfilling their perceived moral duties and/or acting in accordance with autonomously chosen moral standards. As a result, there is likely to be a general breakdown in compliance with moral rules and principles, and a general erosion of individual moral responsibility and accountability. It takes little to imagine what would happen to the moral fabric of the community at large if all its members were forced, say, by order of the state, constantly to violate their reasoned moral judgments or consciences. No less consideration is due to what may ultimately happen to the moral fabric of the nursing profession if its individual members are constantly forced to abandon their reasoned moral judgments and consciences in favour of preserving the prescriptions and proscriptions of law and convention.

Related to this is a third consideration — that moral duty 'is mainly concerned with the avoidance of intolerable results' (Urmson 1958, p. 72). If fulfilling one's supposed duty does not avoid or prevent intolerable results, it seems reasonable to question whether in fact it was one's duty in the first place. As with the case of supererogatory acts (that is, acts above the call of duty, such as those performed by saints and heroes), care must be taken to distinguish those deeds which can be reasonably expected of 'ordinary' persons (or 'ordinary' nurses) from those which it would merely be *nice* of 'ordinary' persons (nurses) to perform, but which could never be reasonably *expected* of them (Urmson 1958, p. 68). On this point, Urmson (1958, p. 71) argues: '… a line must be drawn between what we can expect and demand of others and what we can merely hope for and receive with gratitude when we get it'.

Fourth, those who coerce others to act against their conscience erroneously presume that coercion vitiates moral responsibility. This, however, is not so. Just as more sophisticated claims of duty cannot be escaped or deceived, neither can claims of conscience. It is a mistake to hold that, if a person is forced to perform an act to which they are conscientiously opposed, they are less morally culpable for that act, and that they will feel less morally guilty for having performed it. What users of force fail to understand is that an instance of moral violation still stands, regardless of whether it has been caused by an act of coercion or an act of free will.

Fifth, nurses are not automata or robots, but thinking, reasoning, feeling, responsible human beings. Legal law recognises this by the very fact that it can and does hold nurses independently accountable for their actions (Johnstone 1994). Given this, it is a mistake to hold that nurses have an *unqualified* duty to obey the directives of a superior.

Lastly, it is ultimately more desirable than not to have a health care system comprised of conscientious nurses. Nurses comprise 70 per cent of the health care workforce. The prospect of 70 per cent of health care providers being morally unconscientious is a bleak one. Since most of us cannot be saints, but can be conscientious, we need to preserve and cultivate conscientiousness (Nowell–Smith 1954, p. 259; Garnett 1965, p. 91). Only by doing this can we be assured of achieving and maintaining some sort of moral order in health care domains. As Seeskin (1978) argues, '… we have no guarantee that our deliberations will be perfect or our moral sensibilities adequate' (p. 299); it is for this reason, among others, that conscience and moral conscientiousness should be given a place among the moral virtues. We might be condemned as fanatics if we hold conscience to be infallible, but if we do not at least acknowledge its ultimateness in the scheme of moral reasoning, we might be guilty of moral negligence and moral irresponsibility (Seeskin 1978; Kordig 1976).

The consequences of such views have interesting implications for policy makers attempting to respond to the conscientious objection problem. These views seem to suggest that, even if nurses' consciences are mistaken, on balance there are moral benefits to be gained by permitting their conscientious objections — not least, the benefits of fostering moral sensitivity and moral responsibility in the workplace. These views also suggest that, if nurses are not permitted conscientiously to object, then health care contexts, not to mention the community at large, will be morally worse off by virtue of being more at risk of suffering moral harms on account of receiving care that is not informed or guided by conscientious ethical beliefs and standards.

It might be objected here that permitting conscientious objection is not conducive to the efficient running of hospitals and other health services. There is, however, little support for this kind of claim. In the case of military service, for example, it has been found that objectors are rarely amenable to threats and usually make unsatisfactory soldiers if coerced, and that in fact there are generally not enough objectors to frustrate the community's purpose (Benn and Peters 1959, p. 193). I would suggest that something similar is probably true of objectors in nursing. As many examples in the nursing literature have shown, nurses have preferred to resign and risk dismissal than perform acts which they find morally offensive. Further to this, those nurses who have been coerced have not wholly complied with given orders. (For example, I know of nurses who have resuscitated patients in cases of controversial DNR directives, and not resuscitated patients in the case of controversial CPR orders.) It is also unlikely that there are enough objecting nurses to obstruct the efficient running of the hospital system.

Where lawful directives entail a demand to perform morally controversial proced-ures, there is considerable scope for suggesting that a nurse has a firm moral basis upon which to conscientiously object. Issues such as abortion, organ transplants, electroconvulsive therapy, the enforced and involuntary treatment of psychiatric patients and euthanasia are all morally controversial, and, as yet, no morally clear–cut grounds exist for resolving them. Until these issues can be resolved satisfactorily, it would be morally indefensible and unjust to insist that nurses must, when directed, assist with abortion, organ transplantation, electroconvulsive therapy and euthanasia work — or any other work which is morally controversial. In other words, where a so–called 'standard' or 'reasonable' medical or nursing procedure is morally questionable, nurses cannot decently be forced to perform or participate in that procedure. Further, it is worth noting once again that what we have in a situation of conscientious objection is moral disagreement — something which, as discussed in Chapter 6, may not be resolvable. The most amenable solution seems to be to permit conscientious objection.

CONSCIENTIOUS OBJECTION AND THE PROBLEM OF CONFLICT IN PERSONAL VALUES

Between nurse and patient

The International Council of Nurses' (2000) *Code for Nurses* states that 'the nurse's primary professional responsibility is to people who require nursing care'. It further states that: 'In providing care, the nurse promotes an environment in which the human rights, values, customs and spiritual beliefs of the individual, family and community are respected' (International Council of Nurses 2000). Sometimes, however, a nurse may find it genuinely difficult to respect a person's (or a family's or a community's) values, customs and spiritual beliefs, and for this reason may decline to be involved in caring for such entities. Consider the following cases.

CASE STUDIES

Case 1

A registered nurse working in a general medical ward was assigned a male patient who was known to be an orthodox Muslim. Upon learning of the man's religion, the nurse refused to care for him, stating that she could not accept the attitudes of Muslim males towards women, and that if she cared for him she would be as good as condoning his (and his community's) views.

Case 2

A registered nurse working in an infectious diseases unit was assigned a male patient in the end stages of AIDS. Upon learning that the patient was a homosexual and prior to his illness had been actively involved in the gay community, the nurse refused to accept the assignment. He argued that as a Christian he could not condone homosexuality, and therefore it would be against his religious beliefs to care for the patient.

Case 3

A registered nurse working in a country hospital was asked to admit and care for a patient injured in a fight. When she recognised the patient as a member of a family who had been engaged in a feud with her own family for years, she declined to care for him. She stated as her reason that, were she to care for the man, she would be violating the loyalties she owed to her own family.

There is little doubt that all three registered nurses in the cases just given have sincere motivations behind their refusals to care for the patients in question. What is not so clear, however, is whether these motivations have a moral basis. For instance, their refusals to care for these patients seem to be based more on, for example, non-moral personal dislike, prejudice, fear, disdain or mere disapproval than on sincere moral motivation and the desire to achieve morally desirable ends. Second, it is not clear whether, by refusing to care for these patients, the nurses will preserve their moral integrity. In fact, it may be quite the reverse, since they have allowed personal interests to override the significant moral interests of their patients. Lastly, the professional demand to care for the patients in question is not *itself* morally controversial — at least, not in the same way that, say, the demand to care for and stabilise a 'brain dead' patient for organ donation is (see Johnstone 1989, pp. 302–18). While it may be imprudent to compel the nurses in these cases to care for the patients assigned to them, it is not immediately apparent that it would be immoral to do so. It might be concluded then that their refusals can, at least from a moral perspective, be justly overridden. Nevertheless, there may still exist pragmatic grounds for permitting their refusals. If they cannot be relied upon to give adequate care, for example, it might be better to allow their refusal. If their prejudices and personal feelings are of such a nature as to seriously cloud their prudential judgments and indeed their ability to care and engage in an effective therapeutic relationship, it may be that they should not be allocated the patients in question. This, however, may be more a practical consideration rather than a moral one — although, granted, one which will probably have a significant moral dimension; namely, the patient's wellbeing.

CONSCIENTIOUS OBJECTION, THE FEAR OF CONTAGION, AND HOMOPHOBIA

The question of if, and when, and under what circumstances nurses may refuse to care for certain patients has become a particularly important and challenging one over recent years, largely because of the worldwide HIV/AIDS epidemic.

Questions have been asked, both in Australia and overseas, about whether nurses can rightly refuse to care for HIV/AIDS patients (including infected newborns) (for an exhaustive discussion of this issue, see Crock 2001). Overseas research studies and opinion polls have suggested, for example, that some nurses would rather abandon their practices and nursing careers than place themselves at risk by caring for HIV/AIDS patients (Huerta and Oddi, 1992; Jemmott et al. 1992; Melby et al. 1992; Beard et al. 1988; Lester and Beard 1988). In one United States opinion poll, published in *Nursing 88*, it was revealed that 73 per cent of nurses surveyed were concerned about their own safety, and 47 per cent believed they had a right to refuse to care for HIV/AIDS patients; interestingly, an overwhelming majority (93 per cent) stated that they had never refused to care for an HIV/AIDS patient, despite their fears (Brennan et al. 1988). The poll also revealed that a staggering 80 per cent of nurses surveyed stated that their own families were concerned about their (the nurses') safety when caring for HIV/AIDS patients.

Other studies have found that nurses caring for HIV/AIDS patients have actually been shunned by family, friends and neighbours, and even by other health care workers, who apparently feared association 'with one who provides direct care' (Huerta and Oddi 1992, p. 221; *Nursing Times*, 1986a, p.10). This further demonstrates the complexity of the refusal to care issue, and the difficulties associated with answering the question: To what extent should nurses be expected to sacrifice their own important interests for the sake of those for whom they care?

Significantly, two of the most commonly cited reasons for refusing to care for HIV/AIDS patients are fear of contagion, and disapproval of patients' lifestyles (especially those involving either homosexuality or intravenous drug use) (Crock 2001; Huerta and Oddi 1992, p. 223). A poignant example of how fear of contagion and disapproval of a patient's lifestyle can affect the ability of nurses to care and, in turn, the patient's overall wellbeing, is given below.

CASE STUDIES

Case 4

A client was diagnosed as having AIDS upon his admission to hospital. During his inpatient stay, nurses often cracked open the door and called in to him to learn of his condition, but would not enter the room. The hospital staff would not bathe him, and he was not allowed to shower. Bloody linens were not removed from the room. His emergency bedside signal [call bell] was left unanswered for as long as eight hours. A pamphlet was left at his bedside that described homosexuality as a sinful practice (Staff of the National Health Law Program 1991, p. 260).

Although this is an American case, the prejudicial attitudes it demonstrates are not restricted to the national borders of the United States. In 1989, for example, a respected major hospital in Melbourne caused a public outcry when it imposed a ban on treating all people who had AIDS or who carried the HIV virus (Miller 1989). The decision to impose the ban was made by the hospital's medical advisory board, and was allegedly supported by both doctors and nurses working at the hospital, as well as by the Victorian branch of the Australian Medical Association (AMA) (Athersmith 1989a; Price 1989). As a point of interest, it was later revealed that nurses had not in fact been consulted about the decision to effect the ban (Curtis 1989). The hospital's ban was the first case of its kind in Australia (Allender and Robinson 1989). Subsequently the Victorian Government took steps to outlaw hospital policies which effectively discriminated unjustly against HIV/AIDS patients. (For a more recent example of discriminatory attitudes against patients who are HIV/AIDS positive, see Case Scenario 2 in Chapter 6 of this book.)

It is doubtful whether HIV/AIDS (and/or other cases of infectious diseases — for example, hepatitis B and C, and drug resistant tuberculosis) presents a situation in which conscientious objection claims would be valid. Certainly, claims in these sorts of cases do not seem to satisfy all the five criteria of genuine conscientious objection listed earlier. For example, it is not clear that claims in these cases are based on a distinctive moral motivation aimed at maintaining sound moral standards or achieving a desired moral end. Nor is it clear that claims in these cases are based on informed and critically reflective choice (many may, in fact, be based on misinformed, fearful and arbitrary self-interested choice). It is also not clear that the claims of conscientious objection in these cases are necessary as a 'last resort' in 'the defence of one's moral integrity'. For one thing, it has yet to be shown how, if at all, caring for someone who is HIV positive threatens the moral integrity or standards of a caregiver (a point to be examined further shortly). Finally, it is far from clear that these cases involve a situation that is characteristically 'morally uncertain'. (It has yet to be shown convincingly that it is unethical to care for someone who is seriously ill with an infectious disease.) While the objector may recognise that others' conscientious claims are equally deserving in these cases, and thereby satisfy at least one of the five criteria listed, this is not enough to uphold a genuine claim of conscientious objection.

It should be noted, however, that, even though a claim of genuine conscientious objection might fail in cases of caring for people with potentially life-threatening infectious diseases, this does not necessarily mean that a given refusal to care by a nurse should not be permitted. One set of circumstances under which this might be so is where nurses are so distracted and so disturbed by their fear of contagion that they can no longer be relied upon to give safe, appropriate and therapeutically effective care. In such instances, it would obviously be better for the patient who has an infectious disease not to be cared for by such nurses. One reason for this is that the patient's sense of wellbeing and self-worth — not to mention, his/her health outcomes — are not going to be maximised by nurses who are so overwhelmed by their own fear that they would neglect the patient (as happened in the case cited above). It needs to be noted, however, that nurses whose practice is 'impaired' by a personal fear of contagion have an obligation to seek remedial education and counselling to help address the problem of their 'impaired practice' (Johnstone 1998). In some jurisdictions, it might even result in a nurse's deregistration. In 1990, for example, a nurse was deregistered by the United Kingdom Central Council (UKCC) for refusing to care for people who were 'HIV, AIDS and hepatitis B positive' (Young 1994, p. 103).

Another problem which needs to be addressed is that of homophobia (the 'irrational fear of homosexuality'), which, as Huerta and Oddi (1992, p. 223) argue, can further compound the fear of caring for HIV/AIDS patients. Significantly, attitudinal studies have found that some nurses feel uncomfortable with caring for male homosexuals and exhibit avoidance behaviour towards HIV/AIDS patients who belong to this group (Crock 2001; Huerta and Oddi 1992, p. 223). Nurses opposed to homosexuality also tend to believe that HIV/AIDS patients are 'responsible' for their disease, and, accordingly, these nurses 'blame the victim' (Crock 2001; Viele et al. 1984). Equally significant are research findings which show that nurses who are homophobic manifest 'the greatest fear of HIV/AIDS and the least empathy for AIDS patients' (Huerta and Oddi 1992, p. 224).

While these studies are not conclusive, they nevertheless point to a need for nurses to examine their attitudes towards homosexuality and to explore ways in which prejudicial attitudes towards and fear of HIV/AIDS patients can be overcome (Crock 2001). One study has found, for example, that nurses can be helped to gain a more positive attitude towards and less fear of homosexuality by participating in sexuality workshops where opportunities can be provided to explore and share feelings about the issue, and to engage in other learning activities (Crock 2001; Young 1988).

One group of people who may not be amenable to this kind of education, however, are those who are fundamentally opposed to homosexuality on religious grounds. I have, for instance, heard some nurses who hold conservative religious beliefs express the view that they 'could not possibly care for a homosexual patient with HIV/AIDS, since to do so would be tantamount to condoning homosexuality, and thereby sup-porting a sinful practice'. (Similar arguments are used in the case of abortion; some nurses have expressed the view, for example, that caring for women who have had abortions is tantamount to condoning abortion.) The reasoning used here is, however, flawed. It is a fallacy to hold that caring for a particular class of patients is tantamount to condoning the lifestyles or life circumstances of those patients. If we were to accept this line of reasoning, we would be committed to accepting that, for example, caring for poor people is tantamount to condoning poverty, or that caring for unemployed people is tantamount to condoning unemployment, or that caring for homeless people is tantamount to condoning homelessness. We would, I think, reject the view that caring for these latter groups of people is tantamount to condoning their respective lifestyles, or to providing grounds upon which a morally defensible refusal to care for them could be based. Since the acts of caring for HIV/AIDS patients are demonstrably remote from the sexual acts to which some nurses are opposed on religious grounds, and since caring for patients who are homosexual does not entail performing acts proscribed by religious doctrine, it is not clear that a refusal to care for patients who are homosexual can be sustained. (Readers may also find Fitzpatrick's discussion of the Catholic principles of cooperation/complicity helpful [1988, pp. 128–34].)

It might be objected here, however, that, unlike homosexuality, poverty, unemployment and homelessness are not 'sins' and therefore nurses opposed to sinful practices can care for people in these latter groups without compromising their religious beliefs and moral integrity. In fact, caring for these people might even be construed as 'virtuous'. This, however, is not a satisfactory reply, since it fails to show *why* caring for these groups of people is *not* tantamount to condoning their lifestyles, which, significantly, can be shown to be injurious to these groups of people's wellbeing and moral interests. Let us explore this further.

Why, for instance, is caring for a homosexual patient regarded as tantamount to condoning homosexuality, yet caring for an unemployed person *is not* regarded as tantamount to condoning unemployment? If we take out the descriptive statements referring to these groups whose respective lifestyles are in question, what we end up with is something like this: *caring for members of group X is tantamount to condoning their lifestyles, but caring for members of group Y is not tantamount to condoning their lifestyles.* No reasons are given why this is the case, however, demonstrating that the thinking being used here is at best arbitrary and at worst fallacious. Even if it is conceded that what makes a morally significant difference in this case is the 'sinful' nature of homosexuality, this will not help, since this seems to say that what makes caring for a particular group of people tantamount to condoning their lifestyles is the fact that what they do is 'sinful'. If nurses holding conservative religious beliefs were to accept this, however, they would be committed logically to accepting that caring for a whole range of people would be tantamount to condoning their 'sinful' lifestyles, and thus that there exists a whole range of people for whom they should refuse to care. Nurses holding conservative religious beliefs would, for instance, be obliged to refuse to care for people who work on Sundays, bear false witness, steal, murder, covet their neighbours' goods, fornicate, commit adultery, blaspheme, do not fear God, worship other gods, tell lies, take contraception, have attempted suicide, and have performed a whole range of other acts deemed sins in the Bible or other religious texts. Clearly, if nurses were to accept the view that caring for people who commit sins is tantamount to condoning the sins in question, they would probably have to give up nursing altogether, since many (if not most) people have committed the 'sinful' acts given above.

While the arguments presented here have had as their focus male homosexuals, they could, of course, be applied equally to the cases of other groups of people whose lifestyles some nurses regard as being problematic or sinful — for example, intravenous drug users and prostitutes.

CONSCIENTIOUS OBJECTION AND THE PROBLEM OF UNSAFE WORK CONDITIONS

A final type of situation to be considered here involves the common problem of nurses being expected to work in unsafe working conditions, most notably those caused by severe staff shortages. Typically, nurses might be ordered to work in an area with which they are unfamiliar and/or in which they are not educated to work, such as in an intensive care unit. They might also be expected to work at a staffing level which places patient safety and quality of care at risk. These two situations are inextricably linked. For example, if there was not a shortage of properly educated intensive care nurses, nurse administrators would not have to order an inexperienced nurse to go and 'help out' in the hospital's intensive care unit. A nurse's obligation to object to working under certain conditions may not only be morally imperative, however, but a legal requirement under 'duty of care' and the demand to exercise 'due care' provisions.

Conscientious objection and policy considerations

For a conscientious objection policy to be effective and reliable, it must carry at least two minimal requirements (see Childress 1979). First, conscientious objectors must demonstrate that their claims are sincere. A given proof need not be religious in nature, nor necessarily absolute. As we have seen throughout this book, it is not always inconsistent for nurses (or for anyone) to have a 'moderate' position on the moral permissibility of certain procedures, such as abortion and euthanasia/assisted suicide. Thus, it would not necessarily be inconsistent of nurses to, say, support abortion and to participate in most abortion procedures at their place of employment, yet nevertheless be opposed to a 'particular case' of abortion where the procedure in question fails to satisfy certain autonomously chosen moral standards. The same applies in the case of euthanasia/assisted suicide. Conscientious objection policies, then, must recognise and make provision for the moderate's position, and accept that sometimes conscientious objectors might refuse to assist with a type of procedure they have previously assisted with, such as abortion.

A second minimal requirement is that employers must carry the burden of proof that no alternative is available when not permitting nurses to refuse on conscientious grounds to assist with a given procedure. It is difficult to accept that a claim of conscientious objection cannot be accommodated in cases where nurses have used rightful means in expressing a conscientious refusal — that is, superiors have been given advance notice of an intention to refuse, reasons for refusal have been made explicit, replacement or other attending personnel have not been unduly compromised, other interests of comparable moral worth have not been sacrificed, and patients have not been stranded. Where an administrator does not accept a nurse's genuine conscientious objection claims, serious questions need to be asked about whether the administrator has sincerely tried to find viable alternatives which would make it possible for conscientiously objecting nurses to withdraw from situations they deem morally troubling or intolerable.

The key to settling the conscientious objection debate does not lie only in having enforceable mechanisms for protecting genuine conscientious objection claims, but also in having a demonstrable threshold beyond which nurses can base their claims. However, this threshold is one which can only be supplied by sound ethics education and agreed ethical standards within the profession.

Can superiors decently order nurses to perform tasks to which they are genuinely conscientiously opposed? The answer is 'no'. To compel nurses to act against their conscience is to risk weakening their moral conscientiousness and hence their ability to be moral. To deny moral conscientiousness in health care domains is also to risk the moral interests of those requiring health care. Furthermore, superiors simply do not have the moral authority to dictate to another which moral standards ought and ought not to be appealed to in a given situation.

There is much to support the view that a health care system comprised of morally conscientious and sensitive nurses would be much better than one without such nurses. This seems to support the conclusion that genuine conscientious objection is not only morally permissible, but may even be, in the ultimate analysis, morally required.

The issue of conscientious objection in nursing is at last receiving the attention that is warranted by professional nursing organisations. One notable example of this can be found in the Royal College of Nursing, Australia, which, in February 1998, issued its first position statement on conscientious objection (and subsequently revised it in 2000).

Clinical ethics committees

In health care organisations around the world, clinical ethics committees (also called hospital/health care ethics committees or institutional ethics committees) are increasingly playing a role in assisting both clinicians and managers to deal with and respond effectively to ethical issues in the workplace. Their development and operationalisation, however, is a relatively recent phenomenon and indeed varies markedly across and even within different countries (de Vries and Forsberg 2002; Wenger et al. 2002; Doyal 2001; McNeill 2001; Nelson et al. 2001; Simon 2001a; Slowther et al. 2001a, 2001b; van der Kloot Meijburg and ter Meulen 2001; Reiter-Theil 2000). In North America, for example, clinical ethics committees (or health care ethics committee as they are known there) are well established and have become a 'standard vehicle for the education of health professionals about biomedical ethics, for drafting and review of hospital policy, and for clinical case consultation' (Nelson et al. 2001, p. 205). In Europe and the United Kingdom, however, clinical ethics committees are at an 'emerging' stage only, with questions concerning their ultimate role and function still being very much a matter of debate (Slowther et al. 2001a, 2001b; Simon 2001a; van der Kloot Meijburg and ter Meulen 2001; Reiter-Theil 2000). Israel, meanwhile, has the distinction of hospital ethics committees being a statutory require-ment under its *Patients' Rights Act*, which came into effect in 1996 (Wenger et al. 2002). Under the Act, Israeli ethics committees have four legal functions:

- to allow provision of treatment against a patient's will;
- to allow withholding of information important for informed consent from a patient;
- to allow disclosure of medical information against a patient's wishes to protect public health or the health of a third party;
- to review documentation in a case handled by the control and quality committee.

(Wenger et al. 2002, p. 177)

In Australia, clinical ethics committees have been functioning since the mid-to-late 1980s and in some cases have been involved in approving medico-moral decisions to remove life-sustaining treatment (see, for example, the much publicised 1988 case of Mrs N — Cossar 1988; Pirrie 1988; Wilmoth and Pirrie 1988). The main function of Australian clinical ethics committees, however, has been found to be primarily that of *policy formation* (notably on issues such as informed consent and patient competency, withdrawal of treatment, resource allocation, and issues concerning the use of reproductive technology), with some committees also playing an educational role (McNeill 2001). Significantly, only a few clinical ethics committees are playing a direct role in advising on the ethics of medical treatment options and management of individual patients — and then, only in exceptional circumstances (McNeill 2001). This observation has lead one researcher to conclude with concern that Australian clinical ethics committees have, at best, only a limited scope and function in the organisations where they have been established (McNeill 2001).

The limited role and function of clinical ethics committees in Australia is not unique. In North America, for example, where health care (clinical) ethics committees have long been established, there is some evidence that 'case consultation requests are rare' and that many ethics committees are not functioning effectively (Hofman 2001, p. 58; see also Doyal 2001; DuVal et al. 2001). Likewise in the United Kingdom and Europe (Reiter-Theil 2000). Even in Israel where, as noted above, hospital ethics committees are a statutory requirement, committee function has been impeded due to a variety of processes and accordingly committee activity levels have been 'low' (Wenger et al. 2002). Despite these failings (and the resistance by some medical practitioners who fear that clinical ethics committees will undermine their clinical authority), there is a strong body of opinion as well as philosophical arguments for supporting the role and function of clinical ethics committees (Doyal 2001). There is also an emerging view that the role of clinical ethics committees should, in fact, be expanded; for example, as a critical component of effective clinical governance and of 'organisational ethics' as well — particularly in regard to managed-care, integrated systems, quality assurance, and risk management (clinical and legal) (Rudd 2002; Wenger et al. 2002; Hofman 2001; Nelson et al. 2001; see also Spencer et al. 2000). In light of this, it is evident that a key challenge facing health care organisations today is not how their clinical ethics committees might 'best decide difficult cases' (as is sometimes assumed), but how they might 'best function at all'; that is, how their clinical ethics committees might best be made *more effective*.

Members of the nursing profession have a vested moral interest in clinical ethics committees functioning effectively. In order to understand the challenges facing clinical ethics committees and how their effectiveness might be improved, it is necessary for nurses to have a good working knowledge and understanding of the nature, role and function of clinical ethics committees. It is to addressing these issues that this section now turns. In particular attention will be given to addressing the following nine questions:

1. What is a clinical ethics committee?
2. What processes have influenced the rise of clinical ethics committees across the globe?
3. What role and function should a clinical ethics committee have?
4. What authority and power should clinical ethics committees generally have?

5. Who should serve on clinical ethics committees?
6. How should clinical ethics committees approach moral decision-making?
7. Who should have access to them?
8. Do clinical ethics committees really work (i.e. what are their merits and demerits)?
9. Of what significance are clinical ethics committees to the nursing profession?

What is a clinical ethics committee?

In discussing the issue of clinical ethics committees, it is important first to be quite clear about what is being referred to. For example, the term 'institutional ethics committee' is sometimes incorrectly used as a generic term for other health care institutional committees (e.g. research committees or institutional review boards [IRBs]). Using such a generic term, however, risks muddling the issues at hand (Brodeur 1984) and can also give the false and misleading impression that a health care organisation has a committee process in place for dealing specifically with clinical cases and the ethical problems associated with such cases, when it does not. In short, as McNeill (2001, p. 444) has observed, it can lead to the 'over-reporting' or 'inflation' of the number and function of effective clinical ethics committees. What then is a clinical (or hospital) ethics committee?

Carol Levine defines (1984, p. 9) a clinical or hospital ethics committee as:

a group established by a hospital or health care institution formally charged with advising, consulting, discussing, or otherwise being involved in ethical decisions and policies that arise in *clinical care* ... The committee may serve the entire hospital or a special unit, such as a neonatal intensive care nursery or a cardiac intensive care unit [emphasis added].

While this is not the only definition of a clinical or hospital or health care ethics committee, it is nevertheless an apt one, and the one which will tentatively be relied upon in this discussion. As a point of clarification, the notion of a 'clinical ethics committee' is to be distinguished from what I shall later refer to as a 'patient care ethics committee'.

Factors influencing the rise of clinical ethics committees

There are many processes which have contributed to the rise of clinical/health care ethics committees. Special health care ethics committees were formed in the United States as early as the 1920s to review sterilisation decisions, and in the 1950s to review abortion decisions (Levine 1984, p. 9). It was not until the mid-1970s, however, owing to the much publicised *Karen Quinlan case* (Muir 1978; Hughes 1978; Ross et al. 1986, pp. 5–8), that interest in health care ethics committees began in earnest. This interest was primarily sparked by the New Jersey Supreme Court's decision in the Quinlan case, which made it clear:

that the issue at stake was not definition of death, but rather the decision to stop treatment on one who has suffered serious neurological injury.

(Veatch 1977, p. 22)

The next few years saw interest in health care ethics committees heighten as physicians began to be charged with first degree murder for removing, at the request of the family or patients, life-supporting care and treatment (Cranford and Doudera 1984, p. 13). As doctors increasingly began to recognise their legal vulnerability (La Puma et al. 1988), and as nurses began to feel increasingly frustrated with having 'nowhere to go when confronted by ethical dilemmas' (Cranford and Doudera 1984, p. 15), so too the health care ethics committee movement gained support, and eventually saw the establishment of working ethics committees in hospitals across the United States (see also Ross et al. 1986).

Factors influencing the rise of clinical ethics committees in Australia, Europe and the United Kingdom are similar to those that have influenced the North American scene. With the increasing sophistication of medical technology has come increasing legal and public pressure to meet perceived legal and moral standards of care. Underscoring this pressure has been the patients' rights movement, which has not only given rise to a public more willing and able to assert its rights to, in and against health care, but also the passage of major legislative reforms to protect these rights (Consumers' Health Forum of Australia 1990). A more liberally educated health care professional workforce and the expression of cultural values less tolerant of paternalism, meanwhile, have seen a major shift in attitude towards patients' rights, with a related increase in demands (in the form of professional requirements and expectations) for moral/ethical considerations to be given at least as much attention, if not more, as scientific considerations when making health care and medical treatment decisions. Inquiries into options for dying with dignity, patients' rights, medical malpractice, psychiatric care, the care of the aged and the disabled, and similar issues, have also created a greater awareness in both the professional and the lay communities of the need for developing reliable mechanisms for ensuring just decision-making in health care contexts, and particularly in cases involving patient/ client care.

The role and function of clinical ethics committees

There has been much debate on what the proper function or role of a clinical ethics committee should be (see, for example Rudd 2002; Wenger et al. 2002; Doyal 2001; McNeill 2001; Nelson et al. 2001; Simon 2001a; van der Kloot Meijburg and ter Meulen 2001; Blake 1992; Cranford and Doudera 1984; McCormick 1984; Youngner et al. 1984; Caplan 1982; Freedman 1981; Levine 1977, 1984; Veatch 1977). Debate has centred on whether its function should be *decisional* (i.e. deciding morally hard cases); *prognostic* (i.e. establishing prognostic criteria and determining what a patient's actual prognosis is); *monitoring* (i.e. establishing quality assurance programs and evaluating health care practices); *advisory* (i.e. advising and supporting others on how and what to decide); *educational* (i.e. running workshops, seminars and conferences aimed at addressing ethical issues arising in clinical practice and preparing health providers to deal with these better); or a combination of all five.

Interestingly, the response in both the philosophical and health care professional literature has been almost unanimously supportive of the clinical ethics committee having a multi-purpose/multi-faceted role:

- *as a consultative/advisory/supportive mechanism* for assisting individuals (whether caregivers or care receivers) to make their own moral decisions, and to help ensure that the decisions they make are reasonable and fair;
- *as an education and resource facility* aimed at preparing individuals and groups to better deal with moral problems and moral conflict in clinical practice (activities

to be undertaken here include grand round discussions, seminars, workshops, and conferences, with a particular focus on ethical issues arising from clinical practice);
- *as a mechanism for policy formulation, development and review* (i.e. scrutinising past and existing policies for their moral adequacy and acceptability, and identifying areas where policy is lacking or where new policy is required, as in such areas as DNR procedures, the use and withdrawal of life-saving treatment, conscientious objection, and the like);
- *as a forum* where individuals can express their concerns and views without fear of ridicule or repercussions, and where moral disagreements among staff, patients and families can be aired and resolved; and
- *as a reviewer of morally troubling (hard) cases*, offering advice and viewpoints to all those involved.

Whatever the role the clinical ethics committees in fact play, it should never be viewed as being absolute or static in nature, and should always be subject to review as ethics and experience demand.

The authority and power of clinical ethics committees

As with the question of function, there has also been considerable debate on the kind of power and authority that clinical ethics committees should have. Attention has mainly focused on whether the use of these committees and the demand to follow their findings should be voluntary/optional or compulsory/mandatory.

John Robertson (cited in Levine 1984, p. 11), of the University of Texas Law School, suggests that four possibilities are available to a committee:

1. *optional–optional* (it is optional for individuals to approach the ethics committee for consultation and advice, and optional to follow its recommendations);
2. *optional–mandatory* (it is optional for individuals to approach the ethics committee for consultation and advice, but if they do they must carry out its recommendations);
3. *mandatory–optional* (it is mandatory for individuals to approach the ethics committee for consultation and advice, but optional to follow its recommendations);
4. *mandatory–mandatory* (it is mandatory for individuals to approach the ethics committee for consultation and advice, and mandatory to follow its recommendations).

(Reproduced by permission © The Hastings Centre)

Levine (1984) points out that very few in the United States favour the *mandatory–mandatory* model, and that, in fact, many committees operate on the *optional–optional* model, although not altogether effectively. She also points out that there is mounting political pressure to make some cases the subject of mandatory review — particularly those involving severely disabled newborns, and the chronically and terminally ill from whom doctors wish to withhold life-supporting treatment — a pressure which continues to this day (see, in particular, the discussion on the 'fetal police' in Macklin 1993, pp. 77–103). In Australia, clinical ethics committees (unlike research ethics committees) also tend to operate on the optional–optional model.

During the 1980s and 1990s, cases typically brought before clinical ethics committees involved moral controversies arising from treating the rationally incompetent, the critically ill and the hopelessly ill (i.e. those with poor prognoses), or in situations where health professionals (most notably treating doctors) were 'uncomfortable' with family demands (Brennan 1988, p. 803). Today, little has changed. North American research, for example, has found that cases being presented to a clinical ethics committee for consultation tend to involve those in which 'no one intervention is clearly preferable, when there are conflicts about the value of an intervention, or when communication breaks down' (Nelson et al. 2001, p. 205). A survey of 190 physicians by DuVal et al. (2001) likewise found that the most common reasons for seeking ethics consultation from a committee related to ethical dilemmas and 'ethical impasses' or 'stand off' concerning end of life decision-making, patient autonomy issues, and conflict. The most common triggers (or 'moral catalysts') leading to consultation requests were:

1. wanting help resolving a conflict;
2. wanting assistance interacting with a difficult family, patient, or surrogate;
3. wanting help making a decision or planning care; and
4. emotional triggers (including intimidation, fear, frustration, feeling at a loss about what to do, feeling uncomfortable about a situation, or encountering patient pain and suffering (DuVal 2001, pp. i24, i27).

Interestingly, DuVal and his team found that 'conflicts and other emotionally charged concerns triggered consultation requests more commonly than other cognitively based concerns', leading them to conclude that ethics consultants (whether individuals or committees) needed to be prepared as much to 'mediate conflicts and handle sometimes difficult emotional situations', as they were to provide 'ethics advice' (DuVal et al. 2001, p. i24).

Composition of clinical ethics committees

A third major issue to receive considerable attention in the bioethics and health care professional literature is that pertaining to just who should rightly serve on a clinical ethics committee.

During the early days of the establishment and functioning of clinical ethics committees, many worried that they would become dominated by those representing the interests of the medical profession and hospital administrators — a fear that, at the time, was not without some grounds. For example, a 1984 study in the United States found that 57 per cent of institutional ethics committee members were physicians (Levine 1984, p. 12). Almost two decades later, another United States study has found that although the membership composition of institutional ethics committees has improved and is more representative (i.e. in terms of gender balance and professional disciplines), white males with a medical background continue to be disproportionately represented (e.g. made up 34 per cent of all members). (The next largest group represented was behavioural scientists at 24 per cent; interestingly, the least represented group were professional ethicists at just 2 per cent, followed by clergy at 3 per cent, and lawyers at 5 per cent; nurse representation was just 8 per cent [DeVries and Forsberg 2002, pp. 253–4].) Consistent with other 'snap shots' of clinical ethics committees, 77 per cent of the committees surveyed did not have a member who was a professional ethicist (DeVries and Forsberg 2001, p. 255). (In a study of hospital ethics committees in Germany, Simon [2001a, p. 227], likewise found only a small number of hospital ethics committees — i.e. 2 out of the 29 — had a professional medical ethicist as a member).

Despite the above discrepancies, there is nevertheless general agreement in both the philosophical and health professional literature that clinical ethics committees should at least be interdisciplinary and should include persons independent of the institution. Clinical ethics committees in the United States, the United Kingdom, the Netherlands and Australia typically include doctors, nurses, lawyers, social workers, hospital administrators, psychologists, members of the clergy, and at least one non-staff member (Rudd 2002; Doyal 2001; Nelson et al. 2001; Szeremeta et al. 2001; van der Kloot Meijburg and ter Meulen 2001; Ross et al. 1986; Levine 1984). Whether these people are the most appropriate to serve on the committees is a matter of some controversy.

Kuhse and Singer argue, for example, that the typical composition of clinical ethics committees tends to give 'too much power to the institution' (1985, p. 183). Thus, even if 'outsiders' are represented on the committee, there is still the risk of the committee deciding in favour of the hospital's or the institution's interests. Another problem is that there is no guarantee that the kind of composition outlined above will in fact result in appropriate and effective moral decision-making. While the people represented may well be technically expert, this in no way guarantees their expertise as moral decision-makers. As Veatch has argued in relation to another matter, 'technical competency does not a value judgment expert make' (1972, p. 536). Thus, rather than pooled moral knowledge and competence, such a committee may only yield pooled moral ignorance and incompetence. Even if all members were 'morally competent', the composition may nevertheless be self-defeating; for example, if all members have radically different (though equally valid) views on the matters brought before the committee, they may be quite unable to offer constructive advice and guidance to the people seeking assistance. This problem (i.e. of moral impasse) may be very difficult to resolve. Last, it is not clear why some of these entities should be on an ethics committee at all. While the need for a lawyer can be appreciated (e.g. legal representatives can provide helpful advice on the legal aspects of a given ethical issue [Hendrick 2001]), and while the need for clinical practitioners (such as doctors, nurses and social workers) can be appreciated (insofar as these people are in a unique position to contribute relevant clinical and other factual information to the decision-making process), it is far from clear that the presence of a theologian or clergyman is needed. As Dr Swan, producer and presenter of ABC Radio's 'Health Report', is reported as saying:

> I would love to hear a good reason why a Jew should be subjected to an Anglican's view even though he [sic] may try to hide his [sic] dogma behind an objective gloss. Why should a Catholic be subject to a rabbi or a Hindu to the local priest?
>
> (Voumard 1988, p. 17)

Further to this, Kuhse and Singer point out that, while 'some experienced ethicists are also members of the clergy', it is not the case that 'all members of the clergy are knowledgeable about ethics' (1985, p. 182). In light of these and similar comments, it seems that there is no compelling reason for a member of the clergy to be included in the composition of an ethics committee.

Many of the difficulties identified here can be overcome by ensuring that those who are included in the committee's membership are morally sensitive and responsible (Freedman 1981), are respectful of the other committee members' views, have good communication skills, have at least a working knowledge of bioethics (Levine 1984) and are able to think critically and use a 'problem-solving approach that is primarily reflective' (Ross et al. 1986, p. 37). Humility and a willingness and ability 'to work cooperatively with people who come from different levels within the hospital hierarchy' are also essential attributes (Ross et al. 1986, p. 38). Youngner et al. (1984) argue further that full cooperation between members is essential if 'resentment, political discord, and dysfunction' are to be avoided. More recently, Hendrick has argued (2001, p. i52) that members must have at least the 'fundamentals' necessary for effective clinical ethics committee work, notably:

> an ability: to identify and analyse clinical ethical problems; to use and model reasonable clinical judgements; to communicate with and educate team, patient and family; to negotiate and facilitate negotiations, and to teach and assist in problem resolution.

Even if all these things are attended to, however, there remains the uneasy feeling that the typical composition of institutional ethics committees might still not be *right*, particularly in terms of their role in advising, and possibly even deciding on behalf of a patient, what is to count as an ultimate 'good' (see, for example, Youngner et al. 1984).

Some argue that, in cases of specific patient care dilemmas, perhaps what is called for is not a committee comprised of *hospital and health care agency* caregivers, but rather one which is comprised of persons belonging to the *patient's own support group*. Levine (1977), for example, suggests that patients' interests might, in the end, be better served by a committee (a true patient care ethics committee) made up of the patient's own family, friends, clergyman, lawyers, and the like. This seems a plausible possibility, as long as conditions are carefully defined, and one which should be seriously considered by policy makers and law reformers. Attending health professionals and hospital administrators need not feel threatened by this suggestion, since there need be nothing stopping them from declaring their concerns and interests and imparting their clinical knowledge and other relevant clinical facts to the patient committee. Indeed, there is room to suggest that the only role that attending health professionals and administrators should play is that of giving the relevant clinical information necessary for the patient committee to make an informed choice.

In some respects the role of the public advocate has given legitimacy to the notion of patient representatives (usually family members or friends) assuming some or all of the burden of decision-making in hard cases, rather than this task falling solely into the hands of doctors or the health care team or some other intrusive bureaucratic mechanism such as the court. In cases where there is no one to assume the burden of decision-making, clearly the need exists for a facility, such as an interdisciplinary clinical ethics committee, to help to decide the most morally appropriate course of action to take.

Moral decision-making by clinical ethics committees

The question of how a clinical ethics committee should approach moral decision-making when dealing with the matters brought before it has received surprisingly little attention over the years. While attention has been given to the nature and processes of ethics consultation (see, for example, Fine and Mayo 2003; Schneiderman et al. 2003; La Puma and Schiedermayer 1994) — something which *ethics committees* can and do offer — and to the *accountability* of clinical ethics committees *apropos* the decisions they make (see, in particular, Hendrick 2001; Fry-Revere 1992), little has been written on the actual decision-making processes that committee members might use to decide issues and cases brought before them. (A notable exception to this oversight is Jonathan Moreno's (1995) work *Deciding together: bioethics and moral consensus* in which a consensus approach to bioethical decision-making is articulated and advocated.) Thus an important question to be raised here is: How might clinical ethics committees best approach moral thinking and moral decision-making on the issues brought before them — particularly when these issues involve 'hard cases'?

There is of course a variety of ways in which members of a clinical ethics committee could approach the task of moral decision-making; not least, by using traditional meeting procedures and deciding issues by 'negotiation and agreement' and/or where that fails, deciding by majority vote. Another approach, already discussed in Chapter 5 of this book, is that which is informed by the relatively new moral perspective called 'quantum morality' or 'quantum ethics' (Zohar 1991; Zohar and Marshall 1993). As previously explained, quantum ethics views ethical decision-making as a shared and cooperative venture, where people take time to communicate and to negotiate choices that strike 'a creative balance between more fixed attitudes of control at the one extreme or total receptiveness at the other' (Zohar and Marshall 1993, p. 102). It will be recalled, however, that for this approach to work, participants must come to the moral deliberating process with a willingness to: (1) 'let go' their own point of view as the *only* point of view, and (2) to put their own views alongside others 'as one of many to be compared, contrasted and considered' (Zohar and Marshall 1993, p. 235). Through cooperative and creative communication, the differing viewpoints of all participants can evolve into a new 'synthesised' view. In so far as evaluating whether the 'correct' choices have been made, the following applies: if the values and meanings of the choices break down 'and the moral equivalent of physical chaos sets in', the participants may conclude that 'everything has fallen apart' and that a morally good outcome has not been achieved (Zohar 1991, p.182). Conversely, if the values and meanings of the choices made do not break down, and the moral equivalent of physical order and unity sets in, the participants may conclude that everything has stayed together as a harmonious whole evolving toward a viable futurity, and that a morally good outcome has been achieved.

Access to clinical ethics committees

The question of who should have access to institutional ethics committees has not been as widely addressed as the other more complex questions have been. Nevertheless, this in no way implies that the question of accessibility is any less important. In North America, the general view is fairly unanimous, with arguments tending to favour committees being accessible to virtually anyone (patients, staff, families) who requires assistance in working through a moral problem and making moral decisions. In the United Kingdom, however, views about patients and families having access to clinical ethics committees are more circumspect, with at least one bench mark clinical ethics committee not accepting referrals from patients or their families at all (Rudd 2001). This is likely to be an ongoing issue.

Can clinical ethics committees help?

There is evidence that clinical ethics committees and related consultations have been very helpful – at least for physicians – in resolving conflicts and disputes, particularly concerning the provision of life-sustaining treatment at the end stage of life (see, for example, Schneiderman et al. 2003; Simon 2001b; La Puma et al. 1988). Significantly, there is a paucity of research on the subject of whether nurses have access to and use ethics consultation services, and, if so, whether they have found them beneficial.

A number of other 'indirect' benefits have also been postulated in the bioethics literature. Brodeur (1984), for example, suggests that clinical ethics committees help to ensure good decision-making, which in turn will help to limit the risk of legal liability. More importantly, from a moral perspective, the committees help to re-emphasise *patient care* as *the* central goal of health care practice. Cranford and Doudera (1984), like Brodeur, see clinical ethics committees as ensuring better and more systematic moral decision-making. They also see the committees as helping to identify previously unrecognised moral issues on which there is no general consensus, thus paving the way for moral negotiation and the realisation of just moral outcomes. Caplan (1982), on the other hand, sees the benefit of allowing moral expertise to have a place in technical domains as, quite simply, that of improving moral understanding (see also Moreno 1991).

Clinical ethics committees are not without their problems, however. They are obviously unable to *guarantee* the quality and appropriateness of their moral analyses and decision-making, and are at risk of merely replacing, rather than changing and improving, the traditional loci of decision-making. They are also vulnerable to breeding what McCormick (1984, p. 154) calls 'in house protectionism' (i.e. where committee members 'operate protectively for the institution and its practitioners'), 'legal accommodationism' (i.e. where the committee becomes too narrowly focused on the law to the point that ethical considerations become diluted and even lost), and 'oversensitivity' (i.e. where committees become 'oversensitive to the felt need of consensus' to the point where they lose all the moral ingredients which otherwise distinguish them as ethically imperative). McCormick identifies the further concern that clinical and other institutional ethics committees, by their very nature, may also provide the ultimate breeding ground for 'whistleblowers', particularly if the committee keeps minutes of its activities and findings or documents them in some other way. Just why this should be any more of a problem for clinical ethics committees than it is for any other kind of committee whose proceedings are confidential and yet not subject to statutory immunity provisions is not clear; it may even be, as one colleague has suggested, a *benefit*. Another problem is that clinical ethics committees can be rather cumbersome and clumsy — particularly in situations demanding 'a quick response, without prior notice, at any hour of the day or night' (Kuhse and Singer 1985, p. 183). Such problems are not insurmountable, however, and with careful forethought and planning can be prevented and/or overcome. The use of information technology and electronic communication systems as an adjunct to face-to-face meetings (particularly in 'urgent cases') is also emerging as a solution (Eiser et al. 2001).

Implications of clinical ethics committees for the nursing profession

The last question to be addressed here is: What are the implications of clinical ethics committees for members of the nursing profession?

Possible answers to this question will depend very much on the function, power, composition and accessibility of any given ethics committee. If committees take on a multi-purpose role, as outlined earlier, it is likely that the implications for nurses will be positive. Nurses will have somewhere to go to air their concerns and will gain the opportunity of resolving moral disagreement formally. They will also gain the opportunity of developing a deeper awareness and understanding of moral issues arising from clinical practice and developing their moral problem-solving skills. And they will have the unique opportunity of gaining insights into and understanding of the kinds of moral problems and personal difficulties that other members of the health care team also experience, which will pave the way for more harmonious and interdependent working relationships. If ethics committees adopt only a narrow and singularly focussed role, however, the implication for nurses might not be so positive; indeed, the position of nurses will probably be just as frustrating as it was before thought was first given to the establishment and development of clinical ethics committees.

A committee's power and authority perhaps stand to have the most serious implications of all for the nursing profession — particularly in cases involving mandatory review and mandatory compliance. Where mandatory decisions stand to impinge on and infringe agreed and accepted standards of nursing care (for example, in cases involving the withholding of food and fluids, physician assisted suicide), the nursing profession could be faced with some serious problems (see, for example, Daverschot and van der Wal 2001).

The degree of accessibility also has the potential to affect nurses. If accessibility means that the committee is literally open to all who need it, nurses need not fear suffering any undue burdens or disadvantages. If access is restricted, however, this would pose a different situation altogether. In the unlikely event of access being restricted, nurses might well suffer disproportionate burdens and disadvantages through not having the opportunity to experience the kinds of benefits that a multi-purpose ethics committee could offer.

If nurses are finding that they are not achieving fair representation on established ethics committees, or are being denied access commensurate with their needs, one solution is for nurses to establish their own working ethics committees. Indeed, some nurses have already established their own organisational *nursing ethics committees*. There are sound justifications for doing this. As I have discussed elsewhere (Johnstone 1998, pp. 97–107), unlike the broader institutional or clinical ethics committees, which have as their focus more general concerns relating to patient care and institutional activities, nursing ethics committees focus specifically on the moral concerns and experiences of *nurses*, and on the kinds of moral problems that nurses encounter when planning and delivering nursing care to patients. One of the major advantages of establishing nursing ethics committees is that these can provide nurses with a unique opportunity to identify and examine bioethical issues from a *nursing* point of view, and not from the point of view of those whose dominant interests tend to dictate which ethical issues will be addressed by a broader institutional ethics committee, and how, when, and by whom. This means that nurses can have the 'space' to identify what *they* consider to be important ethical issues, and to determine how, when and by whom they consider these issues should be addressed. Another major advantage of nursing ethics committees is that these can provide an opportunity for nurses to identify what their (educational, support, policy reform and other) needs are and how these needs can best be met. With broader-based institutional ethics committees, these kinds of opportunities to nurses might not always be available.

Nursing ethics committees are not without disadvantages, however. In fact, they can fall prey to exactly the same kinds of problems that clinical and other more general institutional ethics committees can experience. For example, a nursing ethics committee may be lacking in institutional authority, may be lacking in direction, may have a membership which serves the interests more of the institution than of nurses and patients, may be dominated by a particular faction of nurses (for example, nursing administrators), may lack the expertise necessary for dealing with the kinds of ethical problems nurses face in their day-to-day practice, may be plagued by radical moral disagreement among committee members, may be unable or powerless to implement its decisions, may be reluctant to 'rock the boat', and so on. Despite these and like problems, however, the establishment of nursing ethics committees are a worthy initiative and deserve support.

Clinical ethics committees — some further considerations

Clinical ethics committees have an important role to play in assisting health care institutions or, more accurately, the health professionals working within them, to address a range of ethical issues (including 'morally hard cases') encountered during the course of their work. The rise of clinical ethics committees has, however, had a paradoxical cost: they have become thoroughly implicated in the bureaucratisation and institutionalisation of moral decision-making (Jennings 1991, pp. 451–2; see also Bauman 1993, p. 125). As Jennings explains (1991, p. 452), this is evident by the lived reality that:

> ethical choice and agency are now embedded as never before in a network of explicit rules and formal procedures and processes for making decisions. These rules stipulate (within certain limits) what types of decisions may be made, how they may be made, by whom, and with the assistance of what resources.

> Equally important, these rules are increasingly becoming institutionalised: they are embedded in the organisational form of statutes, court opinions, administrative mandates, and institutional protocols; in decisions regarding terminal care, these rules inform counselling and educational mechanisms encouraging individual patients and their families to choose surrogate decision-makers and to give prior statements about wanted and unwanted treatment. As a necessary adjunct to this bureaucratisation and institutionalisation of moral decision-making, hospitals are being strongly encouraged ... to establish ethics committees to support and provide technical assistance to this process.

Whistleblowing

The International Council of Nurses (2000) *Code of Ethics* makes plain that nurses have a stringent responsibility to 'take appropriate action to safeguard individuals when their care is endangered by a co-worker or any other person'. The codes of ethics ratified by other peak nursing organisations (e.g. the Australian Nursing Council, the New Zealand Nursing Council, the Nursing and Midwifery Council (UK), the American Nurses Association and the Canadian Nurses Association) likewise obligate nurses to take appropriate action to safeguard individuals when placed at risk by the incompetent, unethical or illegal acts of others — including 'the system'. Despite being a professional and ethical requirement, however, reporting acts that place others at risk may not be an easy thing to do and, as the nursing and legal literature amply demonstrates, may even be hazardous to the nurses who make such reports. Some notable examples of this are given below.

The Moylan case (Australia)

In 2002, the *Australian Nursing Journal* carried a feature article detailing the story of Kevin Moylan, a senior psychiatric nurse, who experienced a six year 'journey into hell' after he exposed the poor quality practices at a psychiatric clinic in the Australian state of Tasmania (Armstrong 2002, pp. 18–20). Moylan's ordeal began after he reported a range of workplace safety issues to hospital management. His concerns included what he believed to be the legal and ethical abuse of patients, inadequate training of staff and the provision of incompetent services, and serious problems with workplace health and safety — including:

> the employment of a temporary psychiatrist who was not registered, police reluctance to provide support to protect staff from dangerous patients, and the sexual harassment of patients.
>
> (Armstrong 2002, p. 19)

The employment of the unregistered psychiatrist caused Moylan particular concern and provided the catalysts for him deciding that he 'could not remain silent as patients were diagnosed, prescribed medication, and given electro-convulsive therapy by someone he considered a "fraud" ' (Armstrong 2002, p. 19). The workplace safety issues provided a further catalyst for action after these 'reached a critical level when Kevin [Moylan] himself was attacked by a patient' (Armstrong 2002, p. 19). Significantly, when Moylan reported his concerns, rather than 'being praised and rewarded for his advocacy role' he was reportedly 'isolated and intimidated into silence' (Armstrong 2002, p. 19).

Concerned about the lack of response to the issues he had reported, Moylan decided to take the matter further and wrote to the then Tasmanian Minister for Heath outlining his concerns. In a chain of circumstances remarkably similar to the Pugmire case (cited below) and the Pink case (referred to in Chapter 5 of the book), a copy of the letter was delivered to the Tasmanian Shadow Minister for Health who subsequently raised the matter in Parliament, and named Moylan as the 'whistleblower'. Unfortunately, this single act of naming removed Moylan's anonymity and privacy and, in his own words, 'changed his life forever' (Armstrong 2002, p. 19). Over the next six years he lost his home, his farm, his livelihood, and his health. Although the psychiatric clinic was eventually closed and Moylan received some compensation, his lost health, reputation and livelihood remain largely unaddressed. Now a campaigner against what he calls the 'suppression of dissent in the system', Moylan reflects:

> I have been threatened, isolated, intimated and abused [...] My actions were motivated by a desire to see justice done. I tried to protect my patients, but no-one protected me.
>
> (quoted in Armstrong 2002, p. 19)

As a consequence of not being protected, at the time the *Australian Nursing Journal* report was published, Moylan was suffering from a post-traumatic stress disorder (PTSD) and unable to work. He was reported as having 'nothing left but his car and his dog' (Armstrong 2002, p. 19).

The Pugmire case (New Zealand)

In 1993, Neil Pugmire, a registered psychiatric nurse, wrote in confidence to the then Minister of Health outlining concerns he had about the *Mental Health (Compulsory Assessment and Treatment) Act 1992* (New Zealand) and its failure to provide for the compulsory detainment of patients whom responsible mental health professionals strongly believed were 'very dangerous' (Liddell 1994, p. 14). To support his concerns, Pugmire used as an example a named patient whom mental health professionals thought was 'highly likely' to commit very serious sexual crimes against young boys. This concern was based on admissions by the named patient (who, seven years previously, had attempted to rape and strangle two boys) that he had continual feelings of 'wanting to commit sexual acts with little boys' (Liddell 1994, p. 15). The Minister, however, reputedly took the position that 'mental health legislation should not be used to justify the detention of difficult or dangerous individuals' (Liddell 1994, p. 14). Dissatisfied with this response, Pugmire sent a copy of his letter to a member of the opposition, Mr Goff (Liddell 1994, p. 14). In a chain of events, similar to those that occurred in the Moylan case (referred to above), Mr Goff subsequently released the letter publicly, but with the patient's name deleted. However, the patient's name was eventually revealed by other sources thus breaching his confidentiality. Consequently, Pugmire was suspended by his employer for 'serious misconduct' involving the 'unauthorised disclosure of confidential patient information' (Liddell 1994, p. 16).

The Bardenilla case (United States of America)

In 1988, in what has been described as 'one of the most influential whistleblowing incidents ever to be initiated by a nurse during [the twentieth] century', Sandra Bardenilla, a registered nurse, was awarded damages for wrongful dismissal (involuntary resignation) from her place of employment (*American Journal of Nursing* 1988, p. 1576; Fry 1989c, p. 56; Anderson 1990, pp. 5–6). Bardenilla lost her employment as a result of reporting her concerns about two physicians whom she believed had directed 'unethical and potentially illegal nursing care to a comatose patient who later died' (Fry 1989, p. 56).

It is reported that during the course of attempting to have the matter addressed, Bardenilla was 'sharply criticised and accused of overstepping her role as a nurse' (Fry 1989, p. 56). She was also instructed by her director of nursing to 'be quiet and to apologise' to the physicians concerned (Fry 1989, p. 56). She was also advised to 'adopt a more realistic attitude about the hospital system, and she was warned against taking her concerns outside the hospital' (Veatch and Fry 1987, p. 176). Bardenilla did not accept these directives, however, and resigned from her position instead. Following her resignation, Bardenilla formally reported the two physicians to the local county health department who initiated an investigation into the matter (Veatch and Fry 1987, p. 176; *American Journal of Nursing* 1988, p. 1576). Following the investigation into the death of the patient, the two attending physicians were charged with murder. Although the physicians were both subsequently acquitted of the charges against them, 'the case had a strong influence on subsequent termination-of-treatment decisions across the US' (Fry 1989, p. 56). The consequences to Bardenilla, however, were extremely burdensome at both a personal and professional level. As Sara Fry notes (1989, p. 56), although Bardenilla eventually received financial compensation for her employment losses, she nevertheless:

> received a great deal of recrimination as a result of her actions. While she received the support of many individual nurses, she did not receive formal professional support or find reemployment an easy matter. She suffered personal harm and the matter dragged through the courts for a long time.

The MacArthur Health Service case (Australia)

In 2002, four nurses met with the then New South Wales (NSW) Minister for Health to draw to his attention certain management and clinical practices that they believed were placing patients' safety at risk — and had already resulted in patient deaths — at two hospitals that were part of the MacArthur Health Service (MHS) in NSW. These nurses, together with three other nurses who later came forward in the formal investigation that was to follow, had between 13 and 30 years nursing experience, and included clinical nurse specialists and nurse unit managers. As one report put it:

Their professional experience enabled them to identify deficiencies in patient care and to alert the management of the hospital to problems.

(Health Care Complaints Commission 2003, p. 2)

The Health Minister referred the matter to the Director-General of the NSW Department of Health; the Director-General, in turn, made a formal complaint to the NSW Health Care Complaints Commission who then formally investigated the matter. The Commission's investigation included an analysis of 47 specific clinical incidents that occurred between June 1999 and February 2003, in the emergency departments, the intensive care unit (of one hospital), the operating suite (of one hospital) and on the medical wards of both of the hospitals involved. Significantly, 'the evidence obtained about the incidents strongly supported the allegations by the nurse informants about the standard of care' (Health Care Complaints Commission 2003, p. 4). Some examples of the clinical incidents verified are:

- no surgical review of a patient with very poor blood supply to her foot — an urgent surgical problem (an ischaemic foot), for more than two days;
- unacceptable delay in triage of a severely ill newborn baby;
- a patient with severe chest pain was discharged from in [sic] an emergency department when a bed with a cardiac monitor could not be found — she died a few hours later;
- a critically ill cardiac patient who was in shock was left untreated in emergency department for many hours;
- failure to diagnose a patient with serious post birth infection (puerperal sepsis) in the emergency department;
- a delay of over 12 hours in the transfer of a critically ill woman;
- post operative intra-abdominal infection not diagnosed for four days;
- an agitated psychotic patient who waited unsupervised in an emergency department for five hours and subsequently absconded.

(Health Care Complaints Commission 2003, p. 4)

The nurses' 'whistleblowing' actions in this case cost them dearly. Not only were they vilified and isolated by some of their colleagues ('because of the criticism of the health service brought about by the investigation' that followed their allegations being made public), but all four of the nurses were also disciplined by the health service — one of whom was suspended. Of these nurses, two were disciplined after they had intervened on the behalf of a child patient in the operating theatres. Following an investigation into this particular matter, the health service recommended that the nurses be disciplined 'over the way they had addressed a medical officer' (Health Care Complaints Commission 2003, p. 5).

The matter did not end with the Health Care Complaints Commission's investigation, however. In what arguably stands as the most significant nurse whistleblowing case to occur in Australia, following the release of the Commission's report, the current NSW Health Minister sacked the head of the NSW Health Care Complaints Commission and announced a new inquiry — to be headed by an eminent barrister at law (Saunders 2003a; Tobler 2003). This sacking came amid claims by the informant nurses that 'many more deaths were yet to be investigated' and that the Commission's report did not go far enough in holding people accountable (Saunders 2003a, p. 1; AAP 2003). Meanwhile, it was reported by the media that the NSW Coroner would be investigating 19 patient deaths at the health service in question (Saunders 2003; Tobler 2003). In addition to the sacking of the Commission's head, two doctors were suspended, nine other doctors were refereed to the NSW Medical Board for investigation and possible disciplinary action, and disciplinary action was initiated against four senior administrative staff at the health service (Saunders 2003). As well, an investigation was commenced into two further allegations, notably, that the former Minister for Health threatened and bullied two of the nurses who first went to him with their allegations, and that crucial documents pertinent to the allegations had been shredded at the two hospitals involved (Saunders 2003a, 2003b).

Despite having their concerns vindicated and receiving an apology from the current Minister for Health, two of the nurses have left their nursing careers for good, one is currently working as a sales representative selling medical supplies, one is working in the private health care sector, and one is unemployed. One of the nurses who has left nursing for good is reported to have explained that 'she could not return to her former job because she would either have to become part of the cover-up or keep blowing the whistle' (Tobler 2003, p. 4).

The above cases and other examples demonstrating the consequences to nurses who 'blow the whistle' (see also the UK cases of Graham Pink and Dr Nigel Cox given respectively in Chapters 5 and 10 of this book) are just some among many that show that deciding whether to report unsafe practices or to remain silent is not a straightforward matter. Here questions arise of: Why is whistleblowing problematic? And what, if anything, can be done to improve the status quo? It is to answering these questions that the remainder of this discussion now turns. Before proceeding, however, some clarification is required on what the term 'whistleblowing' refers to.

The notion of whistleblowing/whistleblowers

The term 'whistleblowing' is a colloquial term that is used to refer to:

> The voluntary release of nonpublic information, as a moral protest, by a member or former member of an organization outside the normal channels of communication to an appropriate audience about illegal and/or immoral conduct in the organization or conduct in the organization that is opposed in some significant way to the public interest.
>
> (Boatright 1993, p. 133)

Citing Elliston et al. (1985), Vinten (1994, pp. 256–7) argues that in order for an act to count as whistleblowing, the following conditions must be met:

- an individual performs an action or series of actions intended to make information public;
- the information is made a matter of public record;
- the information is about possible or actual, nontrivial wrongdoing in an organization;
- the individual who performs the action is a member or former member of the organization.

Vinten (1994) further clarifies that whistleblowing disclosures lack authorisation, and can apply to both internal and external whistleblowing (see also Coyne 2003; McDonald 2002; Rosen 1999). Others contend that whistleblowing reports are also usually made to a person in a position of authority (i.e. who has the power to stop the wrong), or to some other entity who, if not having the direct power to stop the wrong, nevertheless is perceived to have the capacity to exert pressure on those who do have the power to stop the wrong — for example, the media (Rosen 1999).

A key reason people resort to whistleblowing is to cause other people to pay attention and to take action immediately. Like the siren of an ambulance or a police car, or the fire alarm in a building, the sound of the 'whistleblower' seeks to alert people *immediately* to the fact 'that something is either happening or is about to happen [and] there is a need to pay attention to the alarm that has been sounded' (Erlen 1999, p. 67). Erlen (1999, p. 67) explains:

> Just as the ring of the alarm clock arouses people from sleep, so, too, does an act of whistleblowing. While other sounds and their respective messages do not always signal danger or caution, whistleblowing within the context of a health care situation says that something is seriously wrong.

Deciding to 'go public'

A key question facing members of the nursing profession is: *Are there situations in which nurses should 'go public'?* The short answer to this is yes, no, maybe — depending on the circumstances at hand and whether there genuinely are no other avenues for having the situation addressed.

There is no question that if and when encountering a situation in which the care of individuals is being — or is at risk of being – endangered by a co-worker or any other person, nurses have a stringent responsibility to take appropriate action. The issue here is not *whether* nurses should take action, but rather what *kind* of action they should take.

In situations involving an exceptionally serious failing that, in turn, is placing the public or the public interest at serious risk, and no other means exist for having the situation remedied, it is understandable that a nurse (or nurses) might consider whistleblowing as an option (Erlen 1999). Even so, every effort should be made to first try and correct the situation internally before 'going public' (Rosen 1999, p. 41). There are two reasons for this: first, as we have seen, there are significant risks associated with whistleblowing; second, given the recent developments in clinical governance and clinical risk management, new and more effective processes are now being put in place in health care organisations across the globe that are enabling staff to raise issues of safety and quality within their organisations without having to resort to the extreme measure of whistleblowing. Let us consider these claims further.

Risks of whistleblowing

As the Moylan, Pugmire, Hart, Pink, Bardenilla and MacArthur Health Service cases have each shown, whistleblowing can be an extremely traumatic (and costly) method of 'putting to right a wrong' (see also Lee 2002). Rather than seeing a whistleblower's report as an opportunity to improve the system and protect those whose interests have been placed at risk by questionable practices, an organisation whose conditions have been exposed may take a defensive stance and seek, instead, to protect itself (Erlen 1999). Equally troubling is the reality that whistleblowing offers 'no guarantee that the individual or the system will make the necessary changes to improve the situation' (Erlen 1999, p. 69).

Whistleblowing always upsets the status quo and accordingly is commonly perceived as 'rocking the boat' (Erlen 1999) — something which, in bureaucratic organisations, is generally regarded as taboo. Thus, even though a nurse might have done the 'right thing', whistleblowing can nevertheless result in him or her being portrayed as a disloyal 'troublemaker' and a 'Judas', and stigmatised and shunned accordingly (Erlen 1999; Rosen 1999). Employers and co-workers may retaliate by also: trying to discredit whistleblowing nurses; intimidating them by overly scrutinising the standards of their practice; threatening to terminate or actually terminating their jobs; and taking legal action against them for defamation (Erlen 1999; Rosen 1999). Furthermore, this retaliation can continue long after the situation has been corrected (Rosen 1999). In sum, as the experience of Stephen Bolsin (the UK anaesthetist who famously blew the whistle on problems in paediatric cardiac surgery at the United Bristol Healthcare Trust [UBHT]) warns: speaking out *outside* of an organisation will always make a whistleblower unpopular *inside* that organisation (Bolsin 2003, p. 294).

Nurses who blow the whistle can also experience serious and significant adverse effects on their health as a result of their experience (it will be recalled that Kevin Moylan now suffers from PTSD as a result of his ordeal). In a small but important study on the physical and emotional effects of whistleblowing, McDonald (2002) has found that, as a result of identifying and 'blowing the whistle' on misconduct in the workplace, the majority (70 per cent and 94 per cent respectively) of the nurses surveyed suffered from significant physical and emotional health problems (McDonald 2002). The problems experienced included (but were not limited to): lethargy, sleep disturbances, headaches, backaches, weight loss/gain, increased substance use (e.g. drugs and alcohol intake, smoking), colds, influenza, gastrointestinal problems, cardiac symptoms, anger, anxiety, depression, disillusionment, fear, poor self-esteem, and the breakdown of personal relationships (including separations and divorce) (McDonald 2002). Many nurses suffered multiple health problems, with four nurses suffering 18 or more physical symptoms and one nurse suffering from 24 physical complaints (McDonald 2002, p. 18).

Clinical governance and clinical risk management

Health care systems around the world are adopting and implementing new models of clinical governance and clinical risk management as part of a global strategy aimed at improving safety and quality in health care and reducing the incidence and impact of human error (see Vincent 2001a; Kohn et al. 2000). To this end, it is being increasingly recognised and accepted by all concerned that:

> Safety is everyone's responsibility. Almost everyone working in health care cares about patient safety, in the sense of wanting to do their best for patients. However patient safety needs to be embedded in the *culture* of health care, not just in the sense of individual high standards, but of a widespread acceptance of a *systematic understanding* of risk and safety and the need for *everyone to actively promote patient safety*.
>
> (Vincent 2001b, p. 6, emphasis added)

Clinical governance and clinical risk management frameworks are now enabling all staff within the health care sector to raise issues within their organisation as part of their everyday practice and responsibility for ensuring patient safety and quality in health care (Lee 2002). As these frameworks become embedded in the culture of health care organisations, the identification and management of risks to safety and quality will become 'normalised' and the need for staff to have to resort to the extreme measure of whistleblowing will be substantially reduced if not removed altogether; accordingly, there will be no place (if ever there was) for 'naming, blaming and shaming' those individuals who have had the courage to speak out and to report 'wrong acts'.

Given that reporting incompetent, illegal and/or unethical practices in health care is both a professional requirement and responsibility, it is curious why making such reports has been labelled 'whistleblowing'. As Robbins (1983) points out, reporting improprieties on the part of colleagues, co-workers or associates is not whistleblowing, but rather a matter of professional ethics. By this view, there is room to contend that the term 'whistleblowing' not only has no place in health care contexts, but that in fact it is a misnomer (a wrong name) that should be abandoned altogether. Likewise, the term whistleblower. This term is grossly misleading and serves little more than to damn as immoral the acts of those who have had the moral courage to damn the immoral acts of others.

Whistleblowing as a last resort

Whistleblowing should only ever be considered as a last resort; that is, after all other avenues have been exhausted. The risks and benefits of engaging in such action should also be considered carefully. As with any moral decision-making (refer to the model presented in Chapter 5 of this book), any nurse contemplating 'going public' should first carefully assess the situation and ensure that they have access to all the relevant facts of the matter (this may include seeking advice from other colleagues or a supervisor); they should also ensure that they have 'back up' support to assist dealing with the aftermath of their actions (see also Coyne 1999). Finally, careful consideration should be given to the moral consequences of such an act and whether it would achieve the desirable moral outcomes intended.

Conclusion

Conscientious objection, clinical ethics committees and whistleblowing are all important processes which nurses can use to 'take a stand' on important ethical issues affecting their practice. Being able to use these processes in a just and effective way, however, requires knowledge and understanding of ethics and its application to and in nursing care contexts. It also requires political savvy, astuteness, and a willingness to take 'moral risks' in the interests of questioning and calling into question 'things as they are'.

CASE SCENARIO AND CRITICAL QUESTIONS

Case scenario

A psychiatric nurse, working as a case manager in a major psychiatric hospital in a country area, initiated a relationship with a former client. The nurse and the former client arranged to meet outside of work hours and, as a result of these meetings, the relationship progressed to a sexual relationship between the two. The nurse subsequently ended the relationship resulting in the former client requiring further psychiatric care, including two further admissions into a psychiatric unit.

The nurse's conduct was reported to the relevant nurse registering authority by the Director of Nursing of the hospital after the nurse's conduct had been reported to her. During the disciplinary proceedings that followed the nurse stated in her defence that, 'She had not been given guidelines about professional boundaries in her education, or in her employment' (Peisley 2001, 15). She further stated that under 'normal circumstances' she 'would have recognised that starting a relationship with a former client of hers was unprofessional, but that 'a number of stressors made her make a serious error in judgment' (Peisley 2001, 15).

The nurse registering authority hearing the disciplinary case found that the nurse had engaged in unprofessional conduct of a serious nature. The nurse was subsequently restricted from practising as a psychiatric nurse and required to undergo professional counselling for at least six months or until the registering authority received a satisfactory report from her counsellor. It was also acknowledged by the registering authority that the hospital in question 'had no written policies for professional boundaries and there appeared to be little supervision of a relatively inexperienced psychiatric nurse in a case manager role' (Peisley 2001, 15). It was further acknowledged that the nurse had been given 'inadequate support during [and] after the situation occurred with the former client, with no in-service training about dealing with challenging situations' (Peisley 2001, 15).

Critical questions

1. What professional standards of conduct did the nurse breach in this scenario?
2. If you were a nurse working in a hospital or community health care setting and you suspected that a nurse was having a relationship with a former client, what, if any, action would you take?
3. Upon what basis would you justify your actions (or non-actions)?
4. Would you report the nurse to the Nurses Board or other appropriate authority – e.g. a statutory health complaints office (whether yes or no, give reasons for your answer)?
5. If, after reporting your concerns to an appropriate authority, nothing were done about the matter, what would you do? Would you blow the whistle'?
6. If you decided to 'blow the whistle' on the nurse and the appropriate authorities for not taking action, what steps would you take to ensure you were doing the 'right thing'?
7. To what extent are nurses responsible for ensuring that they are informed about, know and understand the standards of ethical professional conduct and guidelines about professional boundaries in nurse–client relationships?
8. To what extent do nurses have a responsibility to report colleagues who breach professional standards to a nurse regulating authority (e.g. a Nurses Board)?

---

1 An earlier version of the discussion of conscientious objection was presented as a paper entitled 'Conscientious objection and professional obligation — a contradiction in terms?' at Nursing Law and Ethics, 2nd Victorian State Conference, *Dealing with dilemmas*, Monash University, 5 May 1989 (organised by the School of Nursing, Phillip Institute of Technology). The paper has been revised for publication in this text.

Chapter 14

Nursing ethics futures, moral activism and meeting the challenge to be involved

LEARNING OBJECTIVES

Upon the completion of this chapter and with further self-directed learning you are expected to be able to:

- Discuss critically how members of the nursing profession might challenge and change the moral status quo in regard to health promotion and health care.
- Discuss possible barriers and incentives to nurses engaging in moral activism aimed at assisting vulnerable populations.
- Explore some of the 'small' things that nurses could do that might make a positive difference to the life of another made vulnerable by life circumstances beyond his or her control.

KEYWORDS

- Health care ethics
- Moral activism
- Moral passivism
- Nursing ethics futures

Introduction

The field and practice of nursing ethics has developed enormously in modern times. Nevertheless, it is evident that the ethical challenges ahead are as great as they have ever been and that there is no room for complacency. Ironically, one of the biggest challenges facing the nursing profession at this time is not how best to deal with the complex ethical issues facing nurses, but how to get nurses involved *at all* and to take the action necessary to improve the moral status quo. In this final chapter, attention is given to two key issues: nursing ethics futures, and the need for nurses to engage in moral activism in order to challenge and change the moral status quo – particularly in regard to promoting and protecting the public's health.

Nursing ethics futures[1]

As I have argued at length elsewhere (Johnstone 2002b), contemporary health care ethics/bioethics has become preoccupied with the issue of people's rights to and in health care (e.g. the rights to informed consent, confidentiality, quality of life, death with dignity, and so forth). There is no question (as the preceding chapters in this book have amply demonstrated) that this preoccupation has achieved some morally significant and beneficial outcomes in health care domains. Nevertheless, it is equally evident that health care ethics has not achieved its most basic task, namely, to promote and protect the genuine wellbeing and welfare interests of those who are among the most vulnerable people in society and whose health is at risk.

It has long been recognised that although access to health care is an important determinant in ensuring the health of people, it is not the *only* or even the most important determinant (McMurray 1999, p. 40). The health of people rests on a much more complex array of conditions and processes. For instance, it is known that the public's health is deeply rooted in social, cultural, economic, and political circumstances and that if the health of people is to be achieved, these conditions need to be understood and considered (McMurray 1999; Baume 1998). It is also known that, to achieve the goal of heath, people need to be situated in a 'strong, mutually supportive and non-exploitative community' (World Health Organization 1995, p. 4). Over the past four decades this knowledge has seen cycles of public attention given to such things as poverty, unemployment, poor housing, racial discrimination, homophobia, cultural dispossession, social isolation, and the impact these conditions have had on the health of people. But, as commentators observed as early as 1975, 'this attention and interest rapidly wane when it becomes clear that solving these problems requires painful costs that the dominant interests in society are unwilling to pay. Our public ethics do not seem to fit our public problems' (Beauchamp 1975, p. 20; see also Beauchamp and Steinbock 1999).

In several respects the emergence of the bioethics movement in the early 1970s was an attempt to challenge and change the status quo and to redress the lack of 'fit' between 'public ethics' and 'public problems'. The development of the contemporary health care ethics movement (a correlative of bioethics and often treated as being synonymous with bioethics) sought similarly to challenge and change the status quo. Today, however, it is evident that neither the bioethics movement nor the health care ethics movement has succeeded at their most basic task, namely, to promote and protect the public's moral interest in *health*. It is also evident that if health care ethics is to 'fit' the world's health problems — and if it is to succeed in promoting the moral interests that are inherent in a positive health status — then a shift in its focus is required (Johnstone 2002b).

Members of the nursing profession are in a good position to challenge and champion a change in direction in health care ethics. This, however, would fundamentally require the nursing profession to take responsibility for the future by developing an 'ethics of the future'; that is, an ethics that focuses on anticipating and preventing the mistakes that will become future problems (Mayor and Binde 2001). Leading and operationalising a strategic program of nursing ethics futures, in turn, would also require nurses to become involved, in a genuine individual participatory sense, to challenge and change the moral status quo in the domain of health promotion and health care.

Nursing activism[2]

The need for nurses to take action to secure morally just outcomes in professional, social and political domains has perhaps never been greater on account of the complex array of social, cultural, economic and political processes that are increasingly eroding the health and wellbeing of people around the world. Despite this need, and the mandate of the nursing profession to promote and protect health, moral activism by nurses seems conspicuously absent or, if it is present, remains largely invisible, prompting important questions concerning why this situation has occurred and what can be done about it.

As already stated in this book, the modern nursing profession worldwide has a rich and distinctive history of devising and upholding exemplary ethical standards of conduct and of taking action to address ethical issues arising in contexts relevant to the profession and practice of nursing. Furthermore, as the nursing literature dating back to Florence Nightingale's classic text *Notes of nursing* demonstrates, over the past 150 years, nurses have been just as concerned with fulfilling their ethical responsibilities associated with promoting the wellbeing and welfare of people in nursing, health care and other related domains as they are today (Johnstone 1999a, 1994).

Building on its rich and distinctive history, nursing ethics today has arguably never been more informed, more developed or more visible. Neither has it had more authority as a political discourse in both health care and social domains to challenge the status quo, nor a greater capacity to fulfil its task of promoting human welfare and wellbeing. There exists a plethora of literature on the topic (which is growing day-by-day), and opportunities to research and to study nursing ethics abound. Accordingly, nurses are now better prepared and better positioned than they perhaps have ever been to fulfil one of their most stringent moral responsibilities, namely, to advocate the health interests of the individuals, groups and the communities they serve.

Ironically, the development of nursing ethics and the improved capacity of the nursing profession generally to engage in people advocacy is at risk of leading to less activism, rather than more. One reason for this, as I have discussed elsewhere, is that we have entered into an age of 'moral paradox': on the one hand there exists an unprecedented moral activism in the world, with various people fighting all sorts of battles on a whole range of moral causes (such as the right to life, the right to die, and so forth). On the other hand, there also exists an unprecedented moral passivism — imported, paradoxically, by the moral activism of the times (Johnstone 2002b). The moral paradox, in this instance, lies in the reality of individuals subscribing to the highest moral ideals yet never lifting a finger to help another human being or to support in a *personal* and *individual* way reform movements aimed at improving the status quo (Hoff 1982). Equally ironical is the moral complacency (another form of moral passivism) that seems to be emerging among some health care professionals who believe that because they have 'done' ethics (meaning, have studied ethics as part of a formal professional or continuing education program) they have discharged their moral responsibilities to stakeholders and need take no further action as morally accountable professionals.

The nursing profession is at no lesser risk than are others of being sucked into the vortex of moral passivism. Those participating in debates on ethical issues in nursing and health care thus must take care to ensure that their knowledge and words are distilled into action with desirable outcomes, and not left standing merely as substitutes for action and outcomes. As Florence Nightingale once cautioned in a letter to a friend:

> I think one's feelings waste themselves in words, they ought all to be distilled into actions and into actions *which bring results.*
>
> (cited in Woodham-Smith 1964, emphasis added)

Nurses should never underestimate their capacity, as individuals, to achieve good moral outcomes in the contexts in which they live and work (Johnstone 2002a, 2002c). Importantly, nurses also need to be aware that taking moral action need not necessarily involve some 'great startling heroic deed' on their part, and may include 'simple' acts such as showing kindness and compassion toward another, or merely questioning why something is being done one way rather than another. Although 'basic', these latter acts often stand as catalysts for change in people and the environments in which they live and work.

Nurses can also achieve a great deal collectively. Indeed, collective action can often be more powerful and more successful than individual action (Johnstone 2002c). One reason for this is that collective action can help to reduce the vulnerability of individual nurses who, when acting alone, might otherwise be 'martyred by the system' and consequently left to carry a disproportionate burden of loss that others, who merely look on as morally passive bystanders, do not have to suffer (Johnstone 2002c).

In their book *From Silence to Voice: What Nurses Know and Must Communicate to the Public*, Buresch and Gordon (2000) challenge nurses to 'envision how things would be if the voice and visibility of nursing were commensurate with the size and importance of nursing in health care'. Taking up this challenge, we might also envisage how things would be if the *volition* (acts of will) of nursing — in addition to its *voice* and *visibility* — was commensurate with the size and importance of nursing in health care.

In 2003, the ICN Florence Nightingale International Foundation (FNIF) awarded Carol Etherington, a registered nurse from Nashville, Tennessee in the USA, the International Achievement Award for her outstanding work with some of the worlds most desperate populations, notably people living with the aftermath of war and natural disaster and for whom she had designed and implemented community-based support programmes (*International Nursing Review* 2003). The *International Nursing Review* reports that in selecting Ms Etherington for the award, the FNIF Board acknowledged 'the international impact of her outstanding contribution in advocacy for vulnerable and victimised populations'. Her work within the United States in child abuse, ethics and human rights was also identified as being extremely important 'since these are topics on nursing's agenda worldwide'. Etherington is also credited with forging the path for nursing 'into criminal justice and social services by initiating programs serving victims of crime, citizens in crises, social and rescue personnel, and victims of disasters' (*International Nursing Review* 2003).

Etherington and others like her stand as moral exemplars on the horizon of moral possibility across a range of challenging circumstances, including those that are overwhelming and beyond human control. Her story, like the stories of others before and alongside of her, is a story not only of *the power of one* but *the power of all* to make a difference to the world and to the lives of people who live within it — even when the odds are stacked high against them.

We may not all be able to engage in the exemplary levels of activism and advocacy that recipients of the ICN Florence Nightingale International Foundation and other merit awards deservedly receive. However, neither can we rest content that just because *others* are undertaking such work, nothing further needs to be done on our own part and accordingly we can slip silently to the sidelines of human endeavour and passively watch as the world goes by. So long as we chose to work and interact with other human beings in our capacity as nurses and as moral human beings, it is fundamentally within our power and indeed our responsibility to act in ways 'which bring results' that, even when 'small' and seemingly insignificant, may nevertheless have a significant impact on the welfare and wellbeing of others. The challenge before us is to accept this power and to use it wisely and effectively to enable morally just outcomes to be achieved in the world of human affairs. If we elect not to take up this challenge then we risk failing not only ourselves, but the individuals, groups and communities that have come to rely on the nursing profession for care and its global promise to 'walk the talk' of respecting human rights, promoting health, preventing illness, restoring health, and alleviating suffering — particularly among vulnerable populations.

Conclusion

The nursing profession has never been in a better position professionally, socially, or politically to take the action necessary to achieve its moral goals. By using its position and moral capacity to achieve just outcomes in the contexts in which nurses work, the nursing profession will not only demonstrate the fulfilment of its responsibilities to the individuals, groups and communities it aims to serve, but will provide an important example of what it means to *be* moral in a world that is increasingly willing to allow rhetoric rather than reality and words rather than deeds to stand as the hallmarks of moral responsibility and enterprise.

CASE SCENARIO AND CRITICAL QUESTIONS

Case scenario

Present a small case study of a nurse (either of someone you know or have read about in the nursing literature) who has 'made a difference' to the lives of others on account of taking action and 'walking the talk' of respecting human rights, promoting health, preventing illness, restoring health, and/or alleviating suffering — particularly among vulnerable populations.

Critical questions

1. What stands out about the nurse's actions you have chosen to focus on?
2. In what way has his or her moral activism influenced the lives of others?
3. Could you do what this nurses did (whether your answer is yes or no, give reasons for your answer)?

---

1   This section has been taken from Johnstone, M (2002b) 'The changing focus of health care ethics: implications for health care professionals', *Contemporary Nurse* 12(3), pp. 213–24 (reprinted with permission). Website: *www.contemporarynurse.com*

2   This discussion is an expanded version of Johnstone, M. (2003) 'Guest editorial: Moral activism and the nursing profession: meeting the challenge to become involved', *International Nursing Review*, 50(4), pp. 193–4 (reprinted with permission).

Chapter 15

Indigenous perspectives

It might be said that, in a book such as this, perspectives from the world's First Peoples should be included. This expectation might also be said to be underscored by the fact that although 'there are more than 300 million indigenous peoples in the world, on every continent and representing many cultures', these peoples are grossly over represented 'among the world's vulnerable groups, suffering low incomes, living in poor condition and lacking adequate access to employment, education, safe water, food and health care services' (International Council of Nurses 2003b, p. 1). Furthermore, although epidemiological data is 'scanty', what data do exist point to the following health impacts on indigenous peoples:

- Life expectancy at birth is 10–20 years less than for the overall population in a country.
- Infant mortality rates are 1.5 to 3 times greater than the national average.
- Malnutrition, often associated with land displacement and contamination of food supplies, and communicable diseases (malaria, yellow fever, dengue fever, cholera, tuberculosis affect a larger proportion of indigenous peoples).
- Substance abuse (smoking, alcohol, drugs), cardiovascular diseases, diabetes, unintentional injuries and domestic violence are significant health and social problems. Many are associated with lifestyle changes resulting from acculturation.
(International Council of Nurses 2003b, p. 1)

In writing and revising this book, however, I have been mindful of a number of things. First, I have been mindful that no matter how well intended I am and how well informed I might be about indigenous issues, I do not have the legitimated authority to situate myself as *the* voice (or even a voice) of indigenous peoples around the world. Second, I have been mindful that while many of the issues contained in this book are of interest to nurses — and may even constitute a priority area of concern for some nurses — they are not necessarily of interest to or represent a priority area of concern for indigenous peoples (e.g. given their poor life expectancy relative to the overall population in a country, it is not difficult to imagine that a more pressing concern for indigenous peoples is how to *live a full lifespan at all*, not how to die with assistance — be euthanased — at the end of it). Third, I have been mindful (as indicated above) that indigenous peoples are among the most stigmatised and discriminated against group in the world and accordingly are vulnerable to what Martha Minow (1990, p. 20) calls the 'stigma of difference' and the moral pathology of prejudice that underpins it. (According to Minow, the stigma of difference is so potent that it 'may be created both by ignoring it and by focusing on it'.) Thus, ironically, by providing a focus on indigenous issues in this work I might have inadvertently fuelled the 'stigma of difference' and a moral pathology of prejudice against indigenous peoples, rather than progress a 'respect of difference' and a 'moral therapy' of inclusiveness and a 'pro-attitude' toward indigenous peoples. Fourth, and in respect of the views of the late Irihapeti Ramsden (2002), an influential Maori nurse leader and activist in New Zealand, I have been mindful that including material relevant to indigenous communities carried the risk of making indigenous peoples 'exotic' to bioethics and nursing ethics and as 'subjects' of discussion, rather than as equal co-participants in a discourse aimed at challenging and changing the status quo. Fifth, I have been mindful that there are persons who are members of various indigenous communities who are willing and able powerfully to 'speak for themselves' on the issues that matter to them and their communities, and that such people must have the opportunity to speak on their own behalf.

Sixth, I am mindful that we reached mid-point in the Decade of the World's Indigenous Peoples (1994–2003) and that, as shown above, the health of indigenous peoples remains in a state of scandalous compromise. I am also acutely aware that, despite the 'progress' of our thinking in modern times and our ethics, indigenous peoples the world over continue to suffer enormously from the legacies of colonisation, continue to bear the impact of policies 'seeking to assimilate them into the dominant population' (and culture), and continue to 'suffer significantly from the effects of environmental degradation, armed conflict and the application [of] western development models' (International Council of Nurses 2003b, p. 1).

Last, but not least, as the granddaughter of a woman who was a decedent of the Ngati Raukawa (Tainui) people in New Zealand, I am reminded that *the personal is also political*. My grandmother's story, once told to me when I was a young child, of her being smacked by her Anglo-teachers for speaking ('being') Maori at school has left a lasting impression on my mind and soul, as has her premature and suffocating death from pulmonary tuberculosis when I was just 12 years old. Thus, in my case, the political is also personal. When reflecting on my own personal story (and the loss not only of my grandmother, but of her mother's and her grandmother's culture and language) I am reminded that 'personal and intimate experience is not isolated, individual, or undetermined, but rather is social, political, and systematic' and that 'no life-area is too trivial for political analysis' (Kramarae and Treichler 1985, p. 333). By this view I am mindful that the life experiences and 'voices' of indigenous peoples stand (and ought to be recognised) as the methodological starting point for engaging in 'a positive project of constructing and developing alternative models, methods, procedures [and] discourses' (adapted from Gross 1986, p. 195). Likewise in the case of bioethics and nursing ethics: the lived experiences of indigenous peoples should also be taken as the methodological starting point for identifying and addressing what indigenous peoples regard as the 'paramount' ethical issues affecting their communities and how they think these issues can best be addressed.

Because of the above considerations, indigenous perspectives have not been 'woven' into the chapters of this book. Nevertheless, this is not to say that no voice at all should be given to the issues of concern to indigenous peoples. The question is how best to 'voice' these concerns.

In recognition of the above points it seems appropriate that, in concluding this work, an indigenous person should 'voice' the issues at stake and should have the 'last word' on what matters. There are two reasons for this: first, the interests of indigenous peoples have often (too often) been left hanging on the last words of culturally dominant non-indigenous spokespersons who have had no real regard or commitment in promoting or protecting the interests of indigenous peoples. Second, by providing the last word, an indigenous spokesperson will also be at the forefront of providing the 'first word' of a whole new conversation on what I think could be appropriately described as a 'new indigenous ethics', and how nursing ethics might evolve in the future and find ('fit') this with new indigenous ethics and thereby reflect better the needs and interests of the worlds First Peoples. To this end, the concluding remarks of an invited honorary address given by Dr Sally Goold, OAM, a distinguished and widely respected Australian Indigenous nurse, are reprinted below.

Indigenous health, political will and social responsibility[1]

There is a lack of political motivation or will, and also a lack of the acceptance, that we all have responsibility for indigenous Australians who are our most disadvantaged and vulnerable people. While the reasons for distress of the soul have been recognised for many years, little has been done to address the problems. The impact of this on indigenous health continues to be unrecognised. The effects of the overwhelming feelings of hopelessness and helplessness, demoralisation and despair, due to chronic deprivation and persistent loss and low self esteem, combined with a lack of social justice has had — and continues to have — a devastating impact on the everyday lives of the Australian Indigenous peoples of this country. Without the necessary tools to meet their most basic needs, is it any wonder that their health is poor? I believe that we are all responsible for demonstrating political will and accepting social responsibility and standing up to be counted for the healthcare needs of the Australian Indigenous peoples.

So what needs to be done? Before any sort of healing can take place, the history of this country and settlement must be acknowledged. The wounds of injustices inflicted on Aboriginal and Torres Strait Islander people that have caused so much grief and distress must be accepted as having happened, that they are not stories made up, but fact. This acceptance of history is not to engender feelings of guilt. Those reality factors must be addressed, however. The provision of grief counsellors to provide support for those in need will assist in addressing those reality factors.

Social justice issues must be addressed. These social justice issues are in fact human rights issues that apply to everyone in this country: adequate housing, clean water, sewerage disposal, good access to health care and education. These are not 'practical reconciliation' measures, as the Prime Minister states, but are basic human rights that should be available to all.

Abolish racism and racial discrimination. The International Convention on the Elimination of all forms of Racial Discrimination (CERD) was adopted by the UN General Assembly in 1966 and entered into force for Australia in September 1975. But unfortunately, racism is still alive and well in this country. We need, therefore, to look at what can be done on an individual level to combat racism — to provide culturally appropriate care, and to embrace the true spirit of reconciliation in that we can all walk together in peace and harmony. We need to remove the barriers to accessing mainstream health services: people will not go where they are not made to feel welcome. Racist attitudes are alive and well in the health care system with judgmental values and attitudes very obvious on the part of many health care professionals. Aboriginal and Torres Strait Islander people are often treated as if they are invisible and/or as non-persons. There are many good caring people working in health care facilities, but often their good work is undermined by the negative attitudes and behaviours of others.

The education of health professionals needs to be improved. All universities providing education for medical students, nurses and allied health professionals must review their curricula to include the history of Aboriginal and Torres Straight Islander people; cultural awareness and the concept of cultural safety must also be included.

There needs to be increased recruitment and retention of Aboriginal and Torres Straight Islander health care professionals and recognition of the role they play as health care providers. A diverse workforce can only assist with caring for of Aboriginal and Torres Straight Islander people as well as non-Aboriginal and non-Torres Straight Islander people, with the sharing of ideas and experiences.

We as nurses need to and *must* work together and accept and respect each other's views if we hope to provide appropriate care for Aboriginal and Torres Straight Islander people with 'soul distress'. We need to have the capacity and the compassion to acknowledge that Aboriginal and Torres Straight Islander people are actually human beings, and to listen to and hear what the person is saying. If we are able to do these things, we will ensure that Indigenous peoples enjoy the same level of health care services as others, and we will be able to see and be able to hear them and, in doing so, acknowledge that they are not in fact invisible. We as nurses may be able to demonstrate political will and that, in accordance with our social responsibility, we can do something with the power we have.

I leave you with this quote from Sir William Deane (2001): 'The ultimate test of a nation is how we treat the most vulnerable and disadvantaged of our people', and from Ann Deveson (1991), 'A thing is not impossible merely because it is inconceivable'.

Sally Goold[2] OAM
RMIT University, 8 May, 2000

1   Address given by Dr Sally Goold, OAM, at Storey Hall, RMIT University, Melbourne, 8 May, 2000. Reprinted with permission from Dr Sally Goold.

2   Dr Sally Goold is also the Chair Person of the Council for Aboriginal and Torres Straight Islander Nurses (CATSIN). Further information about CATSIN can be obtained by visiting its website at: *www.indiginet.com.au/catsin*

Bibliography

AAP (2003). *Health watchdog* head sacked. [Available at: *www.news.com.au 11 December* — accessed: 16 December 2003.]

Abel, E.K. and Nelson, M.K. (eds) (1990). *Circles of care: work and identity in women's lives.* State University of New York Press, Albany.

Adams, M. (1984). On life .... and death .... and dots. *Nursing 84*, 14(6), June, pp. 53–8.

Addelson, K. (1994). *Moral passages: toward a collectivist moral theory.* Routledge, New York.

Admiraal, P.V. (1991). Is there a place for euthanasia? *Bioethics News*, 10(4), pp. 10–23.

Affara, F. (2000). When traditions maim. *American Journal of Nursing*, 100(8), pp. 52–61.

AFP (1989). Toronto Court has rethink to allow women's abortion. *Australian*, 13 July, p. 8.

AFP, DPA (1999). Dr Death reaps grim fate for murder. *The Australian*, 15 April, p. 10.

Ahronheim, J. and Gasner, R. (1990). The sloganism of starvation. *The Lancet*, 335(8684), pp. 278–9.

Aikens, C. (1943). *Studies in ethics for nurses.* W.B. Saunders, Philadelphia (first published 1916).

Alec, M. (1986). *Hypatia's heritage.* The Women's Press, London.

Allen, R.E. (ed.) (1966). *Greek philosophy: Thales to Aristotle.* The Free Press, New York.

Allender, J. and Robinson, P. (1989). Hospital AIDS ban to be outlawed. *The Australian*, 8 March, p. 1.

Allmark, P. (1995). Can there be an ethics of care? *Journal of Medical Ethics*, 21(1), pp. 19–24.

Almond, B. (ed.) (1990). *AIDS — a moral issue: the ethical, legal and social aspects.* Macmillan, Houndmills, Basingstoke, Hampshire.

Alvarez, A. (1980). The background. In Battin, M. Pabst and Mayo, D., *Suicide: the philosophical issues.* Peter Owen, London, pp. 7–32.

Aly, G. and Roth, K. (1984). The legalization of mercy killings in medical and nursing institutions in Nazi Germany from 1938 until 1941: a commented documentation, *International Journal of Law and Psychiatry* 7, pp. 145–63.

Amato, J.A. (1990). *Victims and values: a history and theory of suffering.* Praeger, New York.

American Journal of Nursing (1988). Court backs nurse fired for questioning an MD, 88(11), p. 1576.

Amundsen, D. (1989). Suicide and early Christian values. In Brody, B. (ed.), *Suicide and euthanasia: historical and contemporary themes.* Kluwer Academic Publishers, Dordrecht, pp. 77–153.

Andersen, S. (1990). Patient advocacy and whistleblowing in nursing: help for the helpers. *Nursing Forum*, 25(3), pp. 5–13.

Anderson, W. Truettt (1990). *Reality isn't what it used to be: Theatrical politics, ready-to-wear religion, global myths, primitive chic, and other wonders of the postmodern world.* Harper San Francisco, New York.

Andolsen, B. Hilkert, Gudorf, C.E. and Pellauer, M.D. (eds) (1987). *Women's consciousness, women's conscience.* Harper & Row, San Francisco (first published by Winston Press, 1985).

Andrews, K. (1985). Informed consent: adrift on a trans–Atlantic crossing. *Lawyer*, 3(6), August, pp. 12–16 (published by Victorian Young Lawyers).

Andrews, M. and Fargotstein, B. (1986). International nursing consultation: a perspective on ethical issues. *Journal of Professional Nursing*, 2(5), pp. 302–8.

Angelucci, P. (2003). Ethics committees: guidance through gray areas. *Nursing Management*, 34(6), pp. 30–3.

Annas, G. (1982a). CPR: the beat goes on. *Hastings Center Report*, 12(4), August, pp. 24–5.

—— (1982b). CPR: when the beat should stop. *Hastings Center Report*, 12(5), October, pp. 30–1.

Anonymous (1983). AMA judicial chairman sees emergence of hospital ethics panels as an inevitability. *Federation of American Hospitals Review*, 16, November/ December, pp. 30–2.

Anonymous. (2000). Blowing the whistle. *Nursing*, 30(4), p. 28.

Ansell, K. (1988). Nile's abortion bill would jail doctors. *The Age*, 28 June, p. 21.

Appelbaum, P. and Grisso, T. (1988). Assessing patients' capacities to consent to treatment. *New England Journal of Medicine*, 319(25), pp. 1635–8.

Aquinas, St Thomas (1978). Whether it is lawful to kill oneself. Reprinted from *Summa Theologica* in Beauchamp, T. and Perlin, S. (eds), *Ethical issues in death and dying*. Prentice Hall, Englewood Cliffs, New Jersey, pp. 102–5.

Archard, D. (1993). *Children: rights and childhood*. Routledge, London/New York.

Aristotle (1957 edn). *The politics*. Penguin Books, Harmondsworth, Middlesex.

—— (1976 edn). *Ethics*. Penguin Books, Harmondsworth, Middlesex.

—— (1976 edn). *Nicomachean ethics* (translated by J.A.K. Thomson). Penguin, Harmondsworth, Middlesex.

Armstrong, F. (2000). Dope 'em up and ship 'em out: Issues in mental health care. *Australian Nursing Journal*, 8(5), pp. 26–9.

—— (2002). Blowing the whistle: the cost of speaking out. *Australian Nursing Journal*, 9(7), pp. 18–20.

—— (2003). Out of hospital, out of mind: the state of mental health. *Australian Nursing Journal*, 11(1), pp. 20–4.

Aroskar, M.A. (1986). Are nurses' mind sets compatible with ethical practice? In P.L. Chinn (ed.), *Ethical issues in nursing*. Aspen Systems, Rockville, Maryland, pp. 69–79.

Asch, D. (1996). The role of critical care nurses in euthanasia and assisted suicide. *New England Journal of Medicine*, 334(21), pp. 1374–9.

Asch, D., Hansen-Flaschen, J. and Lanken, P. (1995). Decisions to limit or continue life-sustaining treatment by critical care physicians in the United States: conflicts between physicians' practices and patients' wishes. *American Journal of Respiratory Critical Care Medicine*, 151, pp. 288–92.

Ashby, M. and Mendelson, D. (2003). Natural death in 2003: are we slipping backwards? *Journal of Law and Medicine*, 10(3), pp. 260–4.

Ashby, M. and Stoffell, B. (1991). Therapeutic ration and defined phases: proposal of ethical framework for palliative care. *British Medical Journal*, 302(1 June), pp. 1322–4.

—— (1995). Aritifical hydration and alimentation at the end of life: a reply to Craig. *Journal of Medical Ethics*, 21(3), pp. 135–40.

Athersmith, F. (1986). Euthanasia could be abused by selfish relatives, says doctor. *The Age*, 3 July, p. 10.

—— (1989a). Hospital's ban on AIDS to be made illegal. *The Age*, 8 March, p. 3.

—— (1989b). Four per cent of nurses hurt by needles, survey finds. *The Age*, 5 May, p. 3.

Atkinson, R.L., Atkinson, R.C. and Hilgard, E.R. (1983). *Introduction to psychology* (8th edn). Harcourt Brace Jovanovich, New York.

Attig, T. (1996). *How we grieve: relearning the world*. Oxford University Press, New York.

Australasian Nurses Journal (1912). The right to die, 19(9), 16 September, pp. 304–8.

Australian Broadcasting Corporation (2002). Media Watch: 'Tampering with Defence PR', 22 April [available at: *www.abc.net.au/mediawatch/stories/220402_s2.htm* — accessed: 25 April 2003]

Australian Consumers' Association (1988). *Your health rights*. Australasian Publishing Company and Australian Consumers' Association, Sydney.

Australian Dr Weekly (1990). Mercy killing survey, 10 August, p. 10.

Australian Health Ministers (1995). *National Mental Health Policy*, Australian Government Publishing Service, Canberra.

Australian Institute of Health and Welfare (AIHW) (1998). *Child protection, Australia 1996–97*. AIHW cat. no. CWS 4, Canberra (Child Welfare Series no. 20).

Australian Medical Association (2003). *AMA Code of Ethics 2003*. AMA, Barton, ACT.

Australian Nurses Journal (1988). A costly misjudgment. Anonymous. *Australian Nurses Journal*, 17(6), December/January, p. 3.

Australian Nursing Council (2002). *National competency standards for the registered nurse and the enrolled nurse*. ANC, Canberra

—— (2002). *Code of ethics for nurses in Australia.* ANC, Canberra.

—— (2003). *Code of professional conduct for nurses in Australia.* ANC, Canberra.

Australian Nursing Council Inc. (1993). *Code of ethics for nurses in Australia.* Australian Nursing Council, Inc., Canberra.

—— (1994). *National Competencies for the Registered and Enrolled Nurse in Recommended Domains.* ANCI, Canberra.

—— (1997). *National Competency Standards for the Registered and Enrolled Nurse.* ANCI, Canberra.

Ayres, S. (1991). Who decides when care is futile? *Hospital Practice*, 26(30 September), pp. 41–53.

Badham, P. (1987). Christian belief and the ethics of in vitro fertilization and abortion. *Bioethics News* 6(2), January, pp. 7–18.

Baier, A. (1985). *Postures of the mind: essays on mind and morals.* Methuen, London, Chapter 6: 'Caring about caring: a reply to Frankfurt'.

Baier, K. (1978a). Deontological theories. In Reich, W.T. (ed.), *Encyclopedia of bioethics.* The Free Press, New York, pp. 413–17.

—— (1978b). Teleological theories. In Reich, W.T. (ed.), *Encyclopedia of bioethics.* The Free Press, New York, pp. 417–21.

Bailey, S. (1994). Critical care nurses' and doctors' attitudes to parasuicide patients. *Australian Journal of Advanced Nursing*, 11(3), pp. 11–17.

—— (1998). An exploration of critical care nurses' and doctors' attitudes towards psychiatric patients. *Australian Journal of Advanced Nursing*, 15(3), pp. 8–14.

Baltimore Sun (1993). US abortion clinics lose civil rights protection, in *The Age*, 15 January, p. 6.

Baly, M. (1984). *Professional responsibility* (2nd edn). H.M. & M. Nursing Publications, Division of John Wiley & Sons, Chichester, UK.

Bandman, E.L. and Bandman B. (1985). *Nursing ethics in the life span.* Appleton-Century-Crofts, Norwalk, Connecticut.

Barnard, D. (1988). 'Ship? What ship? I thought I was going to the doctor!': patient-centred perspectives on the health care team. In King, N.M.P., Churchill, L.R. and Cross, A.W. *Physician as captain of the ship.* D. Reidel, Dordrecht, pp. 89–111.

Barrett, G. (1992a). Ireland abortion law poll likely. *The Age*, 20 February, p. 9.

—— (1992b). Abortion ruling is threat to EC treaty. *The Age*, 21 February, p. 8.

—— (1992c). Parents of girl in abortion row to appeal against ban. *The Age*, 22 February, p. 7.

—— (1992d). Pressure for change in Irish abortion ban. *The Age*, 24 February, p. 8.

—— (1992e). Court rules against Ireland on abortion. *The Age*, 31 October, p. 8.

—— (1992f). Election, abortion vote in Ireland. *The Age*, 26 November, p. 7.

Barrett, L.I. (1992). Abortion: the issue Bush hopes will go away. *Time Magazine*, 13 July, pp. 54–5.

Barrington, M. (1983). Apologia for suicide. In Gorovitz, S., Macklin, R., Jameton, A.L., O'Connor, J.M. and Sherwin, A. (eds), *Moral problems in medicine.* Prentice Hall, Englewood Cliffs, New Jersey, pp. 472–6.

Barritt, E.R. (1973). Florence Nightingale's values and modern nursing education. *Nursing Forum*, 12(1), pp. 7–47.

Barry, V. (1982). *Moral aspects of health care.* Wadsworth, Belmont, California.

Bates, E. and Linder-Pelz, S. (1987). *Health care issues.* Allen & Unwin, Sydney.

Battin, M. Pabst (1982). *Ethical issues in suicide.* Prentice Hall, Englewood Cliffs, New Jersey.

—— (1983). The least worst death. *Hastings Center Report*, 13(2), April, pp. 13–16.

—— (1991). The way we do it, the way they do it. *Journal of Pain and Symptom Management*, 6(5), pp. 298–305.

—— (1996). *The death debate: ethical issues in suicide.* Prentice-Hall, Upper Saddle River, New Jersey.

Battin, M. Pabst and Mayo, D. (1980). *Suicide: the philosophical issues.* Peter Owen, London.

Baum, F. (1998). *The new public health: an Australian perspective.* Oxford University Press, Melbourne.

Bauman, Z. (1993). *Postmodern ethics.* Blackwell, Cambridge, Mass.

Baume, P. (1988). Perspectives on youth suicide. *Australian Journal of Advanced Nursing*, 5(3), pp. 40–8.

—— (1996). Voluntary euthanasia and law reform. *Australian Quarterly*, 68(3), pp. 17–25.

Bayles, M.D. (1981). *Professional ethics.* Wadsworth, Belmont, California.

Beals, A.R. (1979). *Culture in process.* Holt, Rinehart & Winston, New York.

Beard, B., Lester, L., Ivy, S. and Prince, N. (1988). Obstetrical nurses' attitudes about AIDS: an international study. *4th International Conference on AIDS. Book 1: Final program.* Abstracts, Monday June 13, Tuesday June 14. Stockholm International Fairs, Stockholm, Sweden, p. 505 (no. 9116).

Beardshaw, V. (1982). A question of conscience. *Nursing Times*, 78(9), pp. 349–51.

Beauchamp, D. (1975). Public health as social justice. In Teays, W. and L. Purdy (eds) (2001), *Bioethics, justice, & health care*. Belmont, Ca: Wadsworth:20-23. (Reprinted with permission of the Blue Cross and Blue Shield Association. Inquiry, 13:1-14).

Beauchamp, D. and Steinbock, B. (ed.) (1999). *New ethics for the public's health*. Oxford University Press, New York.

Beauchamp, T. (1978). Paternalism. In Reich, W.T. (ed.), *Encyclopedia of bioethics*. The Free Press, New York/Collier Macmillan, London, UK, pp. 1194–201.

—— (1978a). What is suicide? In Beauchamp, T. and Perlin, S. (eds), *Ethical issues in death and dying*. Prentice Hall, Englewood Cliffs, New Jersey, pp. 97–102.

—— (1978b). An analysis of Hume and Aquinas on suicide. In Beauchamp, T. and Perlin, S. (eds), *Ethical issues in death and dying*. Prentice Hall, Englewood Cliffs, New Jersey, pp. 111–22.

—— (1980). Suicide. In Regan, T. (ed.), *Matters of life and death: new introductory essays in moral philosophy*. Random House, New York, pp. 67–108.

—— (1989). Suicide in the age of reason. In Brody, B. (ed.), *Suicide and euthanasia: historical and contemporary themes*. Kluwer Academic Publishers, Dordrecht, pp. 183–219.

—— (1995). Paternalism. In Reich, W.T. (ed.), *Encyclopedia of Bioethics*, revised edition. Simon & Schuster Macmillan, New York/Simon & Schuster and Prentice Hall International, pp. 1914–20.

—— (1997). Justifying physician-assisted deaths. In LaFollette, H. (ed.), *Ethics in practice: an anthology*. Blackwell Publishers, Cambridge, Mass., pp. 33–41.

Beauchamp, T. and Childress, J. (1983). *Principles of biomedical ethics* (2nd edn). Oxford University Press, New York.

—— (1989). *Principles of biomedical ethics* (3rd edn). Oxford University Press, New York.

—— (1994). *Principles of biomedical ethics* (4th edn). Oxford University Press, New York.

—— (2001) *Principles of biomedical ethics* (5th edn). Oxford University Press, New York.

Beauchamp, T.L. (1982). What philosophers can offer. *Hastings Center Report* 12(3), June, pp. 13–14.

Beauchamp, T.L. and Davidson, A.I. (1979). The definition of euthanasia. *Journal of Medicine and Philosophy*, 4(3), pp. 294–312.

Beauchamp, T.L. and Perlin, S. (1978). *Ethical issues in death and dying*. Prentice Hall, Englewood Cliffs, New Jersey.

Beauchamp, T.L. and Walters, L. (eds) (1982). *Contemporary issues in bioethics* (2nd edn). Wadsworth, Belmont, California.

Beecher, H. (1966). Ethics and clinical research. *New England Journal of Medicine*, 274(2), June, pp. 1354–60.

Belcher, N. (1990). Pulling out the drip: an ethical decision in the terminally ill. *Geriatric Medicine*, 20(6), pp. 22–3.

Beloff, J. (1992). Do we have a duty to die? In *Voluntary Euthanasia Society*, 'Your ultimate choice: the right to die with dignity'. Souvenir Press, London. pp. 52–6.

Benhabib, S. and Dallmayr, F. (eds) (1990). *The communicative ethics controversy*. MIT Press, Cambridge, Mass.

Benjamin, M. (2001). Between subway and spaceship: practical ethics at the outset of the twenty-first century. *Hastings Center Report*, 31(4), pp. 24–31.

Benjamin, M. and Curtis, J. (1986). *Ethics in nursing* (2nd edn). Oxford University Press, New York.

Benn, S.I. (1971). Privacy, freedom, and respect for persons. *Nomos* 13 (J.R. Pennock and J.W. Chapman (eds) American Society for Political and Legal Philosophy: Privacy, Artherton Press, New York), pp. 1–21.

Benn, S.I. and Peters, R.S. (1959). *Social principles and the democratic state*. George Allen & Unwin, London.

Benner, P. (1984). *From novice to expert: excellence and power in clinical nursing practice*. Addison-Wesley, Nursing Division, Menlo Park, California.

—— (1991). The role of experience, narrative, and community in skilled ethical comportment. *Advances in Nursing Science*, 14(2), pp. 1–21.

—— (ed.) (1994). *Interpretive phenomenology: embodiment, caring, and ethics in health and illness*. Sage, Thousand Oaks.

Benner, P. and Wrubel, J. (1989). *The primacy of caring*. Addison-Wesley, Menlo Park, California.

Bentham, J. (1962). An introduction to the principles of morals and legislation (reprinted from 1789 edition). In Warnock, M. (ed.), *Utilitarianism*. Fontana Library/Collins, London, pp. 33–77.

Bergman, R. (1973). Ethics — concepts and practice. *International Nursing Review* 20(5), pp. 140–2.

Berkowitz, M. (1982). The role of discussion in ethics training. *Topics in Clinical Nursing*, 4(1), April, pp. 33–48.

Beyer, L. (1989). The globalization of the abortion debate. *Time Magazine*, 21 August, pp. 60–1.

Bickley, J. (1988). What the cervical cancer inquiry report means for nurses. *New Zealand Nursing Journal*, 81(9), pp. 14–15.

—— (1988). Why NZNA supports direct action. *New Zealand Nursing Journal*, 81(3), March, p. 6.

—— (1993). Watchdogs or wimps? Nurses' response to the Cartwright Report. In Coney, S. (ed.), *Unfinished business: what happened to the Cartwright Report? Writings on the aftermath of 'the unfortunate experiment' at National Women's Hospital.* Women's Health Action, Auckland, NZ, pp. 125–36.

Bilton, M. and Sim, K. (1992). *Four hours in My Lai: a war crime and its aftermath.* Viking, London.

Bindels, P., Krol, A., van Ameijden, E., Mulder-Folkerts, D., van den Hoek, J., van Griensven, G. and Coutinho, R. (1996). Euthanasia and physician-assisted suicide in homosexual men with AIDS. *The Lancet*, 347 (24 February), pp. 499–504.

Bioethics News (1985). Request to die. *Bioethics News*, 5(1), October.

Bioethics News (1988). The fetal brain cell debate. *Bioethics News*, 7(4), July, pp. 10–11.

—— (1991). National Bioethics Consultative Committee disbanded. 10(4), July, p. 1.

—— (1992). 'Not for resuscitation' orders — Britain. 12(1), October, p. 4.

—— (1993). Pope: rape victims should not have abortions. 12(3), April, p. 3.

Birnbach, N. and Lewenson, S. (eds) (1991). *First words: selected addresses from the national League for Nursing 1894–1933.* National League for Nursing, New York.

Birnbauer, B. (1986). Government wants to hire 500 UK nurses to ease waiting lists. *The Age*, 30 January, p. 3.

Birrell, R. and Birrell, J. (1966). The 'maltreatment syndrome' in children. *Medical Journal of Australia*, 2, pp. 1134–138.

—— (1968). The 'maltreatment syndrome' in children: a hospital survey. *Medical Journal of Australia*, 2, pp. 1023–29.

Bishop, A.H. and Scudder, J.R. (1987). Nursing ethics in an age of controversy. *Advances in Nursing Science*, 9(3), pp. 34–43.

—— (1990). *The practical, moral and personal sense of nursing: a phenomenological philosophy of practice.* State University of New York Press, Albany.

—— (1991). *Nursing: the practice of caring.* National League for Nursing Press, New York.

Blackburn, S. (1984). *Spreading the word.* Clarendon Press, Oxford.

Blake, D.C. (1992). The hospital ethics committee: health care's moral conscience or white elephant? *Hastings Center Report*, 22(1), pp. 6–11.

Bloch, S. and Chodoff, P. (eds) (1991). *Psychiatric Ethics* (2nd edn). Oxford University Press, New York.

Blum, J.D. (1984). The code of nurses and wrongful discharge. *Nursing Forum* 21, pp. 149–51.

Blum, L. (1980). *Friendship, altruism and morality.* Routledge & Kegan Paul, London/Boston.

—— (1988). Moral exemplars: reflections on Schindler, the Trocmes, and others. *Midwest Studies in Philosophy*, 13, pp. 196–221.

—— (1994). *Moral perception and particularity.* Cambridge University Press, Cambridge, UK/New York.

Blustein, J. (1991). *Care and commitment: taking the personal point of view.* Oxford University Press, New York.

Boatright, J. (1993). *Ethics and the conduct of business.* Prentice-Hall, New Jersey.

Bock, A. (1992). Nurses in call for euthanasia inquiry. *The Age*, 3 March, p. 6.

Boddy, J. (ed.) (1985). *Health: perspectives and practices.* The Dunmore Press, Palmerston North, New Zealand.

Bohm, D. (1989). Meaning and information. In Pylkkanen, P. (ed.), *The search for meaning: the new spirit in science and philosophy.* Crucible, an imprint of The Acquarian Press. Wellingborough, Northamptonshire, UK, pp. 43–85.

Bok, S. (1978). *Lying: moral choice in public and private life.* Vintage Books, New York.

—— (1980). *Lying: moral choice in public and private life.* Quartet Books, London.

—— (1983). *Secrets: on the ethics of concealment and revelation.* Vintage Books, New York.

Bolsin, S. (2003). Whistle blowing. *Medical Education*, 37, pp. 294–6.

Bolton, M. Brandt (1983). Responsible women and abortion decisions. In Gorovitz, S., Macklin, R., Jameton, A.L., O'Connor, J.M. and Sherwin, A. (eds), *Moral problems in medicine*, (2nd edn). Prentice Hall, Englewood Cliffs, New Jersey, pp. 330–8.

Bond, E. (1996). *Ethics and human wellbeing.* Blackwell, Cambridge, Massachusetts/Oxford, UK.

Bone, P. (1987). Pelvic check 'by patient's consent' only. *The Age*, 18 September, p. 5.

Boseley, S. and Dyer, C. (1999). Girl gets a heart against her will. *The Age*, 17 August, p. 19.

Boulware-Miller, K. (1985). Female circumcision: challenges to the practice as a human rights violation. *Harvard Women's Law Journal*, 8, pp. 155–77.

Bowden, P. (1994). The ethics of nursing care and 'the ethic of care'. *Nursing Inquiry*, 2, pp. 10–21.

Bowman, J. (1995). Genetics and racial minorities. In Reich, W.T. (ed.), *Encyclopedia of Bioethics*, revised edition. Simon & Schuster Macmillan, New York, p. 982.

Boyle, J. (1989). Sanctity of life and suicide: tensions and developments within common morality. In Brody, B. (ed.), *Suicide and euthanasia: historical and contemporary themes*. Kluwer Academic Publishers, Dordrecht, pp. 221–50.

—— (1994). Radical moral disagreement in contemporary health care: a Roman Catholic perspective. *Journal of Medicine and Philosophy* 19(2), pp. 183–200.

Brabeck, M.M. (ed.) (1989). *Who cares? Theory, research, and educational implications of the ethic of care*. Praeger, New York.

Braidotti, R. (1986). Ethics revisited: Women and/in philosophy. In C. Pateman and E. Gross (eds), *Feminist challenges*. Allen & Unwin, Sydney.

Brandt, R. (1959). *Ethical theory*. Prentice Hall, Englewood Cliffs, New Jersey (see in particular Chapter 4, 'The use of authority in ethics').

Brandt, R. (1978). The morality and rationality of suicide. In Beauchamp, T. and Perli, S. (eds), *Ethical issues in death and dying*. Prentice Hall, Englewood Cliffs, New Jersey, pp. 122–33.

—— (1980). The rationality of suicide. In Pabst Battin, M. and Mayo, D., *Suicide: the philosophical issues*. Peter Owen, London, pp. 117–32.

Brennan, L. and the editors of *Nursing 88* (1988). The battle against AIDS: a report from the nursing front. *Nursing 88*, (18)4, pp. 60–4.

Brennan, T.A. (1988). Ethics committees and decisions to limit care. *Journal of the American Medical Association*, 260(6), 12 August, pp. 803–7.

Bridges, D.C. (1968). 'International Nursing Review' past, present — and progress? *International Nursing Review* 15 (1), pp. 9–17.

Bridston, E. (1982). An educational strategy for enhancement of moral–ethical decision making. *Topics in Clinical Nursing*, 4(1), April, pp. 57–65.

Briere, J. (1992). *Child abuse trauma: theory and treatment of the lasting effects*. Sage, Newbury Park, Ca.

Briggs, P. and McDonald, B. (1992). 'Straw Men' in the euthanasia debate. *The Age*, 24 March, p. 12.

Brink, D.O. (1989). *Moral realism and the foundations of ethics*. Cambridge University Press, Cambridge.

British Medical Association (1986). *News Review* 11(1), pp. 22–3.

Broad, C.D. (1940). Conscience and conscientious action. First published in *Philosophy*, volume 15; reprinted in J. Feinberg, *Moral concepts*, Oxford University Press, Oxford, 1969, pp. 74–9.

Brock, D. (1993). *Life and death: philosophical essays in biomedical ethics*. Cambridge University Press, New York.

Brodeur, Rev. D. (1984). Towards a clear definition of ethics committees. *Linacre Quarterly*, 51(3), August, pp. 233–47.

Brody, B. (1982). The morality of abortion. In T.L. Beauchamp and L. Walters, *Contemporary issues in bioethics* (2nd edn). Wadsworth, Belmont, California, pp. 240–50.

—— (1986). Should there be a distinctively Jewish medical ethics? *Isaac Frank Memorial Lecture*, Kennedy Institute of Ethics, Georgetown University, Washington DC, ICC Auditorium, 2 June.

—— (ed.) (1989a). *Suicide and euthanasia: historical and contemporary themes*. Kluwer Academic Publishers, Dordrecht.

—— (1989b). A historical introduction to Jewish casuistry on suicide and euthanasia. In Brody, B. (1989a) *Suicide and euthanasia: historical and contemporary themes*. Kluwer Academic Publishers, Dordrecht. pp. 39–75.

Brody, B. and Halevy, A. (1995). Is futility a futile concept? *Journal of Medicine and Philosophy*, 20(2), pp. 123–44.

Brody, H. (1992). Assisted death — a compassionate response to a medical failure. *New England Journal of Medicine*, 327(19), pp. 1384–8.

Broekhuijse, P. (1988). Nurse loses job over abortion. *Sunday Telegraph*, 21 February, p. 13.

Bromberger, B. and Fife-Yeomans, J. (1991). *Deep Sleep: Harry Bailey and the Scandal of Chelmsford*. Simon & Schuster, Sydney.

Broughton, J.M. (1983). Women's rationality and men's virtues: a critique of gender dualism in Gilligan's theory of moral development. *Social Research*, 50(3), Autumn, pp. 597–642.

Brovins, J. and Oehmke, T. (1993). *Dr Death: Dr Jack Kevorkian's Rx: Death*. Lifetime Books, Hollywood.

Brown, J.M., Kitson, A.L. and McKnight, T.J. (1992). *Challenges in caring: explorations in nursing and ethics*. Chapman & Hall, London.

Browne, A. (1990). Assisted suicide and active voluntary euthanasia. *Bioethics News*, 9(4), pp. 9–38.

Bruera, E., Legris, M., Kuehn, N. and Miller, M. (1990). Hypodermoclysis for the administration of fluids and narcotic analgesia in patients with advanced cancer. *Journal of Pain and Symptom Management*, 5, pp. 218–20.

Buchanan, A (1984). The right to a decent minimum of health care. *Philosophy and Public Affairs*, 13(1), Winter, pp. 55–78.

—— (1978). Medical paternalism. *Philosophy and Public Affairs*, 7(4), pp. 371–90.

Buchanan, A.E. and Brock, D.W. (1989). *Deciding for others: the ethics of surrogate decision making.* Cambridge University Press, Cambridge.

Buchanan, F. (1983). Resuscitation procedures. Letter to the Editor, *Nursing Times*, 79(34), p. 7.

Buckle, S. and Dawson, K. (1988). Individuals and syngamy. *Bioethics News*, 7(3), April, pp. 15–30.

Bullivant, B.M. (1981). *Race, ethnicity and curriculum.* Macmillan, Melbourne.

—— (1984). *Pluralism, cultural maintenance and evolution.* Bank House, Clevedon, Avon.

Burdekin, B., Guilfoyle, M. and Hall, D. (1993). *Human rights & mental illness: Report of the National Inquiry into the Human Rights of People with Mental Illness.* Australian Government Publishing Service, Canberra.

Buresch, B. and Gordon, S. (2000). *From Silence to Voice: What Nurses Know and Must Communicate to the Public.* Canadian Nurses Association, Ottawa.

Bynom, S. (1999). When is blowing the whistle not whistle blowing? *British Journal of Perioperative Nursing*, 9(6), pp. 265–8.

Byrne, M. (2002). The use of advanced directives. *Nursing Monograph.* St Vincent's Health Care Campus, Melbourne, pp. 13–16.

Cahn, M. (1989). *The nurse as moral hero: a case for required dissent.* Thesis component of the Doctor of Nursing Sciences degree in the School of Nursing, Indiana University. UMI Dissertation Services, Ann Arbor, Michegan (no. 8822134).

Callahan, J. (ed.) (1995). *Reproduction, ethics and the law: feminist perspectives.* Indiana University Press, Bloomington and Indianapolis.

Callahan, S. (1988). The role of emotion in ethical decision-making. *Hastings Center Report*, 6 (June/July), pp. 9–14.

Campbell, C.S. (1992). Religious ethics and active euthanasia in a pluralistic society. *Kennedy Institute of Ethics Journal* 2(3), pp. 253–77.

Campbell, E.J., Baker, M.D. and Crites-Silver, P. (1988). Subjective effects of humidification of oxygen for delivery by nasal cannula: a prospective study. *Chest*, 93(2), February, pp. 289–93.

Canadian Press (1988). Abortion ruling: What does it mean? *Leader Post*, 29 January, p. 1.

Cannold, L. (1994). Consequences for patients of health care professional's conscientious actions: the ban on abortion in South Australia. *Journal of Medical Ethics*, 20(2), pp. 80–6.

—— (1998). *The abortion myth: feminism, morality and the hard choices women make.* Allen & Unwin, Sydney.

Cantor, N. (1995) Quality of life in legal perspective, in Reich, W.T. (ed.) *Encyclopedia of bioethics*, revised edition. Simon and Schuster MacMillan, New York, pp. 1361–6.

Caplan, A. (ed.) (1992). *When medicine went mad: bioethics and the holocaust.* Humana Press, Totowa, New Jersey.

Caplan, A.L. (1982). Mechanics on duty: the limitations of a technical definition of moral expertise for work in applied ethics. *Canadian Journal of Philosophy*, supplementary vol. 8, pp. 1–17.

Capron, A. (1974). Informed consent in catastrophic disease and treatment. *University of Pennsylvania Law Review* 123, December, pp. 364–76 (cited in T.L. Beauchamp and J.F. Childress [1983], *Principles of biomedical ethics* (2nd edn). Oxford University Press, New York, pp. 67, 102).

Card, C. (ed.) (1991). *Feminist ethics.* University of Kansas Press, Lawrence, Kansas.

Carlton, W. (1978). '*In our professional opinion . . .': the primacy of clinical judgment over moral choice.* University of Notre Dame Press, Notre Dame.

Carper, B. (1986). The ethics of caring. In P. Chinn (ed.), *Ethical issues in nursing.* Aspen Systems, Rockville, Maryland.

Carr, E.H. (1961). *The romantic exiles: a nineteenth-century portrait gallery.* Beacon Press, Boston.

Carrick, P. (1985). *Medical ethics in antiquity.* D. Reidel, Dordrecht.

Carson, R. (1982). Commentary. *Hastings Center Report*, 12(5), October, p. 28.

Carter, W.J. (1991). *Report of the Commission of Inquiry into the Care and Treatment of Patients in the Psychiatric Unit of the Townsville General Hospital between 2nd March, 1975 and 20th February, 1988*, (2 volumes). Government Printing Services, Brisbane.

Cassell, E. (1991). *The nature of suffering and the goals of medicine.* Oxford University Press, New York.

—— (1982). The nature of suffering and the goals of medicine. *New England Journal of Medicine*, 306, pp. 639–45.

Cattanach, J.F. (1985). The distinction between membership of the human species and characteristics of the human being. *Bioethics News* 5(1), October, pp. 28–30.

Centre for Human Bioethics (1986). *Proceedings of the conference, 'AIDS: Social Policy, Ethics and Law'*. Centre for Human Bioethics, Monash University, Melbourne.
—— (1987a). *Proceedings of the conference, 'The role of the nurse: doctors' handmaiden, patients' advocate, or what?* Centre for Human Bioethics, Monash University, Melbourne.
—— (1987b). *Proceedings of the conference, 'IVF: the Current Debate'*. Centre for Human Bioethics, Monash University, Melbourne.
Chaboyer, W. (2000). The use of proxy-generated health status assessments in ICU survivors: the issue of quality of life. *Journal of Law and Medicine*, 8(2), pp. 157–63.
Chandler, J. (1993). Doctors might relent on abuse reporting. *The Age*, 27 March, p. 28.
—— (2001). Transplant row widens. *The Age*, 9 February, p. 9.
Chapell, A. (1994). Protecting the public. *Nursing New Zealand*, August, pp. 28–9.
Char, W.F. and McDermott, J.F. (1972). Abortions and acute identity crisis in nurses. *American Journal of Psychiatry*, 128(8), pp. 952–7.
Cheng-tek Tai, M. and Chung Seng Lin. (2001). Developing a cultural relevant bioethics for Asian people. *Journal of Medical Ethics*, 27(1), pp. 51–4.
Cherniack, E. (2002). Increasing use of DNR orders in the elderly worldwide: whose choice is it? *Journal of Medical Ethics*, 28(5), pp. 303–7.
Chesler, P. (1987). *Mothers on trial: the battle for children and custody*. Harcourt Brace Jovanovich, New York.
Child Protection Victoria (1993). *Reporting Child Abuse*. Health and Community Services, Melbourne.
Childress, J.F. (1979). Appeals to conscience. *Ethics* 89, pp. 315–35.
—— (1982). Who should decide? *Paternalism in health care*. Oxford University Press, New York.
Ching, M. (1993). The use of touch in nursing practice. *Australian Journal of Advanced Nursing*, 10(4), pp. 4–9.
Chinn, P.L. (ed.) (1991). *Anthology on caring*. National League for Nursing Press, New York.
Chodoff, P., Green, S. and Bloch, S. (1999). *Psychiatric ethics* (3rd edn). Oxford University Press, New York.
Chopra, D. (1989). *Quantum healing: exploring the frontiers of mind/body medicine*. Bantam Books, New York.
Chrisman, N.J. (1981). Nursing in the context of social and cultural systems. In P. Mitchell and A. Loustau, *Concepts basic to nursing*. McGraw-Hill, New York, pp. 37–52.

Christensen, C., Bohmer, R. and Kenagy, J. (2001). Will disruptive innovations cure health care? *Harvard Business Review*, September–October, pp. 102–12.
Christensen, R. 1997. Ethical issues in community mental health: cases and conflicts. *Community Mental Health Journal*, 33(1), pp. 5–11.
Christian, M. (1997). No suicide dollars. Letter to the Editor. *BrotherSister*, 25 December (no. 148), p. 9.
Churcher, S. (1999). Mum tests professor of death, *Herald-Sun*, 15 September, p. 19.
Churchill, L. (1989). Reviving a distinctive medical ethic. *Hastings Center Report*, May–June, 19(3), pp. 28–34.
Clarkeburn, H. (2000). Parental duties and untreatable genetic conditions. *Journal of Medical Ethics*, 26(5), pp. 400–403.
Clay, T. (1987). *Nurses: power and politics*. Heinemann Nursing, London.
Clemons, J. (ed.) (1990). *Perspectives on suicide*. Westminster/John Knox Press, Louisville, Kentucky.
Clinical Ethics Committee, Council of Physicians and Dentists (1984). *Use of life support systems: ethical guidelines relating to use of life support systems*. Royal Victoria Hospital, Montreal, Quebec.
Clouser, K. Danner (1978). Bioethics. In Reich, W.T. *Encyclopedia of bioethics*, pp. 115–27.
—— (1995). Common morality as an alternative to principlism. *Kennedy Institute of Ethics Journal*, 5(3), pp. 219–36.
Coady, C. (1996). On regulating ethics. In Coady, M. and Bloch, S. (eds), *Codes of ethics and the professions*. Melbourne University Press, Melbourne, pp. 269–87.
Code, L. (1991). *What can she know? Feminist theory and the construction of knowledge*. Cornell University Press, Ithaca and London.
Code, L., Mullett, S. and Overall, C. (eds) (1988). *Feminist perspectives: philosophical essays on methods and morals*. University of Toronto Press, Toronto.
Coffey, M. (1996). 100 children die in care. *Herald Sun*, 31 October, pp. 1, 4.
Cohen, Y.A. (1968). *Man in adaptation: the cultural present*. Aldine, Chicago.
Cole, E.B. and Coultrap-McQuin, S. (eds) (1992). *Explorations in feminist ethics: theory and practice*. Indiana University Press, Bloomington and Indianapolis.
Cole-Adams, P. (1986). As public support fades, the nurses reach a turning point. *The Age*, 12 December, p. 1.
Collier, K. (1999), Nurse fired over patient's death. *Herald Sun*, 18 May, p. 2.

Colt, G. Howe (1991). *The enigma of suicide*. Simon & Schuster, New York.

Coney, S. (1988). *The unfortunate experiment*. Penguin Books, Auckland.

—— (1990). *Out of the frying pan: inflammatory writing 1972–89*. Penguin Books, Auckland, NZ.

—— (ed.) (1993). *Unfinished business: what happened to the Cartwright Report? Writings on the aftermath of 'the unfortunate experiment' at National Women's Hospital*. Women's Health Action, Auckland, NZ.

Coney, S. and Bunkle, P. (1987). An 'unfortunate experiment' at National Women's. *Metro*, June, pp. 47–65.

Conley, J. (1987). AMA will consider secret AIDS tests. *The Age*, 4 July, p. 1.

Connelly, R. (1991). Nursing responsibility for the placebo effect. *Journal of Medicine and Philosophy*, 16(3), pp. 325–41.

Consumers' Health Forum of Australia (1990). *Legal recognition and protection of the rights of health consumers*. Consumers' Health Forum of Australia, Curtin, ACT.

Cook, D., Guyatt, G., Rocker, G., Sjokvist, P., Weaver, B., Dodek, P., Marshall, J., Leasa, D., Levy, M., Varon, J., Fisher, M. and Cook, R., for the Canadian Critical Care Trial Group (2001). Cardiopulmonary resuscitation directives on admission to intensive-care unit: an international observational study. *The Lancet*, 358(9297), pp. 1941–5.

Cooper, J. (1989). Greek philosophers on euthanasia and suicide. In Brody, B. (ed.), *Suicide and euthanasia: historical and contemporary themes*. Kluwer Academic Publishers, Dordrecht, pp. 9–38.

Cooper, M. (1988). Covenantal relationships: grounding for the nursing ethic. *Advances in Nursing Science* 10(4), pp. 48–59.

—— (1990). Reconceptualizing nursing ethics. *Scholarly Inquiry for Nursing Practice: An International Journal*, 4(3), pp. 209–18.

—— (1991). Principle-orientated ethics and the ethic of care: a creative tension. *Advances in Nursing Science*, 14(2), pp. 22–31.

Corby, B. (2000). *Child abuse: towards a knowledge base*. Open University Press, Buckingham.

Corlett, D. (1993). Former Yugoslavia. *Victorian Foundation for Survivors of Torture Newsletter*, published by VFST, Melbourne, Spring, p. 4.

Corley, M and Raines, D. (1993). Environments that support ethical nursing practice. *AWHONN's Clinial Issues*, 4(4), pp. 611–19.

Cornwell, R. (1993). US plans to reverse abortion, labor laws. *The Age*, 2 April, p. 8.

Cortese, A. (1990). *Ethnic ethics: the restructuring of moral theory*. State University of New York Press, Albany.

Cosic, M. (2003). *The right to die? An examination of the euthanasia debate*. New Holland Publishers, Sydney.

Cossar, L. (1988). Hospital helps woman to die. *The Herald*, 22 March, p. 1.

Cossar, L. and Evans, J. (1986). Nurses: wider role closer for 'aides'. *The Herald*, 12 December, p. 1.

Coster, P. (1986). After 39 days in a crisis the doctors battle for patients — the nurses to keep their patience. *The Herald*, 8 December, p. 1.

Cotterhill, D. (1992). Views not representative. *Australian Nurses Journal*, 21(10), p. 4.

Coulter, C. (1987). Women, infertility and IVF. In *Proceedings of the conference, 'IVF: the Current Debate'*. Centre for Human Bioethics, Monash University, Melbourne, pp. 156–68.

Council for Science and Society (1982). *Expensive medical techniques*. Calvert's Press, London.

Council on Ethical and Judicial Affairs, American Medical Association (1999). Medical futility in end-of life care: report of the Council on Ethical and Judicial Affairs. *JAMA*, 281(10), pp. 937–41.

—— (1991). Guidelines for the appropriate use of Do-Not-Resuscitate orders. *Journal of American Medical Association* 265(14), pp. 1868–71.

Courier-Mail (1995). 13 May, Queenslander supports killing doctors who perform abortion. Reprinted in *Monash Bioethics Review*, 14(3), p. 11.

Coutinho, R. (1996). Euthanasia and physician-assisted suicide in homosexual men with AIDS. *The Lancet*, 347, 24 February, pp. 499–504.

Cowles, K. (1984). Definitions of life and death continue to elude us. *Nursing Outlook*, 32(3), May/June, pp. 169–72.

Cox, D. (1993). *Hemlock's cup: the struggle for death with dignity*. Prometheus Books, New York

Coyler, V. (1986). Why not get tough about child abuse? *The Age*, 15 October.

Coyne, C. (2003). Whistleblowing & problem solving: a 5-step approach. *Physiotherapy*, 11(2), pp. 42–8.

Crabbe, G. (1988). The lonely dilemma. *Nursing Times*, 84(9), p. 18.

Craig, G. (1994). On withholding nutrition and hydration in the terminally ill: has palliative medicine gone to far? *Journal of Medical Ethics*, 20(3), pp. 139–43.

—— (1996). On withholding artificial hydration and nutrition from terminally ill: sedated patients. The debate continues. *Journal of Medical Ethics*, 22(3), pp. 147–53.

Craig, O. (1989). Life or death? How doctors decide which patient gets a 'black dot'. *Sun-Herald* (Sydney), 12 March.

Cranford, R.E. and Doudera, J.D. (1984). The emergence of institutional ethics committees. *Law, Medicine and Health Care*, 12(1), February, pp. 13–20.

Crittenden, B. (1979). The limitations of morality as justice in Kohlberg's theory. In D.B. Cochrane, C.M. Hamm and A.C. Kazepides (eds), *The domain of moral education*. Paulist Press, New York, pp. 251–66.

Crock, E. (2001). *Nursing, ethics and HIV/AIDS: a philosophical investigation*. PhD Thesis, held RMIT University, Melbourne.

—— (1998) Breaking (through) the law — coming out of the silence: nursing, HIV/AIDS and ethanasia. *AIDS Care*, 10, Suppl 2, pp. S137–145

Crosweller, A. and McGilvary, A. (2001). Ban on transplants has smokers gasping. *The Age*, 9 February, p. 4.

Curtin, L. (1979). CPR policies: the art of the possible — optimal care vs maximal treatment. *Supervisor Nurse*, 10, August, pp. 16–18.

—— (1986). The nurse as advocate: a philosophical foundation for nursing. In P. Chinn (ed.), *Ethical issues in nursing*. Aspen System, Rockville, Maryland, pp. 11–20.

—— (1993). Creating moral space for nurses. *Nursing Management*, 24(3), pp. 18–19.

Curtin, L. and Flaherty, M.J. (1982). *Nursing ethics: theories and pragmatics*. Prentice Hall, Bowie, Maryland, p. 61.

Curtis, M. (1989). Nurse AIDS anger. *The Sun*, 10 March, p. 3.

Curzer, H. (1993). Is care a virtue for health care professionals. *Journal of Medicine and Philosophy*, 18(1), pp. 51–69.

Cushing, M. (1981). No code orders: current developments and the nursing director's role. *Journal of Nursing Administration*, 11(26), April, pp. 22–9.

Daley, D.W. (1983). Tarasoff and the psychotherapist's duty to warn. In Gorovitz, S., Macklin, R., Jameton, A.L., O'Connor, J.M. and Sherwin, A. (eds), *Moral problems in medicine* (2nd edn). Prentice Hall, Englewood Cliffs, New Jersey, pp. 234–46.

Dalla-Vorgia, P., Katsouyanni, K., Garanis, T.N., Touloumi, G., Drogari, P. and Koutselinis, A. (1992). Attitudes of a Mediterranean population to the truth-telling issue. *Journal of Medical Ethics*, 18(2), pp. 67–74.

Daly, M. (1978). *Gyn/ecology: the metaethics of radical feminism*. The Women's Press, London.

Daly, M., Farouque, F. and Adams, D. (1996). Children left in danger by care workers:

report. *The Age*, 26 October, p. 1.

Damasio, A. (1994). *Descartes error: emotion, reason, and the human brain*. Avon Books, New York.

Dancy, J. (1993). *Moral reasons*. Blackwell, Oxford, UK and Cambridge, USA.

Daniels, N. (1984). Understanding physician power: a review of the social transformation of American medicine. *Philosophy and Public Affairs*, 13(4), Fall, pp. 347–57.

—— (1996). *Justice and justification: reflective equilibrium in theory and practice*. Cambridge University Press, Cambridge, UK/New York.

Das, S. (1996). Lawyer calls for euthanasia acquittal. *The Age*, 19 December, p. 7.

Daverschot, M. and Van der Wal, H. (2001). The position of Nurses in the new Dutch euthanasia bill: a report of legal and political developments. *Ethics & Medicine*, 17(2), pp. 85–92.

Davies, J. (2002). Unafraid to die, scared to live; Nancy states her case. *The Age*, 27 March, pp. 1 & 8.

—— (2003). Tube woman can die, court rules. *The Age*, 30 May, p. 5.

Davis, A. (1982). Helping your staff address ethical dilemmas, *Journal of Nursing Administration* 12(2), February, pp. 9–13.

Davis, A. (1992). Suicidal behaviour among adolescents: its nature and prevention. In Kosky, R., Eshkevari, H. and Kneebone, G. (eds), *Breaking out: challenges in adolescent mental health in Australia*. Australian Government Publishing Service, Canberra.

Davis, A. and Aroskar, M. (1983). *Ethical dilemmas and nursing practice* (2nd edn). Appleton-Century-Crofts, Norwalk, Connecticut.

Davis, M. (1986a). Use nursing aides, AMA urges. *The Age*, 11 December, p. 10.

—— (1986b). Unions plan strike to support nurses. *The Age*, 26 November, p. 5.

—— (1986c). Casualty nurses to walk out today. *The Age*, 8 December, p. 1.

Davis, M. and Menagh, C. (1986a). Bans threat as unions back nurses' strike. *The Age*, 19 November, p. 1.

—— (1986b). Nurses angered by aides plan. *The Age*, 13 December, p. 1.

Davis M. and Noble, T. (1986). Threats to nurses upset police. *The Age*, 5 November, p. l.

Davis-Floyd, R. and Arvidson P. Sven (eds) (1997). *Intuition: the inside story. Interdisciplinary perspectives*. Routledge, New York.

de Beauvoir, S. (1964 [1987 edn]). *A very easy death*. Penguin, Harmondsworth, Middlesex.

de Bono, E. (1985). *Conflicts: a better way to resolve them*. Penguin Books, London.

—— (1990). *I am right — you are wrong*. Penguin Books, London.

De Vries, R. and Forsberg, C. (2002). Who decides? A look at ethics committee membership. *HEC Forum*, 14(3), pp. 252–8.

de Wachter, M.A.M. (1992). Euthanasia in the Netherlands. *Hastings Center Report* 22(2), pp. 23–30.

Deane, J. (1992). Teen suicide. *Sunday Herald-Sun* (Melbourne), 2 February, p. 81.

Deane, Sir William. (2001). Sir William farewells Government House. *ABC News Online*, Thursday 28 June, 2001 [available at: *http://www.abc.net.au/news/2001/06/item20010628125057_1.htm* — accessed 7 November 2003].

Debelle, P. (1991). Ethics in embryo. *Good Weekend, The Age magazine*, 9 January, pp. 18–24.

Dembner, A. (2003). 'Do Not Resuscitate' instructions often ignored, overlooked. *Boston Globe*, 11 September, p. A.1.

Demopolous, H. (1968). Suicide and Church canon law. Unpublished doctoral dissertation, Claremont School of Theology, California.

Densford, J. and Everett, M. (1947). *Ethics for modern nurses: professional adjustments 1*. W.B. Saunders, Philadelphia.

Derry, R. (1991). How can an organisation support and encourage ethical behaviour? In Freeman, R. (ed.), *Business ethics: the state of the art*. Oxford University Press, New York, pp. 121–36.

Deveson, A. (1991). *Tell me I'm here*. Penguin, Ringwood, Victoria.

Dimond, B. (1999). Confidentiality 9: the law relating to whistle blowing. *British Journal of Nursing*, 8(19), pp. 1322–3.

Dix, A., Errington, M., Nicholson, K. and Powe, R. (1996). *Law for the medical profession in Australia* (2nd edn). Butterworth-Heinemann, Melbourne.

Dixon, N. (1998). On the difference between physician-assisted suicide and active euthanasia. *Hastings Center Report*, 28(5), pp. 25–9.

Dock, L.L. (1900). Ethics — or a Code of Ethics? In Dock, L.L., *Short papers on nursing subjects*, M. Louise Longeway, New York, pp. 37–56 (p. 57 missing).

Doder, D. (1993). Balkans rape babies face life of shame, rejection. *The Age*, 5 July, p. 8.

Dolan, J.A., Fitzpatrick, M.L. and Herrmann, E.K. (1983). *Nursing in society: an historical perspective* (15th edn). W.B. Saunders, Philadelphia.

Dolan, M.B. (1988). Coding abuses hurt nurses, too. *Nursing 88*, 18(12), December, p. 47.

Donnelly, J. (ed.) (1990). *Suicide: right or wrong?* Prometheus Books, Buffalo, New York.

Donovan, M., Dillon, P. and McGuire, L. (1987). Incidence and characteristics of pain in a sample of medical–surgical inpatients. *Pain* 30, pp. 68–78.

Donovan, P. (1996). Murder-charge nurse bailed. *The Age*, 10 May, p. 2.

Dossey, L. (1982). *Space, time and medicine*. New Science Library, Boston, Mass.

—— (1991). *Meaning & medicine: a doctor's tales of breakthrough and healing*. Bantam Books, New York.

—— (1993). *Healing words: the power of prayer and the practice of medicine*. HarperSanFrancisco, New York.

Downie, R.S. and Calman, K.C. (1987). *Healthy respect: ethics in health care*. Faber & Faber, London.

Doyal, L. (2001). Clinical ethics committees and the formulation of health care policy. *Journal of Medical Ethics*, 27(Supplement 1), i44–i49.

Drane, J. (1995). Alternative therapies: ethical and legal issues. In Reich, W.T. (ed.), *The encyclopedia of bioethics*, revised edition. Simon & Schuster Macmillan, New York, pp. 135–43.

Drengson, A.R. (1985). Critical notice. *Canadian Journal of Philosophy*, 15(1), March, pp. 111–31.

Dresser, R. and Roberston, J. (1989). Quality of life and non-treatment decisions: a critique of the orthodox approach. *Law, Medicine & Health Care*, 17(3), pp. 234–44.

Dreyfus, H. and Dreyfus, S. (1991). Towards a phenomenology of ethical expertise. *Human Studies*, 14, pp. 229–50.

Dunleavey, R. (1992). An adequate response to a cry for help? Parasuicide patients' perceptions of their nursing care. *Professional Nurse*, January, pp. 213–15.

Dunnum, L. (1990). Life satisfaction and spinal cord injury: the patient perspective. *Journal of Neuroscience Nursing*, 22, pp. 43–7.

Durkheim, E. (1952). *Suicide*. Routledge & Kegan Paul, London.

DuVal, G., Sartorius, L., Clarridge, B., Gensler, G. and Danis, M. (2001). What triggers requests for ethics consultations? *Journal of Medical Ethics*, 27 (Supplement 1), pp. i24–i29.

Dworkin, G. (1972). Paternalism. *Monist*, 56(1), pp. 64–84.

—— (1988). *The theory and practice of autonomy*. Cambridge University Press, New York.

Dworkin, R. (1977). *Taking rights seriously*. Duckworth, London.

—— (1993). *Life's dominion: an argument about abortion and euthanasia*. HarperCollinsPublishers, London, UK.

Dyck, A. (1984). Ethcal aspects of care for the dying incompetent. *Journal of American Geriatric Society*, 32, pp. 661–4.

Eberst, R.M. (1984). Defining health: a multidimensional model. *JOSH*, 54(3), March, pp. 99–104.

Edwards, J.C. (1982). *Ethics without philosophy: Wittgenstein and the moral life.* University Presses of Florida, Tampa.

Ehrenreich, B. (1985). After two abortions, a clear choice and few regrets. *The Age* 'Saturday Extra', 23 March, p. 7.

Eisenstein, Z.R. (1988). *The female body and the law.* University of California Press, Berkeley.

Eiser, A., Schade, S., Anderson-Shaw, L. and Murphy, T. (2001). Electronic communication in ethics committees: experience and challenges. *Journal of Medical Ethics*, 27(Supplement 1), pp. i30–i32.

Elliott, C. (1992). Where ethics comes from and what to do about it. *Hastings Center Report*, 22(4), pp. 28–35.

Elliott, M. (ed.) (1993). *Female sexual abuse of children: the ultimate taboo.* Longman, Harlow, Essex.

Elliston, F., Keenan, J., Lockhart, P. and van Schaick, J. (1985). *Whistleblowing research: methodological and moral issues.* Praeger, New York.

Else, A. (1991). *A question of adoption: closed stranger adoption in New Zealand 1944–1974.* Bridget Williams Books, Wellington.

Emanuel, E. (2000). Justice and managed care: four principles for the just allocation of health care resources. *Hastings Center Report*, 30(3), pp. 8–16.

Engelhardt, H.T Jr (1986). *The foundations of bioethics.* Oxford University Press, New York.

—— (ed.) (1989). *Journal of Medicine and Philosophy*, 14(1). Special edition: Harvesting cells, tisssues, and organs from fetuses and anencephalic newborns.

—— (1996). *The foundations of bioethics* (2nd edn). Oxford University Press, New York.

Engstrom, B. (1986). Communication and decision-making in a study of multidisciplinary team conference with the registered nurse as conference chairman. *International Journal of Nursing Studies*, 23(4), pp. 299–314.

Erlen, J. (1999). What does it mean to blow the whistle? *Orthopaedic Nursing*, 18(6), pp. 67–70.

Ewing, T. (1994). Spinal damage: scientists cross the frontier. *The Age*, 13 January, p. 1.

—— (1998). Abortion crusader fights for just one political cause, *The Age*, 23 March, p. 8.

Faden, R.R. and Beauchamp, T.L. (1986). *A history and theory of informed consent.* Oxford University Press, New York.

Fader, A.M., Gambert, S.R., Nash, M., Gupta, K.L. and Escher, J. (1989). Implementing a 'Do-Not-Resuscitate' (DNR) policy in a nursing home. *Journal of the American Geriatrics Society*, 37(6), pp. 544–6.

Fagin, C.M. (1975). Nurses' rights. *American Journal of Nursing* 75 (1), pp. 82–5.

Farber, M. (1975). Psychological variables in Italian suicide. In Farberow, N. (ed.), *Suicide in different cultures.* University Park Press, Baltimore, pp. 179–84.

Farberow, N. (1975b). Cultural history of suicide. In Farberow (1975a), pp. 1–15.

—— (ed.) (1975a). *Suicide in different cultures.* University Park Press, Baltimore.

Farouque, F. (1993a). Inquest told of boy's bruises. *The Age*, 11 November, p. 3.

—— (1993b). Doctor left Valerio's mother to get advice. *The Age*, 12 November, p. 3.

Fasching, D. (1993). *The ethical challenge of Auschwitz and Hiroshima: apocalypse or utopia?* State University of New York Press, Albany.

Feather, R.B. (1985). The institutionalised mental health patient's right to refuse psychotropic medication. *Perspectives in Psychiatric Care*, 23(2), pp. 45–68.

Feinberg, J. (1969), *Moral concepts*, Oxford University Press, Oxford, pp. 60–73.

—— (1971). Legal paternalism. *Canadian Journal of Philosophy*, 1, pp. 105–24.

—— (1978). Rights. In Reich, W.T. (ed.), *Encyclopedia of bioethics.* The Free Press, New York, pp. 1507–11.

—— (1979). The rights of animals and unborn generations. In Wasserstrom, R.A. (ed.), *Today's moral problems*, Macmillan, New York, pp. 581–601.

—— (1984). *Harm to others: the moral limits of the criminal law.* Oxford University Press, New York.

Ferngren, G. (1989). The ethics of suicide in the Renaissance and Reformation. In Brody, B. (ed.), *Suicide and euthanasia: historical and contemporary themes.* Kluwer Academic Publishers, Dordrecht, pp. 155–81.

Field, M. (1997). NZ health uproar after life fight fails. *The Age*, 13 October, p. 10.

Fieldhouse, P. (1986). *Food and nutrition: customs and culture.* Croom Helm, London.

Fine, R. and Mayo, T. (2003). Resolution of futility by due process: early experience with the Texas Advance Directives Act. *Annals of Internal Medicine*, 138(9), pp. 743–6.

Fineman, M.A. and Thomadsen, N.S. (eds) (1991). *At the boundaries of law: feminism and legal theory.* Routledge, New York and London.

Firestone, R. (1997). *Suicide and the inner voice: risk assessment, treatment, and case management.* Sage Publications, Thousand Oaks.

Fisher, A. and Buckingham, J. (1985). *Abortion in Australia*. Dove Communications, Melbourne.

Fisher, B. and Tronto, J. (1990). Toward a feminist theory of caring. In Abel, E.K. and Nelson, M.K. (eds), *Circles of care, work and identity in women's lives*. State University of New York Press, Albany, pp. 35–62.

Fitzpatrick, F.J. (1988). *Ethics in nursing practice: basic principles and their application*. The Linacre Centre, London.

Flanagan, O. and Jackson, K. (1987). Justice, care, and gender: the Kohlberg–Gilligan debate revisited. *Ethics*, 97, April, pp. 622–37.

Fletcher, J. (1966). *Situation ethics*. SCM Press, Bloomsbury Street, London.

—— (1973). Ethics and euthanasia. *American Journal of Nursing*, 73(4), April, pp. 670–5.

Flew, A. (ed.) (1979). *A dictionary of philosophy*. Pan Books, London.

Fogarty, J. (1993). *Protective services for children in Victoria: a report* (July). Melbourne.

Fogarty, J. and Sargeant, D. (1989). *Protective services for children in Victoria — an interim report* (February). Melbourne.

Folks, H. (1902). *Care of the destitute, neglected, and delinquent children*. Macmillan, New York.

Foltz, A.T. (1987). The influence of cancer on self-concept and life quality. *Seminars in Oncology Nursing*, 3(4), November, pp. 303–12.

Fordham, J. (1988). *Doctors' orders or patient choice?* Leo Cussen Institute, Melbourne.

Forrell, C. (1986). Concerned nurses should walk out on their leadership. *The Age*, 10 December, p. 13.

Forrester, K. and Griffiths, D. (2001). *Essential of law for health professionals*. Harcourt Australia, Sydney.

Forrow, L., Arnold, R. and Frader, J. (1991). Teaching clinical ethics in the residency years: preparing competent professionals. *Journal of Medicine and Philosophy*, 16(1), pp. 93–112.

Foucault, M. (1973). *The birth of the clinic*. Tavistock Publications, London.

—— (1977). *Discipline and punish: the birth of the prison*. Penguin, London.

Frankena, W. (1973). *Ethics*, (2nd edn). Prentice-Hall, Englewood Cliffs, New Jersey.

Franklin, M., Stolz, G. and Griffith, C. (2002). She died cancer free. *Herald Sun*, 25 May, pp. 1–2.

Frazer, E., Hornsby, J. and Lovibond, S. (eds) (1992). *Ethics: a feminist reader*. Blackwell, Oxford.

Freckelton, I. (1996). Enforcement of ethics. In Coady, M. and Bloch, S. (eds), *Codes of ethics and the professions*. Melbourne University Press, Melbourne, pp. 130–65.

Fredette, S. LaFortune and Beattie, H.M. (1986). Living with cancer: a patient education program. *Cancer Nursing*, 9(6), pp. 308–16.

Free v Holy Cross Hospital 505 NE2d 1188 (Ill App 1 Dist 1987).

Freedman, B. (1978). A meta-ethics for professional morality. *Ethics*, 89, pp. 1–19.

—— (1981). One philosopher's experience on an ethics committee. *Hastings Center Report*, 11(2), April, pp. 20–2.

Freeman, J. and McDonnell, K. (1987). *Tough decisions: a casebook in medical ethics*. Oxford University Press, New York.

Freire, P. (1970). *Cultural action for freedom*. Penguin Books, Harmondsworth, Middlesex.

—— (1972). *Pedagogy of the oppressed*. Penguin Books, London.

French, M. (1985). *Beyond power: on women, men and morals*. Abacus, London.

—— (1998). *A season in hell: a memoir*. Ballantine Books, New York.

Fried, C. (1982). Equality and rights in medical care. In Beauchamp, T.L. and Walters L. (eds) (1982). *Contemporary issues* in bioethics, (2nd edn). Wadsworth, Belmont, California, pp. 395–401.

Friedman, J. (1994). *Cultural identity and global process*. Sage Publications, London.

Fry, S. (1988a). The ethic of caring: can it survive in nursing? *Nursing Outlook*, 36(1), p. 48.

—— (1988b). Response to 'Virtue, ethics, caring and nursing'. *Scholarly Inquiry for Nursing Practice: An International Journal*, 2(2), pp. 97–101.

—— (1989a). Toward a theory of nursing ethics. *Advances in Nursing Science*, 11(4), pp. 9–22.

—— (1989b). The role of caring in a theory of nursing ethics. *Hypatia*, 4(2). Reprinted in Holmes, H.B. and Purdy, L.M. (eds) (1992). *Feminist perspectives in medical ethics*. Indiana University Press, Bloomington and Indianapolis, pp. 93–106.

—— (1989c). Whistleblowing by nurses: a matter of ethics. *Nursing Outlook*, 37(1), p. 56.

Fry, S. and Johnstone, M-J. (2002). *Ethics in Nursing Practice: A Guide to Ethical Decision making* (2nd edn). Blackwell Science Publishers, London.

Fry-Revere, S. (1992). *The accountability of bioethics committees and consultants*. University Publishing Group Inc., Frederick, Maryland.

Fuchs, V.R. (1983). *Who shall live? Health, economics and social choice*. Basic Books, New York.

Fullinwider, R. (1996). Professional codes and moral understanding. In Coady, M. and Bloch, S. (eds), *Codes of ethics and the professions*. Melbourne University Press, Melbourne, pp. 72–87.

Gallagher, J. (1995). Collective bad faith: 'Protecting' the fetus. In Callahan, J. (ed.) *Reproduction, ethics, and the law: feminist perspectives.* Indiana University Press, Bloomington and Indianapolis, pp. 343–79.

Gandevia, B. (1978). *Tears often shed: child health and welfare in Australia from 1788,* Charter, Gordon.

Garbutt, S. (2003). Protecting our children: the endless challenge. *The Age,* 6 June, p. 13.

Gardner, H. and McCoppin, B. (1986). Vocation, career or both? Politicization of Australian nurses, Victoria 1984–1986. *Australian Journal of Advanced Nursing,* 4(1), September–November, pp. 25–35.

Garner, H. (1993). How we lost Daniel's life. *Time Magazine,* 8 March (10), pp. 23–25.

Garnett, A.C. (1965). Conscience and conscientiousness. First published in *Rice University Studies,* volume 51; reprinted in Kolenda, K. (ed.) (1966), *Insight and vision,* Trinity University Press, pp. 71–83; subsequently reprinted in Feinberg, J. (1969), *Moral concepts,* Oxford University Press, Oxford, pp. 80–92.

Gartland, S. (1992). Nurses death aid 'no shock'. *Herald-Sun,* 3 March, p. 5.

Gastmans, C., Dierckx de Casterle, B. and Schotsmans, P. (1998). Nursing considered as moral practice: a philosophical-ethical interpretation of nursing. *Kennedy Institute of Ethics Journal,* 8(1), pp. 43–69.

Gatens, M. (1986). Feminism, philosophy and riddles without answers. In C.O. Pateman and E. Gross (eds), *Feminist challenges.* Allen & Unwin, Sydney, pp. 13–29.

Gaut, D.A. (ed.) (1992). *The presence of caring in nursing.* National League for Nursing Press, New York.

Gaut, D.A. and Leininger, M.M. (eds) (1991). *Caring: the compassionate healer.* National League for Nursing Press, New York.

Gauthier, D.P. (1986). *Morals by agreement.* Clarendon Press, Oxford.

Gawler, I. (2001). *You can conquer cancer: prevention and management* (revised edn). Michelle Anderson Publishing, Melbourne (1st edn published 1984).

Geary, P. and Hawkins, J. (1991). To cure, to care, or to heal. *Nursing Forum,* 26(3), pp. 5–13.

Georgaki, S., Kalaidopoulou, O., Liarmakopoulos, I. and Mystakidou, K. (2002). Nurses' attitudes towards truthful communication with patients with cancer: a Greek study. *Cancer Nursing,* 25(6), pp. 436–41.

Gergen, K. (1994). *Realities and relationships: soundings in social construction.* Harvard University Press, Cambridge, Mass.

Gerhart, K., Koziol-McLain, J., Lowenstein, S. and Whiteneck, G. (1994). Quality of life following spinal cord injury: knowledge and attitude of emergency care providers. *Annals of Emergency Medicine,* 23(4), pp. 807–12.

Germino, B.B. (1987). Symptom distress and quality of life. *Seminars in Oncology Nursing,* 3(4), November, pp. 299–302.

Gert, B. (1984). Moral theory and applied ethics. *The Monist,* 67(4), October, pp. 532–48.

Gert, B. and Culver, C. (1976). Paternalistic behaviour. *Philosophy and Public Affairs,* 6(1), pp. 45–57.

Gert, B., Culver, C. and Clouser, K. Danner. (1997). *Bioethics: a return to fundamentals.* Oxford University Press, New York.

Gert, H. (2002). Avoiding suprises: a model for imforming patients. *Hastings Center Report,* 32(5), pp. 23–32.

Gibbs, N. (1990). Dr Death's suicide machine. *Time Magazine,* 18 June, pp. 70–1.

—— (1990). The gift of life — or else. *Time Magazine,* 10 September, p. 49.

—— (1993). Death giving. *Time Magazine,* 31 May, pp. 49–53.

Gibson, M. (1976). Rationality. *Philosophy and Public Affairs,* 6(3), pp. 193–225.

Gibson, P. (1994). Gay male and lesbian youth suicide. In Remafedi, G. (ed.), *Death by denial: studies of suicide in gay and lesbian teenagers.* Alyson Pubs, Boston, pp. 15–68.

Gilbert, S. (1997). *Wrongful death: a memoir.* WW Norton & Co., New York.

Gillam, L. (ed.) (1989). Proceedings of the conference 'The Fetus as Tissue Donor: Use or Abuse?', Centre for Human Bioethics, Monash university, Melbourne.

Gillard-Glass, S. and England, J. (2002). *Adoption New Zealand: the never-ending story.* HarperCollinsPublishers, Auckland.

Gilligan, C. (1982). *In a different voice: psychological theory and women's development.* Harvard University Press, Cambridge, Mass (see in particular Chapter 3, 'Concepts of self and morality').

—— (1987). Moral orientations and moral development. In E.F. Kittay and D.T. Meyers (eds), *Women and moral theory.* Rowman & Littlefield, Totowa, New Jersey, pp. 19–33.

Gillon, R. (1994). Palliative care ethics: non-provision of artificial nutrition and hydration to terminally ill sedated patients. *Journal of Medical Ethics,* 20(3), pp. 131–2, 187.

—— (2001). Is there a 'new ethics of abortion'? *Journal of Medical Ethics,* 27(SuppII), pp. ii5–9.

Gilmore, K. (nd). Proforma letter from the National Director of Amnesty International

Australia, addressed to 'Friends' (distributed with an attached information leaflet on female genital mutilation via membership list, April, 1998).

Gilmour, J. (1992). *Michael: a mother's battle for the rights of her child.* Little Hills Press, Sydney.

Giovannoni, J. (1982). Mistreated children. In Yelaja, S. (ed.), *Ethical issues in social work.* Charles C. Thomas, Springfield, Illinois, pp. 105–20.

Gladwin, M. (1930). *Ethics talks to nurses,* W.B. Saunders, Philadelphia.

Glaser, R.J. (1975). A time to live and a time to die: the implications of negative euthanasia. In J.A. Behnke and S. Bok (eds), *The dilemmas of euthanasia.* Anchor Books, Anchor Press/ Doubleday, Garden City, New York, pp. 133–50.

Glass, J. (1989). *Private terror/public life: psychosis and the politics of community.* Cornell University Press, Ithaca, New York

Glick, H. (1992). *The right to die: public policy innovation and its consequences.* Columbia University Press, New York.

Glover, J. (1977). *Causing deaths and saving lives.* Penguin Books, Harmondsworth, Middlesex.

Goddard, C. (1996). *Child abuse and child protection: a guide for health, education and welfare workers.* Churchill Livingstone, Melbourne.

Goffman, E. (1963). *Stigma: notes on the management of spoiled identity.* Penguin Books, London, UK.

Goldberg, P. (1983). *The intuitive edge.* Jeremy Tarcher, Los Angeles.

Goldman, A.H. (1980). *The moral foundations of professional ethics.* Rowman & Littlefield, Totowa, New Jersey.

Gonsalves, M. A. (1985). *Right and reason: ethics in theory and practice* (8th edn). Times Mirror/Mosby College, St Louis.

Gordon, M. and Singer, P. (1995). Decisions and care at the end of life. *The Lancet,* 346(8968), 15 July, pp. 163–6.

Gorovitz, S., Macklin, R., Jameton, A., O'Connor, J. and Sherwin, S. (eds) (1983). *Moral problems in medicine* (2nd edn). Prentice Hall, Englewood Cliffs, New Jersey.

Graham, K.Y. and Longman, A.J. (1987). Quality of life and persons with melanoma. *Cancer Nursing,* 10(6), December, pp. 338–46.

Grassi, G., Giraldi, T., Messina, E., Magnani, K., Valle, E and Cartei, G. (2000). Physicians' attitudes to and problems with truth-telling to cancer patients. *Support Care Cancer,* 8(1), pp. 40–45.

Graycar, R. and Morgan, J. (1990). *The hidden gender of law.* Federation Press, Sydney.

Green, O.H. (1980). Killing and letting die. *American Philosophical Quarterly,* 17(3), July, pp. 195–204.

Greenwood, J. (2001). The new ethics of abortion. *Journal of Medical Ethics,* 27(SuppII), pp. ii2–4.

Greenwood, M. and Nunn, P. (1992). *Paradox and healing: medicine, mythology and transformation.* Paradox Publishers, Victoria, BC.

Greipp, M. (1992). Undermedication for pain: an ethical model. *Advances in Nursing Science,* 15(1), pp. 44–53.

Grennan, E. (1930). The Somera case. *International Nursing Review* 5 (December/ January), pp. 325–33.

Griffith, C. (2002). Killing me softly. *Herald Sun,* 24 May, p. 4.

Griffiths, L. (1988). Fetal transplants spark controversy. *Australian Dr Weekly,* 20 May.

Grimshaw, J. (1986). *Feminist philosophers.* Wheatsheaf Books, Brighton, Sussex.

Grisez, G. and Boyle, J. (1979). *Life and death with liberty and justice.* University of Notre Dame Press, Indiana.

Grisso, T. and Appelbaum, P. (1998). *Assessing competence to consent to treatment: a guide for physicians and other health professionals.* Oxford University Press, New York.

Grodin, M. and Glantz, L. (1994). *Children as research subjects: science, ethics & law.* Oxford University Press, New York/Oxford.

Groom, G. and Hickie, I. (2003). *Out of hospital, out of mind! A review of mental health services in Australia – 2003* [Executive Summary]. Mental Health Council of Australia, Canberra [available at: *www.mhca.com.au* — accessed 19 September 2003].

Groom, G., Hickie, I. And Davenport, T. (2003). *Out of hospital, out of mind! A report detailing mental health services in Australia in 2002 and community priorities for national metnal health policy 2003-2008.* Mental Health Council of Australia, Canberra [available at: *www.mhca.com.au* — accessed 19 September 2003].

Gross, E. (1986). Conclusions: what is feminist theory? In C. Pateman and E. Gross (eds), *Feminist challenges: social and political theory.* Allen & Unwin, Sydney, pp. 190–204.

Gross, P.F. (1985). Nursing care in the 1980s and beyond: the challenge to be relevant, ethical and accepted. *Australian Nurses Journal,* 15(1) July, pp. 46–8.

Gruzalski, B. (1981). Killing by letting die. *Mind* 90, pp. 91–8.

Guimón, J. (2001). *Inequity and madness: psychosocial and human rights issues.* Kluwer Academic/Plenum Publishers. New York.

Gunn, M.J. and Smith, J.C. (1985). *Arthur's Case and the right to life of a Down's Syndrome child. Criminal Law Review*, November, pp. 693–756.

Habermas, J. (1990). *Moral consciousness and communicative action*. The MIT Press, Cambridge, Mass.

Hadley, J. (1996). *Abortion: between freedom and necessity*. Virago Press, London, UK.

Hager, C. (2002). Termination of pregnancy with a prenatal diagnosis of cleft lip: cultural differences and ethical analysis. *Plastic Surgical Nursing*, 22(1), pp. 24–8.

Haines, I.E., Zalcberg, J. and Buchanan, J.D. (1990). Not-for-resuscitation orders in cancer patients — principles of decision-making. *Medical Journal of Australia*, 153(4), pp. 225–9.

Hamel, R. and Panicola, M. (2003). Are futility policies the answer? *Health Progress*, 84(4), pp. 21–4.

Hamilton, H. (1995). *Euthanasia: an issue for nurses*. Royal College of Nursing, Australia, Canberra.

Hammes, B. and Rooney, B. (1998). Death and end-of-life planning in one Midwestern community. *Archives of Internal Medicine*, 158(4), pp. 383–90.

Harari, F. (1987). Death can't be legislated, euthanasia committee finds. *The Age*, 1 May, p. 1.

Harari, F. and Clarke, S. (1987). Criticism for bill on rights of dying. *The Age*, 14 October, p. 3.

Harding, S. (ed.) (1987). *Feminism and methodology: social science issues*. Indiana University Press, Bloomington and Indianapolis, and Open University Press, Milton Keynes.

—— (ed.) (1991). *Whose Science? Whose knowledge? Thinking from women's lives*. Open University Press, Milton Keynes.

Harding, S. and Hintikka, M.B. (eds) (1983). *Discovering reality*. D. Reidel, Dordrecht.

Hardwig, J. (1997). Dying at the right time: reflections on (un)assisted suicide. In H. LaFollette (ed.), *Ethics in practice: an anthology*. Blackwell Publishers, Cambridge, Mass., pp. 53–65.

Hare, R.M. (1963). *Freedom and reason*. Oxford University Press, London (see in particular Chapter 9, 'Toleration and fanaticism').

—— (1964). *The language of morals*. Oxford University Press, Oxford.

Hare, R.M. (1981). *Moral thinking*. Clarendon Press, Oxford (see in particular Chapter 10, 'Fanaticism and amoralism').

Harmon, G. (1977). *The nature of morality*. Oxford University Press, New York.

Harper, P. (1983). Lost, but still alive — the natural parents' need to know. *In Proceedings of the Conference: Adoption and AID: Access to Information?* Centre for Human Bioethics, Monash University, Melbourne, 2 November, pp. 29–38.

Harrison, J. (1954). When is a principle a moral principle? *Aristotelian Society*, supplementary vol. 28, July 9–11, pp. 111–34.

Hart, H. (1963). *Law, liberty, and morality*. Stanford University Press, Stanford, Cal.

Hart, H.L.A. (1958). Positivism and the separation of law and morals. *Harvard Law Review*, 71(1–4), pp. 593–629.

—— (1961). *The concept of law*. Oxford University Press (Clarendon Law Series), Oxford.

Hart, R. and Snell, J. (1992). Dr Cox: the nurse's story. *Nursing Times*, 7(88), p. 19.

Haslem, B. (1998). Failed mercy-killer walks free. *The Weekend Australian*, November 21–22, p. 3.

Hastings Center (1982). Does 'doing everything' include CPR? *Hastings Center Report* 12.(5), October, pp. 27–8.

Hauerwas, S. (1986). *Suffering presence*. University of Notre Dame Press, South Bend, Indiana.

Hawes, R. and Honeysett, S. (1996). State accused over child abuse deaths. *The Australian*, 31 October, p. 3.

Health and Community Services (1992). *Adoption: myth and reality. The Adoption Information Service in Victoria*. Health and Community Services Promotions and Media Unit, Melbourne.

Health Call (1987). *Health complaints advisory link line annual report, 1 May, 1986–30 April, 1987*. Health Call, Melbourne.

—— (1988). *Health Call annual report 1988*. Health Issues Centre, Melbourne.

Health Care Committee Expert Panel on Mental Health. (1991). *Homelessness and Severe Mental Disorders*. Australian Government Publishing Service, Canberra.

Health Care Complaints Commission. (2003). *Investigation report: Campbelltown and Camden Hospitals MacArthur Health Service*. Health Care Complaints Commission, Sydney.

Health Issues Centre (1991). *Our better health: getting it together*. Health Issues Centre, Melbourne.

—— (1992). *Casemix: quality and consumers*. Health Issues Centre, Melbourne.

Heckler, R. (1994). *Waking up alive: the descent to suicide and return to life*. Piatkus, London.

Heisenberg, W. (1990). *Physics and philosophy*. Penguin Books, London.

Heitman, L. and Robinson, B. (1997). Developing a nursing ethics round table. *American Journal of Nursing,* 97(10), pp. 36–8.

Hekman, S. (1995). *Moral voices, moral selves: Carol Gilligan and feminist moral theory.* Polity Press, Cambridge, UK.

Held, V. (1987). Feminism and moral theory. In Kittay, E.F. and Meyers, D.T. (eds), *Women and moral theory.* Rowman & Littlefield, Totowa, New Jersey, pp. 111–28.

Helft, P., Siegler, M. and Lantos, J. (2000). The rise and fall of the futility movement. *The New England Journal of Medicine,* 343(4), pp. 293–6.

Helman, C. (1990). *Culture, health and illness.* Wright, London.

Henderson, B. (1975). *Abortion: the Bobigney affair.* Wild & Woolley, Sydney.

Hendin, H. (1998). *Seduced by death: doctors, patients, and assisted suicide.* W.W. Norton & Co, New York.

Hendrick, J. (2001). Legal aspects of clinical ethics committees. *Journal of Medical Ethics,* 27(Supplement 1), i50–53.

Herald-Sun (1992). Nurses admit death role. 2 March, p. 3.

—— (2002). Woman wins right to die. *Herald Sun,* 23 March, p. 7.

Herdman, E. and Kippax, S. (1995). *Institutional discrimination: critical ethnography of HIV/AIDS related discrimination in a hospital setting.* National Centre in HIV Social Research, Macquarie University, Sydney.

Herman, J. (1992). *Trauma and recovery: the aftermath of violence — from domestic abuse to political terror.* Basic Books, a Division of HarperCollins, New York.

Hewson, B. (2001). Reproductive autonomy and the ethics of abortion. *Journal of Medical Ethics,* 27(Supplement), pp. ii10–14.

Heyd, D. and Bloch, S. (1981). The ethics of suicide. In Bloch, S. and Chodoff, P. (eds), *Psychiatric ethics.* Oxford University Press, Oxford, pp. 185–202.

Hickie, J.B. (1990). Guidelines for the decision making process for treatment with cardiopulmonary resuscitation. *Reflections* (an occasional publication of the Bioethics Committee of St Vincent's Hospital, University Campus, Sydney), November, p. 1.

Hicks, C. (1982). Why I am opposing the doctors. *Nursing Times,* 76(36), pp. 1579–80.

Higgins, G. O'Connell. (1994). *Resilient adults: overcoming a cruel past.* Jossey-Bass Publishing, San Franciso.

Hill, C. Stratton (1992). Suffering as contrasted to pain, loss, grief, despair, and loneliness. In Starck, P. and McGovern, J. (1992), *The hidden dimension of illness: human suffering.* National League for Nursing Press, New York, pp. 69–80.

Himsworth, Sir Harold (1953). Change and permanence in education for medicine. *The Lancet,* 6790, 17 October, pp. 789–91.

Hinman, L. (1994). *Ethics: a pluralistic approach to moral theory.* Harcourt Brace Jovanovich, Fort Worth, Texas.

Hirschler, B. (1993). Dying with dignity in Holland. *The Age,* 11 February, p. 7.

Hiskey, E. (1980). Child protection in Victoria, Part 1. *Australian Child and Family Welfare,* 5(3), pp. 6–10.

Hoagland, S.L. (1988). *Lesbian ethics: toward new value.* Institute of Lesbian Studies, Palo Alto, California.

Hobbes, T. (1968). *Leviathan* (reprinted from 1651 edition with notes by C.B. Macpherson). Pelican Books, Harmondsworth, Middlesex.

Hodge, B. (1993a). Practising within an ethic of care. *Newsletter, Bioethics Research Centre,* 2(3), September, pp. 6–8 (Otago University, Dunedin, Wellington NZ).

—— (1993b). Uncovering the ethic of care. *Nursing Praxis in New Zealand,* 8(2), pp. 13–22.

Hoff, C. (1982). When public policy replaces private ethics. *Hastings Center Report,* 12(4), pp. 13–14.

Hoffman, M. (2000). *Empathy and moral development: implications for caring and justice.* Cambridge University Press, Cambridge.

Hofman, P. (2001). Improving ethics committee effectiveness. Healthcare Executive, 16(1), pp. 58–9.

Holden, W. (1994). *Unlawful carnal knowledge: the true story of the Irish 'X' case.* HarperCollins Publishers, London, UK.

Holmes, H.B. and Purdy, L.M. (eds) (1992). *Feminist perspectives in medical ethics.* Indiana University Press, Bloomington and Indianapolis.

Holmes, P. (1988). Over the limit? *Nursing Times,* 20(84), p. 19.

Holy Bible (new King James version). Thomas Nelson, Nashville, Tennessee.

Honan, S., Helseth, C., Bakke, J., Karpiuk, K., Krsnak, G. and Torkelson, R. (1991). Perception of 'No Code' and the role of the nurse. *Journal of Continuing Education in Nursing,* 22(2), pp. 54–61.

Horan, D.J. (1982). Infanticide: when doctor's orders read 'murder'. *Registered Nurse,* 45(1), pp. 75–82.

Howe, D., Sawbridge, P. and Hinings, D. (1992). *Half a million women: mothers who lose their children by adoption.* Penguin, London.

Hudson, F. (2002). 21 Clap as Nancy dies. *Herald Sun*, 24 May, pp. 1, 4.

Huerta, S.R. and Oddi, L.F. (1992). Refusal to care for patients with human immunodeficiency virus/acquired immunodeficiency syndrome: issues and responses. *Journal of Professional Nursing*, 8(4), pp. 221–30.

Hughes, J. (1995). Ultimate justification: Wittgenstein and medical ethics. *Journal of Medical Ethics*, 21, pp. 25–30.

Hughes, Judge C.J. (1978). In the matter of Karen Quinlan. In T.L. Beauchamp and S. Perlin (eds), *Ethical issues in death and dying*. Prentice Hall, Englewood Cliffs, New Jersey, pp. 290–8.

Hume, D. (1888 edn). *Treatise of human nature* (edited by L.A. Selby-Bigge). Oxford University Press, London.

—— (1947). Of the original contract (reprinted from 1748 edition). In Sir Ernest Barker, *Social contract*. Oxford University Press, London, pp. 209–36.

—— (1983). Essay on suicide. In Gorovitz, S., Macklin, R., Jameton, A.L., O'Connor, J.M. and Sherwin, A. (eds), *Moral problems in medicine*. Prentice Hall, Englewood Cliffs, New Jersey, pp. 437–42.

Humphries, D. (1983). Poll shows most favour voluntary euthanasia. *The Age*, 26 November, reprinted in *The Age reprint booklet, no. 44: Euthanasia*, The Age Education Unit, Melbourne, p. 14.

Humphry, D. and Wickett, A. (1986). *The right to die: understanding euthanasia*. Collins/Harper & Row, Sydney.

Hunt, G. (ed.) (1994). *Ethical issues in nursing*. Routledge, London and New York.

Huntington, A. (2002). Working with women experiencing mid-trimester termination of pregnancy: the integration of nursing and feminist knowledge in the gynaecological setting. *Journal of Clinical Nursing*, 11, pp. 273–9.

Hutton, B. (1987). The oft-forgotten grandmothers of Western philosophy. *The Age*, 23 September, p. 20.

Hyun, I. (2002). Waiver of informed consent, cultural sensitivity, and the problem of unjust families and traditions. *Hastings Center Report*, 32(5), pp. 14–22.

Ilffe, J. (2002). Whistleblowing: a difficult decision. *Australian Nursing Journal*, 9(7), p. 1.

In re alleged unfair dismissal of Ms K. Howden by the City of Whittlesea 6/9/90 (Case No 90/3672, Decision D90/1933) IRCV (unreported)).

Independent (1992). Jubilation in Ireland as abortion ban lifted. *The Age*, 28 February, p. 6.

Independent, New York Times (1992). Abortion trip ban on rape victim, 14. *The Age*, 19 February, p. 9.

Inlander, C.B., Levin, L.S. and Weiner, E. (1988). *Medicine on trial: the appalling story of ineptitude, malfeasance, neglect, and arrogance*. Prentice Hall, New York.

International Code of Medical Ethics (1983). In Amnesty International, *Ethical codes and declarations relevant to the health professions*. Amnesty International, London, 1985.

International Council of Nurses (1973). *Code for Nurses*. International Council of Nurses, Geneva, Switzerland.

—— (1977). *The nurse's dilemma*. International Council of Nurses, Florence Nightingale International Foundation, Geneva, Switzerland.

—— (2000a). *Code for nurses*. ICN, Geneva.

—— (2000b). *Position statement: Nurses' role in providing care to dying patients and their families*. ICN, Geneva

—— (2003a). *Framework of Competencies for the Generalist Nurse*. ICN, Geneva.

—— (2003b). *Nursing matters fact sheet: The health of indigenous peoples: a concern for nursing*. ICN, Geneva [available at *www.icn.ch* — accessed 30 October 2003].

International Nursing Review (2003). International perspectives: Advocate for world's most vulnerable people wins top nursing award. *International Nursing Review*, 50(2), 69.

Jackson, A. (2002). Nitschke regrets, as Crick farewelled. *The Age*, 30 May, p. 2.

Jaggar, A.M. (1983). *Feminist politics and human nature*. Rowman & Allanheld, Totowa, New Jersey.

James, S. (1994). Reconciling international human rights and cultural relativism: the case of female circumcision. *Bioethics*, 8(1), pp. 1–26.

Jameton, A. (1984). *Nursing practice: the ethical issues*. Prentice-Hall, Englewood Cliffs, New Jersey.

Jameton, A. and Fowler, M.D.M. (1989). Ethical inquiry and the concept of research. *Advances in Nursing Science*, 11(3), pp. 11–24.

Jecker, N. (1993). Saying 'no' to futile treatment. *8th National Bioethics Conference 1993 Presentation Papers*. Christian Centre for Bioethics at Sydney Adventist Hospital, Sydney, pp. 29–41.

Jecker, N., Jonsen, A. and Pearlman, R. (1997). *Bioethics: an introduction to the history, methods, and practice*. Jones and Bartlett, Sudbury, Massachusetts.

Jecker, N. and Schneiderman, L. (1995). When families request that 'everything possible' be done. *Journal of Medicine and Philosophy*, 20(2), pp. 146–63.

Jemmott, J., Freleicher, J. and Jemmott, L. (1992). Perceived risk of infection and attitudes toward risk groups: determinants of nurses' behavioural intentions regarding AIDS patients. *Research in Nursing and Health*, 15, pp. 295–301.

Jennings, B. (1991). Possibilities of consensus: toward democratic moral discourse. *Journal of Medicine and Philosophy*, 16(4), pp. 447–63.

Jochemsen, H. (1994). Euthanasia in Holland: an ethical critique of the new law. *Journal of Medical Ethics*, 20(4), pp. 212–17.

Jochemsen, H. and Keown, J. (1999). Voluntary euthanasia under control? Further empirical evidence from the Netherlands. *Journal of Medical Ethics*, 25(1), pp. 16–24.

Johns, G. (1988). The commanding presence of George Herbert Green. *New Zealand Herald*, 6 August, p. 9.

Johns, J. (1996). Advance directives and opportunities for nurses. *Image: Journal of Nursing Scholarship*, 28(2), pp. 149–53.

Johnson v State, 21 Tenn. 291, 292 (1840).

Johnson, M. (1993). *Moral imagination: implications of cognitive science for ethics*. University of Chicago Press, Chicago.

Johnston, P. (1989). *Wittgenstein and moral philosophy*. Routledge, London, UK.

Johnstone, M-J. (1987a). Professional ethics in nursing: a philosophical analysis. *Australian Journal of Advanced Nursing*, 4(3), pp. 12–21.

—— (1987b). Ethics in focus. *Australian Nurses Journal*, 17(3), September, pp. 41–2.

—— (1988). Law, professional ethics and the problem of conflict with personal values. *International Journal of Nursing Studies*, 25(2), pp. 147–57.

—— (1989). *Bioethics: a nursing perspective* (1st edn). W.B. Saunders/Baillière Tindall, Sydney.

—— (1990). Bioethics and the health care economics debate: a nursing perspective. Paper presented at the NSW Nurses' Association's 45th Annual Conference/Professional Seminar Day, Bioethical Considerations and Opportunity Cost, Sydney. Reprinted in full in M.-J. Johnstone (1992), *Module 601E. Ethics and Nursing — Book of Readings*. Distance Education Division of Royal College of Nursing Australia, Melbourne, Reading 2.1.

—— (1993). The development of nursing ethics in Australia: an historical overview. *Papers of the First National Nursing History Conference:*

Australian nursing ... the story, Royal College of Nursing, Australia, Melbourne, pp. 33–51.

—— (1994). *Nursing and the injustices of the law*. W.B. Saunders/Baillière Tindall, Sydney.

—— (1995a). Guest Editorial: The scandalous neglect of mental health care ethics. *Contemporary Nurse*, 4, 142–4.

—— (1995b). *Inaugural Bennett Lecture. Moral controversy and the search for solutions: some critical reflections for the nursing profession*. Faculty of Nursing, RMIT University, Melbourne.

—— (ed.) (1996a). *The politics of euthanasia: a nursing response*. Royal College of Nursing, Australia, Canberra.

—— (1996b). The politics of euthanasia: an introduction. In Johnstone, M-J. (ed.), *The politics of euthanasia: a nursing response*. Royal College of Nursing, Australia, Canberra, pp. 13–19.

—— (1996c). The political and ethical dimensions of euthanasia. In Johnstone, M-J. (ed.), *The politics of euthanasia: a nursing response*. Royal College of Nursing, Australia, Canberra, pp. 21–47.

—— (1998). *Determining and responding effectively to ethical professional misconduct: A report to the Nurses Board of Victoria*, Melbourne.

—— (1999a). *Bioethics: a nursing perspective* (3rd edn). Harcourt/Saunders, Sydney.

—— (1999b). *Reporting child abuse: ethical issues for the nursing profession and nurse regulating authorities: a report to the Nurses Board of Victoria*. Department of Nursing and Public Health, RMIT University, Melbourne.

—— (1999c). Reporting child maltreatment: ethical issues for the nursing profession. *Collegian: Journal of the Royal College of Nursing, Australia*, 6(4), p. 5.

—— (2001). Stigma, social justice and the rights of the mentally ill: challenging the status quo. *Australian and New Zealand Journal of Mental Health Nursing*, 10, pp. 200–9.

—— (2002a). Poor working conditions and the capacity of nurses to provide moral care. *Contemporary Nurse*, 12(1), pp. 7–15.

—— (2002b). The changing focus of health care ethics: implications and challenges for the health care professions. *Contemporary Nurse*, 12(3), pp. 213–24. Website: *www.contemporarynurse.com*

—— (2002c). Taking moral action. In Fry, S. and Johnstone, M., *Ethics in nursing practice: a guide to ethical decision making* (2nd edn). Blackwell Science, London, pp. 173–9.

Johnstone, M. and Crock, E. (2001). Dealing with ethical issues in nursing practice. In E. Chang and J. Daly (eds), *Transitions in nursing:*

preparing for professional practice. MacLennan + Petty, Sydney, pp. 137–52.

Johnstone, M. and Kanitsaki, O. (1991). Some moral implications of cultural and linguistic diversity in health care. *Bioethics News*, 10(2), pp. 22–32.

Johnstone, M-J., Kanitsaki, O., Wallace, M. and O'Connor, M. (1996). Conclusion: taking a position on the euthanasia question. In Johnstone, M-J. (ed.), *The politics of euthanasia: a nursing response.* Royal College of Nursing, Canberra, Australia, pp. 117–28.

Jonsen, A. (1993). The birth of bioethics. *Hastings Center Report, Special Supplement*, 23(6), S1–S4.

—— (1995). Casuistry: an alternative or complement to principles? *Kennedy Institute of Ethics Journal*, 5(3), pp. 237–51.

Jonsen, A. and Toulmin, S. (1988). *The abuse of casuistry: a history pf moral reasoning.* University of California Press, Berkeley and Los Angeles, California.

Joyce, J. (1997). Gay gene abortion slammed. *BrotherSister*, 126 (20 February), p. 3.

Kairys, D. (ed.) (1982). *The politics of law: a progressive critique.* Pantheon Books, New York.

Kamisar, Y. (1978). Euthanasia legislation: some non-religious objections. In Beauchamp, T.L. and Perlin, S., *Ethical issues in death and dying.* Prentice Hall, Englewood Cliffs, New Jersey, pp. 220–31.

Kane, R. (1994). *Through the moral maze: searching for absolute values in a pluralistic world.* North Castle Books. Armonk, New York/London, UK.

Kanitsaki, O. (1983). Acculturation — a new dimension in nursing. *Australian Nurses Journal* 13.(5), November, pp. 42–5, 53.

—— (1988). Cancer and informed consent: a cultural perspective. Paper presented at Seminar on Controversial Ethical Issues in Patients with Cancer, Heidelberg Repatriation General Hospital, 13 October 1988, Melbourne.

—— (1988a). Transcultural nursing: challenge to change. *Australian Journal of Advanced Nursing*, 5(3), March–May, pp. 4–11.

—— (1989a). Health–illness–suffering experiences of a sample of Greek-born members of 12 Greek–Australian families living in Melbourne. Minor thesis completed in partial fulfilment of the requirements for the Degree of Master of Educational Studies, Faculty of Education, Monash University, Melbourne.

—— (1989b). Cross-cultural sensitivity in palliative care. In P. Hodder and A. Turley (eds), *The creative option of palliative care: a manual for health professionals.* Melbourne City Mission, Melbourne, pp. 68–71.

—— (1992). Meeting the challenge of patients' rights: a transcultural perspective. *Proceedings of Fourth Victorian State Conference on Nursing Law and Ethics: 'Meeting the challenge of patients rights — issues for the 1990s'*, held Dallas Brooks Hall, 20 November. Faculty of Nursing, RMIT, Bundoora, Melbourne.

—— (1993). Transcultural human care: its challenge to and critique of professional nursing care. In D. A. Gaut (ed.), *A global agenda for caring.* National League for Nursing Press, New York, pp. 19–45.

—— (1994). Cultural and linguistic diversity. In Romanini, J. and Daly, J., *Critical care nursing: Australian perspectives.* W.B. Saunders/Baillière Tindall, Sydney, pp. 94–125.

—— (1996). Care and caring in a multicultural society: a critical examination. Paper presented at *Patterns of Caring: Universal Connections. 18th International Association of Human Caring Research Conference.* April. Mayo Medical Center, Rochester, Minnesota, USA.

—— (2000). Diverse Cultural care: A critical approach to care and caring. (Book chapter). In Taylor, C. and Crisp, J. (Eds), *Fundamentals of nursing.* Harcourt Australia Pty Limited, Sydney, pp. 114–37.

—— (2003). Transcultural nursing and challenging the status quo. *Contemporary Nurse*, 15(3), pp. v–x.

Kant, I. (1930 edn). *Lectures on ethics* (translated by L. Infield and J. MacMurray). Methuen, London, see in particular 'Conscience', pp. 129–35.

—— (1959 edn). *Fundamental principles of the metaphysics of ethics* (translated by T. Kingmill Abbott). Longmans, London, UK.

—— (1972 edn). *The moral law* (translated by H.J. Paton). Hutchinson University Press, London.

—— (1983 edn). *Suicide.* In Gorovitz, S., Macklin, R., Jameton, A.L., O'Connor, J.M. and Sherwin, A. (eds), *Moral problems in medicine.* Prentice Hall, Englewood Cliffs, New Jersey, pp. 434–7.

Kaplan, K. and Schwartz, M. (1993). *A psychology of hope: an antidote to the suicidal pathology of Western civilization.* Praeger, Westport, Connecticut.

Karim, K. (2002). *A grounded theory study of truth-telling in cancer: perceptions of white British and British South Asian Community Workers.* Thesis completed in fulfilment of the requirements for Master of Science (Health Research), Staffordshire University, Stafford, UK [available at: *www.dissertation.com*].

Kass, L. (1993). Is there a right to die? *Hastings Center Report*, 23(1), pp. 34–43.

Katzenstein, M.F. and Laitin, D.D. (1987). Politics, feminism, and the ethics of caring. In Kittay, E.F. and Meyers, D.T. (eds), *Women and moral theory*. Rowman & Littlefield, Totowa, New Jersey, pp. 261–81.

Keireini, E. (1983). International Council of Nurses, Council of National Representatives Meeting, Brasilia, Brazil, 6–10 June 1983. *New Zealand Nursing Journal*, 76(9), pp. 3–9.

Kellmer, D. (1986). No code orders: guidelines for policy. *Nursing Outlook*, 34(4), July/August, pp. 179–83.

Kelly, L.Y. (1985). *Dimensions of professional nursing* (5th edn). Macmillan, New York.

Kelman, H.C. and Hamilton, V.L. (1989). *Crimes of obedience*. Yale University Press, New Haven and London.

Kennedy, H. (1992). Why do the kids suicide? Kyneton stunned by youth suicides. *Sunday Herald-Sun*, Melbourne, 16 August, pp. 4–5.

Kent, A. (1990). Protecting the public? *Nursing Times*, 86(37), p. 20.

Keown, J. (1988). *Abortion, doctors and the law*. Cambridge University Press, Cambridge.

—— (1992). On regulating death. *Hastings Center Report*, 22(2), pp. 39–43.

—— (ed.) (1995). *Euthanasia examined: ethical, clinical and legal perspectives*. Cambridge University Press, Cambridge, UK.

Keown, J. and Jochemsen, H. (1999). Voluntary euthanasia in the Netherlands. *Journal of Medical Ethics*, 25(4), pp. 351–2.

Kerr, J. Fairbanks (1987). *Don't call a doctor*. Veritas, Bullsbrook, Western Australia.

Kerridge, I., Mitchell, K. and Myser, C. (1994). The decision to withhold resuscitation in Australia: problems, hospital policy and legal uncertainty. *Journal of Law and Medicine*, 2(November), pp. 125–30.

Kevorkian, J. (1991). *Prescription: medicide. The goodness of planned death*. Prometheus Books, Buffalo, New York.

Khushf, G. (1994). Intolerant tolerance. *Journal of Medicine and Philosophy*, 19(2), pp. 161–81.

Kilner, J.F. (1990). *Who lives? Who dies? Ethical criteria in patient selection*. Yale University Press, New Haven and London.

King, N.M., Churchill, L.R. and Cross, A.W. (1988). *The physician as captain of the ship*. D. Reidel, Dordrecht.

King, P.A. (1985). Unprofessional conduct and the nursing profession: the *Tuma* case. *Bioethics Reporter*, 6(7), pp. 159–62.

Kirby, M. (1995). Patients' rights — why the Australian courts have rejected 'Bolam'. *Journal of Medical Ethics*, 21(1), pp. 5–8.

Kirkman, M. and Bell, S. (1989). AIDS and confidentiality. *Nursing Forum*, 24(3/4), pp. 47–51.

Kissane, K. (1993). No place like home. *Time Magazine*, 8 March (10), pp. 24–5.

—— (1995). Falling through a larger net. *The Age*, 4 July, p. 13.

—— (2002). Foetal tissue use attracts support. *The Age*, 13 June, p. 7.

Kissling, F. (2001). The place for individual conscience. *Journal of Medical Ethics*, 27(SupplII), pp. ii24–27.

Kitchener, B. (1998). Nurse characteristics and attitudes to active voluntary euthanasia: a survey in the Australian Capital Territory. *Journal of Advanced Nursing*, 28(1), pp. 70–6.

Kittay, E.F. and Meyers, D.T. (eds) (1987). *Women and moral theory*. Rowman & Littlefield, Totowa, New Jersey.

Kleinman, A. (1980). *Patients and healers in the context of culture*. University of California Press, Berkeley, Los Angeles.

Klemke, E.D. (ed.) (1981). *The meaning of life*. Oxford University Press, New York.

Klimek, M. (1990). Virtue, ethics, and care: developing the personal dimension of caring in nursing education. In Leininger, M.M. and Watson, J. (eds), *The caring imperative in education*. National League for Nursing Press, New York, pp. 177–87.

Klostermaier, K. (1998). The truth & the goodness of nature. *The Quest*, 86(2), Spring, pp. 34–41, 52–3.

Klotzko, A. (1995). CQ Interview: Arlene Judith Klotzko and Dr. Boudewijn Chabot discuss assisted suicide in the absence of somatic illness. *Cambridge Quarterly of Health Care Ethics Journal*, 4(2), pp. 239–49.

Kluckhohn, C. (1962). *Culture and behavior*. The Free Press, New York.

Knight, J. (1992). The suffering of suicide: the victim and family considered. In Starck, P. and McGovern, J. (eds), *The hidden dimension of illness: human suffering*. National League for Nursing Press, New York, pp. 245–68.

Kohlberg, L. (1981). *The philosophy of moral development: moral stages and the idea of justice*. Harper & Row, San Francisco.

Kohn, L., Corrigan, J. and Donaldson, M. (eds) (2000). *To err is human: building a safer health system*. National Academy Press, Washington DC.

Komersaroff, P. (2002). Ethics, death and silence: a comment on the euthanasia debate. *Monash Bioethics Review*, 21(4), pp. 35–40.

Koonz, C. (1987). *Mothers in the Fatherland: women, the family and Nazi politics*. St Martin's Press, New York.

Kopelman, L. (1995). Conceptual and moral disputes about futile and useful treatments. *Journal of Medicine and Philosophy*, 20(2), pp. 109–21.

Kordig, C.R. (1976). Pseudo-appeals to conscience. *Journal of Value Inquiry*, 10, pp. 7–17.

Kramarae, C. and Treichler, P. (1985). *A feminist dictionary*. Pandora Press, London. [Section 'P', entry: 'The personal is the political'].

Kreitman, N. (1969). Parasuicide. *British Journal of Psychiatry*, 115, p. 746.

Kroeger Mappes, E. (1985). Ethical dilemmas for nurses: physicians' orders versus patients' rights. *Bioethics Reporter* 6/7, pp. 408–13.

Kruschwitz, R. and Roberts, R. (1987). *The virtues: contemporary essays on moral character*. Wadsworth, Belmont, California.

Kuczewski, M. (1996). Reconceiving the family: the process of consent in medical decision making. *Hastings Center Report*, 26(2), pp. 30–7.

Kuhse, H. (1982). Commenting on David B. Allbrook's paper, 'Medicine and the prolongation of life: does "can" imply "ought"?' *Issues in ethics. Proceedings of the Conference on Medical Science and the Preservation of Life: Ethical and Legal Dilemmas*, November 1981, Centre for Human Bioethics, Monash University, Melbourne, pp. 35–44.

Kuhse, H. (1984). A modern myth. That letting die is not the intentional causation of death: some reflections on the trial and acquittal of Dr Leonard Arthur. *Journal of Applied Philosophy*, 1(1), pp. 21–38.

—— (1987). *The sanctity-of-life doctrine in medicine: a critique*. Clarendon Press, Oxford.

—— (ed.) (1988). Ethics Committees. *Bioethics News*, 7(4), July, special supplement.

—— (1991). Introduction to the Australian edition. In Humphry, D. (1991). *Final exit: the practicalities of self-deliverance and assisted suicide for the dying*. Penguin Books, Ringwood, Victoria, pp. xi–xv.

—— (1992). Quality of life and the death of 'Baby M'. *Bioethics*, 6(3), pp. 233–50.

—— (1995). Editorial: Oregon — medically assisted suicide becomes law. *Monash Bioethics Review*, 14(1), pp. 1–3.

Kuhse, H. and Singer, P. (1985). *Should the baby live?* Oxford University Press, Oxford.

—— (1988). Doctors' practices and attitudes regarding voluntary euthanasia. *Medical Journal of Australia*, 148(20), pp. 623–7.

—— (1992). Euthanasia: a survey of nurses' attitudes and practices. *Australian Nurses Journal*, 21(9), pp. 21–2.

—— (1993). Voluntary euthanasia and the nurse: an Australian survey. *International Journal of Nursing Studies*, 30(4), pp. 311–22.

Kultgen, J. (1982). The ideological use of professional codes. *Business and Professional Ethics Journal*, 1(3), Spring, pp. 53–69.

La Puma, J. and Schiedermayer, D. (1994). *Ethics consultation: a practical guide*. Jones and Bartlett, Boston.

La Puma, J., Stocking, C.B., Silverstein, M.D., DiMartini, A. and Siegler, M. (1988). An ethics consultation service in a teaching hospital. *Journal of the American Medical Association*, 260(6), 12 August, pp. 808–11.

Ladd, J. (1978). The task of ethics. In Reich, W.T., *Encyclopedia of bioethics*. The Free Press, New York, pp. 400–7.

LaFollette, H (ed.) (1997). *Ethics in practice: an anthology*. Blackwell, Cambridge, Massachusetts/Oxford, UK.

Lagnado, L. and Dekel, S. (1991). *Children of the flames: Dr Josef Mengele and the untold story of the twins of Auschwitz*. Sidgwick & Jackson, London.

Lamont, L. (2003). $727,000 payout for infected wife. *The Age*, 11 June, p. 1.

Lancaster, K. (1983). Secrecy in adoption: a historical perspective. In *Proceedings of the Conference: Adoption and AID: Access to Information?* Centre for Human Bioethics, Monash University, Melbourne, 2 November, pp. 21–8.

Lanham, D. (1993). *Taming death by law*. Longman Professional, Melbourne.

Lantos, J. (1995). Child abuse. In Reich, W.T. (ed.), *The encyclopedia of bioethics*, revised edition. Simon & Schuster Macmillan, New York, pp. 42–6.

Larson, P. and Ferketich, S. (1993). Patients' satisfaction with nurses' caring during hospitalisation. *Western Journal of Nursing Research*, 15(6), pp. 690–707.

Lavin, M. (1986). Ulysses contracts. *Journal of Applied Philosophy*, 3, pp. 89–101.

Law Reform Commission of Victoria, Australian Law Reform Commission, and New South Wales Law Reform Commission (1987). *Informed consent to medical treatment*, discussion paper no.7. Law Reform Commission of Victoria, Melbourne.

Le Grand, C. (1998). Doctors still risk fines for abortion. *Weekend Australian*, 23–24 May, p. 11.

Lee, A. and Wu, H. (2002). Diagnosis disclosure in cancer patients — when the family says 'no!'. *Singapore Medical Journal*, 43(10), pp. 533–8.

Lee, D. (2002). Whistle blowing. *British Journal of Perioperative Nursing*, 12(9), pp. 314–15.

Leenaars, A. (ed.) (1993). *Suicidology: essays in honor or Edwin Shneidman*. Jason Aronson, Northvale, New Jersey.

Leftwich, R. (1993). Care and cure as healing processes in nursing. *Nursing Forum*, 28(3), pp. 13–17.

Leininger, M.M. (ed.) (1988). *Care: the essence of nursing and health.* Wayne State University Press, Detroit.

—— (1990a). *Ethical and moral dimensions of care.* Wayne State University Press, Detroit.

Leininger, M. (1990b). Culture: the conspicuous missing link to understanding ethical and moral dimensions of human care. In M. Leininger (ed.), *Ethical and moral dimensions of care.* Wayne State University Press, Detroit, pp. 49–66.

—— (ed.) (1991). *Culture care diversity and universality: a theory of nursing.* National League for Nursing Press, New York.

Leininger, M.M. and Watson, J. (eds) (1990b). *The caring imperative in education.* National League for Nursing Press, New York.

Lemmon, E.J. (1987). Moral dilemmas. In C.W. Gowans (ed.), *Moral dilemmas.* Oxford University Press, New York, pp. 101–14.

Leo, J. (1983). Sharing the pain of abortion. *Time Magazine*, 26 September, p. 59.

Lester, D. and Tallmer, M. (1994). *Now I lay me down: suicide in the elderly.* The Charles Press, Philadelphia.

Lester, L. and Beard, B. (1988). Student nurses' fear of AIDS. *4th International Conference on AIDS. Book 1: Final program. Abstracts, Monday June 13, Tuesday June 14.* Stockholm International Fairs, Stockholm, Sweden, p. 504 (no. 9113).

Levine, C. (1977). Institutional ethics committees: a guarded prognosis. *Hastings Center Report*, 7(3), June, pp. 25–8.

—— (1984). Questions and (some very tentative) answers about institutional ethics committees. *Hastings Center Report*, 14(3), June, pp. 9–12.

—— (ed.) (1995). *Taking sides: clashing views on controversial bioethical issues* (6th edn). The Dushkin Publishing Group, Guilford, Connecticut.

Lewin, L. (1994). Child abuse: ethical and legal concerns. *Journal of Psychosocial Nursing*, 32(12), pp. 15–18.

Lewins, F. (1996). *Bioethics for health professionals: an introduction and critical approach.* Macmillan Education Australia, Melbourne.

Lewis, P. (2001). Rights discourse and assisted suicide. *American Journal of Law, Medicine & Ethics*, 27(1), pp. 45–99.

Lewy, G. (1970). Superior orders, nuclear warfare, and the dictates of conscience. In R.A. Wasserstrom, R.A., *War and morality.* Wadsworth, Belmont, California, pp. 115–34.

Lichtenberg, J. (1996). What are codes of ethics for? In Coady, M. and Bloch, S. (eds), *Codes of ethics and the professions.* Melbourne University Press, Melbourne, pp. 13–27.

Liddell, G. (1994) Pugmire and the dilemma of disclosure. *Otago Bioethics Report*, 3(2), pp. 14–16.

Lifton, B. (1994). *Journey of the adopted self.* Basic Books, New York.

—— (1979). *The broken connection.* Simon & Schuster, New York.

Lifton, B.J. (1986). *The Nazi doctors: a study of the psychology of evil.* Macmillan, London.

Lindars, J. (1991). Holistic care in parasuicide. *Nursing Times*, 87(15), pp. 30–1.

Lindorff, D. (1992). *Marketplace medicine: the rise of the for-profit hospital chains.* Bantam Books, New York.

Lipton, H.L. (1989). Physicians' Do-Not-Resuscitate decisions and documentation in a community hospital. *Quarterly Review Bulletin*, April, pp. 108–13.

Little, M. (1996). Why a feminist approach to bioethics? *Kennedy Institute of Ethics Journal*, 6(1), pp. 1–18.

—— (2001). On knowing the 'why': particularism and moral theory. *Hastings Center Report*, 31(4), pp. 32–40.

Lloyd, G. (1984). *The man of reason: 'male' and 'female' in Western philosophy.* Methuen, London.

Lo, B. (1991). Unanswered questions about DNR orders. *Journal of the American Medical Association*, 265(14), pp. 1874–5.

Lo, B., McLeod, G.A. and Saika, G. (1986). Patient attitudes to discussing life-sustaining treatment. *Archives of Internal Medicine*, 146, pp. 1613–15.

Locke, J. (1947). An essay concerning the true, original extent and end of civil government (reprinted from 1690 edition). In Sir Ernest Barker, *Social contract.* Oxford University Press, London. pp. 3–206.

Loewy, E. and Carlson, R. (1993). Futility and its wider implications: a concept in need for further examination. *Archives of Internal Medicine*, 153 (22 Feburary), pp. 429–31.

Loewy, E.H. (1991). Involving patients in Do Not Resuscitate (DNR) decisions: an old issue raising its ugly head. *Journal of Medical Ethics*, 17(1), pp. 156–60.

Longdon, C. (1993). A survivor's and therapist's viewpoint. In Elliott, M. (ed.), *Female sexual abuse of children: the ultimate taboo.* Longman, Harlow, Essex, pp. 50–60.

Lord, G. (1997). Untitled. In Mullinar, L. and Hunt, C (eds), *Breaking the silence: survivors of child abuse speak out.* Hodder & Stoughton, Sydney, p. i.

Loring, M. (1994). *Emotional abuse*. Lexington Books (an imprint of Macmillan), New York.

Loudon, B. and Wilson, K. (1997). Doctor in gay gene abort call. *Herald-Sun*, 17 February, p. 3.

Lowther, W. (1988). Father seeks right to stop wife's abortion. *The Age*, 26 August, p. 8.

Luckes, E. (1888). *Hospital sisters and their duties*, J. and A. Churchill, London.

Luker, K. (1984). *Abortion and the politics of motherhood*. University of California Press, Berkeley.

Lynn, J. (ed.) (1989). *By no extraordinary means: the choice to forgo life-sustaining food and water*. Indiana University Press, Bloomington and Indianapolis.

Lynn, J. and Teno, J. (1995). Advance directives. In Reich, W. T. (ed.), *Encyclopedia of bioethics*, revised edition. Simon & Schuster Macmillan, New York/Simon & Schuster and Prentice Hall International, pp. 572–7.

Machan, T. (1983). Individualism and the problem of political authority. *The Monist*, 66(4), October, pp. 500–16.

MacIntyre, A. (1966). *A short history of ethics*. Routledge & Kegan Paul, London.

—— (1985). *After virtue: a study in moral theory* (2nd edn). Duckworth, London.

—— (1988). *Whose justice? Which rationality?* Duckworth, London.

Mackie, J.L. (1962). Omnipotence. *Sophia*, 1(2), July, pp. 14–25.

—— (1977). *Ethics: inventing right and wrong*. Penguin Books, Harmondsworth, Middlesex.

MacKinnon, C.A. (1987). *Feminism unmodified: discourses on life and law*. Harvard University Press, Cambridge, Mass.

Macklin, R. (1993). *Enemies of patients*. Oxford University Press, New York.

—— (1998). Ethical relativism in a multicultural society. *Kennedy Institute of Ethics Journal*, 8(1), pp. 1–22.

MacNair, R. (1992). Ethical dilemmas of child abuse reporting: implications for mental health counsellors. *Journal of Mental Health Counselling*, 14(2), pp. 127–36.

Magazanik, M. (1992a). Nurses back euthanasia, survey finds. *The Age*, 2 March, p. 1.

—— (1992b). When death is part of the quality of life. *The Age*, 4 March, p. 3.

—— (1992c). Euthanasia should be legal, says clergyman. *The Age*, 5 March, p. 3.

—— (1992d). Euthanasia law is unrealistic: doctor. *The Age*, 5 June, p. 1.

—— (1992e). Law Commission supports reform on treatment of sick babies. *The Age*, 6 June, p. 5.

—— (1993). Protecting our children. *The Age*, 27 February, p. 18.

—— (1998). Fatal choice: his wife or his faith. *Weekend Australian*, 28-29 November, pp. 1–2.

Magnusson, R. (2002). *Angels of death: exploring the euthanasia underground*. Melbourne University Press, Melbourne.

Makereti (1986). *The old-time Maori*. New Women's Press, Auckland, New Zealand.

Malcolm, N. (1958). *Ludwig Wittgenstein: a memoir*. Oxford University Press, London.

Malone, B. (2003). The Royal College of Nurisng General Secretary, Dr Beverly Malone ommenting on today's debate on euthanasia says: June 6, 2003. RCN Online, RCN, London [available at: *www.rcn.org.uk/news/media_centre1.html* — accessed 24 September 2003].

Mandel, T.E. (1985). The use of immature pancreas as a source of tissue for transplantation in diabetes. *Bioethics News*, 5(1), October, pp. 14–22.

Mann, S. (2001). Dutch courage or cruelty? *The Age*, 12 April, p. 17.

Mapps, T. (2003). Persistent vegative state, prospective thinking, and advance directives. *Kennedy Institute of Ethics Journal*, 13(2), pp. 119–39.

Margolis, J. (1975). Suicide. Reprinted in Beauchamp, T.L. and Perlin, S. (1978), *Ethical issues in death and dying*. Prentice Hall, Englewood Cliffs, New Jersey, pp. 92–7 (with permission from Charles & Merrill Publishing Company).

—— (1978). Cited in Beauchamp, T.L. and Perlin, S. (1978), *Negatives: the limits of life*. Charles E Merrill Publishing Company, pp. 23–9, 34–5.

Marshall, A. and McDonald, M. (2001). *The many-sided triangle: adoption in Australia*. Melbourne University Press, Melbourne.

Marshall, P.A. (1992). Anthropology and bioethics. *Medical Anthropology Quarterly*, 6(1), pp. 49–73.

Martin, D., Emanuel, L. and Singer, P. (2000). Planning for the end of life. *The Lancet*, 356(9242), pp. 1672–6.

Martin, R. and Nickel, J.W. (1980). Recent work on the concepts of rights. *American Philosophical Quarterly*, 17(3), July, pp. 165–80.

Maslen, G. (1986). Should the baby die? *The Age*, 28 June, Saturday Extra, p. 7.

Mathews, S. (1988). Nurses overlooked. *The Age*, 24 March, p. 12.

Matthews, C. (1991). *Sophia goddess of wisdom: the divine feminine from black goddess to world-soul*. Mandala (an imprint of HarperCollins), London, UK.

May, W.F. (1983). Code and covenant or philanthropy and contract? In Gorovitz, S.,

Macklin, R., Jameton, A.L., O'Connor, J.M. and Sherwin, A. (eds), *Moral problems in medicine* (2nd edn). Prentice Hall, Englewood Cliffs, New Jersey, pp. 83–99.

Mayo, D. and Gunderson, M. (2002). Vitalism revisited: vulnerable populations, prejudice, and physician-assisted suicide. *Hastings Center Report*, 32(4), pp. 14–21.

Mayor, F. and Binde, J. (2001). *The world ahead.* Zed Books, London (UK) & New York/UNESCO Publishing, Paris.

McAlister, L. Lopez (ed.) (1989). *Hypatia.* Special issue, 4(1), Spring, *The history of women in philosophy.*

McCann, R., Hall, W. and Groth-Juncker, A. (1994). Confort care for terminally ill patients. The appropriate use of nutrition and hydration. *Journal of the American Medical Association*, 272(16), pp. 1263–6.

McCloskey, H.J. (1980). Privacy and the right to privacy. *Philosophy*, 55, pp. 17–38.

McCormick, R.A. (1984). Ethics committees: promise or peril? *Law, Medicine and Health Care*, 12(4), September, pp. 150–5.

McCorvey, N. (1994). *I am Roe: My life, Roe v Wade, and the freedom of choice.* HarperCollins*Publishers*, New York.

McCullough, L. (1995). Preventive ethics, professional integrity, and boundary setting: the clinical management of moral uncertainty. *Journal of Medicine and Philosophy*, 20(1), pp. 1–11.

McCullough, L. and Jonsen, A. (1991). Bioethics education: diversity and critique. *Journal of Medicine and Philosophy*, 16(1), pp. 1–4.

McCullough, L.B. (1983). The right to health care. In Gorovitz, S., Macklin, R., Jameton, A.L., O'Connor, J.M. and Sherwin, A. (eds), *Moral problems in medicine* (2nd edn). Prentice Hall, Englewood Cliffs, New Jersey, pp. 536–44.

McDonald, S. (2002). Physical and emotional effects of whistle blowing. *Journal of Psychosocial Nursing and Meantla Health Services*, 40(1), pp. 14–27.

McFarland-Icke, B. (1999). *Nurses in Nazi Germany: moral choices in history.* Princeton University Press, Princeton, New Jersey.

McGuire, C. (1987). Euthanasia without consent. *The Age*, Letter to the Editor, 19 October, p. 12.

McIntosh, P. (1988). Nurses must be more aggressive. *Australian Dr Weekly*, 10 June, pp. 1, 10.

McKenzie, N.F. (ed.) (1991). *The AIDS reader: social, political, ethical issues.* Meridian, New York.

McMillan, C. (1982). *Women, reason and nature: some philosophical problems with feminism.* Princeton University Press, Princeton, New Jersey.

McMurray, A. (1999). *Community health and wellness: a socioecological approach.* Mosby, Sydney.

McNaughton, D. (1988). *Moral vision: an introduction to ethics.* Basil Blackwell, Oxford, UK/New York.

McNeill, P. (1993). *The ethics and politics of human experimentation.* Cambridge University Press, Cambridge, UK.

—— (2001). A critical analysis of Australian clinical ethics committees and the functions they serve. *Bioethics*, 15(5/6), pp. 443–60.

McNeill, P.M., Berglund, C.A. and Webster, I.W. (1990). Reviewing the reviewers: a survey of institutional ethics committees in Australia. *Medical Journal of Australia*, 152 (March), pp. 289–96.

McStay, R. (2003). Terminal sedation: palliative care for intractable pain, post Gluckberg and Quill. *American Journal of Law & Medicine*, 29(1), pp. 45–76.

Mead, G. and Turnbull, C. (1995). Cardiopulmonary resuscitation in the elderly: patients' and relatives views. *Journal of Medical Ethics*, 21, pp. 39–44.

Mead, M. (1955). *Cultural patterns and technical change.* Mentor Books, New York.

Meinke, S.A. (1989). *Anencephalic infants as potential organ sources: ethical and legal issues: Scope Notes 12.* Kennedy Institute of Ethics, Georgetown University, Washington DC.

Melby, V., Boore, J. and Murray, M. (1992) Acquired Immunodeficiency Syndrome: knowledge and attitudes of nurses in Northern Ireland. *Journal of Advanced Nursing*, 17, pp. 1068–77.

Melia, K. (1994). The task of nursing ethics. *Journal of Medical Ethics*, 20(1), pp. 7–11.

Mendelsohn, R.S. (1982). *Male practice: how doctors manipulate women.* Contemporary Books, Chicago.

Mendelson, D. (1997). Quill, Glucksberg and palliative care: does alleviation of pain necessarily hasten death? *Journal of Law and Medicine*, 5(November), pp. 110–13.

Mendes, P. (1996). The historical and political context of mandatory reporting and its impact on child protection practice in Victoria. *Australian Social Work*, 49(4), pp. 25–32.

Mental Health Consumers Outcomes Task Force. (1995). *Mental Health Statement of Rights and Responsibilities.* Australian Government Publishing Service, Canberra.

Messer, E. and May, K.E. (1988). *Back rooms: voices from the illegal abortion era.* Simon & Schuster, New York.

Middleton, K. (1994). Act on suicide's tragic toll: expert. *The Age*, 1 March, p. 3.

Midgley, M. (1980). *Beast and man*. Methuen, London.

—— (1991a). *Can't we make moral judgements?* The Bristol Press, Bristol.

—— (1991b). *The origins of ethics*. In Singer, P. (ed.) *A Companion to ethics*. Basil Blockwell, Cambridge, Mas., pp. 3–13.

Midgley, M. and Hughes, J. (1983). *Women's choices*. Weidenfeld & Nicolson, London.

Milburn, C. (1996). Call for national probe on children. *The Age*, 7 November, p. 3.

Mill, J.S. (1929 edn). The subjection of women. In M. Wollstonecraft, *A vindication of the rights of woman*, and J.S. Mill, *The subjection of women*, Everyman's Library, London, pp. 219–317.

—— (1962a). On liberty (reprinted from 1859 edn). In Warnock, M. (ed.), *Utilitarianism*. Fontana Library/Collins, London. pp. 126–250.

—— (1962b). Utilitarianism (reprinted from 1861 edn). In Warnock, M. (ed.) *Utilitarianism*. Fontana Library/Collins, London. pp. 251–342.

Miller, C. (1988a). 1500 Aboriginals tested for AIDS — 5 positive. *The Herald* (Melbourne), 31 August, pp. 1, 2.

—— (1988b). Nurses told, let sick die. *Herald* (Melbourne), 30 September, p. 3.

—— (1989a). NFR system is 'dangerous'. *Australian Dr Weekly*, 20 January.

—— (1989b). Outrage as hospital bans AIDS. *The Herald* (Melbourne), 7 March, p. 1.

Miller, J. (ed.) (1992). *On suicide: great writers on the ultimate question*. Chronicle Books, San Francisco.

Miller, R. and Weinstock, R. (1987). Conflict of interest between therapist–patient confidentiality and the duty to report sexual abuse of children. *Behavioral Sciences and the Law*, 5(2), pp. 161–74.

Miller, W. (2002). Elderly woman assaulted four times while in aged care. *The Age*, 1 November, p. 3.

Millership, R. (1992). A better way. *Australian Nurses Journal*, 21(10), p. 4.

Milo, R. (1986). Moral deadlock. *Philosophy*, 61, pp. 453–71.

Minow, M. (1990). *Making all the difference: inclusion, exclusion, and American law*. Cornell University Press, Ithaca/London.

MinterEllison (2001). Breathing life into resuscitation policies. *Health Industry Update* (March Issue). MinterEllisons Legal Group and Associated Offices, Melbourne.

Mitchel, K., Kerridge, I. and Lovat, T. (1993). Medical futility, treatment withdrawal and the persistent vegetative state. *Journal of Medical Ethics*, 19(2), pp. 71–5.

Monash Review. (1986). Australia gets serious about battered children. October, 5(86), p. 11.

Monkivitch, A. (1992). Euthanasia result not accurate. *The Age*, 5 March, p. 12.

Mono. (1997). The myth of false memory. In L. Mullinar and C. Hunt (eds), *Breaking the silence: survivors of child abuse speak out*. Hodder & Stoughton, Sydney, p. 40–2.

Moody, H. (1992). *Ethics in an aging society*. The John Hopkins University Press, Baltimore.

Moore, G.E. (1903). *Principia ethica*. Cambridge University Press, London.

Moore, N. and Komras, H. (1993). *Patient-focused healing: integrating caring and curing in health care*. Jossey-Bass Publishers, San Francisco.

Mordacci, R. and Sobel, R. (1998). Health: a comprehensive concept. *Hastings Center Report*, 28(1), pp. 34–37.

Moreno, J. (1991). Ethics consultation as moral engagement. *Bioethics News*, 10(2), January, *Ethics committees: a special supplement*, pp. 3–13.

—— (1995). *Deciding together: bioethics and moral consensus*. Oxford University Press, New York.

Morgan, K.P. (1988). Women and moral madness. In Code, L., Mullett, S. and Overall, C. (eds), *Feminist perspectives: philosophical essays on methods and morals*. University of Toronto Press, Toronto, pp. 146–67.

Morreim, E. (1995). Quality of life in health care allocation. In Reich, W.T. (ed.), *The encyclopedia of bioethics*, revised edition. Simon & Schuster Macmillan, New York/Simon & Schuster and Prentice Hall International.

Morrow, L. (1991). When one body can save another. *Time Magazine*, 17 June, pp. 46–50.

Morse, K. (2001). Case in point? A parasuicide patient's recollection of being nurses: a discourse analysis. *Contemporary Nurse*, 19(3-4), pp. 234–43.

Motto, J. (1983). The right to suicide: a psychiatrist's view. In Gorovitz, S., Macklin, R., Jameton, A.L., O'Connor, J.M. and Sherwin, A. (eds), *Moral problems in medicine*. Prentice Hall, Englewood Cliffs, New Jersey, pp. 443–6.

Moulton, J. (1983). A paradigm of philosophy: the adversary method. In Harding, S. and Hintikka, M.B. (eds) (1983), *Discovering reality*. D. Reidel, Dordrecht, pp. 149–64.

Moyers, B. (1993). *Healing and the mind*. Doubleday, New York.

Muir, Judge R. (1978). Opinion in the matter of Karen Quinlan. In T.L. Beauchamp and S. Perlin (eds), *Ethical issues in death and dying*.

Prentice Hall, Englewood Cliffs, New Jersey, pp. 285–90.

Muir-Cochrane, E., Holmes, C. and Walton, J. (2002). Law and policy in relation to the use of seclusion in psychiatric hospitals in Australia and New Zealand. *Contemporary Nurse*, 13(2–3), pp. 136–45.

Muirden, N. (1993). Palliative care and the terminally ill. *St Vincent's Bioethics Centre Newsletter*, 11(1), pp. 13–19.

Muirden, N., Jackson, K., Pisasale, M., Williams, B., Bingham, J. and Evans, B. (1992). A survey among palliative care nurses would give differing views. *The Age*, 10 March, p. 12.

Mukherjee, S. and Shah, A. (2001). Capacity to consent: issues and controversies. *Hospital Medicine*, 62, pp. 351–4.

Mullett, S. (1988). Shifting perspectives: a new approach to ethics. In Code, L., Mullett, S. and Overall, C. (eds), *Feminist perspectives: philosophical essays on methods and morals*. University of Toronto Press, Toronto, pp. 109–26.

Mulley, A.G. (1984). The triage decision. In S. J. Reiser and M. Anbar (eds), *The machine at the bedside*. Cambridge University Press, Cambridge, pp. 221–6.

Mullinar, L. and Hunt, C. (eds) (1997). *Breaking the silence: survivors of child abuse speak out*. Hodder & Stoughton, Sydney.

Murphy, D., Burrows, D., Santilli, S., Kemp, A., Tenner, S., Kreling, B. and Teno, J. (1994). The influence of the probability of survival on patients' preferences. *The New England Journal of Medicine*, 330(8), pp. 545–49.

Murphy, G. (1983). Suicide and the right to die. In Gorovitz, S., Macklin, R., Jameton, A.L., O'Connor, J.M. and Sherwin, A. (eds), *Moral problems in medicine*. Prentice Hall, Englewood Cliffs, New Jersey, p. 442.

Musgrave, C.F. (1987). The ethical and legal implications of hospice care. *Cancer Nursing*, 10(4), pp. 183–9.

Muyskens, J.L. (1982). *Moral problems in nursing: a philosophical investigation*. Rowman & Littlefield, Totowa, New Jersey.

—— (1982a). Collective responsibility and the nursing profession. In Barry, V. (ed.), *Moral aspects of health care*. Wadsworth, Belmont, California, pp. 120–7.

—— (1982c). Nurses' collective responsibility and the strike weapon. *Journal of Medicine and Philosophy*, 7(1), February, pp. 101–12.

Myers, J. (ed.) (1994). *The backlash: child protection under fire*. Sage, Thousand Oaks, California.

Mystakidou, K., Liossi, C., Vlachos, L. and Padadimitriou, J. (1996). Disclosure of diagnostic information to cancer patients in Greece. *Journal of Palliative Medicine*, 10(3), pp. 195–200.

Nadelson, C.C. and Notman, M.T. (1978). Women as health professionals. In Reich, W.T. (ed.), *Encyclopedia of bioethics*. The Free Press, New York, pp. 1713–20.

Nagel, T. (1991). *Mortal questions*. Canto edition. Cambridge University Press (1979), Cambridge, UK.

National Advisory Council on Youth Suicide Prevention (2000). *Living is for everyone (LIFE): a framework for prevention of suicide and self-harm in Australia: Areas for action*. Commonwealth of Australia, Canberra [available at: http://www.mentalhealth.gov.au — accessed 29 September 2003]

National Health and Medical Research Council (1988). *Discussion paper on the ethics of limiting life sustaining treatment*. NH & MRC, Woden, ACT.

National Mental Health Strategy Evaluation Steering Committee, for the Australian Health Ministers Advisory Council. (1997). *Evaluation of the Mental Health Stratgey: Final Report*. Mental Health Branch, Commonwealth Department of Health and Family Services. Canberra.

National Women's Consultative Council (1988). *Women into action*. CPN Publications, Canberra.

Neimeyer, R. (ed.) (2001). *Meaning reconstruction & the experience of loss*. American Psychological Association, Washington DC.

Nelson. R., Botkin, J., Kodish, E., Levetown, M., Truman, J. and Wilfond, B. (2001). Institutional ethics committees. *Pediatrics*, 107(1), pp. 205–9.

Nelson. S. (2003). 'Do everything!': encountering 'futility' in medical practice. *Ethics & Medicine*, 19(2), pp. 103–13.

New South Wales Health Department (1993). *Dying with dignity: interim guidelines on management*. NSW Health Department, Sydney.

New Zealand Herald (1987a). Cancer cases quoted. 12 August, p. 13.

—— (1987b). 'Absolutely appalled' over tests. 12 November, p. 14.

—— (1987c). Dr Collison denies imposing staff gag. 18 November.

—— (1987d). Inquiry judge seeks more nurses' views. 3 December.

—— (1987e). Consent 'not asked' for samples. 10 December.

—— (1988a). Swabbed girls 'often Maoris and Islanders'. 20 January.

—— (1988b). Dr Green 'Did not treat all cases'. 28 January, p. 3.

New Zealand Nurses Association. (1988). *Code of Ethics*. New Zealand Nurses' Association, Wellington, NZ.

New Zealand Nurses Organisation (1993). *Social Policy Statement*. New Zealand Nurses Organisation, Auckland.

—— (1993). *Standards for Nursing Practice*. New Zealand Nurses Organisation, Auckland.

—— (1995). *Code of Ethics*. New Zealand Nurses Organisation, Auckland.

New Zealand Nursing Journal (1988). Prostitutes support nurses. 81(4), April, p. 5.

Newman, M.A. (1986). *Health as expanding consciousness*. C.V. Mosby, St Louis, Missouri.

Newton, L. (1981). Lawgiving for professional life: reflections on the place of the professional code. *Business and Professional Ethics Journal*, 1(1), Fall, pp. 41–53.

Nexus (1996). Hearings. 2(2), pp. 6–7. (Official newsletter of the Nurses Board of Victoria, Melbourne.)

—— (1996). Formal hearing Summaries: Nurse B. *Nexus*, 2(2), p. 9.

Nicolayev, J. and Phillips, D.C. (1979). On assessing Kohlberg's stage theory of moral development. In Cochrane, D.B., Hamm, C.M. and Kazepides A.C. (eds), *The domain of moral education*. Paulist Press, New York, pp. 231–50.

Nielsen, K. (1989). *Why be moral?* Prometheus Books, Buffalo, New York.

Nietzsche, F. (1972 edn). *Beyond good and evil*. Penguin Books, Harmondsworth, Middlesex.

Nightingale, F. (1970). *Note on Nursing: What It Is, and What it Is Not*. Gerald Duckworth and Co, London (first published in 1859 by Harrison and Sons).

Noble, C.N. (1982). Ethics and experts. *Hastings Center Report*, 12(3), June, pp. 7–9.

Noddings, N. (1984). *Caring: a feminine approach to ethics and moral education*. University of California Press, Berkeley.

Noonan, J.T. (1983). From 'An almost absolute value in history'. In Gorovitz, S., Macklin, R., Jameton, A.L., O'Connor, J.M. and Sherwin, A. (eds), *Moral problems in medicine* (2nd edn). Prentice Hall, Englewood Cliffs, New Jersey, pp. 303–8.

Nordenfelt, L. (1987). *On the nature of health*. D. Reidel, Dordrecht.

Northridge v Central Sydney Area Health Service [2000] NSWSC 1241 revised – 17/01/2001, 50 NSWLR 549.

Nowell-Smith, P.H. (1954). *Ethics*. Penguin Books, Harmondsworth, Middlesex.

Nurses Board of Victoria (2001). *Professional boundaries guidelines for Registered Nurses in Victoria*. Nurses Board of Victoria, Melbourne.

Nurses Registration Board of NSW (1999). *Guidelines for Registered Nurses and Enrolled Nurses regarding the Boundaries of Professional*

Practice (approved for use in Queensland by the Queensland Nursing Council). Nurses Registration Board of NSW, Sydney.

Nurses' Board of the Northern Territory. (1996). *Position Statement on the Nurse's Role in Euthanasia*. Nurses' Board of the Northern Territory, Darwin.

Nursing Council of New Zealand. (2001). *Code of conduct for nurses and midwives*. Nursing Council of New Zealand, Wellington.

Nursing Mirror (1984). ECT nurse loses appeal, 158(24), 20 June, p. 2.

Nursing Times (1982a). MP calls for conscience clause in Bill, 78(42), 20 October, p. 1738.

—— (1982b). Secret Wexham report slams Walsh, 78(38), 22 September, p. 1573.

—— (1983a). RCN slams 'life and death' choice, 79(24), p. 20.

—— (1983b). Sacked ECT student presses for new hearing, 79(32), 10 August, p. 18.

—— (1983c). Third nurse sacked over ECT issue, 79(14), 6 April, p. 17.

—— (1985). Midwives demand 24-week time limit for abortions, 81(30), 24 July, p. 5.

—— (1986a). Health staff avoid nurses tending AIDS patients, 82(44), 29 October, p. 10.

—— (1986b). Nurse loses appeal over refusing to give ECT, 82(52), 31 December, p. 7.

—— (1987). Dutch nurses in euthanasia drama, 83(12), 25 March, p. 8.

—— (1988a). Nurses in abortion row, 84(7), 17 February, p. 8.

—— (1988b). Nurses urged to strike worldwide, 84(14), 6 April, p. 5.

—— (1990). Nurses obliged to lie to cancer patients, 86(28), 11 July, p. 9.

Nussbaum, M. (2001). *Upheavals of thought: the intelligence of emotions*. Cambridge University Press, Cambridge, UK.

O'Brien, M. (1981). *The politics of reproduction*. Routledge & Kegan Paul, London, UK.

O'Brien, N. (1998a). Stop abortions or face charges, nurses told. *The Australian*, 12 February, p. 3.

—— (1998b). Doctors demand abortion overhaul. *The Australian*, 17 February, p. 7.

—— (1998c). Abortion laws 'as bad as Cambodia's'. *The Australian*, 24 February, p. 4.

O'Brien, N. and Price, M. (1998a). Abortion charges create state of panic. *The Australian*, 11 February, p. 5.

—— (1998b). AMA tells doctors to refuse abortions. *The Australian*, 10 February, p. 5.

O'Connor, M. (1992). Representative sample? *Australian Nurses Journal*, 21(10) May, p. 4.

O'Hagan, K. (1993). *Emotional and psychological abuse of children*. Open University Press, Buckingham, UK.

O'Hanlan, K., Cabaj, R., Schatz, B., Lock, J. and Nemrow, P. (1997). A review of the medical consequences of homophobia with suggestion for resolutions. *Journal of Gay and Lesbian Medical Association*, 1(1), pp. 25–39.

Oakley, A. (1986). *Telling the truth about Jerusalem*. Basil Blackwell, Oxford.

Ogilvie, A. and Potts, S. (1994). Assisted Suicide for depression: the slippery slope in action? *British Medical Journal*, 309, 20–27 August, pp. 492–3.

Oliver, K. (1989). Marxism and surrogacy. In H. Holmes and L Purdy (eds) (1992), *Feminist perspectives in medical ethics*. Indiana University Press, Bloomington and Indianopolis, pp. 266–83.

Oliver, N. (1990). Nurse, are you a healer? *Nursing Forum*, 25(2), pp. 11–14.

Ooi, C. (1988). 'Paediatrics — a new version', unpublished paper, Sydney.

Outka, G. (1972). *Agape: an ethical analysis*. Yale University Press, New Haven and London.

PA (1987). Law Lords reject father's plea to stop abortion. *The Age*, 26 February, p. 8.

Packard, J.S. and Ferrara, M. (1988). In search of the moral foundation of nursing. *Advances in Nursing Science*, 10(4), pp. 60–71.

Pappworth, M. (1967). *Human guinea pigs: experimentation on man*. Penguin Books, Harmondsworth, Middlesex, UK.

Parkash, R. and Burge, F. (1997). The family's perspective on issues of hydration in terminal care. *Journal of Palliative Care*, 13(4), pp. 23–7.

Parker, M. (1994). Active voluntary euthanasia and physician assisted suicide. *Monash Bioethics Review*, 13(4), pp. 34–42.

Parker, R. (1974). A definition of privacy. *Rutgers Law Review*, 27(2), pp. 275–96.

—— (1990). Nurses stories: the search for a relational ethic of care. *Advances in Nursing Science*, 13(1), pp. 31–40.

Parliament of Victoria, Legislative Council, 50th Parliament, 2nd Session (1988). *Parliamentary Debates (Hansards)* 6 (3, 4, 5 & 6), May. See in particular the debate on the Medical Treatment Bill (no. 2), 3 May 1988, pp. 1012–44.

Parsons, L. (1982). Why ECT is an ethical issue. *Nursing Times*, 78(9), 3 March, p. 352.

Parsons, S. (1916). *Nursing problems and obligations*, Whitcomb & Barrows, Boston (facsimile, Garland Publishing, New York, 1985).

—— (1986). Feminism and moral reasoning. *Australasian Journal of Philosophy*. Supplement to vol. 64, June, pp. 75–90.

Pateman, C. (1989). *The disorder of woman*. Polity Press, Cambridge.

Peers, Lt Gen. W.R. (1979). *The My Lai Inquiry*. W.W. Norton, New York.

Pegler, T. (1993). Coroner urges tight surveillance of psychiatric patients. *The Age*, 19 June, p. 26.

—— (1996). Life of crime for one in five wards. *The Age*, 21 June, p. 4.

Pegler, T. and Farouque, F. (1996). State fails children: auditor. *The Age*, 21 June, p. 1.

Peisley, R. (2001). Professional Conduct Report in *The Nurses Board of Victoria Annual Report 2001*. Nurses Board of Victoria, Melbourne, pp. 12–15.

—— (2002) Operational Program Reports — Professional conduct. *Sustaining our growth: Nurses Board of Victoria annual report 2001/2002* in Nurses Board of Victoria, Melbourne, pp. 12–15.

Pellegrino, E. (1985). Moral choice, the good of the patient, and the patient's good. In J. Moskop and L. Kopelman (eds), *Ethics and critical care medicine*. D. Reidel, Dordrecht, pp. 117–38.

—— (1992). Is truth telling to the patient a cultural artefact? *Journal of American Medical Association*, 268(13), pp. 1734–5.

—— (1995). Toward a virtue-based normative ethics for the health professions. *Kennedy Institute of Ethics Journal*, 5(3), pp. 253–77.

Pence, G. (1984). Recent work on virtues. *American Philosophical Quarterly*, 21(4), pp. 281–97.

—— (1991). Virtue theory. In Singer, P. (ed.), *A companion to ethics*. Basil Blackwell, Oxford, UK, pp. 249–58.

—— (1997). Why physicians should aid the dying. In LaFollette, H. (ed.), *Ethics in practice: an anthology*. Blackwell Publishers, Cambridge, Mass., pp. 22–32.

Perry, S.W., Schwart, H.I. and Amchin, J. (1986). Determining resuscitation status: a survey of medical professionals. *General Hospital Psychiatry*, 8, pp. 198–202.

Petchesky, R.P. (1986). *Abortion and women's choice: the state, sexuality, and reproductive freedom*. Verso (imprint of New Left Books), London.

Petersen. K. (1997). Medical negligence and wrongful birth actions: Australian developments. *Journal of Medical Ethics*, 23(5), pp. 319–22.

Peterson, C. and Bossio, L. (1991). *Health and optimism*. The Free Press, New York.

Pharr, E. (2003). The hospital ethics committee: bridging the gulf of miscommunication and values. *Trustee*, 56(3), pp. 24–8.

Phillips, K. and Woodward, V. (1999). The decision to resuscitate: older people's views. *Journal of Clinical Nursing*, 8(6), pp. 753–61.

Phillips, M. and Frederick, C. (1995). *Healing the divided self: clinical and Ericksonian hypnotherapy for post-traumatic and dissociative conditions.* WW Norton, New York/London.

Pirrie, M. (1987). A disabled baby's right to live. *The Age,* 28 April, p. 11.

—— (1988). Woman's request to stop respirator had legal basis: hospital. *The Age,* 23 March, p. 3.

Plato (1903 edn). *The trial and death of Socrates, being The Euthyphron, Apology, Crito, and Phaedo of Plato* (translated by F. J. Church). Macmillan, London.

Plato (1955 edn). *The Republic.* Penguin Classics, Harmondsworth, Middlesex.

—— (1966). Euthyphro. In Allen, R.E. (ed.), *Greek philosophy: Thales to Aristotle.* The Free Press, New York, pp. 59–74.

—— (1969 edn). *The last days of Socrates* (translated by H. Tredennick). Penguin, Harmondsworth, Middlesex.

Pojman, L. and Beckwith, F. (eds) (1994). *The abortion controversy: a reader.* Jones and Bartlett, Boston.

Pool, R. (2000). *Negotiating a good death: euthanasia in the Netherlands.* The Haworth Press, New York.

Porter, E. (1991). *Women and moral identity.* Allen & Unwin, Sydney, pp. 19–44.

Porterfield, K. (1993). *Blind faith: recognizing and recovering from dysfunctional religious groups.* CompCare, Minneapolis.

Potter, V. (1971). *Bioethics: bridge to the future.* Prentice-Hall, Englewood Cliffs, New Jersey.

Power, T. (1993). Mother's illness drove six-year-old to commit suicide. *The Age,* 17 June, p. 9.

Price, T. (1989). New fears on AIDS: hospital ban may spread. *The Sun,* 8 March, p. 3.

Proctor, R. (1988). *Racial hygiene: medicine under the Nazis.* Harvard University Press, Cambridge, Mass.

—— (1992). Nazi biomedical politics. In Caplan (ed.), *When medicine went mad: bioethics and the holocaust.* Humana Press, Totowa, New Jersey, pp. 23–42.

Puka, B. (1989). The liberation of caring: a different voice for Gilligan's 'different voice'. In Brabeck, M. (ed.), *Who cares? Theory, research, and educational implications of the ethic of care.* Praeger, New York.

Purdy, L. (1996). *Reproducing persons: issues in feminist bioethics.* Cornell University Press, Ithaca, New York.

Pylkkanen, P. (1989b). Introduction. In Pylkkanen, P. (ed.), *The search for meaning: the new spirit in science and philosophy.* Crucible, an imprint of The Acquarian Press. Wellingborough, Northamptonshire, UK, pp. 13–39.

—— (ed.) (1989). *The search for meaning: the new spirit in science and philosophy.* Crucible (an imprint of The Aquarian Press), Wellingborough, Northamptonshire.

Pyne, R.H. (1981). *Professional discipline in nursing: theory and practice.* Blackwell Scientific Publications, Oxford.

Queensland Nursing Council (2000). *Queensland Nursing Council and Health Practitioners Boards' Statement on Sexual Relationships between Health Practitioners and their Patients.* Queensland Nursing Council, Brisbane.

Quill, T., Cassel, C. and Meier, D. (1992). Care of the hopelessly ill: proposed clinical criteria for physician-assisted suicide. *New England Journal of Medicine,* 327(19), pp. 1381–3.

Quinn, C. (1992). Protection and prevention: an integral approach to child sexual assault. In J. Breckenridge and M. Carmody (eds), *Crimes of violence: Australian responses to rape and child sexual assault.* Allen & Unwin, Sydney, pp. 86–96.

Rabkin, M.T., Gillerman, G. and Rice, N.R. (1979). CPR policies: the art of the possible — orders not to resuscitate. *Supervisor Nurse,* 10, August, pp. 26, 29–30.

Rachels, J. (1975). Active and passive euthanasia. *New England Journal of Medicine* 292, pp. 490–7.

—— (1983). Barney Clark's key. *Hastings Center Report* (April), pp. 17–19.

—— (1986). *The end of life: euthanasia and morality.* Oxford University Press, Oxford.

—— (1988). Can ethics provide answers? In Rosenthal, D. and Shehadi, F. (eds), *Applied ethics and ethical theory.* University of Utah Press, Salt Lake City, pp. 3–24.

Radi, H. (1979). Whose child? Custody of children in NSW 1854–1934. In MacKinolty, J. and Radi, H. (eds), *In pursuit of justice: Australian women and the law 1788–1979.* Hale & Iremonger, Sydney, pp. 119–13.

Radic, L. (1982). Most support the right to die. *The Age,* 23 August, reprinted in *The Age Reprint Booklet, no. 44: Euthanasia,* The Age Education Unit, Melbourne, p. 3.

Ramsden, I. (2002). *Cultural safety and nursing education in Aotearoa and Te Waipounamu.* A thesis submitted to the Victoria University of Wellington in fulfilment of the requirements for the degree of Doctor of Philosophy in Nursing (held Victoria University of Wellington, New Zealand).

Ramsey, P. (1976). Prolonged dying: not medically indicated. *Hastings Center Report,* 6, pp. 14–17.

Randal, J. (1983). Are ethics committees alive and well? *Hastings Center Report,* 13(6), December, pp. 10–12.

Raphael, B. (1995). Foreword, in Mental Health Consumers Outcomes Task Force, *Mental Health Statement of Rights and Responsibilities*. Australian Government Publishing Service, Canberra.

Rasmussen, D. (ed.) (1990). *Universalism vs communitarianism: contemporary debates in ethics*. The MIT Press, Cambridge, Mass.

Rauscher, W. (1981). *The case against suicide*. St Martin's Press, New York.

Rave, E.J. and Larsen, C.C. (eds) (1995). *Ethical Decision Making in Therapy: Feminist Perspectives*. The Guilford Press, New York.

Rawls, J. (1971). *A theory of justice*. Oxford University Press, Oxford.

Rea, K. (1981). Legal semantics. *Nursing Times*, 77(9), p. 351.

—— (1987). Negligence. Nursing. *The Add-on Journal of Clinical Nursing*, 3(14), pp. 533–6.

Read, J. and Reynolds, J. (eds) (1996). *Speaking our minds: an anthology of personal experiences of mental distress and its consequences*. The Open University, London.

Reardon, D. (1998). Pro-life grief over abortion laws. *The Age*, 3 April, p. 7.

Reed, C. (1996). Man sues physician who made him live. *The Age*, 20 June, p. 14.

Reeves, P. (1998). Stakes raised in WA pay campaign. *Australian Nursing Journal*, 5(8), p. 11.

—— (1998). WA nurses caught in abortion row. *Australian Nursing Journal*, 5(8), p. 11.

Regan, K.M. (1983). Life at all costs? Letter to the Editor, *Nursing Times*, 79(26), p. 6.

Reich, W.T. (ed.) (1978). *Encyclopedia of bioethics*. The Free Press, New York.

—— (1978). Quality of life. In Reich, W.T. (ed.), *Encyclopedia of bioethics*. The Free Press, New York, pp. 829–39.

—— (1994). The word 'bioethics': its birth and the legacies of those who shaped it. *Kennedy Institute of Ethics Journal*, 4(4), pp. 319–35.

—— (1995a). *Introduction to the Encyclopedia of Bioethics*, revised edition. Simon & Schuster Macmillan, New York/Simon & Schuster and Prentice Hall International.

—— (1995b). The word 'bioethics': the struggle over its earliest meanings. *Kennedy Institute of Ethics Journal*, 5(1), pp. 19–34.

Reich, W.T. (ed.) (1995). *The encyclopedia of bioethics*, revised edition. Simon & Schuster Macmillan, New York/Simon & Schuster and Prentice Hall International.

Reichlin, M. (1994). Observations on the epistemological status of bioethics. *Journal of Medicine and Philosophy*, 19(1), pp. 79–102.

Reiser, S.J. (1975). The dilemma of euthanasia in modern medical history: the English and American experience. In Behnke, J.A. and Bok, S. (eds), *The dilemmas of euthanasia*. Anchor Books, Anchor Press/Doubleday, Garden City, New York, pp. 27–49.

Reiter-Theil, S. (2000). Ethics consultation on demand: concepts, practical experiences and a case study. *Journal of Medical Ethics*, 26(3), pp. 198–203.

Remafedi, G. (1994b). Introduction: The state of knowledge on gay, lesbian, and bisexual youth suicide. In Remafedi, G. (ed.), *Death by denial: studies of suicide in gay and lesbian teenagers*. Alyson Pubs, Boston, pp. 7–14.

—— (ed.) (1994a). *Death by denial: studies of suicide in gay and lesbian teenagers*. Alyson Pubs, Boston.

Renvoize, J. (1993). *Innocence destroyed: a study of child sexual abuse*. Routledge, London/New York.

Report of the Cervical Cancer Inquiry (1988). Prepared by the Committee of Inquiry into Allegations Concerning the Treatment of Cervical Cancer at National Women's Hospital and into Other Related Matters. Government Printing Office, Auckland, NZ.

Report of the Royal Commission into Deep Sleep Therapy (1990). Government Printer, Sydney.

Report of the Study of Professional Issues in Nursing (1988). Health Department (Vic), Melbourne.

Reuter (1990a). Belgian king steps down over legalising abortion. *The Age*, 5 April, p. 7.

—— (1990b). Abortion issue threatens German treaty. *The Age*, 31 August, p. 7.

Rhode, D.L. (1989). *Justice and gender: sex discrimination and the law*. Harvard University Press, Cambridge, Mass.

Rice, S. (1988). *Some doctors make you sick: the scandal of medical incompetence*. Angus & Robertson, Sydney.

Rich, A. (1979). *On lies, secrets and silence: selected prose 1966–1978*. Virago Press, London.

Rights of the Terminally Ill Act 1995 (NT).

Riley, M. (1998a). Tonight on *60 Minutes*: one man's final seconds. *The Age*, 27 November, p. 15.

—— (1998b). Euthanasia doctor charged with murder. *The Age*, 27 November, p. 13.

—— (1998c). Mercy death doctor to stand trial for murder, *The Age*, 11 December, p. 11.

—— (1999a). Doctor Death jailed for murder of dying patient. *The Age*, 15 April, p. 2.

—— (1999b). A life behind bars for America's 'Dr Death'. *The Age*, 17 April, p. 6.

Rivers, F. (1996). *The way of the owl: succeeding with integrity in a conflicted world*. HarperSanFrancisco, New York.

Roach, M.S. (1987). *The human act of caring: a blueprint for the health professions.* Canadian Hospital Association, Ottawa, Ontario.

—— (1992). *The human act of caring: a blueprint for the health professions* (2nd edn). Canadian Hospital Association, Ottawa, Ontario.

Robb, C.S. (1985). A framework for feminist ethics. In Andolsen, B. Hilkert, Gudorf, C.E. and Pellauer, M.D. (eds) (1987), *Women's consciousness, women's conscience.* Harper & Row, San Francisco, pp. 211–33.

Robb, I. Hampton. (1903). *Nursing ethics: for hospital and private use.* J.B. Savage, Cleveland.

Robbins, D. (1983). Breaking the conspiracy of silence. *Journal of Emergency Nursing*, 9(2), p. 109.

Roberts, J. (1987). Women not told of intimate checks. *Sunday Star* (Auckland), 26 September.

Roberts, M. (1987). The nurse as an advocate between patient and family. *Proceedings of the conference, 'The Role of the Nurse: Doctors' Handmaiden, Patients' Advocate or What?* Centre for Human Bioethics, Monash University, 16 November, pp. 98–111.

Robertson, G. (1981). Informed consent to medical treatment. *The Law Quarterly Review*, 97, January, pp. 102–26.

Robertson, J.A. (1981). Dilemma in Danville. *Hastings Center Report*, 11(5), October, pp. 5–8.

Robinson, G. and Merav, A. (1983). Informed consent: recall by patients tested postoperatively. In Gorovitz, S., Macklin, R., Jameton, A.L., O'Connor, J.M. and Sherwin, A. (eds), *Moral problems in medicine* (2nd edn). Prentice Hall, Englewood Cliffs, New Jersey, pp. 182–6.

Robson, A. (1994). Female circumcision. *Amnesty International Australian Newsletter*, 12(2), March, p. 15.

Rogers, J. (1992). Rights for rapists. *The Age*, 'Access Age', 19 February, p. 12.

—— (2000). Nurse on 59 fraud charges. *Northern Star* (Lismore), 3 March, p. 3.

Rohter, L. (1993). Anti-abortion protester kills doctor. *The Age*, 12 March, p. 7.

Romanin, S. (1988). TV telephone poll was unsatisfactory. *The Age*, 11 February, p. 12.

Rosen, L. (1999). Whistle blowing. *Today's Surgical Nurse*, 21(1), pp. 41–2.

Ross, J., Wilson, Bayley C., Michel, V. and Pugh, D. (1986). *Handbook for hospital ethics committees: practical suggestions for ethics committee members to plan, develop, and evaluate their roles and responsibilities.* American Hospital Publishing, Chicago.

Ross, S.D. (1972). *Moral decision: an introduction to ethics.* Freeman, Cooper & Company, San Francisco, California.

Ross, W.D. (1930). *The right and the good.* Oxford University Press, London.

Roth, L.H., Meisel, A. and Lidz, C.W. (1983). Tests of competency to consent to treatment. In Gorovitz, S., Macklin, R., Jameton, A.L., O'Connor, J.M. and Sherwin, A. (eds), *Moral problems in medicine* (2nd edn). Prentice Hall, Englewood Cliffs, New Jersey, pp. 172–9 (reprinted from *American Journal of Psychiatry*, 134(4), pp. 279–84).

Rothenberg, L.S. (1987). An ethicist urges offering all options in disability cases. *Kennedy Institute of Ethics Newsletter*, 1(8), February/March, pp. 1–2.

Rousseau, J.-J. (1911 edn). *Emile.* Everyman's Library, London.

—— (1947). The social contract (reprinted from 1762 edition). In Sir Ernest Barker, *Social contract.* Oxford University Press, London, pp. 239–440.

Rowland, R. (1988). *Woman herself: a transdisciplinary perspective on women's identity.* Oxford University Press, Melbourne.

—— (1992). *Living laboratories: women and reproductive technologies.* Pan Macmillan, Sydney.

Roy, R. (1998). *Childhood abuse and chronic pain.* University of Toronto Press, Toronto.

Royal Australian Nursing Federation (RANF) (Vic) (1986a). *Newsflash.* 10 November, Melbourne.

—— (1986b). *Nurses Action.* December, RANF, Melbourne.

—— (1987). *Nurses Action.* February, RANF, Melbourne.

Royal Australian Nursing Federation (WA) (1987). Position paper: patients' bill of rights. In Royal Australian Nursing Federation, *Ethics in perspective*, vol. 1. RANF, Melbourne, pp. 119–26.

Royal College of Nursing v DHSS (CA) [1981] AC.800.

Royal College of Nursing, Australia. (1996). *Position Statement on Voluntary Euthanasia/Assisted Suicide.* Royal College of Nursing, Australia, Canberra.

—— (1999). *Position statement: Voluntary euthanasia/assisted suicide.* RCNA, Canberra [available at: *www.rcna.org.au/* — accessed 24 September 2003].

Royal College of Nursing, London (1994). Living Wills: Guidance for Nurses, in *Issues in nursing and health*, Royal College of Nursing, London.

Rozsos, E. (2003). Hungary's 'Black Angel' and her 'dragons'. *Nursing Ethics*, 10(4), pp. 428–32.

Rubin, S. (1998). *When doctors say no: the battleground of medical futility*. Indiana University Press, Bloomington & Indianapolis.

Rudd, P. (2002). The clinical ethics committee at the Royal United Hospital — Bath, England. *HEC Forum*, 14(1), pp. 37–44.

Rudd, S. (1992). Ethics committees — a forum for nurses? *Australian Medicine*, 4(12), July 6, p. 15.

Rudnick, A. (2002). Depression and competence to refuse psychiatric treatment. *Journal of Medical Ethics*, 28(3), pp. 151–5.

Rumbold, G. (1986). *Ethics in nursing practice*. Baillière Tindall, London.

Russell, H. (1987). What you don't know can hurt. *Health Issues*, 11 September, pp. 17–19.

Ryffe, C. and Singer, B. (eds) (2001). *Emotion, social relationships, and health*. Oxford University Press, New York.

Ryle, G. (1993). Suicide deaths outstrip state's road fatalities. *The Age*, 8 January, p. 3.

Sade, R.M. (1983). Medical care as a right: a refutation. In Gorovitz, S., Macklin, R., Jameton, A.L., O'Connor, J.M. and Sherwin, A. (eds), *Moral problems in medicine* (2nd edn). Prentice Hall, Englewood Cliffs, New Jersey, pp. 532–5.

Safranek, J. (1998). Autonomy and assisted suicide: the execution of freedom. *Hastings Center Report*, 28(4), pp. 32–6.

Sage, W.M., Hurst, C. R., Silverman, J.F. and Bortz, W.M. (1987). Intensive care for the elderly: outcome of elective and nonelective admissions. *Journal of the American Geriatrics Society*, 35(4), April, pp. 312–18.

Salladay, S. (2002). New role for conscientious objectors. *Nursing*, 32(12), pp. 65–6.

Sanders, K. (1988). Obeying doctor's orders: professional accountability. In *Proceedings of 'Nursing Law and Ethics'. First Victorian State Conference. Theme: 'Matters of Life and Death'*. School of Nursing, Phillip Institute of Technology, Melbourne.

Sanders, K. and Moore, B. (eds) (1991). *Anencephalics, infants and brain death treatment options and the issue of organ donation. Proceedings of Consensus Development Conference*. Law Reform Commission of Victoria, Royal Children's Hospital, Melbourne, and Australian Association of Paediatric Teaching Centres, Melbourne.

Sanford, L. (1990). *Strong at the broken places: overcoming the trauma of childhood abuse*. Random House, New York.

Sass, H. (1998). Advance directives. In Chadwick, R. (ed.) *Encyclopedia of applied ethics*, vol. 3. Academic Press, a division of Harcourt Brace & Co., San Diego, pp. 41–9.

Saunders, D. (1994). Health officials to supervise circumcised girls, court rules. *The Age*, 1 March, p. 2.

Saunders, J.M. and Valente, S.M. (1986). The question that won't go away. *Nursing*, 86, 16(3), pp. 61–4.

Saunders, M. (2003a). Heads roll over horror hospitals. *The Australian*, 12 December, p. 1.

—— (2003b). No escaping that foul hospital smell. *The Australian*, 12 December, p. 4.

Sawyer, L.M. (1989). Nursing code of ethics: an international comparison. *International Nursing Review*, 36(5), pp. 145–8.

Sax, S. (1984). *A strife of interests: politics and policies in Australian health services*. George Allen & Unwin, Sydney.

Schade, S.G. and Muslin, H. (1989). Do not resuscitate decisions: discussions with patients. *Journal of Medical Ethics*, 15(4), pp. 186–90.

Schauble, J. and Willox, I. (1987). Government reviews law on consent to medical treatment. *The Age*, 21 August, p. 19.

Schneiderman, L. and Jecker, N. (1995). *Wrong medicine: doctors, patients and futile treatment*. The John Hopkins University Press, Baltimore and London.

Schneiderman, L., Gilmer, T. Teetzel, H., Dugan, D., et al. (2003) Effects of ethics consultations on nonbeneficial life-sustaining treatments in the intensive care setting: a randomised controlled trial. *Journal of American Medical Association*, 290(9), pp. 116–1172.

Schnookal, R. (1990). Re-introduction of the Bill to abolish Medicare funding of abortion announced. *Alive and WEL* (official newsletter of the Women's Electoral Lobby), October, p. 2.

Schrag, F. (1995). Rights of children. In Reich, W.T. (ed.), *Encyclopedia of Bioethics*, revised edition. Simon & Schuster Macmillan, New York, pp. 355–7.

Schulz, D. (1999). Baby J, the child who was not supposed to live. *The Age*, 5 November, p. 2.

Schumpeter, P. (1988). No-resuscitation rules are unclear: lecturer. *The Age*, 1 October, p. 21.

Schwartz, R.L. (1993). Autonomy, futility and the limits of medicine. *Bioethics News*, 12(3), pp. 31–6.

Scofield, G. R. (1991). Is consent useful when resuscitation isn't? *Hastings Center Report*, 21(6), pp. 28–36.

—— (1992). The problem of the impaired clinical ethicist. *Quarterly Review Bulletin*, 18(1), pp. 26–32.

Scott, D. and O'Neil, D. (1996). *Beyond child rescue: developing family-centred Practice at St Luke's*. Allen & Unwin in association with Institute of Public Affairs, Sydney.

Seary v State Bar of Texas (1980), 604 SW2d 256 at 258.

Seedhouse, D. (1988), *Ethics: the heart of health care.* John Wiley & Sons, Chichester.

Seeskin, K.R. (1978). Genuine appeals to conscience. *Journal of Value Inquiry*, 12, pp. 296–300.

Segal, L. (1987). *Is the future female? Troubled thoughts on contemporary feminism.* Virago Press, London.

Senate Community Affairs References Committee. (1995). *Psychotherapeutic Medication in Australia: Report of the Senate Community Affairs References Committee.* Commonwealth of Australia, Senate Printing Unit, Parliament House, Canberra.

Senate Legal and Constitutional Legislation Committee (1997). *Consideration of Legislation Referred to the Committee: Euthanasia Laws Bill 1996.* Commonwealth of Australia, Canberra.

Senate Select Committee on a Certain Maritime Incident. (2002). *Report on a Certain Maritime Incident.* Commonwealth of Australia, Canberra.

Senate Select Committee on the Human Embryo Experimentation Bill 1985. (1986). *Human embryo experimentation in Australia.* Australian Government Publishing Service, Canberra.

Severinsson, E. (2003). Moral stress and burnout: qualitative content analysis. *Nursing and Health Sciences*, 5, pp. 59–66.

Shanley, M. (1995). Father's rights, mother's wrongs? Reflections on unwed fathers' rights, patriarchy, and sex equality. In Callahan, J. (ed.), *Reproduction, ethics, and the law: feminist perspectives.* Indiana University Press, Bloomington and Indianapolis, pp. 219–48.

Shapira, A. (1998). 'Wrongful life' lawsuits for faulty genetic counselling: should the impaired newborn be entitled to sue? *Journal of Medical Ethics*, 24(6), pp. 369–75.

Sharkey, A. (1994). Killing for life. *The Age*, Extra, pp. 3–4.

Shawyer, J. (1979). *Death by adoption.* Cicada Press, Auckland.

Sheehan, M. and Wells, D. (1985). The allocation of medical resources. In Buchanan, C.L. and Prior, E.W. (eds), *Medical care and markets: conflicts between efficiency and justice.* George Allen & Unwin, Sydney, pp. 55–69.

Sheldon, T. (1996). Dutch court supports whistle blowing surgeon. *British Medical Journal*, 312(7027), pp. 333–4.

Sherwin, S. (1992). *No longer patient: feminist ethics & health care.* Temple University Press, Philadelphia.

Sherwin, S. (1996). Feminism and bioethics. In Wolf, S. (ed.) *Feminism & bioethics: beyond reproduction.* Oxford University Press, New York, pp. 47–66.

Shneidman, E (1985). *Definition of suicide.* Wiley, New York.

—— (1993). *Suicide as psychache: a clinical approach to self-destructive behaviour.* Jason Aronson, Northvale, New Jersey.

Siegler, M. (1982). Commentary. *Hastings Center Report*, 12(5), October, pp. 28–9.

Silberbauer, G. (1991). Ethics in small-scale societies. In Singer, P. (ed.), *A companion to ethics.* Basil Blackwell, Cambridge, Mass., pp. 14–28.

Simon, A. (2001a). Ethics committees in Germany: an empirical survey of Christian hospitals. *HEC Forum*, 13(3), pp. 225–31.

—— (2001b). Support for ethical dilemmas in individual cases: experiences from the Neu-Mariahilf hospital in Goettingen. *Journal of Medical Ethics*, 27(Supplement 1), pp. i18–i20.

Singer, P. (1979a). Famine, affluence, and morality. In Wasserstrom, R.A. (ed.), *Today's moral problems* (2nd edn). Macmillan, New York, pp. 561–72.

—— (1979b). *Practical ethics.* Cambridge University Press, Cambridge.

—— (1982). How do we decide? *Hastings Center Report*, 12(3), June, pp. 9–11.

—— (ed.) (1991). *A companion to ethics.* Basil Blackwell, Cambridge, Mass.

—— (1993). *Practical ethics* (2nd edn). Cambridge University Press, Cambridge, UK.

—— (1994). *Rethinking life & death: the collapse of our traditional ethics.* The Text Publishing Company, Melbourne.

Singer, P. and Kuhse, H. (1994). Bioethics and the limits of tolerance. *Journal of Medicine and Philosophy*, 19(2), pp. 129–45.

Singer, P., Martin, D., Lavery, J., Thiel, E., Kelner, M. and Mendlessohn, D. (1998). Reconceptualizing advance care planning from the patient's perspective. *Archives of Internal Medicine*, 158(8), pp. 879–84.

Skene, L. (1992). Doctor ending baby's pain should not face risk of jail. *The Age*, 9 June, p. 12.

—— (1996). A legal perspective on codes of ethics. In M. Coady and S. Bloch (eds), *Codes of ethics and the professions.* Melbourne University Press, Melbourne, pp. 111–29.

Skinner, B.F. (1973). *Beyond freedom and dignity.* Penguin Books, Harmondsworth, Middlesex, England.

Slater, E. (1980). Choosing the time to die. In Pabst Battin, M. and Mayo, D., *Suicide: the philosophical issues*. Peter Owen, London, pp. 199–204.

Slowther, A., Bunch, C., Woolnough, B. and Hope, T. (2001). *Journal of Medical Ethics*, 27(Supplement 1), pp. i2–i8.

Slowther, A., Hope, T. and Ashcroft, R. (2001a). Clinical ethics committees: a worldwide development. *Journal of Medical Ethics*, 27(Supplement 1), p. i1.

Smart, C. (ed.) (1992). *Regulating womanhood: historical essays on marriage, motherhood and sexuality*. Routledge, London and New York.

Smart, J.J.C. and Williams, B. (1973). *Utilitarianism: for and against*. Cambridge University Press, Cambridge.

Smith, D. and Perlin, S. (1978). Suicide. In Reich, W.T. (ed.), *Encyclopedia of bioethics*. The Free Press, New York, pp. 1618–27.

Smith, M. (1994). *The moral problem*. Blackwell Publishers, Oxford, UK.

Smith, W.B. and Lew, Y.L. (1968). *Nursing care of the patient*. Dymock, Sydney.

Social Development Committee, Parliament of Victoria (1986). *First report on inquiry into options for dying with dignity*. March, Government Printer, Melbourne.

Social Development Committee, Parliament of Victoria (1987). *Inquiry into options for dying with dignity: second and final report*. April. Government Printer, Melbourne.

Solomon, M., Jennings B., Guilfoy, V., Jackson, R., O'Donnell, L., Wolf, S., Nolan, K., Koch-Weser, D. and Donnelley, S. (1991). Toward an expanded vision of clinical ethics education: from the individual to the institution. *Kennedy Institute of Ethics Journal*, 1(3), pp. 225–45.

Solomon, R.C. and Murphy, M.C. (eds) (1990). *What is justice? Classic and contemporary readings*. Oxford University Press, New York.

Solomon, W.D. (1978). Rules and principles. In Reich, W.T. (ed.), *Encyclopedia of bioethics*. The Free Press, New York, pp. 407–12.

Somerville, M. (1986). Rights to, in and against medical treatment. *Bioethics News*, 5(3), April, pp. 5–17.

—— (1996). Legalising euthanasia: why now? *Australian Quarterly*, 68(3), pp. 1–14.

Sophocles (1911 edn). *Oedipus King of Thebes* (translated by G. Murray). George Allen & Unwin, London.

Sorokin, P. (1957). *Social and cultural dynamics*. Extending Horizons. Books–Porter Sargent, Boston.

Soubrier, J-P. (1993). Definitions of suicide. In Leenaars, A. (ed.), *Suicidology: essays in honor or Edwin Shneidman*. Jason Aronson, Northvale, New Jersey, pp. 35–41.

South East Centre Against Sexual Assault (1994). *Certified Truths: Women Who Have Been Sexually Assaulted — Their Experiences of Psychiatric Services*. South East Centre Against Sexual Assault, Monash Medical Centre, Melbourne.

Spellecy, R. (2003). Reviving Ulysses Contracts, *Kennedy Institute of Ethics Journal*, 13(4), pp. 373–92.

Spelman, E. (1997). *Fruits of sorrow: framing our attention to suffering*. Beacon Press, Boston.

Spencer, E., Mills, A., Rorty, M. and Werhane, P. (2000). *Organization ethics in health care*. Oxford University Press, Oxford.

Spender, D. (1988). *Women of ideas, and what men have done to them*. Pandora Press, London (first published by Routledge & Kegan Paul, 1982). (See in particular essay on Harriet Taylor [1807–58], pp. 184–96.)

Spindler, G.D. (1974). *Education and cultural process: towards an anthropology of education*. Holt, Rinehart & Winston, New York.

Spitzer, R.B. (1988). Meeting consumer expectations. *Nursing Administration Quarterly*, 12(3), pp. 31–9.

Staal, H. (1995). Verpleegkundige veroordeeld voor plegen euthanasie. *NRC Handelsblad*: 7 (translated by W Chenhall).

Staff of the National Health Law Program (1991). Health benefits: how the system is responding to AIDS. In McKenzie, N.F. (ed.), *The AIDS reader: social, political, ethical issues*. Meridian, New York, pp. 247–72.

Stanley, D.P. and Reid, D.P. (1989). Withholding cardiopulmonary resuscitation: one hospital's policy. *Medical Journal of Australia*, 151, 4 September, pp. 257–62.

Stanley, T. (1978). Nursing. In Reich, W.T. (ed.), *Encyclopedia of bioethics*. The Free Press, New York, pp. 1138–46.

Starck, P. and McGovern, J. (eds) (1992). *The hidden dimension of illness: human suffering*. National League for Nursing Press, New York.

Staunton, P. and Whyburn, B. (1997). *Nursing and the law* (4th edn). W.B. Saunders/Baillière Tindall, Sydney.

Steinbock, B. (1983). The intentional termination of life. In Gorovitz, S., Macklin, R., Jameton, A.L., O'Connor, J.M. and Sherwin, A. (eds), *Moral problems in medicine* (2nd edn). Prentice Hall, Englewood Cliffs, New Jersey, pp. 290–5.

Steiner, N. (1998). Methods of hydration in palliative care patients. *Journal of Palliative Care*, 14(2), pp. 6–13.

Stengel, E. (1970). *Suicide and attempted suicide*. Penguin Books, Harmondsworth, Middlesex.

Stephens, P. (1986). Should essential workers lose their right to strike? *The Age*, 12 December, p. 13.

—— (1987). Tolerance of abortion is much wider now. *The Age*, 7 December, p. 5.

Steppe, H. (1991). Nursing in the Third Reich. *History of Nursing Journal*, 3(4), pp. 21–37.

—— (1992). Nursing in Nazi Germany. *Victorian Journal of Nursing Research*, 14(6), pp. 744–53.

Stevens, C. and Hassan, R. (1994). Nurses and the management of death, dying and euthanasia. *Medicine and Law*, 13, pp. 541–54.

Stevens, J. and Herbert, J. (1997). Ageism and nursing practice in Australia. *Nursing Review*. September issue, special section, pp. 17–24.

Stevenson, C.L. (1944). *Ethics and language*. Yale University Press, New Haven.

Stewart, K. and Rai, G. (1989). A matter of life and death. *Nursing Times*, 85(35), pp. 27–9.

Stone, D. (1991). Hospitals forced to use cleaners as interpreters. *The Sunday Age*, 10 February, p. 4.

Stout, J. (1988). *Ethics after Babel: the languages of morals and their discontents*. Beacon Press, Boston.

Strang, H. (1996). Children as victims of homicide. *Trends and issues in crime and criminal justice*, no. 53, Australian Institute of Criminology, Canberra.

Strauss, J. (1994). *Birthright: the guide to search and reunion for adoptees, birthparents, and adoptive parents*. Penguin Books, New York.

Stubbs, D. (1994). Foreword, to Heckler, R., *Waking up alive: the descent to suicide and return to life*. Piatkus, London, pp. xi–xiv.

Sugirtharjah, S. (1994). The notion of respect in Asian traditions. *British Journal of Nursing*, 3(14), pp. 739–41.

Suicide Prevention Victorian Task Force (1997). *Suicide Prevention Victorian Task Force Report*. Melbourne (available from Information Victoria, 1/356 Collins Street, Melbourne).

Sundin-Huard, D. and Fahy, K. (1999). Moral distress, advocacy and burnout: theorising the relationships. *International Journal of Nursing Practice*, 5, pp. 8–13.

Sun-Herald (1990). Medically unfit. 17 June, p. 168.

Surbone, A. (1992). Truth telling to the patient. *Journal of American Medical Association*, 268(13), pp. 1661–2.

Svendsen, I. (1987). Lecturer calls for code of nursing conduct. *The Age*, 17 November, p. 21.

Swanson, K. (1993). Nursing as informed caring for the wellbeing of others. *IMAGE: Journal of Nursing Scholarship*, 25(4), pp. 352–7.

Swanton, C. (1987). The rationality of ethical intuitionism. *Australasian Journal of Philosophy*, 65(2), June, pp. 172–81.

Swenson, D.F. (1981). The dignity of human life. In Klemke, E.D. (ed.), *The meaning of life*. Oxford University Press, New York, pp. 20–30.

Sykes, N. (1990). The last 48 hours of life: caring for patient, family and doctor. *Geriatric Medicine*, 20(9), pp. 22–4.

Sykes, N. and Thorns, A. (2003). Sedative use in the last week of life and the implications for end-of-life decision making. *Archives of Internal Medicine*, 163(3), pp. 341–4.

Syme, R. (1992). A missing voice in euthanasia debate. *The Age*, 21 March, p. 10.

—— (2002). Response to the Nancy Crick case. *Monash Bioethics Review*, 21(4), pp. 32–4.

Szasz, T. (1988). The ethics of suicide. In T. Szasz. *The theology of medicine*. Syracuse University Press, New York, pp. 68–85.

Szeremeta, M., Dawson, J., Manning, D., Watson, A. et al. (2001). Snapshots of five clinical ethics committees in the UK. *Journal of Medical Ethics*, 27(Supplement 1), pp. i9–i17.

Tadd, G. (1998). *Ethics and values for care workers*. Blackwell Science, Oxford, UK.

Tadd, V. (1991). Where are the whistleblowers? *Nursing Times*, 87(1), pp. 42–4.

Tan, S., Chun, B. and Kim, E. (2003). Creating a medical futility policy. *Health Progress*, 84(4), pp. 14–20.

Tanne, J. (1991). Jail for pregnant cocaine users in US. *British Medical Journal*, 303 (6807), p. 873.

Tarasoff v Regents of the University of California 13 Cal. 3d 177, 529 P.2d 553, 118 Cal. Rptr. 129 (1974).

Taylor, B. (1995). Nursing as healing work. *Contemporary Nurse*, 4(3), pp. 100–106.

Taylor, C. (1998). Reflections on 'nursing considered as moral practice'. *Kennedy Institute of Ethics Journal*, 8(1), pp. 71–82.

Taylor, R. and Lantos, J (1995) The politics of medical futility. *Issues in Law and Medicine*, 11(1), pp. 4–12.

Taylor, T. (2001). Surgery ban on smokers. *Herald Sun*, 8 February, pp. 1, 4.

Teays, W. and Purdy, L. (eds) (2001). *Bioethics, justice, and health care*. Wadsworth, Belmont, California.

ten Have, H.A.M. and Welie, J.V.M. (1992). Euthanasia: normal medical practice? *Hastings Center Report*, 22(2), pp. 34–8.

Teo, W. (1975). Abortion: the husband's constitutional rights. *Ethics*, 85(4), pp. 337–42.

Terr, L. (1994). *Unchained memories: true stories of traumatic memories, lost and found*. Basic Books, New York.

Tester, K. (1997). *Moral culture*. Sage, London.

The Age (2003). Editorial: Confidentiality and responsible medicine. 12 June, p. 14

The Herald (1986). The achievement of Irene Bolger. Editorial comment, 2 December, p. 6.

The Leader (1992). Save young lives. 19 August, p. 8.

The Regan Report on Hospital Law (1985). Institution — 'no CPR policy': Constitutional Issue 25.(12) May, p. 1.

Thom, A. (1988). Who decides? *Nursing Times*, 85(2), pp. 35–7.

Thomas, M. (1972). Child abuse and neglect: Part 1. Historical overview, legal matrix, and social perspectives. *North Carolina Law Review*, 50, pp. 293–349.

Thomas, S. (1986). *Genetic risk*. Penguin Books, Harmondsworth, Middlesex.

Thomasma, D. (1990). Establishing the moral basis of medicine: Edmund D. Pellegrino's philosophy of medicine. *Journal of Medicine and Philosophy*, 15(3), pp. 245–67.

Thompson, I., Melia, K. and Boyd, K. (2000). *Nursing ethics* (4th edn). First published in 1983. Churchill Livingstone, Edinburgh.

—— (2000) *Nursing Ethics* (4th edn). Churchill Livingstone, Edingburgh.

Thompson, J.B. and Thompson, H.O. (1981). *Ethics in nursing*. Macmillan, New York.

Thomson, J.J. (1971). A defense of abortion. *Philosophy and Public Affairs*, 1(1), pp. 47–66.

—— (1975). The right to privacy. *Philosophy and Public Affairs*, 4(4), Summer, pp. 295–314.

Thornton, M. (1990). *The liberal promise: anti-discrimination legislation in Australia*. Oxford University Press, Melbourne.

Tiedje, L. (2000). Moral distress in perinatal nursing. *Journal of Perinatal & Neonatal Nursing*, 14(2), pp. 36–43.

Tighe, M. (1992). Slippery slope to killing patients. *The Age*, 21 March, p. 10.

Tilden, V., Schmidt, T., Limandri, B., Chiodo, G., Garland, M. and Loveless, P. (1994). Factors that influence clinicians' assessment and management of family violence. *American Journal of Public Health*, 84(4), pp. 628–33.

Timms, N. (1983). *Social work values: an enquiry*. Routledge & Kegan Paul, London (see in particular Chapter 3, 'Conscience in social work: towards the practice of moral judgment', pp. 33–44).

Tippett, V., Elvy, G., Hardy, J. and Raphael, B. (1994). *Mental Health in Australia: A Review of Current Activities and Future Directions*. Australian Government Publishing Service, Canberra.

Tobler (2003). H. Hundreds more deaths, claims nurse. *The Australian*, 12 December, p. 4.

Tomison, A. (1996). Child maltreatment and mental disorder. *Child Abuse Prevention*, discussion paper no. 3. Australian Institute of Family Studies, Melbourne.

Tomlinson, R. and Brody, H. (1990). Futility and the ethics of resuscitation. *Journal of the American Medical Association*, 264(10), 12 September, pp. 1276–80.

Toner, R. (1993). President in move to reverse policy on abortion. *The Age*, 25 January, p. 6.

Tong, R. (1995). Towards a just, courageous, and honest resolution of the futility debate. *Journal of Medicine and Philosophy*, 20(2), pp. 165–89.

Tooley, M. (1972). Abortion and infanticide. *Philosophy and Public Affairs*, 2(1), Fall, pp. 37–65.

—— (1980). An irrelevant consideration: killing versus letting die. In Steinbock, B. *Killing and letting die*. Prentice Hall, Englewood Cliffs, New Jersey, pp. 56–62.

Torrey, E.F. (1988). *Nowhere to Go: The Tragic Odyssey of the Homeless Mentally Ill*. Harper and Row, New York.

Toy, M. (1998). Heavy burden on women. *The Age*, 4 February, p. 2.

—— (2000). Outspoken nurse sacked over criticism. *The Age*, 21 April, p. 5.

Trammell, R.L. (1978). The presumption against taking life. *Journal of Medicine and Philosophy*, 3(1), pp. 53–67.

Tribe, L. (1985). *Constitutional choices*. Harvard University Press, Cambridge, Mass.

Trollope, S. (1995). Legislating a right to die: the *Rights of the Terminally Ill Act 1995* (NT). *Journal of Law & Medicine*, 3(1), pp. 19–29.

Tronto, J.C. (1993). *Moral boundaries: a political argument for an ethic of care*. Routledge, New York/London.

Tschudin, V. (1986). *Ethics in nursing: the caring relationship*. William Heinemann Medical Books, London.

Tuan, Y-F. (1989). *Morality and imagination: paradoxes of progress*. University of Wisconsin Press, Madison, Wisconsin.

Tuma v Board of Nursing of the State of Idaho 593 P 2d 711 (1979).

Turner, T. (1990). Crushed by the system? *Nursing Times*, 86(49), p. 19.

—— (1992). The indomitable Mr Pink. *Nursing Times*, 88(24), p. 26–9.

Turton, P. (1987). Last rights. *Nursing Times*, 83(17), 29 April, pp. 18–19.

—— (1992). Euthanasia and the nurses: last rights. In Voluntary Euthanasia Society (ed.) (1992), *Your ultimate choice: the right to die with dignity*. Souvenir Press, London, pp. 92–4.

Tweeddale, M. 2002. Grasping the nettle — what to do when patients withdraw their consent for treatment: (a clinical perspective on the case of Ms B). *Journal of Medical Ethics*, 28(4), pp. 236–7.

Twomey, J.G. (1989). Analysis of the claim to distinct nursing ethics: normative and non-normative approaches. *Advances in Nursing Science*, 11(3), pp. 25–32.

Twycross, R.G. and Lack, S.A. (1984). *Therapeutics in terminal cancer*. Churchill Livingstone, Edinburgh.

United Kingdom Central Council for Nursing, Midwifery and Health Visiting [UKCC] (1984). *Code of Professional Conduct for the Nurse, Midwife and Health Visitor* (2nd edn). UKCC, London.

United Nations (1959). *Declaration of the Rights of the Child*. United Nations, New York.

—— (1978). *The International Bill of Human Rights*. United Nations, New York.

Unwin, N. (1985). Relativism and moral complacency. *Philosophy*, 60, pp. 205–14.

Upfront (1988). 'Not for Resuscitation' orders leave nurses in a moral, legal and professional dilemma, 7(4), December, pp. 6, 13.

Urmson, J.O. (1958). Saints and heroes. First published in Melden, A.I. (ed.), *Essays in moral philosophy*, University of Washington Press, pp. 198–216; reprinted in J. Feinberg (1969), *Moral concepts*, Oxford University Press, Oxford, pp. 60–73.

—— (1975). A defence of intuitionism. *Proceedings of the Aristotelian Society*, 65, pp. 111–19.

Uyer, G. (1986). Effect of nursing approach in understanding of physicians' directions, by mothers of sick children in an out-patient clinic. *International Journal of Nursing Studies*, 23(1), pp. 79–85.

Valent, P. (1993). *Child survivors: adults living with childhood trauma*. William Heinemann Australia, Melbourne.

van de Pasch, T. (1995). Letter from the Netherlands. *International Nursing Review*, 42(4), p. 108.

van der Arend, A. (1995). President, International Nursing Ethics (& Midwifery) Network (INEN). Letter-to-Megan-Jane Johnstone, dated 15 August.

Van der Kloot Meijburg, H. and ter Meulen, R. (2001). Developing standards for institutional ethics committees: lessons from the Netherlands. *Journal of Medical Ethics*, 27(Supplement 1), pp. i36–i40.

van der Kolk, B. (1996). The complexity of adaptation to trauma: self-regulation, stimulus, discrimination, and characterological development. In van der Kolk, B., McFarlane, A. and Weisaeth, L. (eds), *Traumatic stress: the effects of overwhelming experience on mind, body, and society*. The Guilford Press, New York/ London, pp. 182–213.

van der Kolk, B., McFarlane, A and Weisaeth, L. (eds) (1996). *Traumatic stress: the effects of overwhelming experience on mind, body, and society*. The Guilford Press, New York/ London.

van der Maas, P., van der Wal, G., Haverkate, I., de Graaff, C., Kester, J., Onwuteaka-Philipsen, B., van der Heide, A., Bosma, J. and Willems, D. (1996). Euthanasia, physician-assisted suicide, and other medical practices involving the end of life in the Netherlands, 1900–1995. *New England Journal of Medicine*, 335(22), pp. 1699–705.

van der Wal, G. and Dillmann, R. (1994). Euthanasia in the Netherlands. *British Medical Journal*, 308, 21 May, pp. 1346–9.

van der Wal, G., van der Maas, P., Bosma, J., Onwuteaka-Philipsen, B., Willems, D., Haverkate, I. and Kostense, P. (1996). Evaluation of the notification procedure for physician-assisted death in the Netherlands. *New England Journal of Medicine*, 335(22), pp. 1706–11.

Van Hooft, S. (1987). Caring and professional commitment. *Australian Journal of Advanced Nursing*, 4(4), pp. 29–38.

Vandeveer, D. (1980). The contractual argument for withholding medical information. *Philosophy and Public Affairs*, 9(2), pp. 198–205.

Vardey, L. (1995). *Mother Teresa: a simple path*. Rider, London.

Vatican (1980). *Declaration on euthanasia*. Vatican Polygot Press, Vatican City, Rome.

Vaughan, F.E. (1979). *Awakening intuition*. Anchor Books/Doubleday, New York.

Veatch, R.M. (1972). Medical ethics: professional or universal? *Harvard Theological Review*, 65, pp. 531–9.

—— (1977). *Death, dying, and the biological revolution*. Yale University Press, New Haven.

—— (1977). Institutional ethics committees: is there a role? *Hastings Center Report*, 7(3), June, pp. 22–5.

—— (1985). Nursing ethics, physician ethics and medical ethics. *Bioethics Reporter* 6, (7), pp. 381–3.

Veatch, R.M. and Fry, S.T. (1987). *Case studies in nursing ethics*. J.B. Lippincott Company, Philadelphia.

Ventura, M. (1999). Where nurses stand on abortion. *RN*, 62(3), pp. 44–7.

Vervoorn, A. (1987). Voluntary euthanasia in the Netherlands: recent developments. *Bioethics News*, 6(2), pp. 19–26.

VES (2003). Choice, dignity: public opinion. Voluntary Euthanasia Society, London [available at: *www.ves.org.uk/pdf/PublicOpinion_Apr03.pdf* — accessed 24 September 2003].

Vessey, J. (1994). The ghost of Tuskegee. *Nursing Research*, 43(2), p. 67.

Vicki, J. (1995). *Sex and the sect*. Essien, Melbourne.

Victorian Health Services Commissioner Annual Report 1991. Flash Print, Melbourne.

Victorian Hospital Association Report (1988). 'Stickers recommended', 42, August–September, p. 3.

Victorian Nursing Council (1988). Resuscitation by the nurse. *Position Statements*, Victorian Nursing Council, Melbourne.

Viele, C., Dodd. M. and Morrison, C. (1984). Caring for acquired immune deficiency syndrome patients. *Oncology Nursing Forum*, 11, pp. 56–60.

Viens, D.C. (1989). A history of nursing's code of ethics. *Nursing Outlook*, 37(1), pp. 45–9.

Vincent, C. (ed.) (2001a). *Clinical risk management* (2nd edn). BMJ Books, London

—— (2001b). Introduction. In Vincent, C. (ed.), *Clinical risk management* (2nd edn). BMJ Books, London, pp. 1–6.

Vinten, G. (1994). Whistle while you work in the health-related professions? *Journal of the Royal Society of Health*, 114(5), pp. 256–62.

Voluntary Euthanasia Society (ed.) (1992). *Your ultimate choice: the right to die with dignity*. Souvenir Press, London.

Von Wright, G.H. (1958). Biographical sketch. In Malcolm, N., *Ludwig Wittgenstein: a memoir*. Oxford University Press, London.

Voumard, S. (1988). Ethics committees out of kilter with public opinion, says doctor. *The Age*, 18 May, p. 17.

Vousden, M. (1985). Swallow your pride, or lose your job? *Nursing Mirror*, 160(1), 2 January, p. 23.

Waikato Times (1984a). Police to lay no charges. 11 July, p. 1.

—— (1984b). Waikato Hospital chief says: morphine off limits to trainee. 16 February, p. 3.

—— (1987a). Patient recall: decision later. 1 September.

—— (1987b). Rape by medical students? 18 September.

—— (1990). Ethical guidelines underway. 15 October, p. 3.

Wainer, J. (1989). Report on the pro-abortion march in Washington. *Alive and WEL* (Women's Electoral Lobby) (May), pp. 4–5.

—— (1990). Abortion funding abolition Bill. *Alive and WEL* (official newsletter of the Women's Electoral Lobby), February, p. 8.

Waithe, M.E. (ed.) (1987). *A history of women philosophers*. Volume I: *Ancient women philosophers, 600 BC–500 AD*, Martinus Nijhoff, Dordrecht.

—— (ed.) (1989a). *A history of women philosophers*. Volume II: *Medieval, Renaissance and Enlightenment women philosophers, AD 500–1600*. Kluwer Academic Publishers, Dordrecht.

—— (1989b). Twenty-three hundred years of women philosophers: toward a gender indifferentiated moral theory. In Brabeck, M.M. (ed.), *Who cares? Theory, research, and educational implications of the ethic of care*. Praeger, New York, pp. 3–18.

—— (ed.) (1991). *A history of women philosophers*. Volume III: *Modern women philosophers, 1600–1900*. Kluwer Academic Publishers, Dordrecht.

—— (ed.) (1995). *A history of women philosophers*. Volume 4: *1900–today*. Kluwer Academic Publishers, Dordrecht.

Waithe, M.E. and Ozar, D.T. (1990). The ethics of teaching ethics. *Hastings Center Report*, 20(4), pp. 17–21.

Walker, A. and Parmar, P. (1993). *Warrior marks: female genital mutilation and the sexual blinding of women*. Jonathan Cape, London, UK.

Walker, M. (1998). *Moral understandings: a feminist study in ethics*. Routledge, New York.

Walker, M.U. (1992). Moral understanding: alternative 'epistemology' for a feminist ethics. In Cole, E.B. and Coultrap-McQuin, S. (eds), *Explorations in feminist ethics: theory and practice*. Indiana University Press, Bloomington and Indianapolis, pp. 165–75.

Walker, Q.J. and Langlands, A.O. (1986). The misuse of mammography in the management of breast cancer. *Medical Journal of Australia*, 145, 1 September, pp. 185–7.

Wallace, M. (1991). *Health care and the law: a guide for nurses*. The Law Book Company, North Ryde.

—— (1992). Meeting the challenge of patients' rights: a legal perspective. Proceedings of the conference '*Meeting the Challenge of Patients' Rights—Issues for the 1990s*', RMIT Faculty of Nursing, Nursing Law and Ethics, 4th Victorian State Conference, held 20 November, Dallas Brooks Hall, Melbourne, Royal Melbourne Institute of Technology, Faculty of Nursing, Melbourne.

—— (1998). Misrepresentation = confusion on abortion in WA. *Newsletter of the Legal Issues Society, Royal College of Nursing Australia*, 2(1), pp. 2–3.

Walsh, B. and Pirrie, M. (1996). Nurse faces murder charge. *Herald Sun*, 8 May, pp. 1, 2.

Walter, J. (1995). Quality of life in clinical decisions. In Reich, W.T. (ed.), *Encyclopedia of bioethics*, revised edition. Simon & Schuster Macmillan, New York/Simon & Schuster and Prentice Hall International, pp. 1352–8.

Walton D.N. (1980). The ethical force of definitions. *Journal of Medical Ethics*, 6, pp. 16–18.

Walton, D. (1986), *Courage: a philosophical investigation*. University of California Press, Berkeley and Los Angeles, California.

Walzer, M. (1987). *Interpretation and social criticism*. Harvard University Press, Cambridge, Mass.

Waring, M. (1988). *Counting for nothing: what men value and what women are worth*. Allen & Unwin, Port Nicholson Press, Wellington (NZ).

Warnock, G.J. (1967). *Contemporary moral philosophy*. Macmillan Education, Houndmills, Basingstoke, Hampshire.

Warnock, M. (ed.) (1962). *Utilitarianism*. Fontana Library/Collins, London.

Warren, M. (1997). On the moral and legal status of abortion. In LaFollette, H. (ed.), *Ethics in practice: an anthology*. Blackwell Publishers, Cambridge, Mass, pp. 79–90.

—— (1973). On the moral and legal status of abortion. *The Monist*, 57(1), January, pp. 43–61.

—— (1977). Do potential people have moral rights? *Canadian Journal of Philosophy*, 7(2), June, pp. 275–89.

—— (1985). *Gendercide: the implications of sex selection*. Rowman & Allanheld, Totowa, New Jersey.

—— (1988). The moral significance of birth. *Bioethics News*, 7(2), January, pp. 32–44.

Warthen v Toms River Community Memorial Hospital 488 A 2d 299 (NJ Super AD 1985).

Warthen v Toms River Community Memorial Hospital, Superior Court of New Jersey, AD, 8/1/85–14/2/85. *In Atlantic Reporter*, 2nd Series, New Jersey, pp. 229–34.

Watkins, S. (1990). The Mary Ellen Myth: correcting child welfare history. *Social Work*, 35(6), pp. 500–3.

Watson, J. (1985). *Nursing: human science and human care*. Appleton-Century-Crofts, Norwalk, Connecticut.

—— (1985a). *Nursing: the philosophy and science of caring*. Colorado Associated University Press, Boulder, Colorado.

—— (1985b). *Nursing: human science and human care: a theory of nursing*. Appleton-Century-Crofts, Norwalk, Connecticut.

Wear, S. (1991). The irreducibly clinical character of bioethics. *Journal of Medicine and Philosophy*, 16(1), pp. 53–70.

Wear, S., Lagaipa, S. and Logue, G. (1994). Toleration of moral diversity and the conscientious refusal by physicians to withdraw life-sustaining treatment. *Journal of Medicine and Philosophy*, 19(2), pp. 147–59.

Webb, S. (1988). Is the hospital system sick? *Sunday Examiner*, Tasmania, 19 June, p. 6.

Weil, A. (1983). *Health and healing: understanding conventional and alternative medicine*. Houghton Mifflin, Boston.

Weinryb, E. (1980). Omissions and responsibility. *Philosophical Quarterly*, 30(118), January, pp. 1–18.

Weinstein, H.M. (1990). *Psychiatry and the CIA: Victims of Mind Control*. American Psychiatric Press, Washington DC.

Welch-McCaffrey, D. (1985). Cancer, anxiety, and quality of life. *Cancer Nursing*, 8(3), June, pp. 151–8.

Wenger, N. Golan, O., Shalev, C. and Glick, S. (2002). Hospital ethics committees in Israel: structure, function and heterogeneity in the setting of statutory ethics committees. *Journal of Medical Ethics*, 28(3), pp. 177–82.

Wennberg, R. (1989). *Terminal choices: euthanasia, suicide, and the right to die*. William B. Eerdmans Publishing Company, Grand Rapids, Michigan, and The Paternoster Press, Exeter, UK.

Werner, R. (1979). Abortion: the ontological and moral status of the unborn. In Wasserstrom, R.A. (ed.), *Today's moral problems* (2nd edn). Macmillan, New York, pp. 51–74.

Wertheimer, M. (1990). Separate roles for doctors and nurses need to be recognised. *Medicine*, 2(7), 16 April, p. 11.

Wicclair, M. (2000). Conscientious objection in medicine. *Bioethics*, 14(3), pp. 205–27.

Widdershoven, G. and Berghmans, R. (2001). Advance directives in psychiatric care: a narrative approach. *Journal of Medical Ethics*, 27(2), pp. 92–7.

Wikler, D. and Barondess, J. (1993). Bioethics and anti-bioethics in light of Nazi medicine: what must we remember? *Kennedy Institute of Ethics Journal*, 3(1), pp. 39–55.

Wildes, K. (1993). Moral authority, moral standing, and moral controversy. *Journal of Medicine and Philosophy*, 18(4), pp. 347–50.

—— (1994). Toleration and moral diversity: Bosnia or Pennsylvania. *Journal of Medicine and Philosophy*, 19(2), pp. 123–8.

Wilkes, E. (1994). On withholding nutrition and hydration in the terminally ill: has palliative medicine gone to far? A commentary. *Journal of Medical Ethics*, 20(3), pp. 144–5.

Wilkinson, J. (1987/1988). Moral distress in nursing practice: experience and affects. *Nursing Forum*, 23(1), pp. 16–29.

Williams, A. (2002). Issues of consent and data collection in vulnerable populations. *Journal of Neuroscience Nursing*, 34(4), pp. 211–17.

Williams, B. (1972). *Morality: an introduction to ethics*. Cambridge University Press, Cambridge.

—— (1973). Ethical consistency. In C.W. Gowans (ed.) (1987), *Moral dilemmas*. Oxford University Press, New York, pp. 115–37.

—— (1981). *Moral luck*. Cambridge University Press, Cambridge.

—— (1985). *Ethics and the limits of philosophy*. Fontana and Collins, London.

Williams, C. (1993). Children of rape in Bosnia trapped by new policy. *The Age*, 26 July, p. 8.

Williams, G. (1988). Industrial Report. *New Zealand Nursing Journal*, 81(3), pp. 6–14.

Williams, M. (1997). *Cry of pain: understanding suicide and self-harm*. Penguin Books, London.

Williams, R. (1989). *Resources of hope: culture, democracy, socialism*. Verso, London.

Willis, E. (1979). Sister Elizabeth Kenny and the evolution of the occupational division of labour in health care. *Australian and New Zealand Journal of Sociology*, 15(3), November, pp. 30–8.

Wilmoth, P. and Pirrie, M. (1988). Whose life is it anyway? *The Age* (Saturday Extra), 23 April.

Wilson, J. and Raphael, B. (1993). *International handbook of traumatic stress syndromes*. Plenum Press, New York/London.

Wilson-Barnett, J. (1986). Ethical dilemmas in nursing. *Journal of Medical Ethics*, 12, pp. 123–6, 135.

Windt, P. (1980). The concept of suicide. In Pabst Battin, M. and Mayo, D., *Suicide: the philosophical issues*. Peter Owen, London, pp. 39–47.

Winkler, R. and van Keppel, M. (1983). The long term adjustment of the relinquishing mothers in adoption: a research summary. Reprinted as an appendix in *Proceedings of the Conference: Adoption and AID: Access to Information?* Centre for Human Bioethics, Monash University, Melbourne, 2 November, pp. 39–40.

Winslade, W. (1995). Confidentiality. In Reich, W.T. (ed.), *The encyclopedia of bioethics*, revised edition. Simon & Schuster Macmillan, New York/Simon & Schuster and Prentice Hall International, pp. 451–59.

Winslow, B. and Winslow, G. (1991). Integrity and compromise in nursing ethics. *Journal of Medicine and Philosophy*, 16(3), pp. 307–23.

Winslow, G.R. (1984). From loyalty to advocacy: a new metaphor for nursing. *Hastings Center Report*, 14(3), June, pp. 32–40.

With AAP. (1998). Most nurses in NSW support voluntary euthanasia. *Australian Nursing Journal*, 5(8), p. 9.

Wittgenstein, L. (1965 edn). A lecture on ethics. *Philosophical Review*, 74, January, pp. 3–12.

Wolf, S. (1996a). Gender and feminism in ethics. In Wolf, S. (ed.), *Feminism & bioethics: beyond reproduction*. Oxford University Press, New York, pp. 3–43.

Wolf, S. (ed.) (1996b). *Feminism & bioethics: beyond reproduction*. Oxford University Press, New York.

Wolff, R.P., Moore, B. and Marcuse, H. (1969). *A critique of pure tolerance*. Beacon Press, Boston.

Wollstonecraft, M. (1929 edn). *A vindication of the rights of woman*. In Wollstonecraft, M., A vindication of the rights of woman, and J.S. Mill, *The subjection of women*, Everyman's Library, London, pp. 3–215.

Women's Electoral Lobby (1987). Comment reported in *Victorian Diary Newsletter* (February), Melbourne.

Wong, B. (1992). Coping with moral conflict and ambiguity. *Ethics*, 102 (July), pp. 763–84.

Woodham-Smith, C. (1964). *Florence Nightingale 1820–1910*. Collins Fontana, London.

World Health Organization (1995). *Twenty Steps for Developing a Healthy Cities Project*. WHO Regional Office for Europe, Copenhagen.

—— (1997). *Fact sheet N150: Child abuse and neglect*. WHO, Geneva. [available at: *www.who.org* —accessed 28 October 2003].

—— (1998). *Female genital mutilation: an overview*. WHO, Geneva.

—— (1999). WHO recognises child abuse as a major public health problem. Press release [available at: *www.who.int/inf-pr-1999/en/pr99-20.html* — accessed 19 January 2004].

—— (2001). *The World Health Report 2001*. Mental Health: New Understanding, New Hope. WHO, Geneva.

—— (2002). World Health Day 1998: Address unsafe abortion (WHD 98.10). WHO, Geneva [available at: *www.who.org* — accessed 22 September 2003].

—— (2003). Preventing unsafe abortion. WHO, Geneva [available at: *www.who.org* — accessed 22 September 2003].

Wuthnow, R., Hunter, J.D., Bergesen, A. and Kurzweil, E. (1984). *Cultural analysis*. Routledge & Kegan Paul, London.

Wyatt, J. (2001). Medical peternalism and the fetus. *Journal of Medical Ethics*, 27 Suppl II, pp. ii15–ii20.

Yarling, R. and McElmurry, B. (1986). Rethinking the nurse's role in 'Do Not Resuscitate' orders: a clinical policy proposal in nursing ethics. In Chinn, P. (ed.), *Ethical issues in nursing*. Aspen Systems, Rockville, Maryland, pp. 123–34.

Yarling, R.R. and McElmurry, B.J. (1986). The moral foundation of nursing. *Advances in Nursing Science*, 8(2), pp. 63–73.

Young, A. (1994). *Law and professional conduct in nursing* (2nd edn). Scutari Press, London.

Young, E.W. (1988). Nurses' attitudes toward homosexuality: analysis of change in AIDS workshops. *Journal of Continuing Education in Nursing*, 19(1), pp. 9–12.

Youngner, S., Coulton, C., Juknialis, B.W. and Jackson, D.L. (1984). Patients' attitudes toward institutional ethics committees. *Law, Medicine and Health Care*, 12(1), February, pp. 21–5.

Zerwekh, J.V. (1983). The hydration question. *Nursing*, 83, 13(1), January, pp. 47–51.

Zink, M. and Titus, L. (1994). Nursing ethics committees — where are they? *Nursing Management*, 25(6), pp. 70–6.

Zohar, D. (1991). *The quantum self*. Flamingo, London.

Zohar, D. and Marshall, I. (1993). *The quantum society*. Flamingo, London.

—— (2000). SQ *Spiritual intelligence: the ultimate intelligence*. Bloomsbury, London.

Zucker, M. and Zucker, H. (eds) (1997). *Medical futility and the evaluation of life-sustaining interventions*. Cambridge University Press, Cambridge, UK.

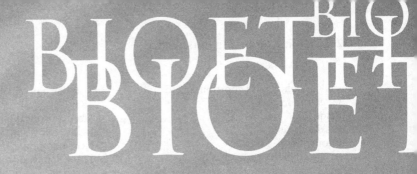

Index